Handbook of Lung Immunity and Inflammation

Handbook of Lung Immunity and Inflammation

Editor: Helen Smith

AMERICAN
MEDICAL PUBLISHERS
www.americanmedicalpublishers.com

AMERICAN
MEDICAL PUBLISHERS
www.americanmedicalpublishers.com

Cataloging-in-Publication Data

Handbook of lung immunity and inflammation / edited by Helen Smith.
p. cm.
Includes bibliographical references and index.
ISBN 979-8-88740-577-3
1. Lungs--Diseases. 2. Pneumonia. 3. Immunity. 4. Lungs--Immunology.
5. Lungs--Diseases--Treatment. I. Smith, Helen.
RC756 .H36 2023
616.24--dc23

American Medical Publishers,
41 Flatbush Avenue,
1st Floor, New York,
NY 11217, USA

ISBN 979-8-88740-577-3 (Hardback)

Contents

Preface

The lungs are essential organs in the human body which facilitate the process of gas exchange. Lung immunity plays a critical role in the prevention of various respiratory diseases characterized by abnormal inflammation. Some of the common lung diseases are asthma, chronic obstructive pulmonary disease (COPD) and fibrosis. Lung inflammation is generally caused by pathogens or by exposure to pollutants, toxins, allergens and irritants. Some common symptoms of lung inflammation are fatigue, extra mucus, wheezing, problem in breathing, gasping for air, etc. Diagnosis of lung inflammation is conducted through several tests, such as CT scan, ventilation or perfusion scan, lung function test, and blood tests. Its treatment involves anti-inflammatory medications, emergency breathing support, and surgery in severe cases. This book includes some of the vital pieces of work being conducted across the world, on various topics related to lung immunity and inflammation. It will also provide interesting topics for research which readers can take up. This book includes contributions of experts and scientists which will provide innovative insights into this field of study.

This book is a comprehensive compilation of works of different researchers from varied parts of the world. It includes valuable experiences of the researchers with the sole objective of providing the readers (learners) with a proper knowledge of the concerned field. This book will be beneficial in evoking inspiration and enhancing the knowledge of the interested readers.

In the end, I would like to extend my heartiest thanks to the authors who worked with great determination on their chapters. I also appreciate the publisher's support in the course of the book. I would also like to deeply acknowledge my family who stood by me as a source of inspiration during the project.

Editor

1

Progress in Model Systems of Cystic Fibrosis Mucosal Inflammation to Understand Aberrant Neutrophil Activity

Daniel R. Laucirica [1,2], Luke W. Garratt [2†] and Anthony Kicic [1,2,3,4†]*

[1] Faculty of Health and Medical Sciences, University of Western Australia, Nedlands, WA, Australia, [2] Telethon Kids Institute, University of Western Australia, Nedlands, WA, Australia, [3] Department of Respiratory and Sleep Medicine, Perth Children's Hospital, Nedlands, WA, Australia, [4] School of Public Health, Curtin University, Bentley, WA, Australia

***Correspondence:**
Luke W. Garratt
luke.garratt@telethonkids.org.au

†These authors share senior authorship

In response to recurrent infection in cystic fibrosis (CF), powerful innate immune signals trigger polymorphonuclear neutrophil recruitment into the airway lumen. Exaggerated neutrophil proteolytic activity results in sustained inflammation and scarring of the airways. Consequently, neutrophils and their secretions are reliable clinical biomarkers of lung disease progression. As neutrophils are required to clear infection and yet a direct cause of airway damage, modulating adverse neutrophil activity while preserving their pathogen fighting function remains a key area of CF research. The factors that drive their pathological behavior are still under investigation, especially in early disease when aberrant neutrophil behavior first becomes evident. Here we examine the latest findings of neutrophils in pediatric CF lung disease and proposed mechanisms of their pathogenicity. Highlighted in this review are current and emerging experimental methods for assessing CF mucosal immunity and human neutrophil function in the laboratory.

Keywords: cystic fibrosis, neutrophil, inflammation, infection, model systems

INTRODUCTION

Polymorphonuclear neutrophils are the most abundant immune cells in human blood and act as first responders to sites of infection. Their function is a key component of host defense against invading pathogens. In the autosomal recessive disorder cystic fibrosis (CF), persistent microbial colonization in the lungs induces abundant and continuous migration of neutrophils to the airways via powerful inflammatory signals of IL-6, IL-8, and leukotriene B4 (1). Recruited CF neutrophils secrete high levels of proteolytic compounds such as neutrophil elastase (NE), which damage airway tissue and highly correlate with disease severity (2, 3). Despite recognition of neutrophils in the progression of CF lung disease, mechanisms modulating their pathological role are not well-characterized. Past investigations have been hampered by a lack of widely available CF animal models and no suitable *in vitro* infection models that effectively incorporate multiple factors driving complex *in vivo* disease. New data from modern clinical studies are changing the view that neutrophils are a fixed population and are revealing a spectrum of functional phenotypes neutrophils employ to address the variety of pathogenic scenarios they encounter (4). Understanding neutrophil phenotypes and mechanisms in early CF disease, when the airway environment is less complex and more responsive to intervention, will require researchers to revisit or adapt many models of CF. With this review, we present new insights, challenges, and considerations for researchers studying neutrophils in early CF lung disease.

PEDIATRIC CF LUNG DISEASE

The clinical picture of early life cystic fibrosis has changed significantly since CF was first identified in the mid twentieth century, when patients rarely survived to the age of 10 (5). Improvements in diagnostics, from sweat tests to genetic testing, and wider screening of newborns by immunoreactive trypsinogen, has permitted earlier detection of CF and management of the disease. Increased antibacterial therapy, mucolytic and osmotic agents, and the advent of CFTR modulators have further increased the lifespan of many CF patients to beyond 40 years of age (6). Despite these advances, signs of airway inflammation and lung damage are still evident in CF from an early age. In 2005, a pioneering study assessing bronchoalveolar lavage fluid (BALF) after CF newborn screening demonstrated that infection in the first year of life is linked to early airway inflammation (7). Subsequent surveillance studies have now established that for most children, inflammation, altered microbiome, active neutrophil proteolytic function, and lung damage all become evident within the first 2 years of life (8–11), before children are old enough to be treated with CFTR modulators (12, 13). Lung function declines can be evident in infants and continue into childhood (14–16). However, early airway disease can occur in the absence of overt respiratory symptoms (17) or infection (18, 19). Computed Tomography (CT) screening has revealed that CF associated structural changes diagnosed in early life persist into childhood and adolescence. Permanent bronchial wall thickening, or bronchiectasis, is detectable in about 8.5% of pediatric CF patients in the first year of life, and this increases to 36% by 4 years (8). In addition to cytokine release, neutrophil influx into early CF airways may be supported by chemotactic fragments from the extracellular matrix (20, 21). Overall, CF lung damage and declines in function are linked to neutrophil counts and levels of neutrophil proteases, that are often a response to early incidence of infection. Understanding the pathology of early lung disease as it appears today will be key to maximizing long-term benefits from subsequent CFTR modulator therapies.

NEUTROPHILS IN CF AIRWAYS

Neutrophil Elastase and Serine Proteases

Early in vertebrate immunity, neutrophils evolved a granule system to separately store enzymes and antimicrobial factors safely until fused with a phagosome (22). Neutrophil elastase (NE) and other serine proteases are a central component of the neutrophil antimicrobial arsenal, stored in the primary granules that are the last granule to mobilize and are highly resistant to fusion with the outer membrane (23). Yet uninhibited NE activity can be detected in over 30% of BALF samples from young children with CF (11, 24). Activity of NE is considered one of the most significant biomarkers in CF lung disease, as activity significantly correlates with lung damage and functional declines at all stages of life with CF (25–28). Unregulated activity is destructive to airway epithelial cells and the lamina propria, and can impede microbial clearance through destruction of host immune factors (29). *In vitro* and *in vivo* studies have demonstrated how elevated NE activity induces epithelial senescence in CF airway cells (30, 31), prevents epithelial repair mechanisms (24), and is a key driver of airway inflammation and mucus production (25–28). Neutrophil Elastase and other serine proteases digest a variety of host proteins, suggesting multiple mechanisms that implicate these compounds in CF airway pathology. Along with neutrophil serine proteases cathepsin G and proteinase 3, NE directly interacts with cytokines, including IL-8 and IL-1α, increasing their potency (32–34). Counter-intuitively, serine proteases also degrade antimicrobial peptides (AMPs), including lactoferrin, midkine, and surfactant protein-A (SP-A) (35–37). In particular, NE has been shown to degrade pattern recognition receptors including toll-like receptor 4 (TLR4), reducing bacterial lipopolysaccharide (LPS) sensitivity and increasing inflammation (38). In addition to modulating mucosal immunity, serine proteases may promote airway epithelial dysfunction in CF. For example, NE cleaves E-cadherin, an important component of adherens junctions, compromising epithelial integrity (39). It also induces CFTR protein degradation by calpain activity in both *in vitro* epithelial cells and *in vivo* mouse models, resulting in impaired channel function as well as increasing sodium transport into cells through proteolytic activation of sodium ion channels (ENaC) (40–42).

Cysteine Proteases, Matrix Metalloproteinases, and Reactive Oxygen Species

In addition to NE and other enzymes found in primary granules, additional neutrophil derived compounds may contribute to CF airway pathology. Crucial for intracellular degradation of pathogens, secreted cysteine proteases have similar deleterious effects as their serine counterparts. Cathepsins B and S positively correlate with clinical markers of inflammation in pediatric CF airways, including NE, IL-8, and TNFα (43, 44). They selectively maintain neutrophil influx through activation of chemokines containing glutamic acid-leucine-arginine (ELR) motifs and inactivation of lymphocyte attracting non-ELR chemokines (45). Similar to serine proteases, cathepsins can compromise immunity through degradation of AMPs such as lactoferrin, LL-37, SP-A, and β-defensins (46–49). Cathepsins B and S are also implicated in airway mucus dehydration through induction of ENaC activity (50, 51). Matrix metalloproteinases (MMPs) are additional proteases implicated in CF associated with airway remodeling following lung injury. They can originate from any tissue, but neutrophil derived MMP-9 is particularly linked to airway damage, inflammation, and lung function decline in early CF (52, 53). Furthermore, MMP-9 sustains airway neutrophilia through potentiation of IL-8 and generation of proline-glycine-proline (PGP) matrikine fragments from breakdown of collagen (21, 54). Upon phagocytosis of pathogens, neutrophils produce large amounts of superoxide radicals for microbial killing. Broadly termed reactive oxygen species (ROS), neutrophils are among the most potent producers of these compounds (55). Oxidative stress as shown by elevated airway ROS is observed in chronic obstructive pulmonary disease (COPD) as well as CF (56–58). Increased ROS production results in destruction of antiproteases, which are crucial for protecting tissue from unregulated proteolysis (59, 60). In the context of CF, ROS may impede the function of antiproteases such as alpha-1-antitrypsin, an important NE inhibitor, prolonging airway neutrophil proteolytic activity (24, 61).

CFTR in Neutrophils

A central conundrum of CF is why proteolytic activity develops in such early, mild stages of CF lung inflammation. One obvious area of investigation has been whether neutrophil dysfunction in CF airways is exclusively influenced by factors in the lung environment or is also a consequence of inherent CFTR defects. Since the discovery of the CFTR gene, there have been studies suggesting CFTR protein is routinely expressed in cells of myeloid origin and has a role in microbial clearance within phagosomes (62–64). Hypochlorous acid (HOCl) is an important antimicrobial component of neutrophil phagosomes whose formation is proposed to be dependent on CFTR-mediated chloride ion transport (65). CFTR is reported to traffic to phagosomal membranes in peripheral blood neutrophils, with CFTR mutation resulting in defective phagosomal chlorination, affecting clearance of microbes such as *P. aeruginosa* (66–68). Contrasting findings have shown normal respiratory burst activity and production of nicotinamide adenine dinucleotide phosphate (NADPH) oxidase components in CF blood neutrophils and no detectable CFTR protein in these cells (69). Additional evidence for the role of CFTR in neutrophils comes from a small number of studies showing restoration of CF neutrophil functions including CFTR phagosomal trafficking (67), leukocyte activation (70), and intracellular ion regulation (71) in response to CFTR modulator treatment. Still, further research is needed to clarify the presence and function of CFTR in neutrophils, and how defects in the gene influence the pathological activity of CF airway neutrophils. One consistent observation is a CFTR mutation dependent effect on *in vivo* neutrophil lifespan, with CF neutrophils displaying delayed apoptosis compared to non-CF neutrophils, possibly preventing resolution of neutrophilic inflammation (72–74). The most recent of these studies demonstrated a link between delayed apoptosis by CF neutrophils and propensity to form neutrophil extracellular traps (74).

Neutrophil Extracellular Traps

The identification of neutrophil extracellular traps (NETs), extracellular networks of DNA containing azurophilic granules, neutrophil elastase and other antimicrobial components, was a significant event in neutrophil biology (75). NET formation was initially viewed as a form of active cell death upon which nuclear and granular membranes were disintegrated, contents ejected and mixed in the cytoplasm, then released upon deterioration of the cell membrane (76). The process was later termed NETosis and proposed to be an alternative strategy used by neutrophils upon failing to clear infection via traditional phagocytosis. While NETs can trap and neutralize invading pathogens, the extent of their microbe killing abilities is debated (77, 78). A significant amount of research into NETosis has been undertaken, as recently reviewed by this journal (79). Multiple studies have described forms of NETosis that result in mitochondrial DNA release rather than nuclear DNA, or allow neutrophils to remain viable and motile after NET formation (80–83). The ability of NETs to harbor NE, the presence of NET derived DNA in CF sputum, and increased pathogen resistance in response to NETs, suggest NETosis is likely to play a role in CF lung disease (84, 85). Yet the question remains on how frequently NETosis occurs during early CF airway inflammation, prior to significant biofilm formation that reduces availability of bacteria to neutrophils.

Neutrophil Exocytosis

Perhaps the most intriguing hypothesis explaining early airway neutrophil proteolytic activity is that upon recruitment to CF airways, neutrophils reprogram toward an aberrant granular-releasing, immunoregulatory, and metabolically distinct (GRIM) phenotype that includes exocytosis of primary granules—as evidenced by high CD63 expression (86–88). The GRIM phenotype is specific to recruited neutrophils as peripheral blood neutrophils from CF patients exhibit a normal phenotype (89). However, when naïve neutrophils from either CF or non-CF donors are stimulated in an *in vitro* transmigration model of neutrophil recruitment by adult CF BALF or sputum, cells from both groups of donors undergo GRIM reprogramming (89). While factors such as tumor necrosis factor-alpha (TNF-α) can prime exocytosis of neutrophil azurophilic granules (90), Forrest and colleagues observed GRIM reprogramming only upon stimulation with *ex vivo* CF samples but not with exogenously added chemokines, suggesting a yet unidentified factor in CF airways is responsible for changes in neutrophil activity (89).

Most significantly, GRIM neutrophils were also found to have reduced bacterial killing capacity, which aligns with the apparent disconnect between NE release and inability to resolve infection in CF airways (89). More recent studies have reported how Staphylococcal superantigen-like protein 13 (SSL13) from *Staphylococcus aureus*, a common early CF pathogen, can induce neutrophil exocytosis (91) and whose production is evident in the CF microbiome (92). In an age related cohort of non-CF children admitted for acute respiratory distress syndrome (ARDS), neutrophil exocytosis and reduced bacterial killing was observed in individuals co-infected with virus and bacteria but not viral infection alone, suggesting that neutrophil exocytosis may be linked to responses against polymicrobial infection (93). This relationship with infection is yet to be established in early CF disease, however neutrophil exocytosis markers correlate positively with disease severity more so than free NE activity (11). Therefore, changes in airway neutrophil functional markers may be more reliable indicators of disease progression in children with CF and should be a focus of early CF lung disease research.

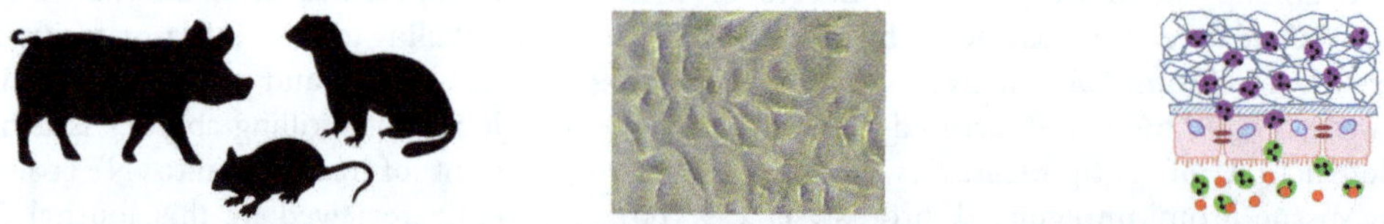

	CF Animals	Primary Airway Cells	Transmigration Models
Current Applications	Observe gross CF disease phenotypes.	Assess CFTR function, effects of modulator therapy, and innate immunity of airway epithelium.	Study PMN recruitment and activity in the airways.
Advantages	Study *in vivo* disease across multiple organ systems. Depending on animal, models full to partial pathology of CF lung (infection, inflammation, mucus plugging, structural changes, etc).	Responses are measured in disease relevant, non-cancerous, human cells. Different ages, sex, and mutation types can be tested in culture systems representative of native airway tissue.	Allows close, controlled, testing and observation of human PMN in response to infectious and non-infectious stimuli.
Disadvantages	Disease phenotype and progression not wholly representative of CF in humans, limited mutation types for testing, care of animals is costly and laborious.	Results are variable depending on sampling and culture of cells among other factors. Limited by access to human donors.	Reliance on cancer cell lines to act as epithelial barrier during migration. Also limited by access to *ex vivo* BALF/sputum.
Potential Applications	Study *in vivo* PMN exocytosis and proteolytic activity? NETosis? CFTR function?	Screen early CF infection scenarios or insults that trigger PMN pathological activity?	Study coordinated CF epithelial/ PMN responses to infection?

FIGURE 1 | Comparison of model systems for studying CF lung disease.

MODELING INFECTION AND INFLAMMATION

Characterizing the early mechanisms that trigger phenotype shifts in airway neutrophils may be key for preventing progressive lung disease. Clinical surveillance gives valuable insights into disease phenotypes *in vivo*, however, basic science is crucial for understanding the biology of CF lung disease and the role of the airway epithelium. Over the years, researchers have developed a variety of approaches for this purpose (**Figure 1**). The following is a summary of some of the more important, biologically relevant models currently in use to study infection and inflammation in CF airways.

Animal Models

While CFTR mutant and knockout mice were developed shortly after discovery of the CFTR gene, their use as animal models for CF lung disease is controversial as they lack a robust CF lung phenotype of spontaneous infection and disease (94–97). Despite extensive similarity, mouse immune cells can behave differently to human counterparts in their response to pathogens, for example, murine neutrophils are not activated by SSL13 (91). Mice also express toll-like receptor 11 (TLR11), a TLR not expressed in humans, that detects profilin and bacterial flagellin (98). Still, mouse models of induced airway infection have provided insights into CF airway inflammation and disease. Studies of acute *Pseudomonas aeruginosa* infection have observed poor growth, increased mortality, and reduced bacterial clearance in CF vs. wild-type mice (99, 100). Additionally, CF mice have exaggerated levels of murine inflammatory cytokines and airway neutrophilia in response to infection, as well as prolonged inflammation compared to wild-type mice (101, 102). Most of these studies have inoculated animals through intratracheal delivery of agarose beads embedded with bacteria, an unrealistic representation of how CF patients normally acquire these organisms. Of interest has been the observation that environmental acquisition of *P. aeruginosa* can be modeled in mice through inoculated drinking water, with CF mice more susceptible to chronic colonization via this route (103). Chronic exposure of CF mice to *P. aeruginosa* LPS also results in increased airway inflammation, neutrophilia and airway remodeling (104, 105). A common theme emerging from these studies, is that neutrophils and their products play a central role in CF lung pathology. With the development of Cre recombinase mice targeting the neutrophil-specific locus Ly6G (106), future studies utilizing this model will continue to play a very useful role in elucidating CF airway neutrophil biology.

The more physiologically relevant animal model for studying CF lung disease include CFTR disrupted pigs and ferrets, as they recapitulate the CF phenotype across all organ systems implicated in human disease (107). Both models were developed just over a decade ago using adenoviral vectors, generating CFTR full or partial knockout animals in both species via exon 10 disruption, as well as a ΔF508 pig (108–110). Pigs are suitable human disease models due to their analogous physiology, and in the case of respiratory disease, similar bronchial structure and distribution of submucosal glands (111). CF pigs have CFTR protein similar to that of humans (112). Neonatal CF pigs have little airway inflammation and normal levels of IL-8 and neutrophil counts in BAL compared to non-CF pigs (109). Neonatal CF pigs also have increased presence of microbes in the lungs as shown by culture from *ex vivo* tissue samples, and are less likely to have sterile BAL samples compared to non-CF pigs (113). In the months following birth, CF pigs develop signs of lung disease such as mucus accumulation, inflammation, infection, and airway remodeling (113). While lung disease progression in the CF pig model reflects progression in humans, there are obvious drawbacks of cost and time of pig husbandry and the need of adequate facilities and resources. Furthermore, virtually all CF pigs develop meconium ileus and require early surgical intervention; in contrast, the condition is present in only 20% of infants with CF (109, 113, 114).

Ferret CFTR protein length, amino acid sequence, and function is also similar to that of humans (115). Like CF humans, CF ferrets are prone to spontaneous airway infection; however, infection in these animals is far more severe, with CF ferrets requiring continuous antibiotic treatment immediately after birth to survive (116). Additionally, CF ferrets demonstrate abnormally high levels of lung inflammation from birth, and lung disease progresses rapidly upon cessation of prophylactic antibiotics (117, 118). As a result, CF ferrets may not be an ideal system to model the slow progressive lung disease observed in humans, as their disease phenotype develops too quickly. However, a recent study developed homozygous $CFTR^{G551D/G551D}$ ferrets to test effects of *in utero* treatment with VX-770 (ivacaftor) (119). Prenatal and early postnatal administration ameliorated CF multi-organ disease, posing new research questions around CFTR in early development, the possibility of prenatal modulator therapy, and disease attenuation in CF animals to further study effects of modulator treatment or model mild disease in humans. While neutrophil counts and elastase activity in CF animals trend similarly to human disease, neutrophil reprogramming has yet to be evaluated. Future studies must assess airway neutrophil exocytosis and lung disease severity in CF animals to determine if they are suitable models for characterizing this process in humans.

Primary Airway Epithelial Cells

While animal models allow observation of gross phenotype of disease, *in vitro* studies permit experimentation in a highly controlled environment and are important for understanding mechanisms of disease at the cellular level. The accepted gold standard for *in vitro* CF research are patient derived primary airway epithelial cells (pAEC). As a barrier that protects the lung from direct environmental exposure, the airway epithelium has long been recognized for its role in host defense and respiratory disease (120–125). Cells are typically isolated from epithelial brushings of the nose or lower airways, or less frequently from explanted lungs (126, 127). Yields from brushings are variable and *ex vivo* pAEC have limited proliferative capacity; they become senescent after only a few passages making them difficult to expand in culture (126, 127). The adaptation of conditionally reprogrammed airway epithelial cells (CRAEC) through co-culture with irradiated fibroblast feeder cells has significantly increased passage number capacity of pAEC, while maintaining lineage specific characteristics (128). Additionally, CRAEC can be seeded from co-culture into air-liquid interface culture (ALI) to form a differentiated pseudostratified epithelial layer (128, 129). This has enabled many CF research groups to look to CF primary airway epithelial cell models in order to understand the cellular drivers of progressive lung disease, and more recently to evaluate the efficacy of CFTR modulators in restoring CFTR function in target cells (130, 131). Nasal pAEC are increasingly being used in epithelial CFTR studies, since their growth, differentiation, CFTR activity, and response to modulators are similar to lower airway cells, and have the advantage of being more readily accessible (129). Nasal cells have also been adapted to three dimensional spheroid cultures that are representative of native epithelium and mature more quickly than traditional ALI cultures (132). These spheroids have then been used to quantify CFTR function via spheroid swelling in cultures from CF patients across different mutation classes, to assess individual responses to modulator treatment (133, 134). As such, they have potential as a preclinical screening tool to identify responses to modulator therapies in a personalized medicine approach.

Despite increased airway inflammation in CF patients, there is still debate as to whether the CF airway epithelium is inherently pro-inflammatory (135–137). Baseline expression of neutrophil chemoattractants including IL-8, IL-6, and IL-1β is reported in some studies to be similar in CF vs. non-CF pAEC (138–140), but others report increases in CF cells at baseline (141, 142). Increased airway inflammation could also be a result of dysfunctional CF epithelial innate immunity, a major topic in CF research, as the airway epithelium has an important role in responding to infection and neutrophil recruitment (143–147). Studies have shown IL-8 release and NF-κB activity are increased in CF vs. non-CF pAEC following *P. aeruginosa* infection (142, 148, 149). CF pAEC have also been shown to display differential gene expression at the transcriptional level compared to non-CF pAEC in response to *P. aeruginosa* infection, which may be further evidence of CF aberrant immune responses (150, 151). In response to infection with respiratory viruses, studies have also observed increased IL-8 production in CF vs. non-CF pAEC (152, 153), which is analogous to *in vivo* findings in pediatric CF patients with rhinovirus infection (154). However, other studies have reported no difference in inflammatory cytokine production as a result of *in vitro* viral infection (155, 156). The filamentous fungi *Aspergillus fumigatus* is emerging as an important early life CF pathogen increasingly detected in pediatric CF airways (157, 158), with *A. fumigatus* infection associated with increased air trapping among 5 year old CF patients (159). Two *in vitro* studies to date have used immortalized cell lines and reported altered cytokine production, though specific data were conflicting (160, 161). Assessing innate immune responses to fungal pathogens in CF will be key to determining treatment priority, but innate immune mechanisms have yet to be corroborated in CF pAEC.

Variability amongst findings from pAEC infection studies could be attributed to the originating cohorts, sampling differences, age and disease severity of subjects, culture methods, and use of differentiated vs. undifferentiated cultures. Additionally, the selection of pathogens can affect outcomes, as pAEC responses can be heterogeneous to individual strains or isolates of the same species (162). Primary cells will continue to be important tools for addressing unanswered questions in CF lung disease, including how epithelial immunity is linked to neutrophil inflammation, how the epithelium responds to fungal and polymicrobial infection, how the airway microbiome affects epithelial homeostasis, and whether CFTR modulators have effects on airway innate immune signaling. Researchers must think carefully about the above factors and how they influence experimental outcomes in pAEC, especially if findings are translated to lung disease pathogenesis in CF patients.

Neutrophil Transmigration to the Airways

The epithelium is not only a barrier to external pathogens, but also presents an obstacle to responding neutrophils. *In vitro* replication of this mucosal physiology was established by early studies assessing neutrophil transmigration across the intestinal mucosa (163–166). These studies established polarized epithelial cultures onto inverted permeable inserts, which were turned over prior to migration for direct loading of naïve isolated neutrophils and thus model basolateral to apical neutrophil migration. It has since been adapted to characterize transmigration across lung epithelium (167), assess the role of neutrophils in β-catenin mediated airway epithelial repair (168, 169), as well as describe responses to infection with respiratory syncytial virus (RSV) and *P. aeruginosa* (170–172). The model previously mentioned in this review uses Alvetex^{TM} 3D scaffolds rather than permeable membranes, which better replicate neutrophil swarming (89, 93), to study neutrophil responses to CF sputum. To understand factors driving early neutrophil fate including exocytosis, this same model could be applied with pediatric BALF. However, pediatric *ex vivo* samples are difficult to obtain, often of limited volume compared to samples from adults. One approach yet to be fully utilized is to apply material from infected CF pAEC as surrogates for human samples. This has multiple benefits. Robust models of pAEC infection responses are well-established and because pAEC can be bio-banked for downstream culture and infection, material can be generated as needed. This approach also facilitates a more focused assessment of factors influencing neutrophil functions, such as epithelial responses to specific infection scenarios.

One caveat of past transmigration studies is the dependence on lung cancer derived cells lines, such as A549, H292, H441, 16HBE, and Calu-3 cells, as a substitute for primary cell derived epithelium. Advantages include easy access to cell lines and robust growth in culture, but at the cost of interpreting epithelial responses during migration through cancer cells. This is critical, since neutrophils directly change airway epithelium via microRNA (173) or exosomes (174) and neoplastic cells may not reproduce CF pAEC responses. As limitations on pAEC culture expansion are overcome, transmigration studies are increasingly incorporating pAEC (175). A remaining challenge is that established methods for differentiating pAEC traditionally employ 0.4 μm pore size inserts, but a 3.0μm pore size or larger is required to permit neutrophil transmigration, which can result in significant loss of primary cells during seeding. One study has managed to address this issue by coating both faces of a transwell insert with extracellular matrix and providing seeded cells with laminins to improve attachment (175). Primary cells differentiated into pseudostratified epithelial layers on a 3.0 μm insert, similar to how they would on a conventional 0.4 μm transwell insert, and permitted neutrophil transmigration upon apical infection with *P. aeruginosa* (175). Future integration of CF pAEC in models of neutrophil transmigration will be required for studying coordinated immune responses of the CF airway

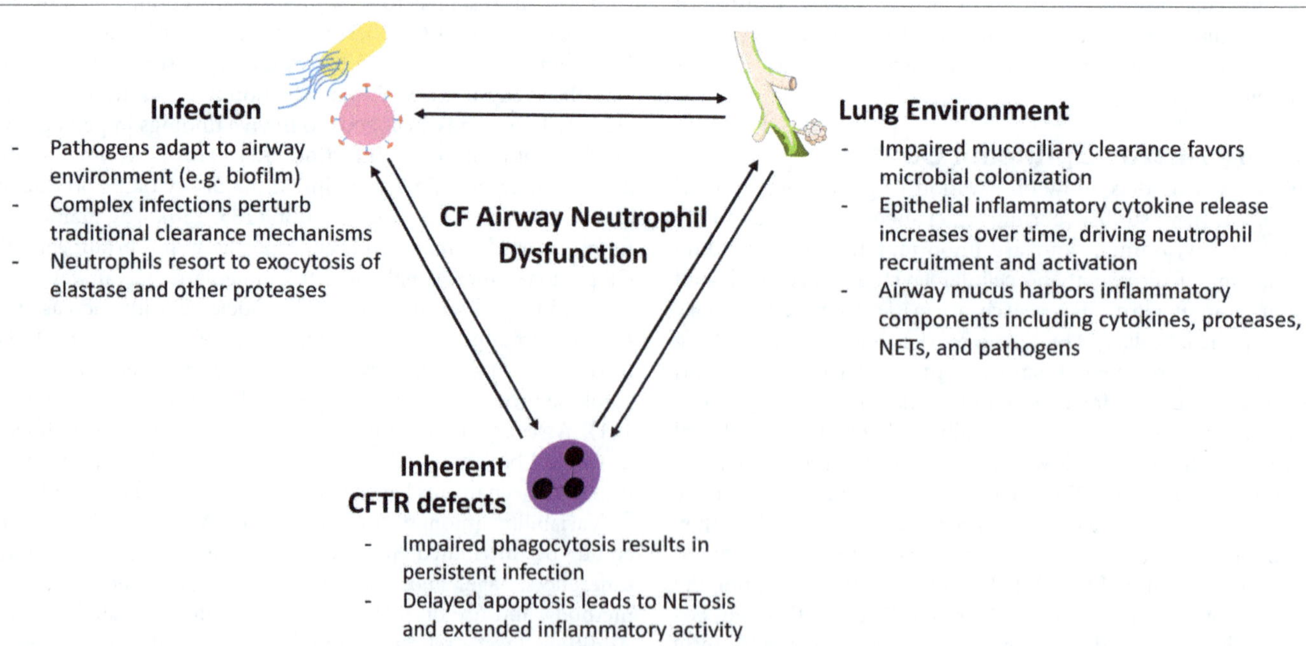

FIGURE 2 | Factors influencing CF airway neutrophil plasticity.

epithelium and recruited neutrophils in a single translational system. If designed with high throughput screening in mind, there is great potential to facilitate much needed pre-clinical testing of anti-inflammatory drugs in CF.

CFTR MODULATOR THERAPY AND AIRWAY INFLAMMATION

Depending on their mechanism of action, CFTR modulators are characterized as correctors that improve defective CFTR trafficking to the cell surface, or potentiators that enhance defective CFTR function. Studies of modulators have shown improvements in patients as measured by sweat chloride levels and FEV_1, however, efficacy against infection and airway inflammation is poorly investigated. In placebo controlled studies of lumacaftor-ivacaftor and tezacaftor-ivacaftor in CF patients $\geq$12 years of age, infective pulmonary exacerbations occurred at similar rates in both treatment and placebo groups (176–178). Phase 3 trials of lumacaftor-ivacaftor in CF patients aged 6–11 also found that incidence of infection associated pulmonary exacerbations was similar between patients receiving treatment (18%) and patients receiving a placebo control (19%) (179). The recently FDA approved elexacaftor-tezacaftor-ivacaftor triple therapy roughly halves the incidence of infective pulmonary excacerbations compared to a placebo (180), but the drug is not yet approved for patients under 12 years of age. Multiple studies have shown that administration of modulators reduces bacterial colonization within the first year of treatment and delays acquisition in uncolonized patients; however, bacterial isolates present in the airways prior to treatment persist and may eventually rebound over longer periods (12, 13, 181, 182). Whether CFTR modulators reduce levels of inflammatory cytokines is still not certain, as there is evidence of both reduction and no effect on clinically relevant biomarkers including NE (12, 13). Altogether, current findings suggest that modulator therapy alone may not be sufficient to manage infection and airway inflammation in this population, especially over the long term.

CONCLUSION

Neutrophils have a major role in CF lung disease but our ability to treat the underlying mechanisms is still limited. Modern approaches are revealing new perspectives on neutrophils as plastic, programmable drivers of airway disease who both respond to and actively shape the local airway environment (**Figure 2**). These novel neutrophil functions are occurring even in mild and largely asymptomatic pediatric CF lung disease and precede structural lung changes. Even with the advent of combination CFTR modulator therapy, which improves lung function but perhaps not infection and inflammation, continued investigation of initial neutrophil pathological activity is necessary to identify much-needed interventions that can address this problem. Researchers now have available a diverse number of tools for understanding the complex interplay between infection, the airway epithelium, and recruited neutrophils (**Figure 1**). Moving forward, basic studies will need to consider the advantages of various approaches, caveats, and carefully select appropriate models when exploring the beginnings of CF airway neutrophilic disease.

AUTHOR CONTRIBUTIONS

DL, LG, and AK conceived the review. DL and LG conducted literature review and wrote the manuscript. LG and AK provided critical review.

REFERENCES

1. Hartl D, Gaggar A, Bruscia E, Hector A, Marcos V, Jung A, et al. Innate immunity in cystic fibrosis lung disease. *J Cyst Fibros.* (2012) 11:363–82. doi: 10.1016/j.jcf.2012.07.003
2. Mayer-Hamblett N, Aitken ML, Accurso FJ, Kronmal RA, Konstan MW, Burns JL, et al. Association between pulmonary function and sputum biomarkers in cystic fibrosis. *Am J Respir Crit Care Med.* (2007) 175:822–8. doi: 10.1164/rccm.200609-1354OC
3. Dittrich AS, Kuhbandner I, Gehrig S, Rickert-Zacharias V, Twigg M, Wege S, et al. Elastase activity on sputum neutrophils correlates with severity of lung disease in cystic fibrosis. *Eur Respir J.* (2018) 51:1701910. doi: 10.1183/13993003.01910-2017
4. Jablonska J, Granot Z. Neutrophil, quo vadis?. *J Leukoc Biol.* (2017) 102:685–8. doi: 10.1189/jlb.3MR0117-015R
5. Davis PB. Cystic fibrosis since 1938. *Am J Respir Crit Care Med.* (2006) 173:475–82. doi: 10.1164/rccm.200505-840OE
6. Bell SC, Mall MA, Gutierrez H, Macek M, Madge S, Davies JC, et al. The future of cystic fibrosis care: a global perspective. *Lancet Respir Med.* (2020) 8:65–124. doi: 10.1016/S2213-2600(19)30337-6
7. Armstrong DS, Hook SM, Jamsen KM, Nixon GM, Carzino R, Carlin JB, et al. Lower airway inflammation in infants with cystic fibrosis detected by newborn screening. *Pediatr Pulmonol.* (2005) 40:500–10. doi: 10.1002/ppul.20294
8. Stick SM, Brennan S, Murray C, Douglas T, von Ungern-Sternberg BS, Garratt LW. et al. Bronchiectasis in infants and preschool children diagnosed with cystic fibrosis after newborn screening. *J Pediatr.* (2009) 155, 623–8 e1. doi: 10.1016/j.jpeds.2009.05.005
9. Schultz A, Stick S. Early pulmonary inflammation and lung damage in children with cystic fibrosis. *Respirology.* (2015) 20:569–78. doi: 10.1111/resp.12521
10. Laguna TA, Wagner BD, Williams CB, Stevens MJ, Robertson CE, Welchlin CW, et al. Airway Microbiota in bronchoalveolar lavage fluid from clinically well infants with cystic fibrosis. *PLoS ONE.* (2016) 11:e0167649. doi: 10.1371/journal.pone.0167649
11. Margaroli C, Garratt LW, Horati H, Dittrich AS, Rosenow T, Montgomery ST, et al. Elastase exocytosis by airway neutrophils is associated with early lung damage in children with cystic fibrosis. *Am J Respir Crit Care Med.* (2019) 199:873–81. doi: 10.1164/rccm.201803-0442OC
12. Rowe SM, Heltshe SL, Gonska T, Donaldson SH, Borowitz D, Gelfond D, et al. Clinical mechanism of the cystic fibrosis transmembrane conductance

regulator potentiator ivacaftor in G551D-mediated cystic fibrosis. *Am J Respir Crit Care Med.* (2014) 190:175–84. doi: 10.1164/rccm.201404-0703OC
13. Hisert KB, Heltshe SL, Pope C, Jorth P, Wu X, Edwards RM, et al. Restoring cystic fibrosis transmembrane conductance regulator function reduces airway bacteria and inflammation in people with cystic fibrosis and chronic lung infections. *Am J Respir Crit Care Med.* (2017) 195:1617–28. doi: 10.1164/rccm.201609-1954OC
14. Kozlowska WJ, Bush A, Wade A, Aurora P, Carr SB, Castle RA, et al. Lung function from infancy to the preschool years after clinical diagnosis of cystic fibrosis. *Am J Respir Crit Care Med.* (2008) 178:42–9. doi: 10.1164/rccm.200710-1599OC
15. Harrison AN, Regelmann WE, Zirbes JM, Milla CE. Longitudinal assessment of lung function from infancy to childhood in patients with cystic fibrosis. *Pediatr Pulmonol.* (2009) 44:330–9. doi: 10.1002/ppul.20994
16. Brumback LC, Davis SD, Kerby GS, Kloster M, Johnson R, Castile R, et al. Lung function from infancy to preschool in a cohort of children with cystic fibrosis. *Eur Respir J.* (2013) 41:60–6. doi: 10.1183/09031936.00021612
17. Sly PD, Brennan S, Gangell C, de Klerk N, Murray C, Mott L, et al. Lung disease at diagnosis in infants with cystic fibrosis detected by newborn screening. *Am J Respir Crit Care Med.* (2009) 180:146–52. doi: 10.1164/rccm.200901-0069OC
18. Montgomery ST, Dittrich AS, Garratt LW, Turkovic L, Frey DL, Stick SM, et al. Interleukin-1 is associated with inflammation and structural lung disease in young children with cystic fibrosis. *J Cyst Fibros.* (2018) 17:715–22. doi: 10.1016/j.jcf.2018.05.006
19. Esther CR Jr, Muhlebach MS, Ehre C, Hill DB, Wolfgang MC, Kesimer M, et al. Mucus accumulation in the lungs precedes structural changes and infection in children with cystic fibrosis. *Sci Transl Med.* (2019) 11:eaav3488. doi: 10.1126/scitranslmed.aav3488
20. Breuer O, Schultz A, Garratt LW, Turkovic L, Rosenow T, Murray CP, et al. Aspergillus infections and progression of structural lung disease in children with cystic fibrosis. *Am J Respir Crit Care Med.* (2020) 201:688–96. doi: 10.1164/rccm.201908-1585OC
21. Turnbull AR, Pyle CJ, Patel DF, Jackson PL, Hilliard TN, Regamey N, et al. Abnormal pro-gly-pro pathway and airway neutrophilia in pediatric cystic fibrosis. *J Cyst Fibros.* (2020) 19:40–8. doi: 10.1016/j.jcf.2019.05.017
22. Fu Z, Thorpe M, Akula S, Chahal G, Hellman LT. Extended cleavage specificity of human neutrophil elastase, human proteinase 3, and their distant ortholog clawed frog PR3-three elastases with similar primary but different extended specificities and stability. *Front Immunol.* (2018) 9:2387. doi: 10.3389/fimmu.2018.02387
23. Jog NR, Rane MJ, Lominadze G, Luerman GC, Ward RA, McLeish KR. The actin cytoskeleton regulates exocytosis of all neutrophil granule subsets. *Am J Physiol Cell Physiol.* (2007) 292:C1690–700. doi: 10.1152/ajpcell.00384.2006
24. Garratt LW, Sutanto EN, Ling KM, Looi K, Iosifidis T, Martinovich KM, et al. Alpha-1 antitrypsin mitigates the inhibition of airway epithelial cell repair by neutrophil elastase. *Am J Respir Cell Mol Biol.* (2016) 54:341–9. doi: 10.1165/rcmb.2015-0074OC
25. Pillarisetti N, Williamson E, Linnane B, Skoric B, Robertson CF, Robinson P, et al. Infection, inflammation, and lung function decline in infants with cystic fibrosis. *Am J Respir Crit Care Med.* (2011) 184:75–81. doi: 10.1164/rccm.201011-1892OC
26. Sagel SD, Wagner BD, Anthony MM, Emmett P, Zemanick ET. Sputum biomarkers of inflammation and lung function decline in children with cystic fibrosis. *Am J Respir Crit Care Med.* (2012) 186:857–65. doi: 10.1164/rccm.201203-0507OC
27. Sly PD, Gangell CL, Chen L, Ware RS, Ranganathan S, Mott LS, et al. Risk factors for bronchiectasis in children with cystic fibrosis. *N Engl J Med.* (2013) 368:1963–70. doi: 10.1056/NEJMoa1301725
28. Rosenow T, Mok LC, Turkovic L, Berry LJ, Sly PD, Ranganathan S, et al. The cumulative effect of inflammation and infection on structural lung disease in early cystic fibrosis. *Eur Respir J.* (2019) 54:1801771. doi: 10.1183/13993003.01771-2018
29. Gifford AM, Chalmers JD. The role of neutrophils in cystic fibrosis. *Curr Opin Hematol.* (2014) 21:16–22. doi: 10.1097/MOH.0000000000000009
30. Tsuji T, Aoshiba K, Nagai A. Alveolar cell senescence exacerbates pulmonary inflammation in patients with chronic obstructive pulmonary disease. *Respiration.* (2010) 80:59–70. doi: 10.1159/000268287
31. Fischer BM, Wong JK, Degan S, Kummarapurugu AB, Zheng S, Haridass P, et al. Increased expression of senescence markers in cystic fibrosis airways. *Am J Physiol Lung Cell Mol Physiol.* (2013) 304:L394–400. doi: 10.1152/ajplung.00091.2012
32. Padrines M, Wolf M, Walz A, Baggiolini M. Interleukin-8 processing by neutrophil elastase, cathepsin G and proteinase-3. *FEBS Lett.* (1994) 352:231–5. doi: 10.1016/0014-5793(94)00952-X
33. Pham CT. Neutrophil serine proteases fine-tune the inflammatory response. *Int J Biochem Cell Biol.* (2008) 40:1317–33. doi: 10.1016/j.biocel.2007.11.008
34. Afonina IS, Tynan GA, Logue SE, Cullen SP, Bots M, Luthi AU, et al. Granzyme B-dependent proteolysis acts as a switch to enhance the proinflammatory activity of IL-1alpha. *Mol Cell.* (2011) 44:265–78. doi: 10.1016/j.molcel.2011.07.037
35. Britigan BE, Edeker BL. Pseudomonas and neutrophil products modify transferrin and lactoferrin to create conditions that favor hydroxyl radical formation. *J Clin Invest.* (1991) 88:1092–102. doi: 10.1172/JCI115408
36. Rubio F, Cooley J, Accurso FJ, Remold-O'Donnell E. Linkage of neutrophil serine proteases and decreased surfactant protein-A (SP-A) levels in inflammatory lung disease. *Thorax.* (2004) 59:318–23. doi: 10.1136/thx.2003.014902
37. Nordin SL, Jovic S, Kurut A, Andersson C, Gela A, Bjartell A, et al. High expression of midkine in the airways of patients with cystic fibrosis. *Am J Respir Cell Mol Biol.* (2013) 49:935–42. doi: 10.1165/rcmb.2013-0106OC
38. Devaney JM, Greene CM, Taggart CC, Carroll TP, O'Neill SJ, McElvaney NG. Neutrophil elastase up-regulates interleukin-8 via toll-like receptor 4. *FEBS Lett.* (2003) 544:129–32. doi: 10.1016/S0014-5793(03)00482-4
39. Boxio R, Wartelle J, Nawrocki-Raby B, Lagrange B, Malleret L, Hirche T, et al. Neutrophil elastase cleaves epithelial cadherin in acutely injured lung epithelium. *Respir Res.* (2016) 17:129. doi: 10.1186/s12931-016-0449-x
40. Caldwell RA, Boucher RC, Stutts MJ. Neutrophil elastase activates near-silent epithelial Na+ channels and increases airway epithelial Na+ transport. *Am J Physiol Lung Cell Mol Physiol.* (2005) 288:L813–9. doi: 10.1152/ajplung.00435.2004
41. Pruliere-Escabasse V, Clerici C, Vuagniaux G, Coste A, Escudier E, Planes C. Effect of neutrophil elastase and its inhibitor EPI-hNE4 on transepithelial sodium transport across normal and cystic fibrosis human nasal epithelial cells. *Respir Res.* (2010) 11:141. doi: 10.1186/1465-9921-11-141
42. Le Gars M, Descamps D, Roussel D, Saussereau E, Guillot L, Ruffin M, et al. Neutrophil elastase degrades cystic fibrosis transmembrane conductance regulator via calpains and disables channel function *in vitro* and *in vivo*. *Am J Respir Crit Care Med.* (2013) 187:170–9. doi: 10.1164/rccm.201205-0875OC
43. Martin SL, Moffitt KL, McDowell A, Greenan C, Bright-Thomas RJ, Jones AM, et al. Association of airway cathepsin B and S with inflammation in cystic fibrosis. *Pediatr Pulmonol.* (2010) 45:860–8. doi: 10.1002/ppul.21274
44. Small DM, Brown RR, Doherty DF, Abladey A, Zhou-Suckow Z, Delaney RJ, et al. Targeting of cathepsin S reduces cystic fibrosis-like lung disease. *Eur Respir J.* (2019) 53:1801523. doi: 10.1183/13993003.01523-2018
45. Repnik U, Starr AE, Overall CM, Turk B. Cysteine cathepsins activate ELR chemokines and inactivate non-ELR chemokines. *J Biol Chem.* (2015) 290:13800–11. doi: 10.1074/jbc.M115.638395
46. Taggart CC, Greene CM, Smith SG, Levine RL, McCray PB Jr, O'Neill S, et al. Inactivation of human beta-defensins 2 and 3 by elastolytic cathepsins. *J Immunol.* (2003) 171:931–7. doi: 10.4049/jimmunol.171.2.931
47. Rogan MP, Taggart CC, Greene CM, Murphy PG, O'Neill SJ, McElvaney NG. Loss of microbicidal activity and increased formation of biofilm due to decreased lactoferrin activity in patients with cystic fibrosis. *J Infect Dis.* (2004) 190:1245–53. doi: 10.1086/423821
48. Lecaille F, Naudin C, Sage J, Joulin-Giet A, Courty A, Andrault PM, et al. Specific cleavage of the lung surfactant protein A by human cathepsin S may impair its antibacterial properties. *Int J Biochem Cell Biol.* (2013) 45:1701–9. doi: 10.1016/j.biocel.2013.05.018
49. Andrault PM, Samsonov SA, Weber G, Coquet L, Nazmi K, Bolscher JG, et al. Antimicrobial peptide LL-37 is both a substrate of cathepsins S and K and a selective inhibitor of cathepsin L. *Biochemistry.* (2015) 54:2785–98. doi: 10.1021/acs.biochem.5b00231
50. Haerteis S, Krappitz M, Bertog M, Krappitz A, Baraznenok V, Henderson I, et al. Proteolytic activation of the epithelial sodium channel (ENaC)

by the cysteine protease cathepsin-S. *Pflugers Arch.* (2012) 464:353–65. doi: 10.1007/s00424-012-1138-3
51. Tan CD, Hobbs C, Sameni M, Sloane BF, Stutts MJ, Tarran R. Cathepsin B contributes to Na+ hyperabsorption in cystic fibrosis airway epithelial cultures. *J Physiol.* (2014) 592:5251–68. doi: 10.1113/jphysiol.2013.267286
52. Sagel SD, Kapsner RK, Osberg I. Induced sputum matrix metalloproteinase-9 correlates with lung function and airway inflammation in children with cystic fibrosis. *Pediatr Pulmonol.* (2005) 39:224–32. doi: 10.1002/ppul.20165
53. Garratt LW, Sutanto EN, Ling KM, Looi K, Iosifidis T, Martinovich KM, et al. Matrix metalloproteinase activation by free neutrophil elastase contributes to bronchiectasis progression in early cystic fibrosis. *Eur Respir J.* (2015) 46:384–94. doi: 10.1183/09031936.00212114
54. Van den Steen PE, Proost P, Wuyts A, Van Damme J, Opdenakker G. Neutrophil gelatinase B potentiates interleukin-8 tenfold by aminoterminal processing, whereas it degrades CTAP-III, PF-4, and GRO-alpha and leaves RANTES and MCP-2 intact. *Blood.* (2000) 96:2673–81. doi: 10.1182/blood.V96.8.2673
55. Winterbourn CC, Kettle AJ, Hampton MB. Reactive oxygen species and neutrophil function. *Annu Rev Biochem.* (2016) 85:765–92. doi: 10.1146/annurev-biochem-060815-014442
56. Brown RK, Kelly FJ. Role of free radicals in the pathogenesis of cystic fibrosis. *Thorax.* (1994) 49:738–42. doi: 10.1136/thx.49.8.738
57. Galli F, Battistoni A, Gambari R, Pompella A, Bragonzi A, Pilolli F, et al. Oxidative stress and antioxidant therapy in cystic fibrosis. *Biochim Biophys Acta.* (2012) 1822:690–713. doi: 10.1016/j.bbadis.2011.12.012
58. Kirkham PA, Barnes PJ. Oxidative stress in COPD. *Chest.* (2013) 144:266–73. doi: 10.1378/chest.12-2664
59. Fischer BM, Pavlisko E, Voynow JA. Pathogenic triad in COPD: oxidative stress, protease-antiprotease imbalance, and inflammation. *Int J Chron Obstruct Pulmon Dis.* (2011) 6:413–21. doi: 10.2147/COPD.S10770
60. Siddiqui T, Zia MK, Ali SS, Rehman AA, Ahsan H, Khan FH. Reactive oxygen species and anti-proteinases. *Arch Physiol Biochem.* (2016) 122:1–7. doi: 10.3109/13813455.2015.1115525
61. McElvaney NG. Alpha-1 antitrypsin therapy in cystic fibrosis and the lung disease associated with alpha-1 antitrypsin deficiency. *Ann Am Thorac Soc.* (2016) 13(Suppl. 2):S191–6. doi: 10.1513/AnnalsATS.201504-245KV
62. Yoshimura K, Nakamura H, Trapnell BC, Chu CS, Dalemans W, Pavirani A, et al. Expression of the cystic fibrosis transmembrane conductance regulator gene in cells of non-epithelial origin. *Nucleic Acids Res.* (1991) 19:5417–23. doi: 10.1093/nar/19.19.5417
63. Painter RG, Valentine VG, Lanson NA Jr, Leidal K, Zhang Q, Lombard G, et al. CFTR Expression in human neutrophils and the phagolysosomal chlorination defect in cystic fibrosis. *Biochemistry.* (2006) 45:10260–9. doi: 10.1021/bi060490t
64. Bonfield TL, Hodges CA, Cotton CU, Drumm ML. Absence of the cystic fibrosis transmembrane regulator (Cftr) from myeloid-derived cells slows resolution of inflammation and infection. *J Leukoc Biol.* (2012) 92:1111–22. doi: 10.1189/jlb.0412188
65. Painter RG, Marrero L, Lombard GA, Valentine VG, Nauseef WM, Wang G. CFTR-mediated halide transport in phagosomes of human neutrophils. *J Leukoc Biol.* (2010) 87:933–42. doi: 10.1189/jlb.1009655
66. Painter RG, Bonvillain RW, Valentine VG, Lombard GA, LaPlace SG, Nauseef WM, et al. The role of chloride anion and CFTR in killing of *Pseudomonas aeruginosa* by normal and CF neutrophils. *J Leukoc Biol.* (2008) 83:1345–53. doi: 10.1189/jlb.0907658
67. Zhou Y, Song K, Painter RG, Aiken M, Reiser J, Stanton BA, et al. Cystic fibrosis transmembrane conductance regulator recruitment to phagosomes in neutrophils. *J Innate Immun.* (2013) 5:219–30. doi: 10.1159/000346568
68. Ng HP, Valentine VG, Wang G. CFTR targeting during activation of human neutrophils. *J Leukoc Biol.* (2016) 100:1413–24. doi: 10.1189/jlb.4A0316-130RR
69. McKeon DJ, Cadwallader KA, Idris S, Cowburn AS, Pasteur MC, Barker H, et al. Cystic fibrosis neutrophils have normal intrinsic reactive oxygen species generation. *Eur Respir J.* (2010) 35:1264–72. doi: 10.1183/09031936.00089709
70. Bratcher PE, Rowe SM, Reeves G, Roberts T, Szul T, Harris WT, et al. Alterations in blood leukocytes of G551D-bearing cystic fibrosis patients undergoing treatment with ivacaftor. *J Cyst Fibros.* (2016) 15:67–73. doi: 10.1016/j.jcf.2015.02.010
71. Pohl K, Hayes E, Keenan J, Henry M, Meleady P, Molloy K, et al. A neutrophil intrinsic impairment affecting Rab27a and degranulation in cystic fibrosis is corrected by CFTR potentiator therapy. *Blood.* (2014) 124:999–1009. doi: 10.1182/blood-2014-02-555268
72. McKeon DJ, Condliffe AM, Cowburn AS, Cadwallader KC, Farahi N, Bilton D, et al. Prolonged survival of neutrophils from patients with Delta F508 CFTR mutations. *Thorax.* (2008) 63:660–1. doi: 10.1136/thx.2008.096834
73. Moriceau S, Lenoir G, Witko-Sarsat V. In cystic fibrosis homozygotes and heterozygotes, neutrophil apoptosis is delayed and modulated by diamide or roscovitine: evidence for an innate neutrophil disturbance. *J Innate Immun.* (2010) 2:260–6. doi: 10.1159/000295791
74. Gray RD, Hardisty G, Regan KH, Smith M, Robb CT, Duffin R, et al. Delayed neutrophil apoptosis enhances NET formation in cystic fibrosis. *Thorax.* (2018) 73:134–44. doi: 10.1136/thoraxjnl-2017-210134
75. Brinkmann V, Reichard U, Goosmann C, Fauler B, Uhlemann Y, Weiss DS, et al. Neutrophil extracellular traps kill bacteria. *Science.* (2004) 303:1532–5. doi: 10.1126/science.1092385
76. Fuchs TA, Abed U, Goosmann C, Hurwitz R, Schulze I, Wahn V, et al. Novel cell death program leads to neutrophil extracellular traps. *J Cell Biol.* (2007) 176:231–41. doi: 10.1083/jcb.200606027
77. Menegazzi R, Decleva E, Dri P. Killing by neutrophil extracellular traps: fact or folklore?. *Blood.* (2012) 119:1214–6. doi: 10.1182/blood-2011-07-364604
78. Rahman S, Gadjeva M. Does NETosis contribute to the bacterial pathoadaptation in cystic fibrosis?. *Front Immunol.* (2014) 5:378. doi: 10.3389/fimmu.2014.00378
79. Delgado-Rizo V, Martinez-Guzman MA, Iniguez-Gutierrez L, Garcia-Orozco A, Alvarado-Navarro A, Fafutis-Morris M. Neutrophil extracellular traps and its implications in inflammation: an overview. *Front Immunol.* (2017) 8:81. doi: 10.3389/fimmu.2017.00081
80. Yousefi S, Mihalache C, Kozlowski E, Schmid I, Simon HU. Viable neutrophils release mitochondrial DNA to form neutrophil extracellular traps. *Cell Death Differ.* (2009) 16:1438–44. doi: 10.1038/cdd.2009.96
81. Pilsczek FH, Salina D, Poon KK, Fahey C, Yipp BG, Sibley CD, et al. A novel mechanism of rapid nuclear neutrophil extracellular trap formation in response to *Staphylococcus aureus*. *J Immunol.* (2010) 185:7413–25. doi: 10.4049/jimmunol.1000675
82. Yipp BG, Petri B, Salina D, Jenne CN, Scott BN, Zbytnuik LD, et al. Infection-induced NETosis is a dynamic process involving neutrophil multitasking *in vivo*. *Nat Med.* (2012) 18:1386–93. doi: 10.1038/nm.2847
83. Byrd AS, O'Brien XM, Johnson CM, Lavigne LM, Reichner JS. An extracellular matrix-based mechanism of rapid neutrophil extracellular trap formation in response to *Candida albicans*. *J Immunol.* (2013) 190:4136–48. doi: 10.4049/jimmunol.1202671
84. Young RL, Malcolm KC, Kret JE, Caceres SM, Poch KR, Nichols DP, et al. Neutrophil extracellular trap (NET)-mediated killing of *Pseudomonas aeruginosa*: evidence of acquired resistance within the CF airway, independent of CFTR. *PLoS ONE.* (2011) 6:e23637. doi: 10.1371/journal.pone.0023637
85. Manzenreiter R, Kienberger F, Marcos V, Schilcher K, Krautgartner WD, Obermayer A, et al. Ultrastructural characterization of cystic fibrosis sputum using atomic force and scanning electron microscopy. *J Cyst Fibros.* (2012) 11:84–92. doi: 10.1016/j.jcf.2011.09.008
86. Tirouvanziam R, Gernez Y, Conrad CK, Moss RB, Schrijver I, Dunn CE, et al. Profound functional and signaling changes in viable inflammatory neutrophils homing to cystic fibrosis airways. *Proc Natl Acad Sci USA.* (2008) 105:4335–9. doi: 10.1073/pnas.0712386105
87. Laval J, Touhami J, Herzenberg LA, Conrad C, Taylor N, Battini JL, et al. Metabolic adaptation of neutrophils in cystic fibrosis airways involves distinct shifts in nutrient transporter expression. *J Immunol.* (2013) 190:6043–50. doi: 10.4049/jimmunol.1201755
88. Mitchell TC. A GRIM fate for human neutrophils in airway disease. *J Leukoc Biol.* (2018) 104:657–9. doi: 10.1002/JLB.5CE0418-162R
89. Forrest OA, Ingersoll SA, Preininger MK, Laval J, Limoli DH, Brown MR, et al. Frontline science: pathological conditioning of human neutrophils recruited to the airway milieu in cystic fibrosis. *J Leukoc Biol.* (2018) 104:665–75. doi: 10.1002/JLB.5HI1117-454RR

90. McLeish KR, Merchant ML, Creed TM, Tandon S, Barati MT, Uriarte SM, et al. Frontline science: tumor necrosis factor-alpha stimulation and priming of human neutrophil granule exocytosis. *J Leukoc Biol.* (2017) 102:19–29. doi: 10.1189/jlb.3HI0716-293RR
91. Zhao Y, van Kessel KPM, de Haas CJC, Rogers MRC, van Strijp JAG, Haas PA. Staphylococcal superantigen-like protein 13 activates neutrophils via formyl peptide receptor 2. *Cell Microbiol.* (2018) 20:e12941. doi: 10.1111/cmi.12941
92. Ibberson CB, Whiteley M. The *Staphylococcus aureus* transcriptome during cystic fibrosis lung infection. *MBio.* (2019) 10:e02774-19. doi: 10.1128/mBio.02774-19
93. Grunwell JR, Giacalone VD, Stephenson S, Margaroli C, Dobosh BS, Brown MR, et al. Neutrophil dysfunction in the airways of children with acute respiratory failure due to lower respiratory tract viral and bacterial coinfections. *Sci Rep.* (2019) 9:2874. doi: 10.1038/s41598-019-39726-w
94. Dorin JR, Dickinson P, Alton EW, Smith SN, Geddes DM, Stevenson BJ, et al. Cystic fibrosis in the mouse by targeted insertional mutagenesis. *Nature.* (1992) 359:211–5. doi: 10.1038/359211a0
95. Snouwaert JN, Brigman KK, Latour AM, Malouf NN, Boucher RC, Smithies O, et al. An animal model for cystic fibrosis made by gene targeting. *Science.* (1992) 257:1083–8. doi: 10.1126/science.257.5073.1083
96. Colledge WH, Abella BS, Southern KW, Ratcliff R, Jiang C, Cheng SH, et al. Generation and characterization of a delta F508 cystic fibrosis mouse model. *Nat Genet.* (1995) 10:445–52. doi: 10.1038/ng0895-445
97. McCarron A, Donnelley M, Parsons D. Airway disease phenotypes in animal models of cystic fibrosis. *Respir Res.* (2018) 19:54. doi: 10.1186/s12931-018-0750-y
98. Hatai H, Lepelley A, Zeng W, Hayden MS, Ghosh S. Toll-like receptor 11 (TLR11) interacts with flagellin and profilin through disparate mechanisms. *PLoS ONE.* (2016) 11:e0148987. doi: 10.1371/journal.pone.0148987
99. Heeckeren A, Walenga R, Konstan MW, Bonfield T, Davis PB, Ferkol T. Excessive inflammatory response of cystic fibrosis mice to bronchopulmonary infection with *Pseudomonas aeruginosa*. *J Clin Invest.* (1997) 100:2810–5. doi: 10.1172/JCI119828
100. McMorran BJ, Palmer JS, Lunn DP, Oceandy D, Costelloe EO, Thomas GR, et al. G551D CF mice display an abnormal host response and have impaired clearance of *Pseudomonas* lung disease. *Am J Physiol Lung Cell Mol Physiol.* (2001) 281:L74 0–7. doi: 10.1152/ajplung.2001.281.3.L740
101. Saadane A, Soltys J, Berger M. Acute Pseudomonas challenge in cystic fibrosis mice causes prolonged nuclear factor-kappa B activation, cytokine secretion, and persistent lung inflammation. *J Allergy Clin Immunol.* (2006) 117:1163–9. doi: 10.1016/j.jaci.2006.01.052
102. van Heeckeren AM, Schluchter MD, Xue W, Davis PB. Response to acute lung infection with mucoid *Pseudomonas aeruginosa* in cystic fibrosis mice. *Am J Respir Crit Care Med.* (2006) 173:288–96. doi: 10.1164/rccm.200506-917OC
103. Coleman FT, Mueschenborn S, Meluleni G, Ray C, Carey VJ, Vargas SO, et al. Hypersusceptibility of cystic fibrosis mice to chronic *Pseudomonas aeruginosa* colonization and lung infection. *Proc Natl Acad Sci USA.* (2003) 100:1949–54. doi: 10.1073/pnas.0437901100
104. Bruscia EM, Zhang PX, Ferreira E, Caputo C, Emerson JW, Tuck D, et al. Macrophages directly contribute to the exaggerated inflammatory response in cystic fibrosis transmembrane conductance regulator-/- mice. *Am J Respir Cell Mol Biol.* (2009) 40:295–304. doi: 10.1165/rcmb.2008-0170OC
105. Bruscia EM, Zhang PX, Barone C, Scholte BJ, Homer R, Krause DS, et al. Increased susceptibility of Cftr-/- mice to LPS-induced lung remodeling. *Am J Physiol Lung Cell Mol Physiol.* (2016) 310:L711–9. doi: 10.1152/ajplung.00284.2015
106. Hasenberg A, Hasenberg M, Mann L, Neumann F, Borkenstein L, Stecher M, et al. Catchup: a mouse model for imaging-based tracking and modulation of neutrophil granulocytes. *Nat Methods.* (2015) 12:445–52. doi: 10.1038/nmeth.3322
107. Rosen BH, Chanson M, Gawenis LR, Liu J, Sofoluwe A, Zoso A, et al. Animal and model systems for studying cystic fibrosis. *J Cyst Fibros.* (2018) 17:S28–34. doi: 10.1016/j.jcf.2017.09.001
108. Rogers CS, Hao Y, Rokhlina T, Samuel M, Stoltz DA, Li Y, et al. Production of CFTR-null and CFTR-DeltaF508 heterozygous pigs by adeno-associated virus-mediated gene targeting and somatic cell nuclear transfer. *J Clin Invest.* (2008) 118:1571–7. doi: 10.1172/JCI34773
109. Rogers CS, Stoltz DA, Meyerholz DK, Ostedgaard LS, Rokhlina T, Taft PJ, et al. Disruption of the CFTR gene produces a model of cystic fibrosis in newborn pigs. *Science.* (2008) 321:1837–41. doi: 10.1126/science.1163600
110. Sun X, Yan Z, Yi Y, Li Z, Lei D, Rogers CS, et al. Adeno-associated virus-targeted disruption of the CFTR gene in cloned ferrets. *J Clin Invest.* (2008) 118:1578–83. doi: 10.1172/JCI34599
111. Rogers CS, Abraham WM, Brogden KA, Engelhardt JF, Fisher JT, McCray PB Jr, et al. The porcine lung as a potential model for cystic fibrosis. *Am J Physiol Lung Cell Mol Physiol.* (2008) 295:L240–63. doi: 10.1152/ajplung.90203.2008
112. Fisher JT, Zhang Y, Engelhardt JF. Comparative biology of cystic fibrosis animal models. *Methods Mol Biol.* (2011) 742:311–34. doi: 10.1007/978-1-61779-120-8_19
113. Stoltz DA, Meyerholz DK, Pezzulo AA, Ramachandran S, Rogan MP, Davis GJ, et al. Cystic fibrosis pigs develop lung disease and exhibit defective bacterial eradication at birth. *Sci Transl Med.* (2010) 2:29ra31. doi: 10.1126/scitranslmed.3000928
114. Sathe M, Houwen R. Meconium ileus in Cystic Fibrosis. *J Cyst Fibros.* (2017) 16(Suppl. 2):S32–9. doi: 10.1016/j.jcf.2017.06.007
115. Fisher JT, Liu X, Yan Z, Luo M, Zhang Y, Zhou W, et al. Comparative processing and function of human and ferret cystic fibrosis transmembrane conductance regulator. *J Biol Chem.* (2012) 287:21673–85. doi: 10.1074/jbc.M111.336537
116. Sun X, Sui H, Fisher JT, Yan Z, Liu X, Cho HJ, et al. Disease phenotype of a ferret CFTR-knockout model of cystic fibrosis. *J Clin Invest.* (2010) 120:3149–60. doi: 10.1172/JCI43052
117. Sun X, Olivier AK, Liang B, Yi Y, Sui H, Evans TI, et al. Lung phenotype of juvenile and adult cystic fibrosis transmembrane conductance regulator-knockout ferrets. *Am J Respir Cell Mol Biol.* (2014) 50:502–12. doi: 10.1165/rcmb.2013-0261OC
118. Keiser NW, Birket SE, Evans IA, Tyler SR, Crooke AK, Sun X, et al. Defective innate immunity and hyperinflammation in newborn cystic fibrosis transmembrane conductance regulator-knockout ferret lungs. *Am J Respir Cell Mol Biol.* (2015) 52:683–94. doi: 10.1165/rcmb.2014-0250OC
119. Sun X, Yi Y, Yan Z, Rosen BH, Liang B, Winter MC, et al. In utero and postnatal VX-770 administration rescues multiorgan disease in a ferret model of cystic fibrosis. *Sci Transl Med.* (2019) 11:eaau7531. doi: 10.1126/scitranslmed.aau7531
120. Mills PR, Davies RJ, Devalia JL. Airway epithelial cells, cytokines, and pollutants. *Am J Respir Crit Care Med.* (1999) 160(5 Pt 2):S38–43. doi: 10.1164/ajrccm.160.supplement_1.11
121. Knight DA, Holgate ST. The airway epithelium: structural and functional properties in health and disease. *Respirology.* (2003) 8:432–46. doi: 10.1046/j.1440-1843.2003.00493.x
122. Lambrecht BN, Hammad H. The airway epithelium in asthma. *Nat Med.* (2012) 18:684–92. doi: 10.1038/nm.2737
123. Weitnauer M, Mijosek V, Dalpke AH. Control of local immunity by airway epithelial cells. *Mucosal Immunol.* (2016) 9:287–98. doi: 10.1038/mi.2015.126
124. Mertens TCJ, Karmouty-Quintana H, Taube C, Hiemstra PS. Use of airway epithelial cell culture to unravel the pathogenesis and study treatment in obstructive airway diseases. *Pulm Pharmacol Ther.* (2017) 45:101–13. doi: 10.1016/j.pupt.2017.05.008
125. De Rose V, Molloy K, Gohy S, Pilette C, Greene CM. Airway epithelium dysfunction in cystic fibrosis and COPD. *Mediators Inflamm.* (2018) 2018:1309746. doi: 10.1155/2018/1309746
126. Randell SH, Fulcher ML, O'Neal W, Olsen JC. Primary epithelial cell models for cystic fibrosis research. *Methods Mol Biol.* (2011) 742:285–310. doi: 10.1007/978-1-61779-120-8_18
127. Garratt LW, Sutanto EN, Foo CJ, Ling KM, Looi K, Kicic-Starcevich E, et al. Determinants of culture success in an airway epithelium sampling program of young children with cystic fibrosis. *Exp Lung Res.* (2014) 40:447–59. doi: 10.3109/01902148.2014.946631
128. Martinovich KM, Iosifidis T, Buckley AG, Looi K, Ling KM, Sutanto EN, et al. Conditionally reprogrammed primary airway epithelial cells maintain

morphology, lineage and disease specific functional characteristics. *Sci Rep.* (2017) 7:17971. doi: 10.1038/s41598-017-17952-4

129. Brewington JJ, Filbrandt ET, LaRosa FJ III, Moncivaiz JD, Ostmann AJ, Strecker LM, et al. Brushed nasal epithelial cells are a surrogate for bronchial epithelial CFTR studies. *JCI Insight.* (2018) 3:99385. doi: 10.1172/jci.insight.99385
130. Awatade NT, Wong SL, Hewson CK, Fawcett LK, Kicic A, Jaffe A, et al. Human primary epithelial cell models: promising tools in the era of cystic fibrosis personalized medicine. *Front Pharmacol.* (2018) 9:1429. doi: 10.3389/fphar.2018.01429
131. Castellani S, Di Gioia S, di Toma L, Conese M. Human cellular models for the investigation of lung inflammation and mucus production in cystic fibrosis. *Anal Cell Pathol.* (2018) 2018:3839803. doi: 10.1155/2018/3839803
132. Brewington JJ, Filbrandt ET, LaRosa FJ III, Moncivaiz JD, Ostmann AJ, Strecker LM, et al. Generation of human nasal epithelial cell spheroids for individualized cystic fibrosis transmembrane conductance regulator study. *J Vis Exp.* (2018) 134. doi: 10.3791/57492
133. Guimbellot JS, Leach JM, Chaudhry IG, Quinney NL, Boyles SE, Chua M, et al. Nasospheroids permit measurements of CFTR-dependent fluid transport. *JCI Insight.* (2017) 2:95734. doi: 10.1172/jci.insight.95734
134. Brewington JJ, Filbrandt ET, LaRosa FJ III, Ostmann AJ, Strecker LM, Szczesniak RD, et al. Detection of CFTR function and modulation in primary human nasal cell spheroids. *J Cyst Fibros.* (2018) 17:26–33. doi: 10.1016/j.jcf.2017.06.010
135. Machen TE. Innate immune response in CF airway epithelia: hyperinflammatory?. *Am J Physiol Cell Physiol.* (2006) 291:C218–30. doi: 10.1152/ajpcell.00605.2005
136. Ratner D, Mueller C. Immune responses in cystic fibrosis: are they intrinsically defective?. *Am J Respir Cell Mol Biol.* (2012) 46:715–22. doi: 10.1165/rcmb.2011-0399RT
137. Murphy SV, Ribeiro CMP. Cystic fibrosis inflammation: hyperinflammatory, hypoinflammatory, or both?. *Am J Respir Cell Mol Biol.* (2019) 61:273–4. doi: 10.1165/rcmb.2019-0107ED
138. Becker MN, Sauer MS, Muhlebach MS, Hirsh AJ, Wu Q, Verghese MW, et al. Cytokine secretion by cystic fibrosis airway epithelial cells. *Am J Respir Crit Care Med.* (2004) 169:645–53. doi: 10.1164/rccm.200207-765OC
139. Wiszniewski L, Jornot L, Dudez T, Pagano A, Rochat T, Lacroix JS, et al. Long-term cultures of polarized airway epithelial cells from patients with cystic fibrosis. *Am J Respir Cell Mol Biol.* (2006) 34:39–48. doi: 10.1165/rcmb.2005-0161OC
140. Schogler A, Blank F, Brugger M, Beyeler S, Tschanz SA, Regamey N, et al. Characterization of pediatric cystic fibrosis airway epithelial cell cultures at the air-liquid interface obtained by non-invasive nasal cytology brush sampling. *Respir Res.* (2017) 18:215. doi: 10.1186/s12931-017-0706-7
141. Sajjan U, Keshavjee S, Forstner J. Responses of well-differentiated airway epithelial cell cultures from healthy donors and patients with cystic fibrosis to burkholderia cenocepacia infection. *Infect Immun.* (2004) 72:4188–99. doi: 10.1128/IAI.72.7.4188-4199.2004
142. Carrabino S, Carpani D, Livraghi A, Di Cicco M, Costantini D, Copreni E, et al. Dysregulated interleukin-8 secretion and NF-kappaB activity in human cystic fibrosis nasal epithelial cells. *J Cyst Fibros.* (2006) 5:113–9. doi: 10.1016/j.jcf.2005.12.003
143. Conese M, Copreni E, Di Gioia S, De Rinaldis P, Fumarulo R. Neutrophil recruitment and airway epithelial cell involvement in chronic cystic fibrosis lung disease. *J Cyst Fibros.* (2003) 2:129–35. doi: 10.1016/S1569-1993(03)00063-8
144. Yamamoto K, Ahyi AN, Pepper-Cunningham ZA, Ferrari JD, Wilson AA, Jones MR, et al. Roles of lung epithelium in neutrophil recruitment during pneumococcal pneumonia. *Am J Respir Cell Mol Biol.* (2014) 50:253–62. doi: 10.1165/rcmb.2013-0114OC
145. Kim ND, Luster AD. The role of tissue resident cells in neutrophil recruitment. *Trends Immunol.* (2015) 36:547–55. doi: 10.1016/j.it.2015.07.007
146. Parkos CA. Neutrophil-epithelial interactions: a double-edged sword. *Am J Pathol.* (2016) 186:1404–16. doi: 10.1016/j.ajpath.2016.02.001
147. Brazil JC, Parkos CA. Pathobiology of neutrophil-epithelial interactions. *Immunol Rev.* (2016) 273:94–111. doi: 10.1111/imr.12446
148. Aldallal N, McNaughton EE, Manzel LJ, Richards AM, Zabner J, Ferkol TW, et al. Inflammatory response in airway epithelial cells isolated from patients with cystic fibrosis. *Am J Respir Crit Care Med.* (2002) 166:1248–56. doi: 10.1164/rccm.200206-627OC
149. Joseph T, Look D, Ferkol T. NF-kappaB activation and sustained IL-8 gene expression in primary cultures of cystic fibrosis airway epithelial cells stimulated with *Pseudomonas aeruginosa. Am J Physiol Lung Cell Mol Physiol.* (2005) 288:L471–9. doi: 10.1152/ajplung.00066.2004
150. Balloy V, Varet H, Dillies MA, Proux C, Jagla B, Coppee JY, et al. Normal and cystic fibrosis human bronchial epithelial cells infected with *Pseudomonas aeruginosa* exhibit distinct gene activation patterns. *PLoS ONE.* (2015) 10:e0140979. doi: 10.1371/journal.pone.0140979
151. Balloy V, Koshy R, Perra L, Corvol H, Chignard M, Guillot L, et al. Bronchial epithelial cells from cystic fibrosis patients express a specific long non-coding RNA signature upon *Pseudomonas aeruginosa* infection. *Front Cell Infect Microbiol.* (2017) 7:218. doi: 10.3389/fcimb.2017.00218
152. Zheng S, De BP, Choudhary S, Comhair SA, Goggans T, Slee R, et al. Impaired innate host defense causes susceptibility to respiratory virus infections in cystic fibrosis. *Immunity.* (2003) 18:619–30. doi: 10.1016/S1074-7613(03)00114-6
153. Sutanto EN, Kicic A, Foo CJ, Stevens PT, Mullane D, Knight DA, et al. Innate inflammatory responses of pediatric cystic fibrosis airway epithelial cells: effects of nonviral and viral stimulation. *Am J Respir Cell Mol Biol.* (2011) 44:761–7. doi: 10.1165/rcmb.2010-0368OC
154. Kieninger E, Singer F, Tapparel C, Alves MP, Latzin P, Tan HL, et al. High rhinovirus burden in lower airways of children with cystic fibrosis. *Chest.* (2013) 143:782–90. doi: 10.1378/chest.12-0954
155. Kieninger E, Vareille M, Kopf BS, Blank F, Alves MP, Gisler FM, et al. Lack of an exaggerated inflammatory response on virus infection in cystic fibrosis. *Eur Respir J.* (2012) 39:297–304. doi: 10.1183/09031936.00054511
156. Dauletbaev N, Das M, Cammisano M, Chen H, Singh S, Kooi C, et al. Rhinovirus load is high despite preserved interferon-beta response in cystic fibrosis bronchial epithelial cells. *PLoS ONE.* (2015) 10:e0143129. doi: 10.1371/journal.pone.0143129
157. King J, Brunel SF, Warris A. Aspergillus infections in cystic fibrosis. *J. Infect.* (2016) (72 Suppl):S50–5. doi: 10.1016/j.jinf.2016.04.022
158. Breuer O, Schultz A, Turkovic L, de Klerk N, Keil AD, Brennan S, et al. Changing prevalence of lower airway infections in young children with cystic fibrosis. *Am J Respir Crit Care Med.* (2019) 200:590–9. doi: 10.1164/rccm.201810-1919OC
159. Harun SN, Wainwright CE, Grimwood K, Hennig S, Australasian Cystic Fibrosis Bronchoalveolar Lavage study G. *Aspergillus* and progression of lung disease in children with cystic fibrosis. *Thorax.* (2019) 74:125–131. doi: 10.1136/thoraxjnl-2018-211550
160. Reihill JA, Moore JE, Elborn JS, Ennis M. Effect of Aspergillus fumigatus and *Candida albicans* on pro-inflammatory response in cystic fibrosis epithelium. *J Cyst Fibros.* (2011) 10:401–6. doi: 10.1016/j.jcf.2011.06.006
161. Chaudhary N, Datta K, Askin FB, Staab JF, Marr KA. Cystic fibrosis transmembrane conductance regulator regulates epithelial cell response to Aspergillus and resultant pulmonary inflammation. *Am J Respir Crit Care Med.* (2012) 185:301–10. doi: 10.1164/rccm.201106-1027OC
162. Schogler A, Stokes AB, Casaulta C, Regamey N, Edwards MR, Johnston SL, et al. Interferon response of the cystic fibrosis bronchial epithelium to major and minor group rhinovirus infection. *J Cyst Fibros.* (2016) 15:332–9. doi: 10.1016/j.jcf.2015.10.013
163. Nash S, Stafford J, Madara JL. Effects of polymorphonuclear leukocyte transmigration on the barrier function of cultured intestinal epithelial monolayers. *J Clin Invest.* (1987) 80:1104–13. doi: 10.1172/JCI113167
164. Madara JL, Colgan S, Nusrat A, Delp C, Parkos C. A simple approach to measurement of electrical parameters of cultured epithelial monolayers: use in assessing neutrophil-epithelial interactions. *J Tissue Culture Methods.* (1992) 14:209–15. doi: 10.1007/BF01409013
165. Parkos CA, Colgan SP, Delp C, Arnaout MA, Madara JL. Neutrophil migration across a cultured epithelial monolayer elicits a biphasic resistance response representing sequential effects on transcellular and paracellular pathways. *J Cell Biol.* (1992) 117:757–64. doi: 10.1083/jcb.117.4.757
166. McCormick BA, Colgan SP, Delp-Archer C, Miller SI, Madara JL. Salmonella typhimurium attachment to human intestinal epithelial monolayers:

transcellular signalling to subepithelial neutrophils. *J Cell Biol.* (1993) 123:895–907. doi: 10.1083/jcb.123.4.895

167. Kidney JC, Proud D. Neutrophil transmigration across human airway epithelial monolayers: mechanisms and dependence on electrical resistance. *Am J Respir Cell Mol Biol.* (2000) 23:389–95. doi: 10.1165/ajrcmb.23.3.4068
168. Zemans RL, Briones N, Suzuki T, Downey GP. Neutrophil migration across cultured lung epithelium induces modulation of the WNT-beta-catenin pathway. *Am J Respir Crit Care Med.* (2009) 179:A5664. doi: 10.1164/ajrccm-conference.2009.179.1_MeetingAbstracts.A5664
169. Zemans RL, Briones N, Campbell M, McClendon J, Young SK, Suzuki T, et al. Neutrophil transmigration triggers repair of the lung epithelium via beta-catenin signaling. *Proc Natl Acad Sci USA.* (2011) 108:15990–5. doi: 10.1073/pnas.1110144108
170. Hurley BP, Siccardi D, Mrsny RJ, McCormick BA. Polymorphonuclear cell transmigration induced by *Pseudomonas aeruginosa* requires the eicosanoid hepoxilin A3. *J Immunol.* (2004) 173:5712–20. doi: 10.4049/jimmunol.173.9.5712
171. Kusek ME, Pazos MA, Pirzai W, Hurley BP. *In vitro* coculture assay to assess pathogen induced neutrophil trans-epithelial migration. *J Vis Exp.* (2014) 83:e50823. doi: 10.3791/50823
172. Deng Y, Herbert JA, Smith CM, Smyth RL. An *in vitro* transepithelial migration assay to evaluate the role of neutrophils in respiratory syncytial virus (RSV) induced epithelial damage. *Sci Rep.* (2018) 8:6777. doi: 10.1038/s41598-018-25167-4
173. Neudecker V, Brodsky KS, Clambey ET, Schmidt EP, Packard TA, Davenport B, et al. Neutrophil transfer of miR-223 to lung epithelial cells dampens acute lung injury in mice. *Sci Transl Med.* (2017) 9:eaah5360. doi: 10.1126/scitranslmed.aah5360
174. Genschmer KR, Russell DW, Lal C, Szul T, Bratcher PE, Noerager BD, et al. Activated PMN exosomes: pathogenic entities causing matrix destruction and disease in the lung. *Cell.* (2019) 176:113–126 e15. doi: 10.1016/j.cell.2018.12.002
175. Yonker LM, Mou H, Chu KK, Pazos MA, Leung H, Cui D, et al. Development of a primary human co-culture model of inflamed airway mucosa. *Sci Rep.* (2017) 7:8182. doi: 10.1038/s41598-017-08567-w
176. Wainwright CE, Elborn JS, Ramsey BW. Lumacaftor-ivacaftor in patients with cystic fibrosis homozygous for Phe508del CFTR. *N Engl J Med.* (2015) 373:1783–4. doi: 10.1056/NEJMoa1409547
177. Taylor-Cousar JL, Munck A, McKone EF, van der Ent CK, Moeller A, Simard C, et al. Tezacaftor-ivacaftor in patients with cystic fibrosis homozygous for Phe508del. *N Engl J Med.* (2017) 377:2013–23. doi: 10.1056/NEJMoa1709846
178. Donaldson SH, Pilewski JM, Griese M, Cooke J, Viswanathan L, Tullis E, et al. Tezacaftor/Ivacaftor in subjects with cystic fibrosis and F508del/F508del-CFTR or F508del/G551D-CFTR. *Am J Respir Crit Care Med.* (2018) 197:214–24. doi: 10.1164/rccm.201704-0717OC
179. Ratjen F, Hug C, Marigowda G, Tian S, Huang X, Stanojevic S, et al. Efficacy and safety of lumacaftor and ivacaftor in patients aged 6-11 years with cystic fibrosis homozygous for F508del-CFTR: a randomised, placebo-controlled phase 3 trial. *Lancet Respir Med.* (2017) 5:557–67. doi: 10.1016/S2213-2600(17)30215-1
180. Middleton PG, Mall MA, Drevinek P, Lands LC, McKone EF, Polineni D, et al. Elexacaftor-tezacaftor-ivacaftor for cystic fibrosis with a single Phe508del Allele. *N Engl J Med.* (2019) 381:1809–19. doi: 10.1056/NEJMoa1908639
181. Heltshe SL, Mayer-Hamblett N, Burns JL, Khan U, Baines A, Ramsey BW, et al. *Pseudomonas aeruginosa* in cystic fibrosis patients with G551D-CFTR treated with ivacaftor. *Clin Infect Dis.* (2015) 60:703–12. doi: 10.1093/cid/ciu944
182. Singh SB, McLearn-Montz AJ, Milavetz F, Gates LK, Fox C, Murry LT, et al. Pathogen acquisition in patients with cystic fibrosis receiving ivacaftor or lumacaftor/ivacaftor. *Pediatr Pulmonol.* (2019) 54:1200–8. doi: 10.1002/ppul.24341

2

Bronchial Epithelial Cells on the Front Line to Fight Lung Infection-Causing *Aspergillus fumigatus*

Jeanne Bigot[1], *Loïc Guillot*[2], *Juliette Guitard*[1], *Manon Ruffin*[2], *Harriet Corvol*[3], *Viviane Balloy*[2*†] *and Christophe Hennequin*[1*†]

[1] Sorbonne Université, Inserm, Centre de Recherche Saint-Antoine, CRSA, AP-HP, Hôpital Saint-Antoine, Service de Parasitologie-Mycologie, Paris, France, [2] Sorbonne Université, Inserm, Centre de Recherche Saint-Antoine, Paris, France, [3] Sorbonne Université, Inserm, Centre de Recherche Saint-Antoine, CRSA, AP-HP, Hôpital Trousseau, Service de Pneumologie Pédiatrique, Paris, France

***Correspondence:**
Viviane Balloy
viviane.balloy@inserm.fr
Christophe Hennequin
christophe.hennequin-sat@aphp.fr

† These authors have contributed equally to this work

Aspergillus fumigatus is an environmental filamentous fungus that can be pathogenic for humans, wherein it is responsible for a large variety of clinical forms ranging from allergic diseases to life-threatening disseminated infections. The contamination occurs by inhalation of conidia present in the air, and the first encounter of this fungus in the human host is most likely with the bronchial epithelial cells. Although alveolar macrophages have been widely studied in the *Aspergillus*–lung interaction, increasing evidence suggests that bronchial epithelium plays a key role in responding to the fungus. This review focuses on the innate immune response of the bronchial epithelial cells against *A. fumigatus*, the predominant pathogenic species. We have also detailed the molecular interactants and the effects of the different modes of interaction between these cells and the fungus.

Keywords: bronchial epithelial cells, *Aspergillus fumigatus*, innate immunity, lung infection, mucociliary machinery

INTRODUCTION

Aspergillus spp. are saprophytic filamentous fungi capable of colonizing different ecological habitats. They are usually isolated from soils, decaying organic matters, and plants but are also present in the air and indoor environments (1). *Aspergillus* spores, or so-called conidia, represent the disseminating form of the fungus that spreads through the air. These conidia are produced through asexual reproduction by differentiated fungal cells called phialides, which are themselves carried on a conidiophore. Conidia remain "dormant" or metabolically inactive until they encounter favorable environmental conditions. In this case, the conidia swell, germinate to produce hyphae that grow into a mycelium that harbor conidiophores, and then form conidia (2).

Aspergillus genus encompasses several hundred of species (3). *Aspergillus fumigatus* is by far the most frequent pathogenic species, responsible for about 90% of the cases of *Aspergillus* diseases, followed by *Aspergillus flavus*, *Aspergillus niger*, *Aspergillus terreus*, and *Aspergillus nidulans* (3, 4). Indeed, *A. fumigatus* is the predominant fungal species isolated from the ambient air able to grow at 37°C, the human body temperature.

Humans inhale around a few hundred conidia daily (5). Due to their small size (2- to 3-μm diameter) they can reach the lower respiratory tract (4) but, in most of cases, this phenomenon does not lead to any symptoms thanks to their evacuation by the mucociliary machinery of the tracheobronchial epithelium. However, depending on the immune status of the host, this contamination can be followed by a wide spectrum of manifestations (1). Concisely, immunocompromised patients are at risk for invasive infection, so-called invasive pulmonary aspergillosis (IPA) and patients with pre-formed lung cavity (typically following previous pulmonary tuberculosis) are prone to chronic pulmonary aspergillosis, of which aspergilloma is one of the main presentations. Finally, patients with altered mucociliary clearance, such as cystic fibrosis (CF) patients, may be colonized which can turn, in patients with exacerbated immune response, into allergic bronchopulmonary aspergillosis (ABPA).

The essential role of neutrophils and monocytes in anti-*Aspergillus* immunity has been emphasized by the high rate of incidence of *Aspergillus* invasive infection in patients with quantitative (neutropenia) or qualitative (corticosteroid therapy, chronic granulomatous disease) deficiency of these cells (6–8). However, the role of the bronchial epithelium should not be underestimated as it represents the first physical and biological barrier preventing fungal implantation.

While studies looking at the interactions between *Aspergillus* and leukocytes (alveolar macrophages and recruited neutrophils) are numerous (6, 9–11), data on the role of bronchial epithelial cells (BECs) in anti-*Aspergillus* defense are still limited. Yet, BECs seem to play a crucial role in the innate immune response against *Aspergillus* particularly in preventing the bronchial colonization. The high prevalence of *Aspergillus* bronchial colonization in patients suffering from CF (12, 13), a disease characterized by the thickening of the bronchial mucus, highlights this phenomenon. Bronchial *Aspergillus* colonization, whose role in the subsequent development of IPA is still debated, may have deleterious consequences as it is the starting point of *Aspergillus* bronchitis and immuno-allergic forms (14, 15). In CF patients, while remaining superficial, bronchial colonization is associated with the occurrence of bronchial exacerbations, a decline in lung function, and ABPA with a prevalence ranging between 1 and 15% (16). Fungal sensitization to *Aspergillus* antigens may also occur in allergic patients (17) but the role of the bronchial epithelium in these diseases won't be analyzed in this review.

Thanks to experimental studies, there is increasing knowledge on the interactions between the different morphotypes of *A. fumigatus* and BECs. This review aims to decipher these interactions at the molecular level and their effect on anti-*Aspergillus* immunity.

STUDY MODELS OF THE INTERACTION BETWEEN *ASPERGILLUS FUMIGATUS* AND BRONCHIAL EPITHELIAL CELLS

The respiratory tract is lined by epithelial cells whose types vary according to the anatomic structure of the airways. Trachea, bronchi, and bronchioles are lined by the pseudostratified epithelium, while type I and II pneumocytes constitute the alveolar epithelium. At the bronchial level, the pseudostratified epithelium is mostly composed of ciliated, secretory, and basal cells from which the first two derive.

To understand the interactions between *Aspergillus* and BECs, different cell lines (immortalized or tumor) have been commonly used. Among the most popular bronchial cell lines used and commercially available, we can cite BEAS-2B and 16HBE, both isolated from normal human bronchial epithelium and secondarily immortalized through transfection of a replication-defective SV40 plasmid (18, 19). NCI-H292 cells derive from a lymph node metastasis sample of a pulmonary mucoepidermoid carcinoma. But other respiratory cell lines are occasionally used in some studies. All these cell lines have major advantages such as easy to maintain (cultured in simple and inexpensive culture media), capable of growing at high densities, and exhibiting an extended life span (20). However, these cells represent only one donor, and many cellular processes are deregulated due to immortalization. Refinement of the model consists of the use of commercially available primary bronchial cells that are free from any genetic modification and whose physiological functions are intact. However, before they are used, those cells must undergo antibiotic, antifungal, and growth factor treatment. Usually, these cells have a limited life span with limited proliferation capacity and are more difficult to culture than cell lines requiring more complex, specialized, and expensive cell culture media. Irrespective of the cell type, cells are usually cultured under submerged conditions, i.e., in flat-bottom plastic wells filled with culture medium, that hamper cells to differentiate. To better mimic physiological conditions, air-liquid interface cell culture (ALI) systems have been developed (21). In this case, primary BECs and also some cell lines such as 16HBE, differentiate until they develop the mucociliary phenotype characteristic of a pseudostratified epithelium and express mucins (20). Basal surface is therefore in contact with the liquid medium and the apical part of the cellular layer is exposed to the air. Obtaining this type of differentiated epithelium is time-consuming and requires specific technical skills but such cell culture systems mimic the required *in vivo* conditions in the best way.

Different approaches can be used to mimic an *Aspergillus* infection. *Aspergillus*, mostly in the form of dormant conidia can be inoculated in cell culture supernatants and then recovered after defined incubation intervals to measure the parameters of interest (such as cytokine level, cytotoxicity, etc.). In these conditions, *A. fumigatus* hyphae are usually obtained after 15 h of incubation. Killed (UV or irradiated for example) resting, swollen conidia and hyphae have also been used as inoculum. Differences between experimental protocols, especially the use of different multiplicity of infection, likely far from reality, could explain some discrepancies in the results obtained in different studies.

In addition to *in vitro* models, *in vivo* models of *Aspergillus* infection have already been used. Mice, rats or rabbits are the animals the most commonly used. They are immunosuppressed or not, and infected with *A. fumigatus* through inhalation of conidia administered either intranasal or *via* intratracheal route. In addition to the measurements of mortality rate and/or fungal

Abbreviations: BECs, Bronchial epithelial cells; IPA, Invasive pulmonary aspergillosis; CF, Cystic fibrosis; PCD, Primary ciliary dyskinesia; ABPA, Allergic bronchopulmonary aspergillosis; ALI, Air-liquid interface; DHN, Dihydroxynaphthalene; HBE cells, papilloma virus-immortalized bronchial epithelial cell line; PAMPs, Pathogen-associated molecular patterns; PRRs, Pathogen recognition receptors; IL-1Ra, Interleukin-1 receptor antagonist; NLRP3, NOD-, LRR-, and pyrin domain-containing 3; ROS, Reactive oxygen species; IL, Interleukin; AMPs, Antimicrobial peptides; hBD, Human β-defensins; NAGase, N-Acetyl-β-d-glucosaminidase.

load in the lungs, more precise descriptions of the immune response have also been reported, looking at the immune cells recruitment or inflammatory response (22). *In vivo* models have the considerable advantage of most closely imitate lung infection and immunity as a whole, however, there is a paucity of *in vivo* models (conditional and inducible transgenic mice targeting bronchial/airway epithelial cells) allowing the study of BECs against *Aspergillus* challenge specifically.

ANTI-*ASPERGILLUS* PHYSICOCHEMICAL ACTIVITY EXHIBITED BY THE BRONCHIAL EPITHELIUM

Inhaled conidia first face the physical barriers of the upper airways that include the mouth, nose, larynx, and pharynx. Mucociliary clearance from the nasal walls and mechanical defenses such as coughing and sneezing help eliminate most of the inhaled particles. If the conidia pass these first barriers, they then arrive in the lower airways consisting of the trachea that divided into two-stem bronchial tubes, which in turn are subdivided into several smaller bronchial tubes, followed by bronchioles that end with the alveoli. The bronchial epithelium participates in the clearance of inhaled conidia to prevent their germination and growth locally. Secretory cells, including serous and goblet cells, together with submucosal glands, participate in the formation of mucus, which protects the epithelium from the inhaled particles. Basically, the mucus traps the inhaled particles, which are then actively transported by the beating of the cilia to the oropharynx where they are swallowed or expectorated. Under healthy conditions, mucus is composed of 97% water and 3% of mucins, non-mucin proteins, salts, lipids, and cellular debris (23). Mucins, namely MUC5AC and MUC5B, are the major macromolecular constituents of the mucus. They are large glycoproteins with serine-/threonine-rich domains linked by their hydroxyl side groups to sugar chains forming a polymeric gel that ensure the properties of the mucus (24). Ciliated cells also play a fundamental role in the elimination of particles engulfed in the mucus because they mechanize the movement of the mucus blanket (25). The role of these physicochemical barriers associated with the bronchial epithelium can be better understood in patients suffering from CF or primary ciliary dyskinesia (PCD) in whom mucus properties and/or ciliary beating are impaired. Hence, CF patients are frequently colonized by *A. fumigatus* (14), and a similar trend has been noticed in patients with PCD (26). This machinery can also be altered by pathogens. Indeed, mycotoxins secreted by *A. fumigatus*, damage epithelial cells and inhibit ciliary beating (27). Among those toxins, gliotoxin has been extensively studied because it is the most abundant one produced by *A. fumigatus* and it exhibits immunosuppressive properties that have been described extensively in a previously reported review (28).

RECOGNITION OF *ASPERGILLUS FUMIGATUS* BY BRONCHIAL EPITHELIAL CELLS

Schematically, the interaction between *Aspergillus fumigatus* and the BECs leads to three main types of cellular response: internalization, synthesis of cytokines/chemokines and release of bioactive molecules potentially active against *Aspergillus*. Specific interactions between *A. fumigatus* and BECs require close contact between the fungus and the cell-surface ligands. Fungal cell-wall polysaccharides and, to a lesser extent, some proteins or the genetic material (ADN or ARN) act as pathogen-associated molecular patterns (PAMPs). They are sensed through pathogen recognition receptors (PRRs), several of which but not all, have been identified in BECs (5) (**Table 1**).

TABLE 1 | Pattern recognition receptors (PRRs) and pathogen-associated molecular patterns (PAMPs) involved in the recognition of *Aspergillus fumigatus* by bronchial epithelial cells and the consequences of their activation.

PRRs	*A. fumigatus* PAMPs	Cellular study model	Role in Anti-*Aspergillus* immunity on BECs	References
Dectin-1	β-D-Glucan	HBE cells	Internalization Pro-inflammatory cytokines and chemokines release Inflammasome activation ROS generation	(29)
TLR2	β-D-Glucan	HBE cells	IL-6 and IL-8 release Increase in Dectin-1 expression	(29)
MR	Mannose-rich polysaccharides		Not elicited	
Unknown	FleA (conidia)	BEAS-2B cells	IL-8 synthesis Inhibition of *Aspergillus fumigatus* germination of extracellular conidia Binding of conidia to mucins and to macrophages	(30–32)
TLR3	dsRNA (resting conidia)	Primary human BECs	Release of inflammatory mediators, interferon (IFN)-β and IFN-γ-inducible protein (IP)-10	(33)
TLR4	Unknown		Not elicited	(34, 35)
TLR9	Hypomethylated DNA		Not elicited	(34, 35)
Pentraxin 3	Galactomannan		Not elicited	(36)

BECs, Bronchial epithelial cells; IL, Interleukin; dsRNA, double stranded RNA; ROS, Reactive oxygen species; HBE cells, Papilloma virus–immortalized bronchial epithelial cell line.

A. fumigatus cell wall encompasses an inner and outer layer whose composition varies along with the fungus' life cycle (**Figure 1**). The outer part of the conidial surface is composed of hydrophobic RodA proteins that conceal an underlying fungal pigment, dihydroxynaphthalene (DHN) melanin (37). This outer layer plays a key role in conidial dispersion, their protection against external stress factors such as desiccation, physical damage, drugs, and UV radiation. They also mask the epitopes present in the underlying layer by inhibiting their recognition by the host's innate immune system (38–40). Whereas, dormant conidia are described as immunologically inert, the FleA lectin, a fucose-binding lectin expressed on their surface (30, 41), has been shown to mediate their binding both to the airway mucins produced by the epithelial cells and also to macrophages (31). Moreover, stimulation of BEAS-2B cells by FleA has been reported to lead to an increase in interleukin (IL)-8 synthesis and contributed to the inflammatory response (30). Thus, FleA acts as a PAMP-like molecule whose cellular ligands remain to be identified.

Under favorable conditions, the dormant conidia become metabolically active and ensue an increased intracellular osmotic pressure followed by water uptake and isodiametric growth (42). The resulting swollen conidia lose their rodlet layer by proteolytic degradation, and consequently, their hydrophobicity. This phenomenon is associated with a rupture of the melanin layer by a still-unknown mechanism (43). Then, the swollen conidia grow in a polarized way that leads to the formation of a germ tube. At this stage, the melanin layer is disrupted but the inner layer of the cell wall remains unchanged and participates in hyphal formation. The hyphae are mainly composed of galactosaminogalactan (GAG) that allows adhesion of the filaments to various biotic or abiotic surfaces (44, 45). Recent studies have also shown that GAG, expressed during conidial germination, exhibits a possible anti-inflammatory effect. Indeed, GAG induces the release of the IL-1 receptor antagonist (IL-1Ra), a potent anti-inflammatory cytokine that blocks IL-1 signaling (46), by macrophages and neutrophils. Furthermore, in a mouse model of aspergillosis, treatment by GAG before and during intranasally induced *A. fumigatus* infection inhibits neutrophil infiltration in the lung at the site of infection (6, 44, 46).

Regardless of the *A. fumigatus* morphotype, the inner layer, the so-called fibrillary core, is continuously composed of branched β-(1, 3)-glucan/β-(1, 4)-glucan, chitin, galactomannan, and α-(1, 3)-glucan (43). A few studies have shown that, as already demonstrated for macrophages and digestive epithelial cells (47), Dectin-1 is a major but not the unique receptor for β-glucan on a papilloma virus-immortalized BEC cell line (HBE cells) (29). Dectin-1 is a transmembrane receptor and member of the C-type lectin receptor family (11). The role of Dectin-1 in the immune response against *A. fumigatus* has been highlighted in different *in vivo* studies. For example, immunocompetent mice lacking Dectin-1 are more sensitive to intratracheal challenge with *A. fumigatus* than control mice (48). In humans, mutations in Dectin-1 are associated with increased susceptibility to IPA (49). It has also been shown that immunocompromised mice, transfected to upregulate Dectin-1 expression in airway epithelial cells, have a lower fungal burden, an increase in the recruitment of neutrophils into the lungs and a greater survival rate in response to intratracheal injection of *A. fumigatus* conidia compared to the controls (50). After ligation of β-glucan to Dectin-1, two distinct signaling pathways are activated through the spleen tyrosine kinase (SYK)-caspase recruitment domain-containing protein 9 (CARD9) or through RAF-1 (51). These pathways act synergistically to induce nuclear factor-κB

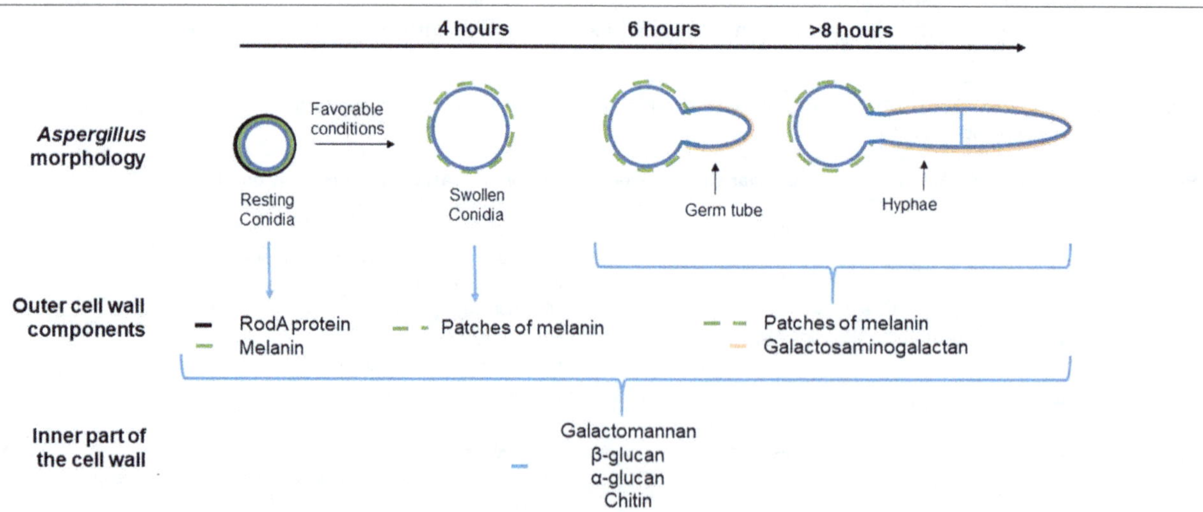

FIGURE 1 | Different morphological stages and compositions of the cell wall during the vegetative cycle of *Aspergillus fumigatus*. The cell wall of the resting conidia consists of (the most external part to the inner) (i) the rodlet layer (black), composed of the hydrophobin RodA, (ii) the melanin layer below (green), and (iii) polysaccharides (blue). Under favorable conditions, the resting conidia begin to swell after 4 h. The rodlet layer is lost by proteolytic degradation and conidium swelling is due to an increase in the internal osmotic pressure. The melanin layer is then disorganized and the inner layer of the swollen conidium forms the mycelium cell wall. After 8 h, hyphae are apparent. Then, an extracellular matrix mainly composed of galactosaminogalactan (GAG) (pink) covers up the hyphae. Specific and universal components of each morphotype are shown below each image.

activation and pro-inflammatory gene expression (52). The SYK–CARD9 pathway also activates the NOD-, LRR-, and pyrin domain-containing 3 (NLRP3) inflammasome, which results in the proteolytic activation of the pro-inflammatory cytokines IL-1β and IL-18 by caspase 1. The role of *A. fumigatus* antigens in this activation cascade has been demonstrated by Jeong et al. They showed that sensitized mice intratracheally challenged with *A. fumigatus* crude antigens displayed an increased in immunofluorescence intensities of NLRP3 and caspase-1 in lung tissue, particularly in epithelial cell layers, leading to an increase in IL1-β concentration in the lung tissue (53). Similar results were obtained by using an *in vitro* model utilizing primary human BECs stimulated with the same *A. fumigatus* antigens (53). The mannose receptor (MR) is another C-type lectin receptor involved in fungal, and notably *Aspergillus* conidia, recognition and is expressed by 16HBE cells and primary BECs (54). The MR recognizes carbohydrates rich in mannose typically produced by many microorganisms including fungi (55) but its immune-specific role against *A. fumigatus* in association with BECs has not been investigated.

Toll-like receptors (TLRs) are another family of conserved PRRs (56). So far 10 different TLRs have been identified and described. TLR2, TLR4, and TLR9 are the main molecules involved in sensing fungal components (11, 57, 58). These receptors possess extracellular leucine-rich repeat ligand-binding domains and a conserved intracellular toll/IL-1R (TIR) signaling domain that induces specific signaling cascades through intracellular TIR containing adaptors such as MyD88. Interestingly, the expression of the 10 TLRs has been detected by reverse transcription–quantitative real-time polymerase chain reaction in two independent studies using human primary BECs (34, 35). Using a silencing method, it has been demonstrated that TLR2, in a heterodimer form with TLR1 or TLR6, is required for the expression of Dectin-1 by HBE cells in response to *A. fumigatus* infection (29). Moreover, blocking TLR2 with antibodies results in the inhibition of the release of IL-6 and IL-8 by BEAS-2B cells infected with *A. fumigatus* hyphal fragments (59). Certain polymorphisms in TLR4, receptor for the bacterial lipopolysaccharide, are clearly associated with increased susceptibility to invasive aspergillosis (60). TLR4 expressed by mouse macrophages, recognizes *A. fumigatus* conidia and hyphae and induces the release of pro-inflammatory molecules. However, after blocking TLR4 with a specific monoclonal antibody, Øya et al. failed to detect any significant change in the levels of IL-6 and IL-8 released by BEAS-2B cells infected with X-ray-treated hyphal fragments of *A. fumigatus* (59). Hypomethylated DNA, the natural ligand of TLR9, has been extracted in *A. fumigatus* hyphae (61). In murine model of invasive aspergillosis, Leiva-Juarez et al. revealed that therapeutic stimulation of lung epithelial defenses by inhalation of a synergistic combination of TLR 2/6 and TLR9 agonists robustly protects against the development of *A. fumigatus* lung infection despite the profound immune dysfunction (62). TLR9 is expressed by BECs (16HBE cells) (63) but its role in response to *Aspergillus* challenge remains to be investigated in the context of these cells. TLR3 is localized onto endosomal membranes and recognizes double-stranded (ds)RNA. It is primarily involved in the recognition of viruses but has also been implicated in the recognition of *A. fumigatus* dsRNA of resting conidia (33). In this study, the infection by *Aspergillus* of human primary BECs cultivated either in submerged or in ALI culture system, induced the release of inflammatory mediators, notably interferon-β and interferon-γ-inducible protein-10, through TLR3 signaling. Interestingly, this induction is internalization dependent, as demonstrated by the use of an actin-polymerization inhibitor and observed only with killed resting conidia (heat- or UV light-inactivated).

Finally, pentraxin 3, a soluble PRR, plays a key role in the recognition, uptake, and killing of *Aspergillus* conidia by macrophages and dendritic cells through binding to galactomannan (64). This molecule can act as an opsonizing factor for activating the complement system and subsequent phagocytosis by macrophages (65). Pentraxin 3 is secreted by both human primary bronchial and BEAS-2B cells but, again, its precise role in these cell types has yet to be determined (36).

INTERNALIZATION OF *ASPERGILLUS FUMIGATUS* CONIDIA BY BRONCHIAL EPITHELIAL CELLS

The alveolar epithelial cell line A549 has been extensively used to study conidia internalization by non-professional phagocytic cells (66–68). Wasylnka and Moore described that internalized conidia fused with lysosomes and colocalized with lysosomal protein (Lysosomal-associated membrane protein 1 and CD63). Nonetheless, a significant percentage of internalized conidia persist and germinate in A549 epithelial cells. Little is known about the internalization by BECs and conflicting results have been published (**Figure 2A**). First, Paris et al., showed by microscopic observations that rabbit tracheal epithelial cells were able to internalize *A. fumigatus* conidia after 6 h of incubation and that conidia were enclosed in membrane-bound vacuoles (69). Then, other studies reported that the conidia of *A. fumigatus* were taken up *in vitro* by a human bronchial epithelial cell line cultured in monolayers (70, 71). Indeed, Clark et al. observed the internalization of 10 to 20% of the conidia in contact with BEAS-2B cells at 6 and 9 h after challenge. In comparison, 70% of conidia in contact with macrophages were internalized after 1 h incubation (71). A 41% internalization rate has also been reported with 16HBE cells after 6 h incubation (70). Overall, these results contrast with those from other studies that have considered the internalization by BECs a very minor phenomenon. By using a model of primary BECs grown in ALI culture system, Toor et al. showed that only 1% of the bound conidia were internalized 6 h after exposure (72). Similarly, Fernandes et al. were unable to demonstrate any case of internalization using primary BECs cultured in ALI (73). However, these authors described the formation, within the cell, of an actin tunnel not altering the viability of the penetrated cells (**Figure 2A**). The authors suggested that this event could explain the penetration of the hyphae into the underlying

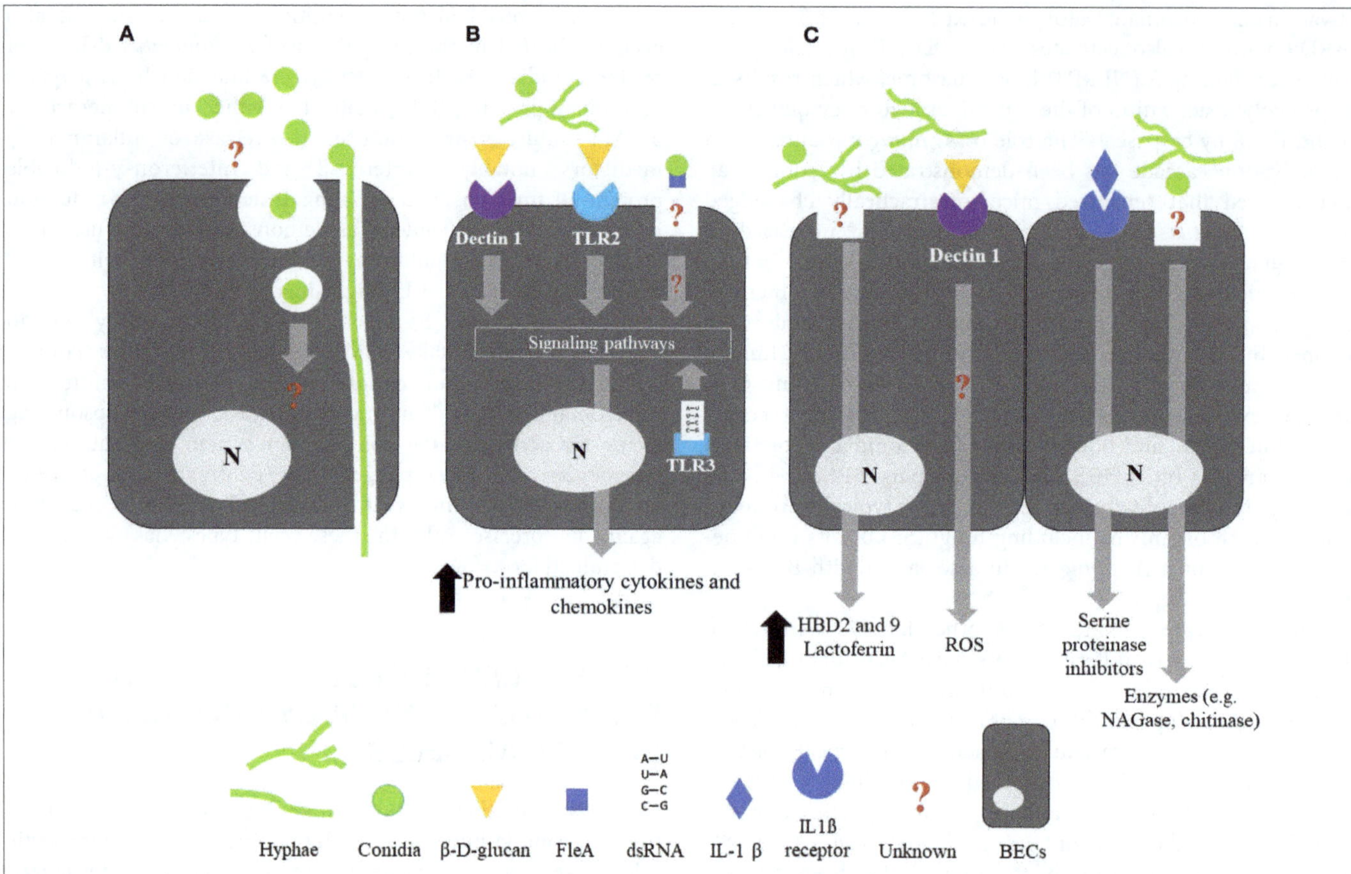

FIGURE 2 | Summary of the interactions between bronchial epithelial cells and *Aspergillus fumigatus*. For clarity, it should be noted that the schematized epithelial cells are not polarized. **(A)** Internalization; BECs are able to internalized *A. fumigatus* conidia but the molecular mechanisms involved in this phenomenon and the fate of the internalized conidia are still unknown. An alternative way of penetration of the hyphae through an actin channel within the cell has been proposed. **(B)** Cytokine/chemokine release; Recognition of β-D-glucan by BECs through the membrane receptors Dectin-1 and TLR2, and recognition of *A. fumigatus* dsRNA by the endosomal receptor TLR3 result in the activation of intracellular signaling pathways and a significant increase in the release of proinflammatory cytokines and chemokines, leading to phagocyte recruitment. FleA lectin, expressed on the surface of *A. fumigatus* conidia, induces IL-8 synthesis by BECs and binding of the conidia to airway mucins. Recognition of FleA by BEC induces the inhibition of conidium germination. **(C)** Bioactive molecules potentially active against *A. fumigatus*; BECs synthetize antimicrobials molecules such as defensins HBD2 and HBD9, lactoferrin, reactive oxygen species (ROS), SLPI, ESI, and chitinase in response to *A. fumigatus* infection or inflammatory challenge. Until now, an antifungal activity has only been described for lactoferrin, ROS, SLPI, ESI, and chitinase. BECs, Bronchial epithelial cells; SLPI, Secretory leukocyte proteinase inhibitor; ESI, Elastase-specific inhibitor; NAGase, N-Acetyl-β-d-glucosaminidase; ROS, Reactive oxygen species; N, nucleus.

parenchyma leading to the development of invasive infection in immunocompromised patients (73). It is noteworthy that the internalization of conidia by BECs was not seen 18 h after an intratracheal challenge in an immunosuppressed mouse model (74). The molecular mechanism(s) involved in the internalization of *Aspergillus* conidia by BECs remains incompletely understood. Adhesion of conidia onto BECs induces actin polymerization (75), a phenomenon dependent on the activity of the human actin reorganization complex 2 and 3, regulated by Wiskott-Aldrich syndrome protein-interacting proteins (76). Using the BEAS-2B cell line, Clark et al. identified 7 host markers—caveolin, flotillin-2, RAB5C, RAB8B, RAB7A, 2xFYVE, and FAPP1—that consistently localized around the internalized conidia (71).

Even if the internalization of *Aspergillus fumigatus* conidia by BECs is a rare event, however, it could represent a starting point of invasive forms in immunosuppressed patients. The fate of the internalized conidia is still unknown and one can postulate that some of them remain quiescent within the cells until they reactivate, thanks to iatrogenic immunosuppression (77). This could explain the breakthrough of some invasive aspergillosis cases occurring in immunocompromised patients otherwise protected from contamination from the ambient air using a high-efficiency particulate air filter chamber (78).

SYNTHESIS AND RELEASE OF BIOACTIVE MOLECULES BY BRONCHIAL EPITHELIAL CELLS INFECTED WITH *ASPERGILLUS FUMIGATUS*

Cytokine/Chemokine Synthesis

One of the most studied consequences of PAMP/PRR interaction is the induction of cytokine/chemokine synthesis. Several studies have shown that infection of BECs with *Aspergillus fumigatus* leads to the release of pro-inflammatory cytokines, mostly IL-6, IL-8, or tumor necrosis factor-α provided that the infection time is more than 6 h and allows conidia germination (79–81) (**Figure 2B**). Hence, after 6 h of incubation, expression (mRNA) of not only tumor necrosis factor-α and IL-8 but also granulocyte macrophage-colony stimulating factor (GM-CSF) in HBE cells exposed to *A. fumigatus* conidia, is significantly increased by 8 to 14 times in regards to non-infected cells (29). Similarly, BEAS-2B cells release an increased amount of IL-8, 8 h after having been infected with *A. fumigatus* conidia, at a time corresponding to the hyphal formation (79) (**Figure 1**). In contrast, IL-8 synthesis was not triggered 15 h post-infection in BEAS-2B cells infected with a mutant strain of *A. fumigatus* unable to germinate (79). Considering the differences in the cell-wall content between the conidial and hyphal stages, these observations strongly suggest a role for some parietal molecules in masking resting conidia, avoiding their recognition by the BECs. RodA hydrophobin, whose masking role toward immune cells has been mentioned above, could be involved but, to the best of our knowledge, this hiding role toward BECs has never been checked.

Inflammatory mediators act synergistically to establish an organized and regulated host response against *Aspergillus fumigatus*. For example, IL-8, also known as CXCL-8, is a chemokine exhibiting a pleiotropic effect on neutrophils: strong chemotactic influence, degranulation of lysosomes with release of enzymes within the phagosome, production of reactive oxygen species (ROS), and increased expression of adhesion molecules (82). GM-CSF acts both as a hematopoietic growth factor favoring the proliferation and differentiation of myeloid cells into mature cells such as neutrophils and macrophages, and as an enhancer of the antimicrobial functions of those cells. Very recently, our group demonstrated that the inflammatory response of BEAS-2B cells and human primary BECs against *A. fumigatus* could be reprogrammed after the first contact with a microbial ligand, in this case *Pseudomonas aeruginosa* flagellin (81). Pre-stimulation with this TLR5 ligand led to a significantly enhanced release of two proinflammatory cytokines, IL-6 and IL-8, after an *A. fumigatus* challenge. This is comparable to the phenomenon called trained immunity or innate immune memory that has been largely studied using monocytes/macrophages (83–85).

Molecules Potentially Active Against *Aspergillus fumigatus*

Antimicrobial peptides (AMPs) are cationic small-peptide chains that exhibit antimicrobial activity against a variety of pathogens including fungi (86). Although membrane permeabilization is the main mechanism of action of AMPs against pathogens, additional mechanisms have been described including inhibition of macromolecular synthesis (87). Under basal conditions, BECs release a number of AMPs or proteins, some of which exhibit potential antifungal activity (**Figure 2C**).

The defensin family, divided into three classes (α-, β-, and θ-defensins), includes broad-spectrum antimicrobial peptides that are evolutionarily conserved across the living world (88). Human β-defensins are a characteristic of epithelial tissues and present a constitutive expression in primary human BECs (89). Human β-defensin 2 and human β-defensin 9 are reported to be highly expressed by BECs (HBE and 16HBE cells) exposed to different morphotypes of *A. fumigatus* (29, 90). Lactoferrin is a protein synthesized and released by 16HBE cells (91). Interestingly, according to Lupetti et al., a synthetic peptide based on the human lactoferrin sequence but containing only the first cationic domain is one of the most potent antimicrobial peptides against *A. fumigatus* hyphae and conidia *in vitro* (92). Lactoferrin can also act by reducing the toxic effect on host cells (cytotoxicity, oxidation level, and DNA damage) of aflatoxin, a mycotoxin synthesized by *Aspergillus* (93). Secretory leukocyte proteinase inhibitor (SLPI), also called anti-leukoprotease or mucus proteinase inhibitor, and elastase-specific inhibitor (or elafin and trappin-2) are two serine proteinase inhibitors constitutively secreted from the airway epithelium (94). Both are secreted by BECs in response to pro-inflammatory cytokines such as IL-1β (95, 96). Different biological functions have been reported for these molecules: protection of the lungs against the damage induced by neutrophil serine proteases and also antimicrobial activity notably against fungi like *A. fumigatus* (97, 98). However, these proteins are not considered as AMPs because their size, 11.7 and 9.9 kDa for SPLI and elastase-specific inhibitor respectively, are too large to be classified as peptides.

Interestingly, BEAS-2B and HBE cells are also able to produce ROS (29, 99). In their study on BECs challenged with *A. fumigatus*, Sun et al. showed that conidia induced ROS generation in a Dectin-1-dependent manner after 6 h of infection (29). ROS are known to be produced by neutrophils thanks to nicotinamide adenine dinucleotide phosphate oxidase produced in response to germinating *A. fumigatus* challenge (100, 101). They are released from granules either into phagosomes or into the extracellular environment, inducing damage to *Aspergillus* (6). But until now, the precise role of ROS produced by BECs in antifungal activity remains undetermined.

The study of the secretome of BEAS-2B cells infected with *A. fumigatus* also gave more insight into the role of some molecules that may possibly act against the fungal infection (102). Among the most significant results, Fekkar et al. found the release of lysosomal enzymes such as N-Acetyl-β-d-glucosaminidase, cathepsin B, and cathepsin D. N-Acetyl-β-d-glucosaminidase is responsible for the hydrolysis of glycosidic bonds. Cathepsin B and D, members of the lysosomal cysteine protease family, are known to acidify the phagosome of macrophages but their role in BECs has not been determined yet. Chitinase, a member of N-Acetyl-β-d-glucosaminidase, degrades the major fungal-wall component chitin and as such could play a role in the control of *Aspergillus* infection (103, 104).

At this time, not all the active molecules may have been described. Recently, Richard et al. reported that BEAS-2B cells prevent the germination of conidia without internalization but failed to demonstrate the role of any soluble compound present in the supernatants of infected cells (32). This antifungal activity of BECs is fungistatic and occurs via a mechanism that is phosphoinositide 3-kinase dependent. The same kind of observation was made by Clark et al. who found that after infecting BEAS-2B cells with *A. fumigatus* conidia, a large subset of conidia is rendered metabolically inactive, as measured with the metabolic marker FUN-1, while not being internalized by the cells (71).

CONCLUSION

The evidence of BECs playing an important role in the innate immunity-based defense mechanism against *Aspergillus fumigatus* is now growing. Recent studies have been able to demonstrate that, in addition to the production of mucus and ciliary beating that allow the clearance of the conidia, BECs are directly involved in an immune response against *A. fumigatus* through the recognition of fungal cell-wall components, mainly polysaccharides, by cellular ligands such as Dectin-1 or TLRs. There is a consensus for a pro-inflammatory response by BECs stimulated by *A. fumigatus*. However, additional studies are needed to better decipher BECs response. Studies focused on the internalization of the conidia by BECs reported divergent results according to the study model. This warrants further studies to clarify this point such as the investigation of the fate of the internalized conidia that could play a role in the future development of invasive aspergillosis. Different types of AMPs are also produced by BECs, some of them being active directly or indirectly against *Aspergillus*, making these molecules appealing for new therapeutic approaches. Overall, the bronchial epithelium appears as a suitable target for novel therapeutic strategies aiming to restore barrier integrity and to enhance defenses against inhaled pathogens.

AUTHOR CONTRIBUTIONS

JB, VB, and CH: drafting of the manuscript. JB, VB, CH, LG, JG, MR, and HC: revision of the manuscript.

ACKNOWLEDGMENTS

The authors would like to dedicate this paper in the honor of their deceased colleague and friend, Michel Chignard.

REFERENCES

1. Latgé JP, Chamilos G. *Aspergillus fumigatus* and aspergillosis in 2019. *Clin Microbiol Rev.* (2019) 33:e00140-18. doi: 10.1128/CMR.00140-18
2. Samson RA, Visagie CM, Houbraken J, Hong SB, Hubka V, Klaassen CHW, et al. Phylogeny, identification and nomenclature of the genus *Aspergillus*. *Stud Mycol.* (2014) 78:141–73. doi: 10.1016/j.simyco.2014.07.004
3. Paulussen C, Hallsworth JE, Álvarez-Pérez S, Nierman WC, Hamill PG, Blain D, et al. Ecology of aspergillosis: insights into the pathogenic potency of *Aspergillus fumigatus* and some other *Aspergillus* species. *Microb Biotechnol.* (2017) 10:296–322. doi: 10.1111/1751-7915.12367
4. Latgé J-P. *Aspergillus fumigatus* and aspergillosis. *Clin Microbiol Rev.* (1999) 12:310–50. doi: 10.1128/CMR.12.2.310
5. van de Veerdonk FL, Gresnigt MS, Romani L, Netea MG, Latgé JP. *Aspergillus fumigatus* morphology and dynamic host interactions. *Nat Rev Microbiol.* (2017) 15:661–74. doi: 10.1038/nrmicro.2017.90
6. Cunha C, Kurzai O, Löffler J, Aversa F, Romani L, Carvalho A. Neutrophil responses to aspergillosis: new roles for old players. *Mycopathologia.* (2014) 178:387–93. doi: 10.1007/s11046-014-9796-7
7. Balloy V, Huerre M, Latgé JP, Chignard M. Differences in patterns of infection and inflammation for corticosteroid treatment and chemotherapy in experimental invasive pulmonary aspergillosis. *Infect Immun.* (2005) 73:494–503. doi: 10.1128/IAI.73.1.494-503.2005
8. Nawada R, Amitani R, Tanaka E, Niimi A, Suzuki K, Murayama T, et al. Murine model of invasive pulmonary aspergillosis following an earlier stage, noninvasive *Aspergillus* infection. *J Clin Microbiol.* (1996) 34:1433–9. doi: 10.1128/JCM.34.6.1433-1439.1996
9. Ibrahim-Granet O, Philippe B, Boleti H, Boisvieux-Ulrich E, Grenet D, Stern M, et al. Phagocytosis and intracellular fate of *Aspergillus fumigatus* conidia in alveolar macrophages. *Infect Immun.* (2003) 71:891–903. doi: 10.1128/IAI.71.2.891-903.2003
10. Philippe B, Ibrahim-Granet O, Prévost MC, Gougerot-Pocidalo MA, Sanchez Perez M, Van der Meeren A, et al. Killing of *Aspergillus fumigatus* by alveolar macrophages is mediated by reactive oxidant intermediates. *Infect Immun.* (2003) 71:3034–42. doi: 10.1128/IAI.71.6.3034-3042.2003
11. Romani L. Immunity to fungal infections. *Nat Rev Immunol.* (2011) 11:275–88. doi: 10.1038/nri2939
12. Brandt C, Roehmel J, Rickerts V, Melichar V, Niemann N, Schwarz C. *Aspergillus* bronchitis in patients with cystic fibrosis. *Mycopathologia.* (2018) 183:61–9. doi: 10.1007/s11046-017-0190-0
13. Zhao J, Cheng W, He X, Liu Y. The Co-colonization prevalence of *Pseudomonas aeruginosa* and *Aspergillus fumigatus* in cystic fibrosis: a systematic review and meta-analysis. *Microbial Pathog.* (2018) 125:122–28. doi: 10.1016/j.micpath.2018.09.010
14. Armstead J, Morris J, Denning DW. Multi-country estimate of different manifestations of aspergillosis in cystic fibrosis. *PLoS ONE.* (2014) 9:e98502. doi: 10.1371/journal.pone.0098502
15. Gago S, Denning DW, Bowyer P. Pathophysiological aspects of *Aspergillus* colonization in disease. *Med Mycol.* (2019) 57(Suppl. 2):S219–27. doi: 10.1093/mmy/myy076
16. Stevens DA, Moss RB, Kurup VP, Knutsen AP, Greenberger P, Judson MA, et al. Allergic bronchopulmonary aspergillosis in cystic fibrosis—state of the art: cystic fibrosis foundation consensus conference. *Clin Infect Dis.* (2003) 37(Suppl. 3):S225–64. doi: 10.1086/376525
17. Agarwal R. Allergic bronchopulmonary aspergillosis. *Chest.* (2009) 135:805–26. doi: 10.1378/chest.08-2586
18. Reddel RR, Ke Y, Gerwin BI, McMenamin MG, Lechner JF, Su RT, et al. Transformation of human bronchial epithelial cells by infection with SV40 or adenovirus-12 SV40 hybrid virus, or transfection via strontium phosphate coprecipitation with a plasmid containing SV40 early region genes. *Cancer Res.* (1988) 48:1904–9.
19. Gruenert DC, Basbaum CB, Welsh MJ, Li M, Finkbeiner WE, Nadel JA. Characterization of human tracheal epithelial cells transformed by an origin-defective Simian virus 40. *Proceedings Natl Acad Sci USA.* (1988) 85:5951–5. doi: 10.1073/pnas.85.16.5951
20. Hiemstra PS, Grootaers G, van der Does AM, Krul CAM, Kooter IM. Human lung epithelial cell cultures for analysis of inhaled toxicants: lessons learned and future directions. *Toxicology In Vitro.* (2018) 47:137–46. doi: 10.1016/j.tiv.2017.11.005
21. Gray TE, Guzman K, Davis CW, Abdullah LH, Nettesheim P. Mucociliary differentiation of serially passaged normal human tracheobronchial epithelial cells. *Am J Respir Cell Mol Biol.* (1996) 14:104–12. doi: 10.1165/ajrcmb.14.1.8534481
22. Desoubeaux G, Cray C. Rodent models of invasive aspergillosis due to *Aspergillus fumigatus*: still a long path toward standardization.

Front Microbiol. (2017) 8:841. doi: 10.3389/fmicb.2017.00841
23. Fahy JV, Dickey BF. Airway mucus function and dysfunction. *N Engl J Med.* (2010) 363:2233–47. doi: 10.1056/NEJMra0910061
24. Cowley AC, Thornton DJ, Denning DW, Horsley A. Aspergillosis and the role of mucins in cystic fibrosis. *Pediatr Pulmonol.* (2017) 52:548–55. doi: 10.1002/ppul.23618
25. Yaghi A, Dolovich MB. Airway epithelial cell cilia and obstructive lung disease. *Cells.* (2016) 5:40. doi: 10.3390/cells5040040
26. Sehgal IS, Dhooria S, Bal A, Agarwal R. Allergic bronchopulmonary aspergillosis in an adult with Kartagener syndrome. *BMJ Case Rep.* (2015) 2015:bcr2015211493. doi: 10.1136/bcr-2015-211493
27. Chotirmall SH, Mirkovic B, Lavelle GM, McElvaney NG. Immunoevasive *Aspergillus* virulence factors. *Mycopathologia.* (2014) 178:363–70. doi: 10.1007/s11046-014-9768-y
28. Arias M, Santiago L, Vidal-García M, Redrado S, Lanuza P, Comas L, et al. Preparations for invasion: modulation of host lung immunity during pulmonary aspergillosis by gliotoxin and other fungal secondary metabolites. *Front Immunol.* (2018) 9:2549. doi: 10.3389/fimmu.2018.02549
29. Sun WK, Lu X, Li X, Sun QY, Su X, Song Y, et al. Dectin-1 is inducible and plays a crucial role in *Aspergillus*-induced innate immune responses in human bronchial epithelial cells. *Eur J Clin Microbiol Infect Dis.* (2012) 31:2755–64. doi: 10.1007/s10096-012-1624-8
30. Houser J, Komarek J, Kostlanova N, Cioci G, Varrot A, Kerr SC, et al. A soluble fucose-specific lectin from *Aspergillus fumigatus* conidia - structure, specificity and possible role in fungal pathogenicity. *PLoS ONE.* (2013) 8:e83077. doi: 10.1371/journal.pone.0083077
31. Kerr SC, Fischer GJ, Sinha M, McCabe O, Palmer JM, Choera T, et al. FleA expression in *Aspergillus fumigatus* is recognized by fucosylated structures on mucins and macrophages to prevent lung infection. *PLoS Pathog.* (2016) 12:e1005555. doi: 10.1371/journal.ppat.1005555
32. Richard N, Marti L, Varrot A, Guillot L, Guitard J, Hennequin C, et al. Human bronchial epithelial cells inhibit *Aspergillus fumigatus* germination of extracellular conidia via FleA recognition. *Sci Rep.* (2018) 8:15699. doi: 10.1038/s41598-018-33902-0
33. Beisswenger C, Hess C, Bals R. *Aspergillus fumigatus* conidia induce interferon-β signalling in respiratory epithelial cells. *Eur Respir J.* (2012) 39:411–8. doi: 10.1183/09031936.00096110
34. Sha Q, Truong-Tran AQ, Plitt JR, Beck LA, Schleimer RP. Activation of airway epithelial cells by toll-like receptor agonists. *Am J Respir Cell Mol Biol.* (2004) 31:358–64. doi: 10.1165/rcmb.2003-0388OC
35. Mayer AK, Muehmer M, Mages J, Gueinzius K, Hess C, Heeg K, et al. Differential recognition of TLR-dependent microbial ligands in human bronchial epithelial cells. *J Immunol.* (2007) 178:3134–42. doi: 10.4049/jimmunol.178.5.3134
36. Han B, Mura M, Andrade CF, Okutani D, Lodyga M, dos Santos CC, et al. TNFα-induced long pentraxin PTX3 expression in human lung epithelial cells via JNK. *J Immunol.* (2005) 175:8303–11. doi: 10.4049/jimmunol.175.12.8303
37. Baltussen TJH, Zoll J, Verweij PE, Melchers WJG. Molecular mechanisms of conidial germination in *Aspergillus* spp. *Microbiol Mol Biol Rev.* (2020) 84:e00049-19. doi: 10.1128/MMBR.00049-19
38. Bayry J, Beaussart A, Dufrêne YF, Sharma M, Bansal K, Kniemeyer O, et al. Surface structure characterization of *Aspergillus fumigatus* conidia mutated in the melanin synthesis pathway and their human cellular immune response. *Infect Immun.* (2014) 82:3141–53. doi: 10.1128/IAI.01726-14
39. Valsecchi I, Dupres V, Stephen-Victor E, Guijarro JI, Gibbons J, Beau R, et al. Role of hydrophobins in *Aspergillus fumigatus*. *J Fungi.* (2018) 4:2. doi: 10.3390/jof4010002
40. Aimanianda V, Bayry J, Bozza S, Kniemeyer O, Perruccio K, Elluru SR, et al. Surface hydrophobin prevents immune recognition of airborne fungal spores. *Nature.* (2009) 460:1117–21. doi: 10.1038/nature08264
41. Kuboi S, Ishimaru T, Tamada S, Bernard EM, Perlin DS, Armstrong D. Molecular characterization of AfuFleA, an l-fucose-specific lectin from *Aspergillus fumigatus*. *J Infect Chemother.* (2013) 19:1021–8. doi: 10.1007/s10156-013-0614-9
42. Taubitz A, Bauer B, Heesemann J, Ebel F. Role of respiration in the germination process of the pathogenic mold *Aspergillus fumigatus*. *Curr Microbiol.* (2007) 54:354. doi: 10.1007/s00284-006-0413-y
43. Latgé JP, Beauvais A, Chamilos G. The cell wall of the human fungal pathogen *Aspergillus fumigatus*: biosynthesis, organization, immune response, and virulence. *Annu Rev Microbiol.* (2017) 71:99–116. doi: 10.1146/annurev-micro-030117-020406
44. Fontaine T, Delangle A, Simenel C, Coddeville B, van Vliet SJ, van Kooyk Y, et al. Galactosaminogalactan, a new immunosuppressive polysaccharide of *Aspergillus fumigatus*. *PLoS Pathog.* (2011) 7:e1002372. doi: 10.1371/journal.ppat.1002372
45. Gravelat FN, Beauvais A, Liu H, Lee MJ, Snarr BD, Chen D, et al. *Aspergillus* galactosaminogalactan mediates adherence to host constituents and conceals hyphal β-glucan from the immune system. *PLoS Pathog.* (2013) 9:e1003575. doi: 10.1371/journal.ppat.1003575
46. Gresnigt MS, Bozza S, Becker KL, Joosten LA, Abdollahi-Roodsaz S, van der Berg WB, et al. A polysaccharide virulence factor from *Aspergillus fumigatus* elicits anti-inflammatory effects through induction of interleukin-1 receptor antagonist. *PLoS Pathog.* (2014) 10:e1003936. doi: 10.1371/journal.ppat.1003936
47. Goyal S, Castrillón-Betancur JC, Klaile E, Slevogt H. The interaction of human pathogenic fungi with C-type lectin receptors. *Front Immunol.* (2018) 9:1261. doi: 10.3389/fimmu.2018.01261
48. Werner JL, Metz AE, Horn D, Schoeb TR, Hewitt MM, Schwiebert LM, et al. Requisite role for the Dectin-1 beta-glucan receptor in pulmonary defense against *Aspergillus fumigatus*. *J Immunol.* (2009) 182:4938–46. doi: 10.4049/jimmunol.0804250
49. Sainz J, Lupiáñez CB, Segura-Catena J, Vazquez L, Ríos R, Oyonarte S, et al. Dectin-1 and DC-SIGN polymorphisms associated with invasive pulmonary aspergillosis infection. *PLoS ONE.* (2012) 7:e32273. doi: 10.1371/journal.pone.0032273
50. Liu ZC, Wang M, Sun WK, Xia D, Tan MM, Ding Y, et al. Up-regulation of Dectin-1 in airway epithelial cells promotes mice defense against invasive pulmonary aspergillosis. *Int J Clin Exp Med.* (2015) 8:17489–97.
51. Drummond RA, Brown GD. The role of dectin-1 in the host defence against fungal infections. *Curr Opin Microbiol.* (2011) 14:392–9. doi: 10.1016/j.mib.2011.07.001
52. Geijtenbeek TB, Gringhuis SI. Signalling through C-type lectin receptors: shaping immune responses. *Nat Rev Immunol.* (2009) 9:465–79. doi: 10.1038/nri2569
53. Jeong JS, Lee KB, Kim SR, Kim DI, Park HJ, Lee HK, et al. Airway epithelial phosphoinositide 3-kinase-δ contributes to the modulation of fungi-induced innate immune response. *Thorax.* (2018) 73:758–68. doi: 10.1136/thoraxjnl-2017-210326
54. Michael CF, Waters CM, LeMessurier KS, Samarasinghe AE, Song CY, Malik KU, et al. Airway epithelial repair by a prebiotic mannan derived from *Saccharomyces cerevisiae*. *J Immunol Res.* (2017) 2017:8903982. doi: 10.1155/2017/8903982
55. Gazi U, Martinez-Pomares L. Influence of the mannose receptor in host immune responses. *Immunobiology.* (2009) 214:554–61. doi: 10.1016/j.imbio.2008.11.004
56. De Nardo D. Toll-like receptors: activation, signalling and transcriptional modulation. *Cytokine.* (2015) 74:181–9. doi: 10.1016/j.cyto.2015.02.025
57. Balloy V, Si-Tahar M, Takeuchi O, Philippe B, Nahori MA, Tanguy M, et al. Involvement of toll-like receptor 2 in experimental invasive pulmonary aspergillosis. *Infect Immun.* (2005) 73:5420–5. doi: 10.1128/IAI.73.9.5420-5425.2005
58. Chignard M, Balloy V, Sallenave JM, Si-Tahar M. Role of toll-like receptors in lung innate defense against invasive aspergillosis. Distinct impact in immunocompetent and immunocompromized hosts. *Clin Immunol.* (2007) 124:238–43. doi: 10.1016/j.clim.2007.05.004
59. Øya E, Becher R, Ekeren L, Afanou AKJ, Øvrevik J, Holme JA. Pro-Inflammatory responses in human bronchial epithelial cells induced by spores and hyphal fragments of common damp indoor molds. *Int J Environ Res Public Health.* (2019) 16:1085. doi: 10.3390/ijerph16061085
60. Bochud PY, Chien JW, Marr KA, Leisenring WM, Upton A, Janer M, et al. Toll-like receptor 4 polymorphisms and aspergillosis

in stem-cell transplantation. *N Engl J Med.* (2008) 359:1766–77. doi: 10.1056/NEJMoa0802629

61. Ramirez-Ortiz ZG, Specht CA, Wang JP, Lee CK, Bartholomeu DC, Gazzinelli RT, et al. Toll-like receptor 9-dependent immune activation by unmethylated CpG motifs in *Aspergillus fumigatus* DNA. *Infect Immun.* (2008) 76:2123–9. doi: 10.1128/IAI.00047-08
62. Leiva-Juárez MM, Ware HH, Kulkarni VV, Zweidler-McKay PA, Tuvim MJ, Evans SE. Inducible epithelial resistance protects mice against leukemia-associated pneumonia. *Blood.* (2016) 128:982–92. doi: 10.1182/blood-2016-03-708511
63. Greene CM, Carroll TP, Smith SG, Taggart CC, Devaney J, Griffin S, et al. TLR-induced inflammation in cystic fibrosis and non-cystic fibrosis airway epithelial cells. *J Immunol.* (2005) 174:1638–46. doi: 10.4049/jimmunol.174.3.1638
64. Garlanda C, Hirsch E, Bozza S, Salustri A, De Acetis M, Nota R, et al. Non-redundant role of the long pentraxin PTX3 in anti-fungal innate immune response. *Nature.* (2002) 420:182–6. doi: 10.1038/nature01195
65. Bozza S, Campo S, Arseni B, Inforzato A, Ragnar L, Bottazzi B, et al. PTX3 binds MD-2 and promotes TRIF-dependent immune protection in aspergillosis. *J Immunol.* (2014) 193:2340–8. doi: 10.4049/jimmunol.1400814
66. Wasylnka JA, Moore MM. *Aspergillus fumigatus* conidia survive and germinate in acidic organelles of A549 epithelial cells. *J Cell Sci.* (2003) 116:1579–87. doi: 10.1242/jcs.00329
67. DeHart DJ, Agwu DE, Julian NC, Washburn RG. Binding and germination of *Aspergillus fumigatus* conidia on cultured A549 pneumocytes. *J Infect Dis.* (1997) 175:146–50. doi: 10.1093/infdis/175.1.146
68. Zhang Z, Liu R, Noordhoek JA, Kauffman HF. Interaction of airway epithelial cells (A549) with spores and mycelium of *Aspergillus fumigatus*. *J Infect.* (2005) 51:375–82. doi: 10.1016/j.jinf.2004.12.012
69. Paris S, Boisvieux-Ulrich E, Crestani B, Houcine O, Taramelli D, Lombardi L, et al. Internalization of *Aspergillus fumigatus* conidia by epithelial and endothelial cells. *Infect Immunity.* (1997) 65:1510–14. doi: 10.1128/IAI.65.4.1510-1514.1997
70. Gomez P, Hackett TL, Moore MM, Knight DA, Tebbutt SJ. Functional genomics of human bronchial epithelial cells directly interacting with conidia of *Aspergillus fumigatus*. *BMC Genomics.* (2010) 11:358. doi: 10.1186/1471-2164-11-358
71. Clark HR, Powell AB, Simmons KA, Ayubi T, Kale SD. Endocytic markers associated with the internalization and processing of *Aspergillus fumigatus* conidia by BEAS-2B cells. *mSphere.* (2019) 4:e00663-18. doi: 10.1128/mSphere.00663-18
72. Toor A, Culibrk L, Singhera GK, Moon KM, Prudova A, Foster LJ, et al. Transcriptomic and proteomic host response to *Aspergillus fumigatus* conidia in an air-liquid interface model of human bronchial epithelium. *PLoS ONE.* (2018) 13:e0209652. doi: 10.1371/journal.pone.0209652
73. Fernandes J, Hamidi F, Leborgne R, Beau R, Castier Y, Mordant P, et al. Penetration of the human pulmonary epithelium by *Aspergillus fumigatus* hyphae. *J Infect Dis.* (2018) 218:1306–13. doi: 10.1093/infdis/jiy298
74. Rammaert B, Jouvion G, de Chaumont F, Garcia-Hermoso D, Szczepaniak C, Renaudat C, et al. Absence of fungal spore internalization by bronchial epithelium in mouse models evidenced by a new bioimaging approach and transmission electronic microscopy. *Am J Pathol.* (2015) 185:2421–30. doi: 10.1016/j.ajpath.2015.04.027
75. Croft CA, Culibrk L, Moore MM, Tebbutt SJ. Interactions of *Aspergillus fumigatus* conidia with airway epithelial cells: a critical review. *Front Microbiol.* (2016) 7:472. doi: 10.3389/fmicb.2016.00472
76. Culibrk L, Croft CA, Toor A, Yang SJ, Singhera GK, Dorscheid DR, et al. Phagocytosis of *Aspergillus fumigatus* by human bronchial epithelial cells is mediated by the Arp2/3 complex and WIPF2. *Front Cell Infect Microbiol.* (2019) 9:16. doi: 10.3389/fcimb.2019.00016
77. Amitani R, Kawanami R. Interaction of *Aspergillus* with human respiratory mucosa: a study with organ culture model. *Med Mycol.* (2009) 47(Suppl. 1):S127–31. doi: 10.1080/13693780802558959
78. Roilides E, Simitsopoulou M. Local innate host response and filamentous fungi in patients with cystic fibrosis. *Med Mycol.* (2010) 48:S22–31. doi: 10.3109/13693786.2010.511286
79. Balloy V, Sallenave JM, Wu Y, Touqui L, Latgé JP, Si-Tahar M, et al. *Aspergillus fumigatus*-induced interleukin-8 synthesis by respiratory epithelial cells is controlled by the phosphatidylinositol 3-kinase, P38 MAPK, and ERK1/2 pathways and not by the toll-like receptor-MyD88 pathway. *J Biol Chem.* (2008) 283:30513–21. doi: 10.1074/jbc.M803149200
80. Tomee JF, Wierenga AT, Hiemstra PS, Kauffman HK. Proteases from *Aspergillus fumigatus* induce release of proinflammatory cytokines and cell detachment in airway epithelial cell lines. *J Infect Dis.* (1997) 176:300–3. doi: 10.1086/517272
81. Bigot J, Guillot L, Guitard J, Ruffin M, Corvol H, Chignard M, et al. Respiratory epithelial cells can remember infection: a proof of concept study. *J Infect Dis.* (2019) 221:1000–5. doi: 10.1093/infdis/jiz569
82. Balloy V, Chignard M. The innate immune response to *Aspergillus fumigatus*. *Microbes Infect.* (2009) 11:919–27. doi: 10.1016/j.micinf.2009.07.002
83. Ifrim DC, Quintin J, Joosten LAB, Jacobs C, Jansen T, Jacobs L, et al. Trained immunity or tolerance: opposing functional programs induced in human monocytes after engagement of various pattern recognition receptors. *Clin Vaccine Immunol.* (2014) 21:534–45. doi: 10.1128/CVI.00688-13
84. Netea MG, Quintin J, van der Meer JW. Trained immunity: a memory for innate host defense. *Cell Host Microbe.* (2011) 9:355–61. doi: 10.1016/j.chom.2011.04.006
85. Netea MG, Joosten LAB, Latz E, Mills KHG, Natoli G, Stunnenberg HG, et al. Trained immunity: a program of innate immune memory in health and disease. *Science.* (2016) 352:aaf1098. doi: 10.1126/science.aaf1098
86. Kang HK, Kim C, Seo CH, Park Y. The therapeutic applications of antimicrobial peptides (AMPs): a patent review. *J Microbiol.* (2017) 55:1–12. doi: 10.1007/s12275-017-6452-1
87. Sierra JM, Fusté E, Rabanal F, Vinuesa T, Viñas M. An overview of antimicrobial peptides and the latest advances in their development. *Expert Opin Biol Ther.* (2017) 17:663–76. doi: 10.1080/14712598.2017.1315402
88. Ganz T, Weiss J. Antimicrobial peptides of phagocytes and epithelia. *Semin Hematol.* (1997) 34:343–54.
89. Arnason JW, Murphy JC, Kooi C, Wiehler S, Traves SL, Shelfoon C, et al. Human β-defensin-2 production upon viral and bacterial co-infection is attenuated in COPD. *PLoS ONE.* (2017) 12:e0175963. doi: 10.1371/journal.pone.0175963
90. Alekseeva L, Huet D, Féménia F, Mouyna I, Abdelouahab M, Cagna A, et al. Inducible expression of beta defensins by human respiratory epithelial cells exposed to *Aspergillus fumigatus* organisms. *BMC Microbiol.* (2009) 9:33. doi: 10.1186/1471-2180-9-33
91. van den Berge M, Jonker MR, Miller-Larsson A, Postma DS, Heijink I. H. Effects of fluticasone propionate and budesonide on the expression of immune defense genes in bronchial epithelial cells. *Pulmon Pharmacol Ther.* (2018) 50:47–56. doi: 10.1016/j.pupt.2018.04.002
92. Lupetti A, van Dissel JT, Brouwer CP, Nibbering PH. Human antimicrobial peptides' antifungal activity against *Aspergillus fumigatus*. *Eur J Clin Microbiol Infect Dis.* (2008) 27:1125–9. doi: 10.1007/s10096-008-0553-z
93. Zheng N, Zhang H, Li S, Wang J, Liu J, Ren H, et al. Lactoferrin inhibits aflatoxin B1- and aflatoxin M1-induced cytotoxicity and DNA damage in Caco-2, HEK, Hep-G2, SK-N-SH cells. *Toxicon.* (2018) 150:77–85. doi: 10.1016/j.toxicon.2018.04.017
94. Williams SE, Brown TI, Roghanian A, Sallenave JM. SLPI and Elafin: one glove, many fingers. *Clin Sci.* (2006) 110:21–35. doi: 10.1042/CS20050115
95. Sallenave JM, Shulmann J, Crossley J, Jordana M, Gauldie J. Regulation of secretory leukocyte proteinase inhibitor (SLPI) and elastase-specific inhibitor (ESI/elafin) in human airway epithelial cells by cytokines and neutrophilic enzymes. *Am J Respir Cell Mol Biol.* (1994) 11:733–41. doi: 10.1165/ajrcmb.11.6.7946401
96. Sallenave JM. Secretory leukocyte protease inhibitor and elafin/trappin-2. *Am J Respir Cell Mol Biol.* (2010) 42:635–43. doi: 10.1165/rcmb.2010-0095RT
97. Baranger K, Zani ML, Chandenier J, Dallet-Choisy S, Moreau T. The antibacterial and antifungal properties of trappin-2 (Pre-Elafin) do not depend on its protease inhibitory function. *FEBS J.* (2008) 275:2008–20. doi: 10.1111/j.1742-4658.2008.06355.x

98. Tomee JF, Hiemstra PS, Heinzel-Wieland R, Kauffman HF. Antileukoprotease: an endogenous protein in the innate mucosal defense against fungi. *J Infect Dis.* (1997) 176:740–7. doi: 10.1086/514098
99. Chan TK, Tan WSD, Peh HY, Wong WSF. Aeroallergens induce reactive oxygen species production and DNA damage and dampen antioxidant responses in bronchial epithelial cells. *J Immunol.* (2017) 199:39–47. doi: 10.4049/jimmunol.1600657
100. Imbert S, Bresler P, Boissonnas A, Gauthier L, Souchet L, Uzunov M, et al. Calcineurin inhibitors impair neutrophil activity against *Aspergillus fumigatus* in allogeneic hematopoietic stem cell transplant recipients. *J Allergy Clin Immunol.* (2016) 138:860–8. doi: 10.1016/j.jaci.2016.02.026
101. Chotirmall SH, Al-Alawi M, Mirkovic B, Lavelle G, Logan PM, Greene CM, et al. *Aspergillus*-associated airway disease, inflammation, and the innate immune response. *Biomed Res Int.* (2013) 2013:723129. doi: 10.1155/2013/723129
102. Fekkar A, Balloy V, Pionneau C, Marinach-Patrice C, Chignard M, Mazier D. Secretome of human bronchial epithelial cells in response to the fungal pathogen *aspergillus fumigatus* analyzed by differential in-gel electrophoresis. *J Infect Dis.* (2012) 205:1163–72. doi: 10.1093/infdis/jis031
103. Karamanos Y. Endo-N-Acetyl-β-D-glucosaminidases and their potential substrates : structure/function relationships. *Res Microbiol.* (1997) 148:661–71. doi: 10.1016/S0923-2508(99)80065-5
104. Chen L, Shen Z, Wu J. Expression, purification and *in vitro* antifungal activity of acidic mammalian chitinase against *Candida albicans, Aspergillus fumigatus* and *Trichophyton rubrum* strains. *Clin Exp Dermatol.* (2009) 34:55–60. doi: 10.1111/j.1365-2230.2008.03092.x

3

Impact of the Local Inflammatory Environment on Mucosal Vitamin D Metabolism and Signaling in Chronic Inflammatory Lung Diseases

Jasmijn A. Schrumpf*, Anne M. van der Does and Pieter S. Hiemstra

Department of Pulmonology, Leiden University Medical Center, Leiden, Netherlands

***Correspondence:**
Jasmijn A. Schrumpf
j.a.schrumpf@lumc.nl

Vitamin D plays an active role in the modulation of innate and adaptive immune responses as well as in the protection against respiratory pathogens. Evidence for this immunomodulatory and protective role is derived from observational studies showing an association between vitamin D deficiency, chronic airway diseases and respiratory infections, and is supported by a range of experimental studies using cell culture and animal models. Furthermore, recent intervention studies have now shown that vitamin D supplementation reduces exacerbation rates in vitamin D-deficient patients with chronic obstructive pulmonary disease (COPD) or asthma and decreases the incidence of acute respiratory tract infections. The active vitamin D metabolite, 1,25-dihydroxy-vitamin D ($1,25(OH)_2D$), is known to contribute to the integrity of the mucosal barrier, promote killing of pathogens (via the induction of antimicrobial peptides), and to modulate inflammation and immune responses. These mechanisms may partly explain its protective role against infections and exacerbations in COPD and asthma patients. The respiratory mucosa is an important site of local $1,25(OH)_2D$ synthesis, degradation and signaling, a process that can be affected by exposure to inflammatory mediators. As a consequence, mucosal inflammation and other disease-associated factors, as observed in e.g., COPD and asthma, may modulate the protective actions of $1,25(OH)_2D$. Here, we discuss the potential consequences of various disease-associated processes such as inflammation and exposure to pathogens and inhaled toxicants on vitamin D metabolism and local responses to $1,25(OH)_2D$ in both immune- and epithelial cells. We furthermore discuss potential consequences of disturbed local levels of 25(OH)D and $1,25(OH)_2D$ for chronic lung diseases. Additional insight into the relationship between disease-associated mechanisms and local effects of $1,25(OH)_2D$ is expected to contribute to the design of future strategies aimed at improving local levels of $1,25(OH)_2D$ and signaling in chronic inflammatory lung diseases.

Keywords: inflammation, airway mucosa, vitamin D, vitamin D metabolism, host defense, COPD exacerbations

INTRODUCTION

Vitamin D is a pleiotropic hormone that is well-known for its role in the regulation of calcium and phosphate homeostasis and bone mineralization. The vitamin D receptor (VDR) acts as the receptor for the active form of vitamin D, i.e., 1,25-dihydroxy-vitamin D [1,25$(OH)_2$D], and is expressed in nearly all tissues and cell-types and regulates a large number of genes (~0.8–5% of the total genome) (1, 2). As a result, vitamin D affects many additional processes including cell proliferation and differentiation, apoptosis, DNA repair, ion transport, metabolism, cell adhesion, and oxidative stress responses (1, 3). Vitamin D deficiency [serum 25-hydroxy-vitamin D [25(OH)D] < 50 nmol/L; 25(OH)D is the main circulating form of vitamin D and its levels are used to assess vitamin D status in the clinic (4, 5) affects more than 30% of the children and adults worldwide and is a major cause of bone diseases such as rickets and osteoporosis (6). Increasing evidence has indicated that vitamin D deficiency is also associated with various other diseases such as cancer, cardiovascular disease, Alzheimer's disease and muscle myopathy, as well as several immune-related diseases such as type 1 diabetes, multiple sclerosis, inflammatory bowel disease (IBD), psoriasis and chronic inflammatory lung diseases including asthma, cystic fibrosis (CF), and chronic obstructive pulmonary disease (COPD) (6–9).

Several studies have now shown that vitamin D deficiency is prevalent in COPD patients and inversely correlated with lung function and severity of the disease (8–12). It is currently unknown whether vitamin D deficiency is a cause or consequence of COPD, since many COPD patients have low physical activity levels and spend most time indoors (13). There are however studies suggesting that low 25(OH)D levels are associated with development of COPD, based on observed associations between polymorphisms in the vitamin D binding protein (VDBP), 25(OH)D serum levels and COPD severity (8, 10, 11, 14). In addition, one study in mice showed that maternal vitamin D deficiency can impair lung -development, -structure and -function in the offspring and suggests that even before birth, maternal 25(OH)D serum levels are important for a healthy lung development (15). This might be relevant, since associations have been found between lower childhood lung function and development of COPD later in life (16). The link between maternal 25(OH)D status and asthma development is however much clearer, since two recent randomized controlled trials (RCTs) have shown that maternal vitamin D supplementation reduces the risk of childhood asthma/recurrent wheeze (17). This might be explained by the fact that multiple vitamin D-regulated genes are transcriptionally active during alveolar maturation and a number of these genes are differentially expressed in asthma (18). Additionally, this protective effect was linked to the GG-genotype of the 17q21 functional SNP rs12936231, which is associated with lower expression of *ORMDL3* and increased sphingolipid metabolism (19). Moreover, maternal circulating 25(OH)D levels affect the gut microbiota and can therefore indirectly modulate immune responses in the lung via the gut-lung-axis (20). Also later in life, optimal 25(OH)D levels remain crucial for keeping the lungs healthy. For example, Heulens et al. showed that subacute and chronic cigarette smoke (CS) exposure decreased lung function and promoted early signs of emphysema and airway inflammation in vitamin D-deficient mice compared to vitamin D-sufficient animals (21). Similarly in an elastase-induced COPD mouse model, topical administration of vitamin D in the lungs counteracted alveolar damage and improved lung function (22). Yet in humans, it is still unclear whether vitamin D status influences COPD development and disease progression. Taken together, these observations suggest an important role for vitamin D during fetal and childhood lung maturation, and indicate that sufficient 25(OH)D levels might contribute to protection against development of childhood asthma and possibly COPD at older age.

Systemic levels of biologically active 1,25$(OH)_2$D are tightly regulated to preserve sufficient levels of calcium (Ca^{2+}) and phosphate (PO_4^{2-}) for optimal bone mineralization, whereas in mucosal tissues locally produced (autocrine) 1,25$(OH)_2$D levels and signaling can be elevated or decreased upon exposure to inflammatory mediators, pathogens or inhaled toxicants (6). This could be important, since the inflamed airway mucosa of patients suffering from chronic inflammatory lung diseases is constantly exposed to these disease-associated factors (8, 23, 24). Impaired local levels of 1,25$(OH)_2$D and VDR signaling might have consequences for disease pathogenesis and progression. Dysregulated host defenses as found in patients with chronic inflammatory airway diseases include aberrant immune responses, altered microbiome composition, impaired epithelial barrier function, and aberrant secretion of host defense molecules (25–27). Adequate 1,25$(OH)_2$D levels may provide protection against these dysregulated processes by maintaining the integrity of the mucosal barrier and promotion of killing of pathogens (e.g., via the induction of the antimicrobial peptide [AMP] hCAP18/LL-37) and via the modulation of both innate and adaptive immune responses (7, 28, 29).

In this review, we first discuss the effects of these disease-associated factors on local synthesis and availability of 1,25$(OH)_2$D and 1,25$(OH)_2$D-induced responses in the lung mucosa. In the second part of the review we will describe the mechanistic links between vitamin D deficiency and the pathogenesis of chronic inflammatory lung diseases such as asthma, CF and COPD, and discuss recent evidence related to the protective effects of vitamin D on COPD and on COPD exacerbations.

MUCOSAL VITAMIN D METABOLISM IN HEALTH

Vitamin D enters the circulation either via food intake (plant-based: vitamin D_2/animal-based: vitamin D_3) or as a result of its synthesis in the skin by UVB radiation. It subsequently binds to the VDBP (30, 31), after which this complex is transported to the liver where it is converted by vitamin D-25-hydroxylases (CYP2RI and CYP27A1) into 25(OH)D. However, recent studies showed that also other cell types such as airway epithelial cells, keratinocytes, intestinal epithelial cells, and monocytes/macrophages express CYP2RI and CYP27A1, and thus are able to (locally) convert vitamin D_3 into $25(OH)D_3$ (32, 33). This inactive 25(OH)D needs to be converted into the active $1,25(OH)_2D$ by 25-hydroxyvitamin D-1α-hydroxylase (CYP27B1) in the kidney and in other cells, including several immune- and epithelial cells (34–40). $1,25(OH)_2D$ regulates expression of several genes by binding the nuclear VDR, which heterodimerizes with the retinoic acid receptor (RXR) to interact with vitamin D response elements (VDREs) that are present on the promoter region of these genes (1, 2). VDR is most abundantly expressed in intestinal enterocytes, pancreatic islets, renal distal tubules and osteoblasts, but is also present at lower levels in most other tissues and several other epithelial- and immune cells (41–45). Expression of VDR is classically regulated by $1,25(OH)_2D$, growth factors and hormones such as FGF-23 and PTH, respectively, circulating calcium levels, bile acids, transcriptional co-activators/repressors, and genetic- and epigenetic modifications, which is tissue specific (46–49). $1,25(OH)_2D$ regulates its own negative feedback by several mechanisms, including induction of expression of the catabolic enzymes 25-hydroxyvitamin D-24-hydroxylase (CYP24A1) and CYP3A4 (50, 51). CYP24A1 is expressed in most tissues and converts both 25(OH)D and $1,25(OH)_2D$ into $23,25(OH)_2D$ or $24,25(OH)_2D$ and $1,23,25(OH)_3D$ or $1,24,25(OH)_3D$, respectively (dependent on whether CYP24A1 hydroxylates at C-23 or at C-24). These are further converted into metabolites that have been found to be excreted into the bile (summarized in **Figure 1**) (50, 52, 56). CYP3A4 is mainly expressed in the liver and small intestines and contributes to the metabolic clearance of 25(OH)D and $1,25(OH)_2D$ by converting 25(OH)D into $4β,25(OH)_2D$, and $1,25(OH)_2D$ into

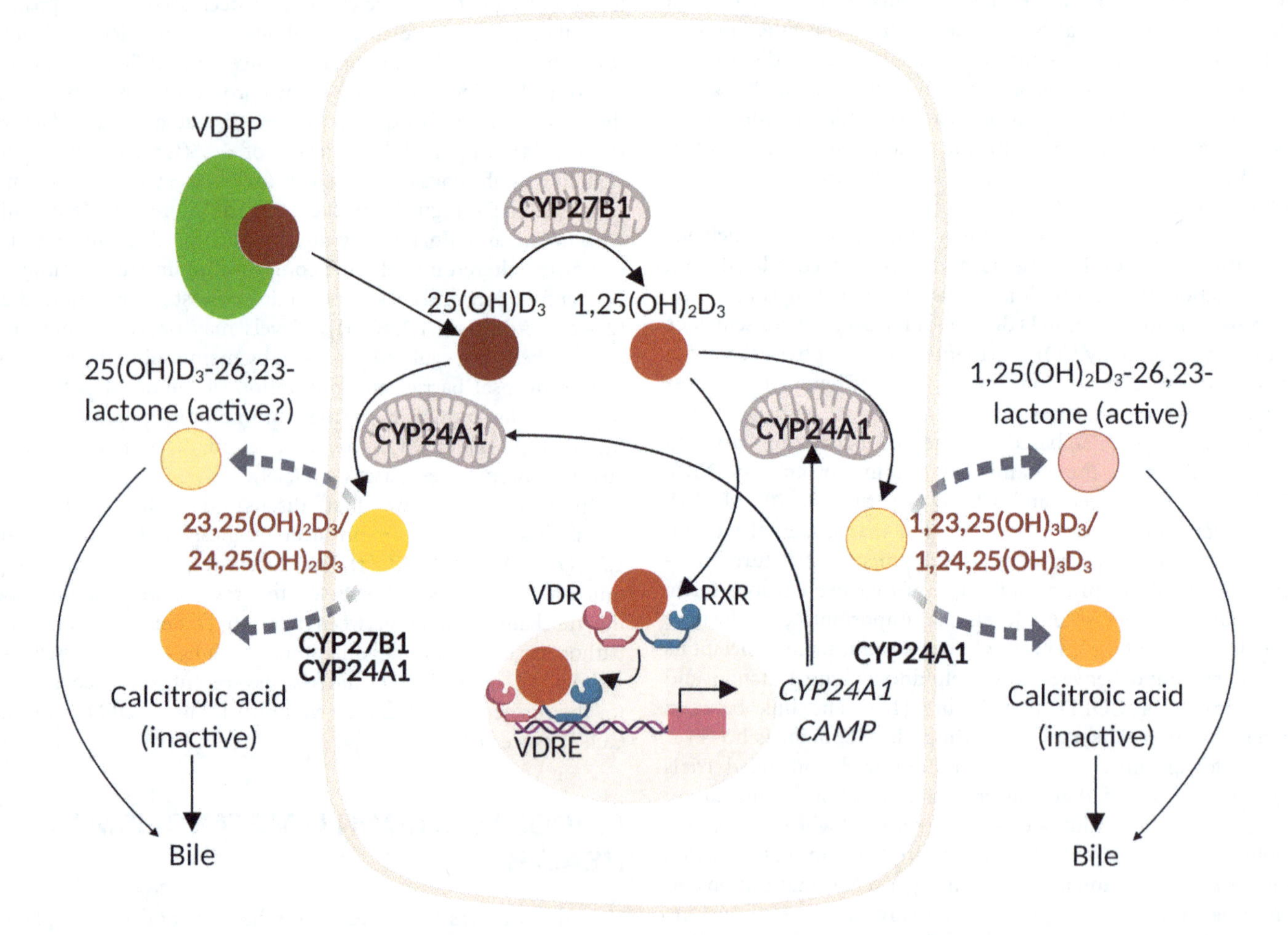

FIGURE 1 | Vitamin D metabolism and expression of hCAP18/LL-37 (*CAMP*) in epithelial cells. The vitamin D binding protein (VDBP)-$25(OH)D_3$ complex enters the epithelial cell from the circulation and $25(OH)D_3^*$ is subsequently released from the complex. In the cytoplasm, $25(OH)D_3$ is hydroxylated by 25-hydroxyvitamin D-1α-hydroxylase (CYP27B1; localized to the inner mitochondrial membrane) into the active metabolite $1,25(OH)_2D_3$. $1,25(OH)_2D_3$ subsequently binds to the nuclear vitamin D receptor (VDR) which heterodimerizes with the retinoic acid receptor (RXR) to interact with vitamin D response elements (VDREs) that are present on the promoter region of numerous genes, including *CAMP* (hCAP18/LL-37) and *CYP24A1* (25-hydroxyvitamin D-24-hydroxylase). $1,25(OH)_2D_3$ thereby regulates its own negative feedback via direct induction of CYP24A1 that hydroxylates both $25(OH)D_3$ and $1,25(OH)_2D_3$ either at the C-23 or at the C-24 to $23,25(OH)_2D_3$ or $24,25(OH)_2D_3$ and $1,23,25(OH)_3D_3$ or $1,24,25(OH)_3D_3$, respectively. These metabolites are further converted by CYP27B1 [that first converts $24,25(OH)_2D_3$ into $1,24,25(OH)_3D_3$] and CYP24A1 into $25(OH)D_3$-26,23-lactone and $1,25(OH)_2D_3$-26,23-lactone or into calcitroic acid, metabolites that are excreted in the bile (50, 52–55). *The metabolism of $25(OH)D_3$ is shown in this figure, since there is more consensus regarding the metabolism of $25(OH)D_3$ and 1,25(OH)2D3 in literature.

1,23R,25(OH)$_2$D or 1,24S,25(OH)$_2$D (51). Expression of both CYP27B1 and CYP24A1 in the kidneys is tightly regulated to maintain optimal Ca^{2+}- and PO_4^{2-} levels in the circulation, which are important for bone mineralization (57). In short, in response to low Ca^{2+} levels, parathyroid hormone (PTH) is secreted by the pituitary glands, which in turn reduces Ca^{2+} excretion and reabsorption of PO_4^{2-} (57). PTH further induces expression of CYP27B1 and represses expression of CYP24A1 in the kidneys (57). This will increase the levels of 1,25(OH)$_2$D in the circulation, which promotes intestinal Ca^{2+} and PO_4^{2-} absorption (57). These elevated circulating Ca^{2+} and PO_4^{2-} levels will subsequently induce expression of fibroblast growth factor 23 (FGF-23) in osteocytes and osteoblasts and impair secretion of parathyroid hormone (PTH) by the parathyroid glands (3). In the kidneys, FGF-23 suppresses expression of CYP27B1 and induces expression of CYP24A1, thereby inhibiting the synthesis and promoting degradation of 1,25(OH)$_2$D (3). These complex mechanisms that explain how vitamin D and its metabolic enzymes maintain sufficient Ca^{2+} and PO_4^{2-} levels in the circulation are more extensively discussed by Quarles et al. (57). In summary, it has become increasingly evident that the effects of vitamin D are not limited to homeostasis of Ca^{2+} and PO_4^{2-} and bone mineralization, because several extra-renal cells such as airway epithelial cells and immune cells express the VDR and are capable of converting circulating 25(OH)D into the active 1,25(OH)$_2$D metabolite.

MUCOSAL VITAMIN D METABOLISM AND VITAMIN D SIGNALING IN CHRONIC INFLAMMATORY AIRWAY DISEASES

Local levels and activity of 1,25(OH)$_2$D are in part determined by expression of VDR and the equilibrium between the vitamin D metabolic enzymes CYP27B1 and CYP24A1. It is important to realize that mucosal expression of CYP24A1, CYP27B1 and also VDR can be affected by several disease-associated inflammatory mediators, toxicants and pathogens, summarized in **Table 1**. As a consequence of this, the local availability of 1,25(OH)$_2$D and/or VDR signaling in tissues such as the inflamed airways of patients that suffer from chronic inflammatory airway diseases might be reduced.

TABLE 1 | Effects of inflammatory mediators on the expression of VDR, CYP24A1, and CYP27B1 in immune cells and epithelial cells.

Cell/tissue type	Stimulus	Effect	References
Primary airway epithelial cells	Poly(I:C); RSV; IL-13; IL-4; PM	CYP27B1 ↑	(38, 58–60)
	TNF-α; IL-1β; IL-17A; TGF-β1; NTHi	CYP24A1 ↑	(61, 62)
	CSE	CYP27B1 ↓	(63, 64)
	A. fumigatus; HRV; RSV	VDR ↓	(58, 65)
BEAS-2B (bronchial epithelial cell line)	HRV; RSV	VDR ↓	(58)
	PM	VDR ↑	(59)
16HBE (bronchial epithelial cell line)	*A. fumigatus*	VDR ↑	(21)
	TGF-β1	CYP27B1 ↑	(60)
	A. fumigatus	CYP27B1 ↑	(21)
A549 (lung carcinoma cell line)	CSE	VDR translocation ↓	(66)
HCT116 (colon cancer epithelial cell line)	LPS; TNF-α	CYP27B1 ↑	(67)
	LPS; TNF-α	VDR ↓	(67, 68)
	LPS	CYP24A1 ↓	(67)
COGA-1A (colon cancer epithelial cell line)	TNF-α ± IL-6	CYP27B1 ↓	(69)
Trophoblasts	TNF-α; IL-1β; IL-6	CYP24A1 ↑	(70)
	IFN-γ	CYP27B1 ↑	(70)
Macrophages	ss-RNA	CYP27B1 ↑ VDR ↑	(71)
Macrophages (derived from THP-1)	CSE	VDR ↑	(72)
Macrophages (derived from THP-1)	BaP	CYP24A1 ↑	(73)
Monocytes	TLR2/1L ± IFN-γ; LPS; IL-15	CYP27B1 ↑ VDR ↑	(39, 74–76)
	IL-4 ± TLR2/1L	CYP24A1 ↑	(39)
Neutrophils	IFN-γ *S. pneumoniae* T4R	CYP27B1 ↑ VDR ↑	(77)
T cells	T cell activators (anti-CD3/anti-CD28; PHA; PMA/ionomycin)	CYP27B1 ↑ VDR ↑	(78)
B cells	B cell activators (anti-IgM/anti-CD40/IL-21)	CYP27B1 ↑ VDR ↑	(79)

Poly(I:C), Polyinosinic:polycytidylic acid; PM, Particulate matter; NTHi, nontypeable Haemophilus influenzae; A. fumigatus, Aspergillus fumigatus; CSE, Cigarette smoke extract; HRV, Human rhinovirus; RSV, Respiratory syncytial virus; ssRNA, Single stranded RNA; BaP, Benzo[a]pyrene; TLR2/1L, Toll like receptor 2/1 Ligand; PHA, Phytohemagglutinin; PMA, Phorbol 12-myristate 13-acetate.

Epithelial Cells

Chronic lung diseases are characterized by airway inflammation and impaired respiratory host defense, which is illustrated by the increased susceptibility for respiratory infections and exacerbations (25, 80, 81). Furthermore, exposure to inhaled toxicants such as cigarette smoke and air pollutants are associated with disease pathogenesis and exacerbations in COPD, CF and in asthma patients (82–84). It would therefore be of great interest to investigate these effects on local 1,25(OH)$_2$D levels and on 1,25(OH)$_2$D-mediated respiratory host defense in the airway mucosa. Studies in airway epithelial cells have shown that exposure to UV-inactivated non-typeable *Haemophilus influenzae* (NTHi) increased expression of the catabolic enzyme CYP24A1, whereas exposure to viral double stranded-RNA analog polyinosinic:polycytidylic acid (Poly[I:C]) increased expression of CYP27B1 and thereby conversion of 25(OH)D into 1,25(OH)$_2$D, the active metabolite (38, 61). On the other hand, in the bronchial cell line BEAS-2B expression of VDR was decreased after infection with respiratory viruses such as human rhinovirus (HRV) and respiratory syncytial virus (RSV) (58). Collectively, these studies have shown in airway epithelial cells that respiratory viral- and bacterial infections can either promote or impair 1,25(OH)$_2$D synthesis and responses.

A local airway inflammatory milieu can also exert differential effects on 1,25(OH)$_2$D synthesis and signaling, dependent on the type of inflammatory mediators that are predominantly present. We have shown in differentiated primary airway epithelial cells that Th2 cytokines such as IL-4 and IL-13, enhance expression of CYP27B1 and expression of hCAP18/LL-37 upon 25(OH)D3 treatment, which suggests that a Th2-inflammatory environment, as found in allergic airway inflammation, increases the conversion of 25(OH)D into the active 1,25(OH)$_2$D (83, 85). The observation that levels of both 1,25(OH)$_2$D and hCAP18/LL-37 were increased in bronchoalveolar lavage (BAL) after allergen challenge is in line with this proposed mechanism (86). This effect of Th2 cytokines was in contrast to the effects (chronic) exposures to the proinflammatory cytokines IL-1β, TNF-α and IL-17A that strongly increased the expression of the 25(OH)D- and 1,25(OH)$_2$D-degrading CYP24A1, even in absence of its inducer 1,25(OH)$_2$D (61). Furthermore, short-term exposures to TGF-β1, a pleiotropic growth factor which is elevated in the lungs of COPD, CF and asthma patients, also increases the expression of CYP24A1 (62). As a consequence, 1,25(OH)$_2$D-mediated expression of the AMP hCAP18/LL-37 was impaired, which was likely the result of the enhanced degradation of both 25(OH)D and 1,25(OH)$_2$D by this enzyme (61, 62). In addition to pathogens and cytokines, exposure to inhaled toxicants such as cigarette smoke (CS) and particulate matter (PM) may also alter expression or activity of VDR and CYP27B1. Studies have demonstrated that cigarette smoking or exposure to CS extract (CSE) decreases expression of CYP27B1 and inhibited membrane bound (m)VDR translocation to the cell membrane in airway epithelial cells and A549 cells (an alveolar tumor cell line), respectively (63, 64, 66). This inhibition reduces the conversion of 25(OH)D to 1,25(OH)$_2$D and 1,25(OH)$_2$D-mediated gene expression as well as non-genomic actions of 1,25(OH)$_2$D-membrane associated, rapid response steroid-binding (MARRS)- signaling (63, 64, 66). This adverse effect of cigarette smoking on the synthesis and effects of 1,25(OH)$_2$D in airway epithelial cells was recently confirmed *in vivo* by Vargas Buonfiglio et al. who demonstrated that vitamin D supplementation increased antimicrobial activity in apical surface liquid (ASL) in the airway of healthy non-smokers, but not in smokers (64). On the other hand, exposure to PM increases the expression of both CYP27B1 and VDR in airway epithelial cells, thereby possibly promoting the synthesis and effects of 1,25(OH)$_2$D (59). It is however important to consider that several retrospective and observational studies have demonstrated that air pollution is an independent risk factor for developing vitamin D deficiency (87). In conclusion, exposure to CS, TGF-β1 and presence of a proinflammatory milieu appeared to most strongly decrease local presence and signaling of 1,25(OH)$_2$D in airway epithelial cells.

Immune Cells

Whereas, various studies show that exposure to proinflammatory stimuli most likely affects local 25(OH)D and 1,25(OH)$_2$D-levels and reduces the effects of 25(OH)D and 1,25(OH)$_2$D in (airway) epithelial cells, the opposite appears to be the case for immune cells. In monocytes, macrophages and neutrophils, effects on 1,25(OH)$_2$D synthesis and antimicrobial responses upon 25(OH)D treatment were generally enhanced by these proinflammatory stimuli as illustrated by increased expression of both VDR and CYP27B1 (39, 71, 74–77). It is therefore tempting to speculate that this apparent increase in antimicrobial responses upon 25(OH)D treatment in immune cells in an inflammatory environment may serve as a second line of defense and compensate for the enhanced epithelial degradation of 25(OH)D and 1,25(OH)$_2$D during inflammation. Inhaled toxicants may also affect 1,25(OH)$_2$D availability and responsiveness of immune cells. This is illustrated by two recent studies studying the effects of cigarette smoke on the human monocyte/macrophage-like cell line THP-1. One study showed that treatment with cigarette smoke extract (CSE) increased the expression of VDR without enhancing 1,25(OH)$_2$D responses (72), while the other study -that focused on the effects of Benzo[a]pyrene (BaP) (a component produced by cigarette combustion)- demonstrated that 1,25(OH)$_2$D -mediated CYP24A1 expression was induced, which was found to further enhance degradation of 1,25(OH)$_2$D (73). In summary, proinflammatory stimuli generally increased the effect of 25(OH)D and 1,25(OH)$_2$D on immune cells, whereas more studies are needed to fully determine the impact of exposure to cigarette smoke and other inhaled toxicants.

Lung Mucosa

Whereas, these studies provide evidence that inflammation and inhaled toxicants may affect 25(OH)D and 1,25(OH)$_2$D metabolism and responsiveness in epithelial cells and immune cells, it is not clear whether this has an impact on these events in lung tissue of patients with chronic lung diseases. Although evidence is limited, we can speculate that levels of 1,25(OH)$_2$D and responses are also affected by disease-associated factors in mesenchymal cells that are present in the lung mucosa. One study that showed in a bleomycin fibrosis model and in primary lung mouse fibroblasts that TGF-β1 reduced expression of the VDR might support this assumption (88). It is currently insufficiently studied whether exposures to disease-associated factors promote or impair levels of 1,25(OH)$_2$D and responses in immune-, mesenchymal and epithelial cells combined to give a better reflection of the *in vivo* situation. Interestingly, one study did already show that nasal CYP27B1- and 1,25(OH)$_2$D-levels are both reduced in chronic rhinosinusitis (CRS) patients with nasal polyps as compared to CRS-patients without nasal polyps, whereas no difference was found in circulating 1,25(OH)$_2$D-levels (89). Since most other studies were performed *in vitro* using monocultures of epithelial cells or immune cells, more complex models are needed to delineate this. Therefore, animal models or preferably more complex animal-free cell culture models using co-cultures or organs-on-chips models of primary fully differentiated epithelial cells, airway-derived fibroblasts or smooth muscle cells and immune cells could be considered in future studies.

PROTECTIVE EFFECTS OF VITAMIN D ON MUCOSAL HOMEOSTASIS

After discussing altered 25(OH)D and $1,25(OH)_2D$ metabolism and responsiveness in the inflamed airway mucosa, it is important to consider the possible consequences of these inflammation-induced changes in the airway mucosa keeping in mind the pleotropic effects of $1,25(OH)_2D$ that were introduced earlier. In several cells, tissues and organs, $1,25(OH)_2D$ regulates multiple cellular processes that affect normal and malignant cell growth and differentiation (90, 91). $1,25(OH)_2D$ displays furthermore protective effects on mucosal host defense by maintaining the integrity of the epithelial barrier, inhibition of epithelial-to-mesenchymal transition (EMT), stimulating production of AMPs and modulating both innate- and adaptive immune functions (7, 29, 92). In addition, $1,25(OH)_2D$ maintains both energetic and survival homeostasis in the mucosal epithelium through the modulation of stress and damage responses, including clearance of disturbing and stressful agents (3, 93) (**Figure 2**).

Epithelial Barrier Function

In chronic inflammatory lung diseases, epithelial barrier function is impaired, and as a consequence the susceptibility toward respiratory infections is increased (94). There is increasing evidence that $1,25(OH)_2D$ promotes epithelial barrier integrity or protects against epithelial barrier destruction. In cells of the bronchial epithelial cell line 16HBE, $1,25(OH)_2D$ inhibited CSE-mediated reduction of the epithelial barrier and expression of

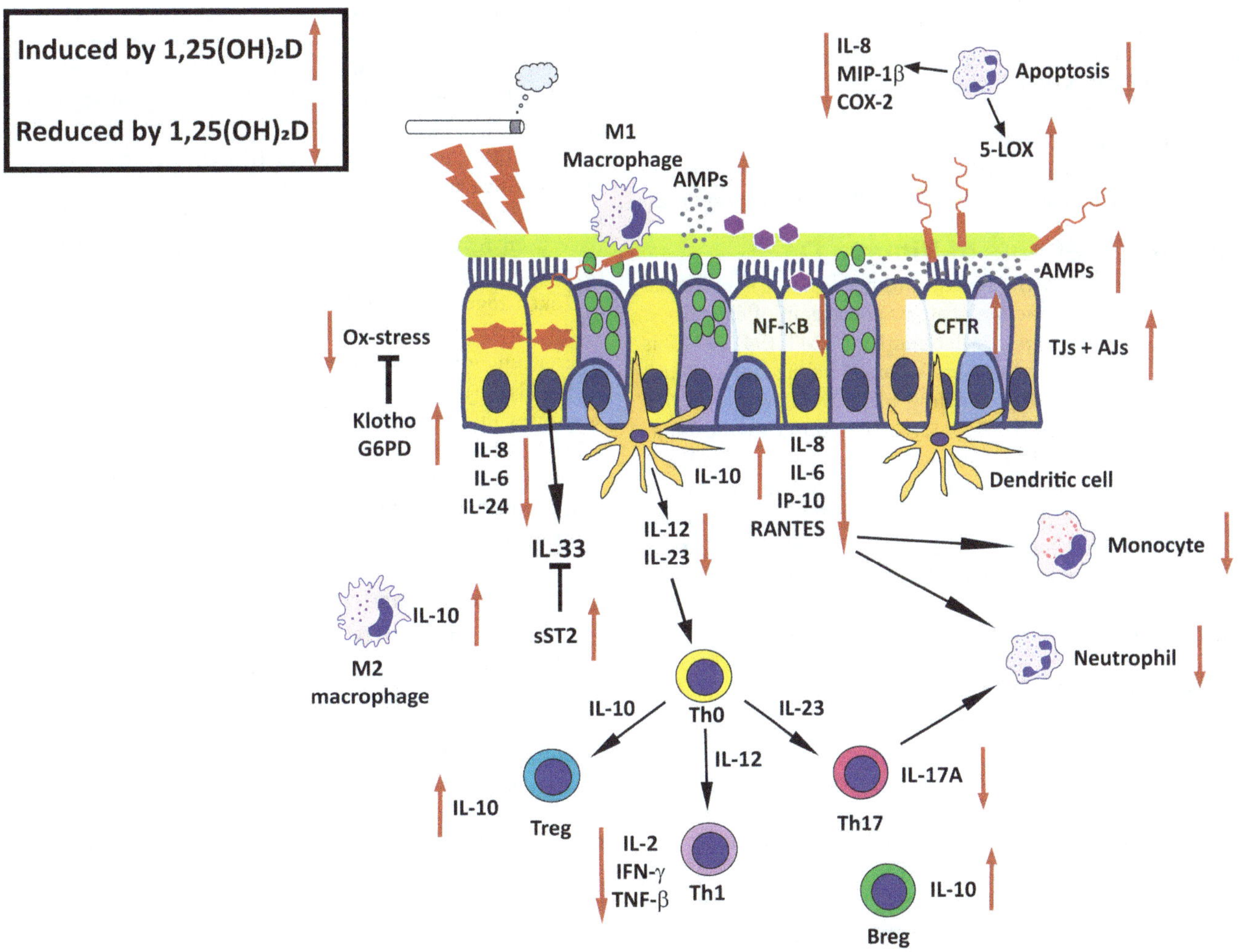

FIGURE 2 | Effects of active $1,25(OH)_2D$ on airway epithelial host defense-mechanisms in chronic airway disease. The promoting or inhibitory effects of $1,25(OH)_2D$ are indicated by the red arrows. AMPs, Antimicrobial peptides; CFTR, Cystic fibrosis transmembrane conductance regulator; Ox-stress, Oxidative stress; SOCS, Suppressor of cytokine signaling proteins; TJs, Tight junctions; AJs, Adherens junctions; G6PD, Glucose-6-phosphate dehydrogenase; sST2, Soluble suppression of tumorigenicity 2; NF-κB, Nuclear factor kappa-light-chain-enhancer of activated B cells; Th0, Naieve T cell; Treg, Regulatory T cell; Th1, T helper type 1 cell; Th2, T helper type 2 cell; Th17, T helper type 17 cell; Breg, Regulatory B cell. See text for details and references.

E-cadherin and β-catenin (95). Recently, two murine studies were published that investigated the effects of vitamin D on pulmonary epithelial barrier function. Shi et al. showed that vitamin D-supplementation alleviated lung injury in LPS-treated mice through maintenance of the pulmonary barrier by inducing expression of Zonula occludens (ZO)-1 and occludin in whole lung homogenates (96), whereas Gorman et al. showed in healthy mice, fed with a vitamin D-poor diet, that vitamin D supplementation had little effect on epithelial integrity (97). Only the first study that used a more severe mouse model with higher levels of inflammation and edema found an effect of vitamin D on epithelial barrier function. Since inflammation is detrimental for epithelial barrier integrity (98), it cannot be excluded that the main protective effects of $1,25(OH)_2D$ on the epithelial barrier in the first study by Shi et al. were in fact exerted through inhibition of inflammation rather than via direct induction of cell junction proteins. $1,25(OH)_2D$ might also promote epithelial barrier function through its ability to increase expression of cystic fibrosis transmembrane conductance regulator (CFTR) in airway epithelial cells (32). CFTR maintains optimal ASL- and mucus hydration, volume and pH that support mucociliary clearance and activity of AMPs (99). Moreover, CFTR is also affected in the airways of smokers and COPD patients (100). In summary, these studies indicate that $1,25(OH)_2D$ promotes both the integrity and function of the epithelial barrier and might additionally protect against epithelial damage by dampening inflammatory responses.

Anti-fibrotic Effects of Vitamin D

The loss of epithelial barrier function with a decrease in epithelial polarization and cell-junction proteins and a gain of expression of mesenchymal markers is a hallmark of EMT (94). EMT is primarily involved in development, wound healing and stem cell differentiation, and TGF-β signaling plays a major role in this process (101). Elevated TGF-β1 levels are found in the lungs of patients with chronic inflammatory lung diseases and this was associated with cigarette smoking, inflammation and fibrosis (80, 102). There are indications that $1,25(OH)_2D$ counteracts various pathways leading to EMT. In mouse models and in airway epithelial cell lines, vitamin D supplementation and $1,25(OH)_2D$, respectively, has been shown to inhibit EMT and fibrosis, in particular when this process is induced by TGF-β1 (88, 103–106).

Effects of Vitamin D on Epithelial Antimicrobial Responses

In addition to maintenance of the epithelial barrier and inhibition of fibrosis as discussed in the previous paragraphs, vitamin D is also actively involved in respiratory host defense by a variety of mechanisms (3, 29). $1,25(OH)_2D$ is an important inducer of AMPs, which are mostly cationic peptides that have a broad-spectrum antimicrobial activity, the ability to modulate immune responses and to promote epithelial wound repair and angiogenesis (107). hCAP18/LL-37 is likely to be the most prominent AMP that is induced by $1,25(OH)_2D$ and is expressed in several types of mucosal epithelial cells and immune cells such as monocytes and neutrophils (38, 77, 108). In macrophages and intestinal epithelial cells, $1,25(OH)_2D$ also increases expression of human β-defensin-2 (hBD-2), whereas in keratinocytes expression of both hBD-2 and human β-defensin-3 (hBD-3) is increased by $1,25(OH)_2D$ (109–112). Collectively these data show that AMPs are modulated by $1,25(OH)_2D$ in mucosal tissues, which could have impact on susceptibility to both bacterial and viral infections and on the composition of the microbiota, which will be discussed in the next section.

Effects of Vitamin D on Innate and Adaptive Immune Responses

Diseases such as COPD and asthma are characterized by chronic inflammation, a low-grade and prolonged inflammation that may result in destruction and aberrant repair of surrounding tissue by growth factors, proteases and cytokines that are released at the site of inflammation (113–115). Cumulative data suggest that vitamin D exerts anti-inflammatory effects via its actions on both innate and adaptive immune responses. Upon viral infection or exposure of pro-inflammatory stimuli such as Poly(I:C) or PM, $1,25(OH)_2D$ attenuates induced expression of cytokines and chemokines e.g., via inhibition of nuclear factor (NF)-κB or oxidative stress, respectively, in (airway) epithelial cells (38, 59, 116). Furthermore, $1,25(OH)_2D$ increases expression of the soluble decoy receptor for IL-33 (sST2) by airway epithelial cells, which in turn inhibits the actions of the type 2 alarmin IL-33 (117). Further effects of $1,25(OH)_2D$ on local innate and adaptive immune responses in the epithelial mucosa are mediated through its actions on immune and structural cells and have been reviewed by Heulens et al. (29) Vanherwegen et al. (118), and Pfeffer et al. (119).

Taken together, these findings suggest that on the one hand $1,25(OH)_2D$ protects against infections by enhancing epithelial barrier function and production of AMPs, and on the other hand $1,25(OH)_2D$ induces tolerance and dampens proinflammatory responses in various cell types of the airway mucosa. Thereby, $1,25(OH)_2D$ may prevent exaggerated inflammatory responses and further damage to the mucosal tissue, qualities that are very relevant in the context of chronic inflammatory (lung) diseases (**Figure 2**).

Effects of Vitamin D on Epithelial Oxidative Stress and Aging

COPD is considered to be a disease of accelerated aging lungs, underscored by markers of aging being increased in these patients partly as a result of oxidative stress (120). Evidence that $1,25(OH)_2D$ may protect epithelial cells from oxidative stress was provided by Pfeffer et al. who demonstrated that $1,25(OH)_2D$ increased expression of the antioxidant gene *G6PD* in airway epithelial cells. Furthermore, $1,25(OH)_2D$ increased the ratio of reduced to oxidized glutathione and decreased the formation of 8-isoprostane after exposure to PM (59). The induction of klotho by $1,25(OH)_2D$ might be another $1,25(OH)_2D$-mediated anti-aging mechanism (121). Klotho is an anti-aging protein that is mainly expressed in the kidney, brain and in the lung by airway epithelial cells and exerts its protective effects through the inhibition of inflammation, insulin/IGF-1 signaling and activation of forkhead transcription factor (FoxO) signaling, which enables removal of reactive oxygen species

(ROS) (122–124). Expression of klotho is impaired in the airways of smokers and further decreased in the airways of COPD patients and in cultures of the bronchial epithelial cell line 16HBE after CSE exposure (124). These studies suggest that $1,25(OH)_2D$ may protect against aging via inhibition of oxidative stress and possibly via its ability to restore klotho expression (**Figure 2**). However, direct evidence showing that $1,25(OH)_2D$ indeed increases expression of klotho in airway epithelial cells is currently lacking.

Effects of Vitamin D on Epithelial Autophagy and Apoptosis

In addition to providing protection against oxidative stress and aging, data from studies using intestinal epithelial cells suggest that $1,25(OH)_2D$ may also promote cellular survival via the induction of autophagy and reduction of apoptosis (125, 126). In chronic inflammatory lung diseases, aberrant activation of autophagy plays a role in disease pathogenesis (127). A recent study showed that club cells and autophagy-related proteins were both decreased in COPD patients and that these proteins were important for club cell structure and function in airways (128). However, the effects of $1,25(OH)_2D$ on autophagy in the airway mucosa of chronic inflammatory lung diseases are still unclear and need to be further evaluated (127).

ROLE OF VITAMIN D IN THE TREATMENT OF CHRONIC AIRWAY DISEASES

Clearly vitamin D has pivotal actions in host defense that are relevant in the context of chronic inflammatory lung diseases, in which vitamin D deficiency may be prevalent. Strategies to promote local levels of $1,25(OH)_2D$ or use it as a treatment itself could be therefore of interest. Here, we will discuss the latest clinical evidence accompanied with functional *in vitro* and animal studies that may explain the effects of vitamin D supplementation on typical hallmarks of chronic airway diseases.

Effect of Vitamin D on Inhaled Corticosteroid Responsiveness in Chronic Airway Diseases

Currently, inhaled corticosteroid (ICS)-use with or without long acting bronchodilators is the most frequently used treatment for COPD and asthma patients[1]. However, the response to corticosteroids is not always effective in many COPD patients and in patients with steroid resistant (SR)-asthma (129). There are several complex mechanisms that underlie the resistance to corticosteroids in both COPD and SR-asthma that include but are not limited to genetic background, impaired glucocorticoid receptor binding, T helper type 17 cell (Th17)-inflammation and oxidative stress (e.g., from air pollution or smoking) and decreased numbers of IL-10 secreting regulator T cells (Tregs), which normally prevent skewing toward Th17-inflammation (129). Direct evidence of the ability of $1,25(OH)_2D$ to reverse SR was provided by a study showing that *ex-vivo* stimulation with $1,25(OH)_2D$ promoted generation of IL-10-secreting Tregs which restored sensitivity toward corticosteroids in CD4+ T cells that were derived from SR-asthma patients (130). A further potential treatment role of $1,25(OH)_2D$ was elegantly illustrated by studies that showed that vitamin D deficiency is associated with decreased steroid responsiveness in asthmatics and by the fact that several potential underlying mechanisms of SR such as oxidative stress and Th17-mediated inflammatory responses could be reversed by vitamin D treatment (59, 131–136). Interestingly, the corticosteroid dexamethasone was shown to increase expression of the 25(OH)D and $1,25(OH)_2D$ degrading enzyme CYP24A1 in renal cells and osteoblasts (137), which suggests a bidirectional interaction between corticosteroids and $1,25(OH)_2D$ and could further limit $1,25(OH)_2D$ levels for patients. Additional research is needed to determine if vitamin D may also improve corticosteroid responsiveness in COPD.

[1]https://goldcopd.org (2019).

Vitamin D and Exacerbations in COPD

Exacerbations are a major burden for COPD patients, they accelerate decline in lung function and frequently result into hospital admissions (138, 139). Exacerbations are often triggered by pollutants or by bacterial- and/or viral infections (82, 140, 141). COPD patients generally have lower serum 25(OH)D levels than age- and smoking-matched controls, which is associated with more and more severe exacerbations (8, 10). Several *in vivo* and *in vitro* studies have provided evidence that explain the protective effects of vitamin D on exacerbations in COPD patients and this will be discussed accordingly.

Air Pollution

First of all, Pfeffer et al. showed that 25(OH)D and $1,25(OH)_2D$ reduce the production of proinflammatory cytokines in part via the ability to enhance antioxidant responses in airway epithelial cells that were exposed to PM (59). This was also demonstrated in human DCs that were matured in presence of PM, where treatment with $1,25(OH)_2D$ counteracted the expansion of proinflammatory IL-17A$^+$ and IFN-γ^+ Th17.1 cells (134). In line with this, Bolcas et al., showed that vitamin D supplementation counteracted the development of airway hyperresponsiveness and accumulation of Th2/Th17 cells in mice that had been repeatedly exposed to both diesel exhaust and house dust mite allergens (142). Vitamin D could therefore exert a protective role in air pollution-triggered exacerbations.

Respiratory Viral Infections

In addition to its protective effects against pollutants, there is also increasing evidence that $1,25(OH)_2D$ may enhance clearance of respiratory viral infections that account for 30–50% as underlying cause of exacerbations in COPD patients (143). Infections with respiratory viruses such as HRV, coronaviruses and to a lesser extend respiratory syncytial virus (RSV) and (para)influenza virus are present during exacerbations and may predispose the host toward secondary bacterial infections that can eventually lead to uncontrolled bacterial outgrowth, more severe exacerbations and neutrophilic inflammation (143, 144). Two recent *in vitro* studies showed that acute exposure to relatively high doses (100–1000 nM) of $1,25(OH)_2D$ reduced

HRV-infection in undifferentiated cultures of airway epithelial cells (58, 145). In those models, 1,25(OH)$_2$D most likely interfered with viral replication by increasing expression of interferon-stimulated genes and expression of hCAP18/LL-37, which has been shown to have direct antiviral activity (58, 145, 146). In fully differentiated airway epithelial cells, treatment with lower concentrations of 1,25(OH)$_2$D (10 nM) during epithelial differentiation had no effect on acute HRV infection (147). As for other viruses than HRV, both Hansdottir et al. and Telcian et al. showed that 1,25(OH)$_2$D did not decrease RSV infection in airway epithelial cells, but did reduce virus-induced inflammatory responses (58, 116). In addition, two other studies reported in influenza (H9N2 and H1N1)-infected A549 cells comparable findings (148, 149). Moreover, inhibitory effects of 1,25(OH)$_2$D on poly(I:C)-induced inflammatory responses were furthermore confirmed in primary airway epithelial cells Hansdottir et al. and by our group (38, 85). Up to now, the afore mentioned studies suggest that higher doses of 1,25(OH)$_2$D might be protective against HRV-infections in undifferentiated airway epithelial cells only, whereas for other respiratory viral infections 1,25(OH)$_2$D mainly reduces inflammatory responses without affecting viral clearance. However, more studies are needed, especially in differentiated airway epithelial cells using multiple HRV-serotypes that use different receptors for infection to verify if 1,25(OH)$_2$D indeed is capable of promoting HRV-clearance. There is more consensus about 1,25(OH)$_2$D reducing virus-induced inflammatory responses and this may certainly help to alleviate the burden of exacerbations in COPD (38, 85).

Bacterial Infections

In addition to viral infections, also bacterial infections are associated with COPD exacerbations and account for ~50% of all exacerbations (150). Due to improved study design and sampling techniques from the lower airways using bronchoscopy in recent decades, the causative role of bacteria in COPD-related exacerbations has become clear (150). This was additionally supported by Sethi et al., who found that acquisition of a new strain of pathogenic bacterial species into the airways was linked to COPD exacerbations (151). Recent developments in assessing the airway microbiota using 16S rRNA sequencing techniques further demonstrated that during exacerbations, the relative abundance of Haemophilus, Pseudomonas, and Moraxella was increased and the microbial composition was shifted toward the Proteobacteria phylum (141). The ability of 1,25(OH)$_2$D to promote antibacterial activity was recently demonstrated in cultures of airway epithelial cells. In differentiated airway epithelial cells, we have shown that both 25(OH)D and 1,25(OH)$_2$D treatment enhances epithelial expression of hCAP18/LL-37 and antibacterial activity against NTHi, a Gram-negative bacterium, which is associated with COPD exacerbations (61, 152). In addition, Yim et al. demonstrated that 1,25(OH)$_2$D treatment increased expression of the AMP hCAP18/LL-37 and killing of *Pseudomonas aeruginosa* and *Bordetella bronchiseptica*, which are both Gram-negative bacteria (153). These observed antibacterial effects of 1,25(OH)$_2$D on airway epithelium *in vitro* were recently confirmed *in vivo* by Vargas Buonfiglio et al. The authors demonstrated that vitamin D supplementation increased antimicrobial activity against the Gram-positive *Staphylococcus aureus* in ASL in healthy non-smokers and was dependent on presence of hCAP18/LL-37 (64).

In murine airways, studies showed no effects of 1,25(OH)$_2$D on the expression of *Defb4* or *mCramp* (the murine homolog for *CAMP*) (154). This can be explained by the fact that both the promotors of *mCramp* and *Defb4* lack VDREs, suggesting that mice might not be suitable for studying the role of 1,25(OH)$_2$D in AMP-mediated host defense in infection (155). Indeed, Niederstrasser et al. showed no effects of vitamin D deficiency on the susceptibility of mice to pulmonary infection with *Streptococcus pneumoniae* or *Pseudomonas aeruginosa* (156). However, in a recently developed mouse model by Lowry et al., who transfected *mCramp* knockout mice with the human *CAMP* gene, topical vitamin D$_3$ treatment increased expression of *CAMP* and promoted antibacterial effects on the mucosa of the skin (157). There are also multiple other murine studies that demonstrate protective effects of vitamin D on bacterial infections in the gut, indicating that 1,25(OH)$_2$D -mediated antibacterial effects are additional modulated by other mechanisms such as via enhancement of epithelial barrier integrity (67, 158). In conclusion, these observations show that 1,25(OH)$_2$D promotes protection against pollutants and enhances clearance of viral– and bacterial infections (both Gram-positive and negative bacteria) in combination with a dampening effect on exaggerated immune responses and these features might explain why vitamin D (deficiency) is linked to COPD exacerbations.

Modulation of Microbiota by Vitamin D

There are strong indications that modulation of immune responses and antibacterial activities by 1,25(OH)$_2$D and/or 1,25(OH)$_2$D-regulated AMPs as well as autophagy have implications for the composition of the microbiota at the epithelial mucosa of the airways and the gut (159). Evidence for a role of AMPs in regulating the composition of the microbiota in the gut came from a variety of studies, including those showing that Paneth cell-derived defensins may modulate the composition of the microbiome (160). This notion is further supported by observations showing that many commensal gut bacteria are protected from killing by AMPs such as the 1,25(OH)$_2$D-inducible hCAP18/LL-37 and hBD-2, whereas pathogens are in general more sensitive (161). Alterations in the gut microbiota have been linked to many diseases of the gut such as IBD but also with diseases affecting the lungs such as COPD and asthma, implicating an important role for the so-called gut–lung axis (162, 163). The mechanisms that explain how gut microbiota affect lung health and disease are complex and include the production of short chain fatty acids (SCFAs). SCFA have a wide range of effects on both immune and structural cells, and the effect of SCFA produced in the intestine on lung immunity may in part be explained by modulation of myeloid cells in the bone marrow, which subsequently migrate to the airways and modulate local immune responses (163). Microbiota that are diverse, rich and contain a higher abundance of SCFA-producing species within these populations are considered to be associated with health (164). In the gut there is strong evidence that both vitamin D deficiency and/or supplementation affect composition of the adult and infant microbiota (164, 165), specifically in relation to disease (166). However, due to the limited number of RCTs and small sample sizes, the precise effects on the microbiota and the mechanisms involved in this are still unclear (164). Alterations in the lung microbiota are also observed in COPD and asthma patients and are likely the result of environmental exposures, airway remodeling, infections and treatments such as the use of antibiotics. This may contribute to disease pathogenesis through altered epithelial innate and adaptive immune responses that damages the airway epithelial barrier and provokes further changes in the lung microbiome that accumulates with increasing disease severity (167, 168). To date only 2 studies describe a possible influence of vitamin D on composition of the microbiota in the airways (169, 170). Toivonen et al. showed an association between low serum 25(OH)D levels and reduced richness of the nasopharyngeal microbiota and bronchiolitis severity in patients with low 25(OH)D levels (169), whereas in another study vitamin D supplementation decreased the abundance of *Staphylococcus aureus*, *Staphylococcus epidermidis* and Corynebacterium species in sputum samples in vitamin D-deficient CF patients compared to sufficient CF patients (170). In summary, there is evidence that alterations in the airway or gut microbiota can affect chronic airway disease and that these changes could be related to both vitamin D deficiency and/or supplementation. However, due to the limited number of RCTs and small sample sizes more RCTs are needed in larger patient populations.

Effect of Vitamin D Supplementation on Chronic Airway Diseases

COPD

The above described protective and therapeutic possibilities of vitamin D, together with observations that many COPD patients are vitamin D deficient, suggest that COPD patients might benefit from vitamin D supplementation. As discussed elsewhere in this review, the link between circulating 25(OH)D levels and the number of exacerbations has been extensively studied (8). So far however, only 4 RCTs have investigated the effect of vitamin D supplementation in the context of COPD: only 2 out of 4 RCTs showed that vitamin D supplementation reduces the number of exacerbations (171–174). However, in a *post-hoc* analysis, selecting those patients that were vitamin D deficient, exacerbations were indeed reduced after vitamin D supplementation. Jolliffe et al. summarized these 4 RCTs and performed a recent individual participant data meta-analysis and concluded that vitamin D supplementation is only protective against exacerbations in COPD patients with baseline serum 25(OH)D levels < 25 nmol/L (175). These important findings suggest that exacerbations in this specific subset of COPD patients are connected to vitamin D deficiency and this part can be resolved with supplementation. In summary, the protective effects of vitamin D in patients suffering from COPD are most prominent in those with vitamin D deficiency and this would indicate that serum levels 25(OH)D in these patients should always be determined before considering using vitamin D supplementation. Since only 4 RCTs with relatively small patient populations have been conducted in both vitamin D-sufficient and -deficient COPD patients, more RCTs are needed, especially in vitamin D-deficient patients. Currently, a multicenter RCT is being conducted by Rafiq et al. in a group of vitamin-deficient COPD patients (25(OH)D < 50 nmol/L), which may reveal whether vitamin D supplementation is indeed protective against exacerbations in this group (176).

Vitamin D Supplementation in Asthma, Cystic Fibrosis and Acute Respiratory Tract Infections

In addition to the effects of vitamin D supplementation in COPD patients, the effects of vitamin D supplementation has also been extensively investigated in other lung diseases (which have associations with vitamin D deficiency) such as asthma, cystic fibrosis, upper respiratory tract infections. Most RCTs that investigated the effects of vitamin D supplementation were performed in acute respiratory tract infections (ARTIs) and asthma. A recent meta-analysis that assessed the effects of vitamin D supplementation in 25 RCTs (11,321 participants) showed that indeed vitamin D supplementation was protective against ATRIs and this effect was again more profound in patients with vitamin D deficiency 25(OH)D < 25 nmol/L at baseline (177). A recent meta-analysis in asthma that included a total of 14 randomized controlled trials (1,421 participants), indicated that vitamin D supplementation reduced the rate of asthma exacerbations and increased lung function, especially in patients with vitamin D insufficiency (25(OH)D < 75 nmol/L) (178). Interestingly, in asthma patients that were supplemented with vitamin D, the frequency of respiratory infections was reduced, and this effect was related to the increase of hCAP18/LL-37 (179). CF patients with vitamin D deficiency had a higher rate of exacerbations as compared to patients with sufficient 25(OH)D levels (180). However, only one recent multicenter RCT was conducted and indicated that vitamin D supplementation did not affect the number of exacerbations in CF patients with serum 25(OH)D concentrations between 25 and 137.5 nmol/L (181). In summary, the protective effects of vitamin D supplementation in patients suffering from COPD, asthma or ARTIs are most prominent in those with vitamin D deficiency and this would indicate the importance of establishing serum levels 25(OH)D in these patients as supplementation could reduce unnecessary aggravated disease pathology as a result of this deficiency.

CONCLUSION AND PERSPECTIVES

Many drivers of COPD pathogenesis such as chronic exposure to noxious particles and gases, which are present in CS and air pollution, proteolytic enzymes, cytokines and chemokines that are released by infiltrating inflammatory cells, are known to harm the epithelial barrier and cause aberrant remodeling of the airway epithelium with important functional consequences for e.g., host defense. A dysfunctional epithelial barrier increases the susceptibility toward bacterial and viral infections, which are important triggers of COPD exacerbations and these exacerbations contribute importantly to disease progression. Sufficient local levels of 1,25(OH)$_2$D may provide partial protection against these effects by reducing the effects of oxidative stress induced by exposure to inhaled oxidants or those derived from recruited inflammatory cells. 1,25(OH)$_2$D furthermore protects against impairment of epithelial barrier function by promoting the integrity of the epithelial barrier, and by modulating both innate and adaptive immune responses. Protection against the detrimental effects of both bacterial and viral infections is provided by the ability of 1,25(OH)$_2$D to promote of antiviral responses, induce expression of AMPs and modulate of inflammatory responses. Taken together, these activities suggest that 1,25(OH)$_2$D may provide protection against development and progression of COPD, and against disease exacerbations.

In addition, the local inflammatory milieu as well as the chronic exposure to noxious particles and gases, which are present in CS and air pollution, may negatively affect synthesis and signaling of 1,25(OH)$_2$D. Here we discussed recent *in vitro* studies that demonstrated that disease-associated factors such as inflammation and exposure to CS and air pollution could interfere with 1,25(OH)$_2$D signaling and its degradation and activation by affecting expression of VDR, CYP24A1 and CYP27B1, respectively. These findings indicate that 1,25(OH)$_2$D levels and its activities on airway mucosa might be impaired especially in patients with COPD with exposures to cigarette smoke and cytokines such as TNF-α, IL-1β, IL-17A and TGF-β1. This suggests that even in patients with sufficient 25(OH)D serum levels the local activity of 1,25(OH)$_2$D in the lungs can be improved. We have to start generating more information on both systemic and local 1,25(OH)$_2$D levels and gene expression signatures related to 25(OH)D and 1,25(OH)$_2$D metabolism or responses in COPD (and other chronic inflammatory diseases that are related to vitamin D deficiency), both at baseline and after vitamin D supplementation. This information could lead to improved treatment strategies that enhance local efficacy of 1,25(OH)$_2$D, using e.g., specific CYP24A1-inhibitors such as VID400 (182). Alternatively, degradation by CYP24A1 could be prevented by using 1,25(OH)$_2$D analogs that are insensitive to CYP24A1-mediated degradation, such as sulfone and sulfoximine derivatives, that also act as a VDR agonist (183). A third option is to entail the use of combination treatment with vitamin D and anti-inflammatory or certain anti-fibrotic drugs that target cytokines/proteins that are known to potentially decrease local levels and signaling of 1,25(OH)$_2$D by inducing expression of CYP24A1 (48, 184, 185). When considering such strategies, it should be noted that these may enhance the calcemic side effects and lead to unwanted inhibition of the immune system. We therefore need to carefully analyze the preclinical *in vivo* and *in vitro* studies and balance the pros and cons of the different strategies. In conclusion, future studies in COPD and but also in other chronic inflammatory diseases that are related to vitamin D deficiency, should be designed with more focus on assessing and improving local levels of 1,25(OH)$_2$D. These new insights may lead to the development of new treatment strategies, such as those targeting CYP24A1 to enhance local 1,25(OH)$_2$D resulting in improved homeostasis and protection of the airway mucosa in patients with chronic inflammatory lung diseases.

AUTHOR CONTRIBUTIONS

JS, AD, and PH: Conception and design. JS: Analyzing literature and drafting the manuscript. AD and PH: Revision of the manuscript. All authors: reviewed the manuscript and agree with its submission.

REFERENCES

1. Bouillon R, Carmeliet G, Verlinden L, van Etten E, Verstuyf A, Luderer HF, et al. Vitamin D and human health: lessons from vitamin D receptor null mice. *Endocr. Rev.* (2008) 29:726–76. doi: 10.1210/er.2008-0004
2. Wang TT, Tavera-Mendoza LE, Laperriere D, Libby E, Burton MacLeod N, Nagai Y, et al. Large-scale *in silico* and microarray-based identification of direct 1,25-dihydroxyvitamin D3 target genes. *Mol Endocrinol.* (2005) 19:2685–95. doi: 10.1210/me.2005-0106
3. Christakos S, Dhawan P, Verstuyf A, Verlinden L, Carmeliet G. Vitamin D: metabolism, molecular mechanism of action, pleiotropic effects. *Physiol Rev.* (2016) 96:365–408. doi: 10.1152/physrev.00014.2015
4. Smith JE, Goodman DS. The turnover and transport of vitamin D and of a polar metabolite with the properties of 25-hydroxycholecalciferol in human plasma. *J Clin Invest.* (1971) 50:2159–67. doi: 10.1172/JCI106710
5. Holick MF, Binkley NC, Bischoff-Ferrari HA, Gordon CM, Hanley DA, Heaney RP, et al. Treatment, and prevention of Vitamin D deficiency: an endocrine society clinical practice guideline. *J Clin Endocrinol Metab.* (2011) 96:1911–30. doi: 10.1210/jc.2011-0385
6. Holick MF. The vitamin D deficiency pandemic: approaches for diagnosis, treatment and prevention. *Rev Endocr Metab Disord.* (2017) 18:153–65. doi: 10.1007/s11154-017-9424-1
7. Herr C, Greulich T, Koczulla RA, Meyer S, Zakharkina T, Branscheidt M, et al. The role of vitamin D in pulmonary disease: COPD, asthma, infection, and cancer. *Respir Res.* (2011) 12:31. doi: 10.1186/1465-9921-12-31
8. Zhu M, Wang T, Wang C, Ji Y. The association between vitamin D and COPD risk, severity, and exacerbation: an updated systematic review and meta-analysis. *Int J Chronic Obstr Pulm Dis.* (2016) 11:2597–607. doi: 10.2147/COPD.S101382
9. Brehm JM. Vitamin D and asthma—life after VIDA? *Curr Allergy Asthma Rep.* (2014) 14:461. doi: 10.1007/s11882-014-0461-5
10. Janssens W, Bouillon R, Claes B, Carremans C, Lehouck A, Buysschaert I, et al. Vitamin D deficiency is highly prevalent in COPD and correlates with variants in the vitamin D-binding gene. *Thorax.* (2010) 65:215–20. doi: 10.1136/thx.2009.120659
11. Persson LJ, Aanerud M, Hiemstra PS, Hardie JA, Bakke PS, Eagan TM. Chronic obstructive pulmonary disease is associated with low levels of vitamin D. *PLoS ONE.* (2012) 7:e38934. doi: 10.1371/journal.pone.0038934
12. Burkes RM, Ceppe AS, Doerschuk CM, Couper D, Hoffman EA, Comellas AP, et al. Associations between 25-hydroxy-vitamin D levels, lung function, and exacerbation outcomes in COPD: an analysis of the SPIROMICS cohort. *Chest.* (2020) 157:856–65. doi: 10.1016/j.chest.2019.11.047
13. Kokturk N, Baha A, Oh YM, Young Ju J, Jones PW. Vitamin D deficiency: what does it mean for chronic obstructive pulmonary disease (COPD)? A

compherensive review for pulmonologists. *Clin Respir J.* (2018) 12:382–97. doi: 10.1111/crj.12588
14. Persson LJ, Aanerud M, Hiemstra PS, Michelsen AE, Ueland T, Hardie JA, et al. Vitamin D, vitamin D binding protein, and longitudinal outcomes in COPD. *PLoS ONE.* (2015) 10:e0121622. doi: 10.1371/journal.pone.0121622
15. Zosky GR, Berry LJ, Elliot JG, James AL, Gorman S, Hart PH. Vitamin D deficiency causes deficits in lung function and alters lung structure. *Am J Respir Crit Care Med.* (2011) 183:1336–43. doi: 10.1164/rccm.201010-1596OC
16. Bui DS, Burgess JA, Lowe AJ, Perret JL, Lodge CJ, Bui M, et al. Childhood lung function predicts adult chronic obstructive pulmonary disease and asthma-chronic obstructive pulmonary disease overlap syndrome. *Am J Respir Crit Care Med.* (2017) 196:39–46. doi: 10.1164/rccm.201606-1272OC
17. Wolsk HM, Chawes BL, Litonjua AA, Hollis BW, Waage J, Stokholm J, et al. Prenatal vitamin D supplementation reduces risk of asthma/recurrent wheeze in early childhood: a combined analysis of two randomized controlled trials. *PLoS ONE.* (2017) 12:e0186657. doi: 10.1371/journal.pone.0186657
18. Kho AT, Sharma S, Qiu W, Gaedigk R, Klanderman B, Niu S, et al. Vitamin D related genes in lung development and asthma pathogenesis. *BMC Med Genomics.* (2013) 6:47. doi: 10.1186/1755-8794-6-47
19. Kelly RS, Chawes BL, Guo F, Zhang L, Blighe K, Litonjua AA, et al. The role of the 17q21 genotype in the prevention of early childhood asthma and recurrent wheeze by vitamin D. *Eur Respir J.* (2019) 54:1900761. doi: 10.1183/13993003.00761-2019
20. Sordillo JE, Zhou Y, McGeachie MJ, Ziniti J, Lange N, Laranjo N, et al. Factors influencing the infant gut microbiome at age 3-6 months: findings from the ethnically diverse Vitamin D Antenatal Asthma Reduction Trial (VDAART). *J Allergy Clin Immunol.* (2017) 139:482–91.e14. doi: 10.1016/j.jaci.2016.08.045
21. Heulens N, Korf H, Cielen N, De Smidt E, Maes K, Gysemans C, et al. Vitamin D deficiency exacerbates COPD-like characteristics in the lungs of cigarette smoke-exposed mice. *Respir Res.* (2015) 16:110. doi: 10.1186/s12931-015-0271-x
22. Horiguchi M, Hirokawa M, Abe K, Kumagai H, Yamashita C. Pulmonary administration of 1,25-dihydroxyvitamin D3 to the lungs induces alveolar regeneration in a mouse model of chronic obstructive pulmonary disease. *J Control Release.* (2016) 233:191–7. doi: 10.1016/j.jconrel.2016.05.006
23. Limketkai BN, Mullin GE, Limsui D, Parian AM. Role of Vitamin D in inflammatory bowel disease. *Nutr Clin Pract.* (2017) 32:337–45. doi: 10.1177/0884533616674492
24. Jolliffe DA, Greenberg L, Hooper RL, Griffiths CJ, Camargo CA, Kerley CP, et al. Vitamin D supplementation to prevent asthma exacerbations: a systematic review and meta-analysis of individual participant data. *Lancet RespirMed.* (2017) 5:881–90. doi: 10.1016/S2213-2600(17)30306-5
25. V. De Rose, Molloy K, Gohy S, Pilette C, Greene CM. Airway epithelium dysfunction in cystic fibrosis and COPD. *Med Inflam.* (2018) 2018:20. doi: 10.1155/2018/1309746
26. Martini E, Krug SM, Siegmund B, Neurath MF, Becker C. Mend your fences: the epithelial barrier and its relationship with mucosal immunity in inflammatory bowel disease. *Cell Mol Gastroenterol Hepatol.* (2017) 4:33–46. doi: 10.1016/j.jcmgh.2017.03.007
27. Heijink IH, Nawijn MC, Hackett TL. Airway epithelial barrier function regulates the pathogenesis of allergic asthma. *Clin Exp Allergy.* (2014) 44:620–30. doi: 10.1111/cea.12296
28. Colotta F, Jansson B, Bonelli F. Modulation of inflammatory and immune responses by vitamin D. *J Autoimmun.* (2017) 85:78–97. doi: 10.1016/j.jaut.2017.07.007
29. Heulens N, Korf H, Janssens W. Innate immune modulation in chronic obstructive pulmonary disease: moving closer toward vitamin D therapy. *J Pharmacol Exp Ther.* (2015) 353:360–8. doi: 10.1124/jpet.115.223032
30. Reboul E. Intestinal absorption of vitamin D: from the meal to the enterocyte. *Food Func.* (2015) 6:356–62. doi: 10.1039/C4FO00579A
31. Holick MF. The cutaneous photosynthesis of previtamin D3: a unique photoendocrine system. *J Invest Dermatol.* (1981) 77:51–8. doi: 10.1111/1523-1747.ep12479237
32. DiFranco KM, Mulligan JK, Sumal AS, Diamond G. Induction of CFTR gene expression by 1,25(OH)2 vitamin D3, 25OH vitamin D3, and vitamin D3 in cultured human airway epithelial cells and in mouse airways. *J Steroid Biochem Mol Biol.* (2017) 173:323–32. doi: 10.1016/j.jsbmb.2017.01.013
33. Vantieghem K, Overbergh L, Carmeliet G, De Haes P, Bouillon R, Segaert S. UVB-induced 1,25(OH)2D3 production and vitamin D activity in intestinal CaCo-2 cells and in THP-1 macrophages pretreated with a sterol Delta7-reductase inhibitor. *J Cell Biochem.* (2006) 99:229–40. doi: 10.1002/jcb.20910
34. Adams JS, Clemens TL, Parrish JA, M.F. Holick Vitamin-D synthesis and metabolism after ultraviolet irradiation of normal and vitamin-D-deficient subjects. *N Engl J Med.* (1982) 306:722–5. doi: 10.1056/NEJM198203253061206
35. Stoffels K, Overbergh L, Giulietti A, Verlinden L, Bouillon R, Mathieu C. Immune regulation of 25-hydroxyvitamin-D3-1α-hydroxylase in human monocytes. *J Bone Min Res.* (2006) 21:37–47. doi: 10.1359/JBMR.0 50908
36. Zehnder D, Bland R, Williams MC, McNinch RW, Howie AJ, Stewart PM, et al. Extrarenal expression of 25-hydroxyvitamin D3-1α-hydroxylase1. *J Clin Endocrinol Metab.* (2001) 86:888–94. doi: 10.1210/jcem.8 6.2.7220
37. Cross HS, Kállay E, Khorchide M, Lechner D. Regulation of extrarenal synthesis of 1,25-dihydroxyvitamin D3—-relevance for colonic cancer prevention and therapy. *Mol Aspects Med.* (2003) 24:459–65. doi: 10.1016/S0098-2997(03)00041-4
38. Hansdottir S, Monick MM, Hinde SL, Lovan N, Look DC, Hunninghake GW. Respiratory epithelial cells convert inactive vitamin D to its active form: potential effects on host defense. *J Immunol.* (2008) 181:7090–9. doi: 10.4049/jimmunol.181.10.7090
39. Edfeldt K, Liu PT, Chun R, Fabri M, Schenk M, Wheelwright M, et al. T-cell cytokines differentially control human monocyte antimicrobial responses by regulating vitamin D metabolism. *Proc Natl Acad Sci USA.* (2010) 107:22593–8. doi: 10.1073/pnas.1011624108
40. Pillai S, Bikle DD, Elias PM. 1, 25-dihydroxyvitamin D production and receptor binding in human keratinocytes varies with differentiation. *J Biol Chem.* (1988) 263:5390–5.
41. Wang Y, Zhu J, DeLuca HF. Where is the vitamin D receptor? *Arch Biochem Biophys.* (2012) 523:123–33. doi: 10.1016/j.abb.2012.04.001
42. Boland RL. VDR activation of intracellular signaling pathways in skeletal muscle. *Mol Cell Endocrinol.* (2011) 347:11–6. doi: 10.1016/j.mce.2011.05.021
43. O'Connell TD, Simpson RU. Immunochemical identification of the 1,25-dihydroxyvitamin D3 receptor protein in human heart. *Cell Biol Int.* (1996) 20:621–4. doi: 10.1006/cbir.1996.0081
44. Chen S, Glenn DJ, Ni W, Grigsby CL, Olsen K, Nishimoto M, et al. Expression of the Vitamin D receptor is increased in the hypertrophic heart. *Hypertension.* (2008) 52:1106–12. doi: 10.1161/HYPERTENSIONAHA.108.119602
45. Gascon-Barré M, Demers C, Mirshahi A, Néron S, Zalzal S, Nanci A. The normal liver harbors the vitamin D nuclear receptor in nonparenchymal and biliary epithelial cells. *Hepatology.* (2003) 37:1034–42. doi: 10.1053/jhep.2003.50176
46. Saccone D, Asani F, Bornman L. Regulation of the vitamin D receptor gene by environment, genetics and epigenetics. *Gene.* (2015) 561:171–80. doi: 10.1016/j.gene.2015.02.024
47. Lee SM, Meyer MB, Benkusky NA, O'Brien CA, Pike JW. The impact of VDR expression and regulation *in vivo*. *J Steroid Biochem Mol Biol.* (2017) 177:36–45. doi: 10.1016/j.jsbmb.2017.06.002
48. Solomon JD, Heitzer MD, Liu TT, Beumer JH, Parise RA, Normolle DP, et al. VDR activity is differentially affected by Hic-5 in prostate cancer and stromal cells. *Mol Cancer Res.* (2014) 12:1166–80. doi: 10.1158/1541-7786.MCR-13-0395
49. Makishima M, Lu TT, Xie W, Whitfield GK, Domoto H, Evans RM, et al. Vitamin D receptor as an intestinal bile acid sensor. *Science.* (2002) 296:1313–6. doi: 10.1126/science.1070477
50. Jones G, Prosser DE, Kaufmann M. 25-Hydroxyvitamin D-24-hydroxylase (CYP24A1): Its important role in the degradation of vitamin D. *Arch Biochem Biophys.* (2012) 523:9–18. doi: 10.1016/j.abb.2011.11.003
51. Wang Z, Schuetz EG, Xu Y, Thummel KE. Interplay between vitamin D and the drug metabolizing enzyme CYP3A4. *J Steroid Biochem Mol Biol.* (2013) 136:54–8. doi: 10.1016/j.jsbmb.2012.09.012
52. Sakaki T, Sawada N, Komai K, Shiozawa S, Yamada S, Yamamoto K, et al. Dual metabolic pathway of 25-hydroxyvitamin D3 catalyzed by human CYP24. *Eur J Biochem.* (2000) 267:6158–65. doi: 10.1046/j.1432-1327.2000.01680.x

53. Jones G, Strugnell SA, DeLuca HF. Current understanding of the molecular actions of vitamin D. *Physiol Rev.* (1998) 78:1193–231. doi: 10.1152/physrev.1998.78.4.1193
54. Veldurthy V, Wei R, Campbell M, Lupicki K, Dhawan P, Christakos S. Chapter six - 25-Hydroxyvitamin D3 24-Hydroxylase: a key regulator of 1,25(OH)2D3 catabolism and calcium homeostasis. In Litwack G, editor, *Vitamins & Hormones*, (Academic Press) (2016). p. 137–150. doi: 10.1016/bs.vh.2015.10.005
55. Ishizuka S, Norman AW. Metabolic pathways from 1 alpha,25-dihydroxyvitamin D3 to 1 alpha,25-dihydroxyvitamin D3-26,23-lactone. Stereo-retained and stereo-selective lactonization. *J Biol Chem.* (1987) 262:7165–70.
56. Zimmerman DR, Reinhardt TA, Kremer R, Beitz DC, Reddy GS, Horst RL. Calcitroic acid is a major catabolic metabolite in the metabolism of 1α-dihydroxyvitamin D2. *Arch Biochem Biophys.* (2001) 392:14–22. doi: 10.1006/abbi.2001.2419
57. Quarles LD. Endocrine functions of bone in mineral metabolism regulation. *J Clin Invest.* (2008) 118:3820–28. doi: 10.1172/JCI36479
58. Telcian AG, Zdrenghea MT, Edwards MR, Laza-Stanca V, Mallia P, Johnston SL, et al. Vitamin D increases the antiviral activity of bronchial epithelial cells *in vitro*. *Antiviral Res.* (2017) 137:93–101. doi: 10.1016/j.antiviral.2016.11.004
59. Pfeffer PE, Lu H, Mann EH, Chen Y-H, Ho T-R, Cousins DJ, et al. Effects of vitamin D on inflammatory and oxidative stress responses of human bronchial epithelial cells exposed to particulate matter. *PLoS ONE.* (2018) 13:e0200040. doi: 10.1371/journal.pone.0200040
60. Wang J, Liu X, Wang H, Li Y, Lan N, Yuan X, et al. Allergen specific immunotherapy enhanced defense against bacteria via TGF-β1-induced CYP27B1 in asthma. *Oncotarget.* (2017) 8:68681–95. doi: 10.18632/oncotarget.19826
61. Schrumpf JA, Amatngalim GD, Veldkamp JB, Verhoosel RM, Ninaber DK, Ordonez SR, et al. Proinflammatory cytokines impair vitamin D–induced host defense in cultured airway epithelial cells. *Am. J. Resp. Cell Mol Biol.* (2017) 56:749–61. doi: 10.1165/rcmb.2016-0289OC
62. Schrumpf JA, Ninaber DK, A.M. van der Does, Hiemstra PS. TGF-beta1 impairs vitamin D-induced and constitutive airway epithelial host defense mechanisms. *J Innate Immun.* (2020) 12:74–89. doi: 10.1159/000497415
63. Mulligan JK, Nagel W, O'Connell BP, Wentzel J, Atkinson C, Schlosser RJ. Cigarette smoke exposure is associated with vitamin D3 deficiencies in patients with chronic rhinosinusitis. *J Allergy Clin Immunol.* (2014) 134:342–9.e1. doi: 10.1016/j.jaci.2014.01.039
64. Vargas Buonfiglio LG, Cano M, Pezzulo AA, Vanegas Calderon OG, Zabner J, Gerke AK, et al. Effect of vitamin D(3) on the antimicrobial activity of human airway surface liquid: preliminary results of a randomised placebo-controlled double-blind trial. *BMJ Open Respir Res.* (2017) 4:e000211. doi: 10.1136/bmjresp-2017-000211
65. Coughlan CA, Chotirmall SH, Renwick J, Hassan T, Low TB, Bergsson G, et al. The effect of aspergillus fumigatus infection on vitamin D receptor expression in cystic fibrosis. *Am J Respir Crit Care Med.* (2012) 186:999–1007. doi: 10.1164/rccm.201203-0478OC
66. Uh ST, Koo SM, Kim YK, Kim KU, Park SW, Jang AS, et al. Inhibition of vitamin d receptor translocation by cigarette smoking extracts. *Tubercul. Respir Dis.* (2012) 73:258–65. doi: 10.4046/trd.2012.73.5.258
67. Du J, Wei X, Ge X, Chen Y, Li YC. Microbiota-dependent induction of colonic Cyp27b1 Is associated with colonic inflammation: implications of locally produced 1,25-dihydroxyvitamin D3 in inflammatory regulation in the colon. *Endocrinology.* (2017) 158:4064. doi: 10.1210/en.2017-00578
68. Bakke D, Sun J. Ancient nuclear receptor VDR with new functions: microbiome and inflammation. *Inflam Bowel Dis.* (2018) 24:1149–54. doi: 10.1093/ibd/izy092
69. Hummel DM, Fetahu IS, Gröschel C, Manhardt T, Kállay E. Role of proinflammatory cytokines on expression of vitamin D metabolism and target genes in colon cancer cells. *J Steroid Biochem Mol Biol.* (2014) 144:91–5. doi: 10.1016/j.jsbmb.2013.09.017
70. Noyola-Martínez N, Díaz L, Zaga-Clavellina V, Avila E, Halhali A, Larrea F, et al. Regulation of CYP27B1 and CYP24A1 gene expression by recombinant pro-inflammatory cytokines in cultured human trophoblasts. *J Steroid Biochem Mol Biol.* (2014) 144:106–9. doi: 10.1016/j.jsbmb.2013.12.007
71. Campbell GR, Spector SA. Toll-like receptor 8 ligands activate a vitamin D mediated autophagic response that inhibits human immunodeficiency virus type 1. *PLoS Pathog.* (2012) 8:e1003017. doi: 10.1371/journal.ppat.1003017
72. Heulens N, Korf H, Mathyssen C, Everaerts S, De Smidt E, Dooms C, et al. 1,25-dihydroxyvitamin D modulates antibacterial and inflammatory response in human cigarette smoke-exposed macrophages. *PLoS ONE.* (2016) 11:e0160482. doi: 10.1371/journal.pone.0160482
73. Matsunawa M, Amano Y, Endo K, Uno S, Sakaki T, Yamada S, et al. The aryl hydrocarbon receptor activator benzo[a]pyrene enhances vitamin d3 catabolism in macrophages. *Toxicolog Sci.* (2009) 109:50–8. doi: 10.1093/toxsci/kfp044
74. Liu PT, Stenger S, Li H, Wenzel L, Tan BH, Krutzik SR, et al. Toll-Like receptor triggering of a vitamin d-mediated human antimicrobial response. *Science.* (2006) 311:1770–3. doi: 10.1126/science.1123933
75. Adams JS, Ren S, Liu PT, Chun RF, Lagishetty V, Gombart AF, et al. Vitamin d-directed rheostatic regulation of monocyte antibacterial responses. *J Immunol.* (2009) 182:4289–95. doi: 10.4049/jimmunol.0803736
76. Krutzik SR, Hewison M, Liu PT, Robles JA, Stenger S, Adams JS, et al. IL-15 links TLR2/1-induced macrophage differentiation to the vitamin D-dependent antimicrobial pathway. *J Immunol.* (2008) 181:7115–20. doi: 10.4049/jimmunol.181.10.7115
77. Subramanian K, Bergman P, Henriques-Normark B. Vitamin D promotes pneumococcal killing and modulates inflammatory responses in primary human neutrophils. *J Innate Immun.* (2017) 9:375–386. doi: 10.1159/000455969
78. Baeke F, Korf H, Overbergh L, van Etten E, Verstuyf A, Gysemans C, et al. Human T lymphocytes are direct targets of 1,25-dihydroxyvitamin D3 in the immune system. *J Steroid Biochem Mol Biol.* (2010) 121:221–7. doi: 10.1016/j.jsbmb.2010.03.037
79. Chen S, Sims GP, Chen XX, Gu YY, Chen S, Lipsky PE. Modulatory effects of 1,25-Dihydroxyvitamin D^3 on human B cell differentiation. *J Immunol.* (2007) 179:1634–47. doi: 10.4049/jimmunol.179.3.1634
80. Thomas BJ, Kan-o K, Loveland KL, Elias JA, Bardin PG. In the shadow of fibrosis: innate immune suppression mediated by transforming growth factor-β. *Am. J. Resp. Cell Mol. Biol.* (2016) 55:759–66. doi: 10.1165/rcmb.2016-0248PS
81. Barnes PJ. Targeting cytokines to treat asthma and chronic obstructive pulmonary disease. *Nat Rev Immunol.* (2018) 18:454–66. doi: 10.1038/s41577-018-0006-6
82. Wedzicha JA, Seemungal TAR. COPD exacerbations: defining their cause and prevention. *Lancet.* (2007) 370:786–96. doi: 10.1016/S0140-6736(07)61382-8
83. Loxham M, Davies DE. Phenotypic and genetic aspects of epithelial barrier function in asthmatic patients. *J Allergy Clin Immunol.* (2017) 139:1736–51. doi: 10.1016/j.jaci.2017.04.005
84. Skolnik K, Quon BS. Recent advances in the understanding and management of cystic fibrosis pulmonary exacerbations. *F1000Res.* (2018) 7:F1000 Faculty Rev—575. doi: 10.12688/f1000research.13926.1
85. Schrumpf JA, van Sterkenburg MA, Verhoosel RM, Zuyderduyn S, Hiemstra PS. Interleukin 13 exposure enhances vitamin D-mediated expression of the human cathelicidin antimicrobial peptide 18/LL-37 in bronchial epithelial cells. *Infect Immun.* (2012) 80:4485–94. doi: 10.1128/IAI.06224-11
86. Liu MC, Xiao HQ, Brown AJ, Ritter CS, Schroeder J. Association of vitamin D and antimicrobial peptide production during late-phase allergic responses in the lung. *Clin Exp Allergy.* (2012) 42:383–91. doi: 10.1111/j.1365-2222.2011.03879.x
87. Barrea L, Savastano S, Di Somma C, Savanelli MC, Nappi F, Albanese L, et al. Low serum vitamin D-status, air pollution and obesity: a dangerous liaison. *Rev Endocr Metab Disord.* (2017) 18:207–14. doi: 10.1007/s11154-016-9388-6
88. Tzilas V, Bouros E, Barbayianni I, Karampitsakos T, Kourtidou S, Ntassiou M, et al. Vitamin D prevents experimental lung fibrosis and predicts survival in patients with idiopathic pulmonary fibrosis. *Pulm Pharmacol Ther.* (2019) 55:17–24. doi: 10.1016/j.pupt.2019.01.003
89. Schlosser RJ, Carroll WW, Soler ZM, Pasquini WN, Mulligan JK. Reduced sinonasal levels of 1alpha-hydroxylase are associated with worse quality of

life in chronic rhinosinusitis with nasal polyps. *Int Forum Allergy Rhinol.* (2016) 6:58–65. doi: 10.1002/alr.21576

90. Souberbielle JC, Body JJ, Lappe JM, Plebani M, Shoenfeld Y, Wang TJ, et al. Vitamin D and musculoskeletal health, cardiovascular disease, autoimmunity and cancer: recommendations for clinical practice. *Autoimmun Rev.* (2010) 9:709–15. doi: 10.1016/j.autrev.2010.06.009
91. DeLuca GC, Kimball SM, Kolasinski J, Ramagopalan SV, Ebers GC. Review: The role of vitamin D in nervous system health and disease. *Neuropathol Appl Neurobiol.* (2013) 39:458–84. doi: 10.1111/nan.12020
92. Dankers W, Colin EM, van Hamburg JP, Lubberts E. Vitamin D in autoimmunity: molecular mechanisms and therapeutic potential. *Front Immunol.* (2017) 7:697. doi: 10.3389/fimmu.2016.00697
93. Berridge MJ. Vitamin D cell signalling in health and disease. *Biochem Biophys Res Commun.* (2015) 460:53–71. doi: 10.1016/j.bbrc.2015.01.008
94. Aghapour M, Raee P, Moghaddam SJ, Hiemstra PS, Heijink IH. Airway epithelial barrier dysfunction in chronic obstructive pulmonary disease: role of cigarette smoke exposure. *Am J RespirCell Mol Biol.* (2018) 58:157–69. doi: 10.1165/rcmb.2017-0200TR
95. Zhang R, Zhao H, Dong H, Zou F, Cai S. 1α,25-Dihydroxyvitamin D3 counteracts the effects of cigarette smoke in airway epithelial cells. *Cell Immunol.* (2015) 295:137–43. doi: 10.1016/j.cellimm.2015.03.004
96. Shi YY, Liu TJ, Fu JH, Xu W, Wu LL, Hou AN, et al. Vitamin D/VDR signaling attenuates lipopolysaccharide-induced acute lung injury by maintaining the integrity of the pulmonary epithelial barrier. *Mol Med Rep.* (2016) 13:1186–94. doi: 10.3892/mmr.2015.4685
97. Gorman S, Buckley AG, Ling K-M, Berry LJ, Fear VS, Stick SM, et al. Vitamin D supplementation of initially vitamin D-deficient mice diminishes lung inflammation with limited effects on pulmonary epithelial integrity. *Physiol Rep.* (2017) 5:e13371. doi: 10.14814/phy2.13371
98. Luissint AC, Parkos CA, Nusrat A. Inflammation and the intestinal barrier: leukocyte-epithelial cell interactions, cell junction remodeling, mucosal repair. *Gastroenterology.* (2016) 151:616–32. doi: 10.1053/j.gastro.2016.07.008
99. Pezzulo AA, Tang XX, Hoegger MJ, Abou Alaiwa MH, Ramachandran S, Moninger TO, et al. Reduced airway surface pH impairs bacterial killing in the porcine cystic fibrosis lung. *Nature.* (2012) 487:109–13. doi: 10.1038/nature11130
100. Rab A, Rowe SM, Raju SV, Bebok Z, Matalon S, Collawn JF. Cigarette smoke and CFTR: implications in the pathogenesis of COPD. *Am J Physiol Lung Cell Mol Physiol.* (2013) 305:L530–41. doi: 10.1152/ajplung.000 39.2013
101. Lamouille S, Xu J, Derynck R. Molecular mechanisms of epithelial-mesenchymal transition. *Nat Rev Mol Cell Biol.* (2014) 15:178–96. doi: 10.1038/nrm3758
102. Milara J, Peiró T, Serrano A, Cortijo J. Epithelial to mesenchymal transition is increased in patients with COPD and induced by cigarette smoke. *Thorax.* (2013) 68:410–20. doi: 10.1136/thoraxjnl-2012-201761
103. Ricca C, Aillon A, Viano M, Bergandi L, Aldieri E, Silvagno F. Vitamin D inhibits the epithelial-mesenchymal transition by a negative feedback regulation of TGF-β activity. *J Steroid Biochem Mol Biol.* (2018) doi: 10.1016/j.jsbmb.2018.11.006
104. Jiang F, Yang Y, Xue L, Li B, Zhang Z. 1α,25-dihydroxyvitamin D3 attenuates TGF-β-induced pro-fibrotic effects in human lung epithelial cells through inhibition of epithelial–mesenchymal transition. *Nutrients.* (2017) 9:980. doi: 10.3390/nu9090980
105. Tan ZX, Chen YH, Xu S, Qin HY, Zhang C, Zhao H, et al. Calcitriol inhibits bleomycin-induced early pulmonary inflammatory response and epithelial–mesenchymal transition in mice. *Toxicol Lett.* (2016) 240:161–71. doi: 10.1016/j.toxlet.2015.10.022
106. Fischer KD, Hall SC, Agrawal DK. Vitamin D Supplementation Reduces Induction of Epithelial-Mesenchymal transition in allergen sensitized and challenged mice. *PLoS ONE.* (2016) 11:e0149180. doi: 10.1371/journal.pone.0149180
107. Hancock REW, Haney EF, Gill EE. The immunology of host defence peptides: beyond antimicrobial activity. *Nat Rev Immunol.* (2016) 16:321–334. doi: 10.1038/nri.2016.29
108. Wang TT, Nestel FP, Bourdeau V, Nagai Y, Wang Q, Liao J, et al. Cutting edge: 1,25-Dihydroxyvitamin D3 is a direct inducer of antimicrobial peptide gene expression. *J Immunol.* (2004) 173:2909–12. doi: 10.4049/jimmunol.173.5.2909
109. Huang FC. The differential effects of 1,25-dihydroxyvitamin D3 on Salmonella-induced interleukin-8 and human beta-defensin-2 in intestinal epithelial cells. *Clin Exp Immunol.* (2016) 185:98–106. doi: 10.1111/cei.12792
110. Wang TT, Dabbas B, Laperriere D, Bitton AJ, Soualhine H, Tavera-Mendoza LE, et al. Direct and indirect induction by 1,25-dihydroxyvitamin D3 of the NOD2/CARD15-Defensin β2 innate immune pathway defective in crohn disease. *J Biol Chem.* (2010) 285:2227–31. doi: 10.1074/jbc.C109.071225
111. Gonzalez-Curiel I, Trujillo V, Montoya-Rosales A, Rincon K, Rivas-Calderon B, deHaro-Acosta J, et al. 1,25-dihydroxyvitamin D3 induces LL-37 and HBD-2 production in keratinocytes from diabetic foot ulcers promoting wound healing: an *in vitro* model. *PLoS ONE.* (2014) 9:e111355. doi: 10.1371/journal.pone.0111355
112. Dai X, Sayama K, Tohyama M, Shirakata Y, Hanakawa Y, Tokumaru S, et al. PPARγ mediates innate immunity by regulating the 1α,25-dihydroxyvitamin D3 induced hBD-3 and cathelicidin in human keratinocytes. *J Dermatol Sci.* (2010) 60:179–86. doi: 10.1016/j.jdermsci.2010.09.008
113. Hou W, Hu S, Li C, Ma H, Wang Q, Meng G, et al. Cigarette smoke induced lung barrier dysfunction, EMT, and tissue remodeling: a possible link between COPD and lung cancer. *Biomed Res Int.* (2019) 2019:2025636. doi: 10.1155/2019/2025636
114. Ito JT, Lourenço JD, Righetti RF, I.Tibério FLC, Prado CM, F.D.Lopes TQS. Extracellular matrix component remodeling in respiratory diseases: what has been found in clinical and experimental studies? *Cells.* (2019) 8:342. doi: 10.3390/cells8040342
115. Shimshoni E, Yablecovitch D, Baram L, Dotan I, Sagi I. ECM remodelling in IBD: innocent bystander or partner in crime? The emerging role of extracellular molecular events in sustaining intestinal inflammation. *Gut.* (2015) 64:367–72. doi: 10.1136/gutjnl-2014-308048
116. Hansdottir S, Monick MM, Lovan N, Powers L, Gerke A, Hunninghake GW. Vitamin D decreases respiratory syncytial virus induction of NF-kappaB-linked chemokines and cytokines in airway epithelium while maintaining the antiviral state. *J Immunol.* (2010) 184:965–74. doi: 10.4049/jimmunol.0902840
117. Pfeffer PE, Chen YH, Woszczek G, Matthews NC, Chevretton E, Gupta A, et al. Vitamin D enhances production of soluble ST2, inhibiting the action of IL-33. *J Allergy Clin Immunol.* (2015) 135:824–7.e3. doi: 10.1016/j.jaci.2014.09.044
118. Vanherwegen AS, Gysemans C, Mathieu C. Regulation of immune function by vitamin D and Its use in diseases of immunity. *Endocrinol Metab Clin North Am.* (2017) 46:1061–94. doi: 10.1016/j.ecl.2017.07.010
119. Pfeffer PE, Hawrylowicz CM. Vitamin D in asthma: mechanisms of action and considerations for clinical trials. *Chest.* (2018) 153:1229–39. doi: 10.1016/j.chest.2017.09.005
120. Mercado N, Ito K, Barnes PJ. Accelerated ageing of the lung in COPD: new concepts. *Thorax.* (2015) 70:482–9. doi: 10.1136/thoraxjnl-2014-206084
121. Haussler MR, Whitfield GK, Kaneko I, Haussler CA, Hsieh D, Hsieh JC, et al. Molecular mechanisms of vitamin D action. *Calcified Tissue Int.* (2013) 92:77–98. doi: 10.1007/s00223-012-9619-0
122. Torres PU, Prié D, Molina-Blétry V, Beck L, Silve C, Friedlander G. Klotho: an antiaging protein involved in mineral and vitamin D metabolism. *Kidney Int.* (2007) 71:730–7. doi: 10.1038/sj.ki.5002163
123. Krick S, Grabner A, Baumlin N, Yanucil C, Helton S, Grosche A, et al. Fibroblast growth factor 23 and Klotho contribute to airway inflammation. *Eur Respir J.* (2018) 52:1800236. doi: 10.1183/13993003.00236-2018
124. Gao W, Yuan C, Zhang J, Li L, Yu L, Wiegman CH, et al. Klotho expression is reduced in COPD airway epithelial cells: effects on inflammation and oxidant injury. *Clin Sci.* (2015) 129:1011–23. doi: 10.1042/CS20150273
125. Li YC, Chen Y, Du J. Critical roles of intestinal epithelial vitamin D receptor signaling in controlling gut mucosal inflammation. *J Steroid Biochem Mol Biol.* (2015) 148:179–83. doi: 10.1016/j.jsbmb.2015.01.011
126. Lu R, Zhang YG, Xia Y, Sun J. Imbalance of autophagy and apoptosis in intestinal epithelium lacking the vitamin D receptor. *FASEB J.* (2019) 33:11845–856. doi: 10.1096/fj.201900727R
127. Racanelli AC, Kikkers SA, Choi AMK, Cloonan SM. Autophagy and inflammation in chronic respiratory disease. *Autophagy.* (2018) 14:221–32. doi: 10.1080/15548627.2017.1389823

128. Malvin NP, Kern JT, Liu TC, Brody SL, Stappenbeck TS. Autophagy proteins are required for club cell structure and function in airways. *Am J Physiol Lung Cell Mol Physiol.* (2019) 317:L259–L70. doi: 10.1152/ajplung.00394.2018
129. Barnes PJ. Corticosteroid resistance in patients with asthma and chronic obstructive pulmonary disease. *J Allergy Clin Immunol.* (2013) 131:636–45. doi: 10.1016/j.jaci.2012.12.1564
130. Xystrakis E, Kusumakar S, Boswell S, Peek E, Urry Z, Richards DF, et al. Reversing the defective induction of IL-10-secreting regulatory T cells in glucocorticoid-resistant asthma patients. *J Clin Invest.* (2006) 116:146–55. doi: 10.1172/JCI21759
131. Sutherland ER, Goleva E, Jackson LP, Stevens AD, Leung DYM. Vitamin D levels, lung function, and steroid response in adult asthma. *Am J RespirCrit Care Med.* (2010) 181:699–704. doi: 10.1164/rccm.200911-1710OC
132. Lan N, Luo G, Yang X, Cheng Y, Zhang Y, Wang X, et al. 25-Hydroxyvitamin D3-deficiency enhances oxidative stress and corticosteroid resistance in severe asthma exacerbation. *PLoS ONE.* (2014) 9:e111599. doi: 10.1371/journal.pone.0111599
133. Konya V, Czarnewski P, Forkel M, Rao A, Kokkinou E, Villablanca EJ, et al. Vitamin D downregulates the IL-23 receptor pathway in human mucosal group 3 innate lymphoid cells. *J Allergy Clin Immunol.* (2018) 141:279–92. doi: 10.1016/j.jaci.2017.01.045
134. Mann EH, Ho TR, Pfeffer PE, Matthews NC, Chevretton E, Mudway I, et al. Vitamin D counteracts an IL-23-dependent IL-17A(+)IFN-γ(+) response driven by urban particulate matter. *Am J Respir Cell Mol Biol.* (2017) 57:355–66. doi: 10.1165/rcmb.2016-0409OC
135. Fawaz L, Mrad MF, Kazan JM, Sayegh S, Akika R, Khoury SJ. Comparative effect of 25(OH)D3 and 1,25(OH)2D3 on Th17 cell differentiation. *Clin Immunol.* (2016) 166–7:59–71. doi: 10.1016/j.clim.2016.02.011
136. Nanzer AM, Chambers ES, Ryanna K, Richards DF, Black C, Timms PM, et al. Enhanced production of IL-17A in patients with severe asthma is inhibited by 1α,25-dihydroxyvitamin D3 in a glucocorticoid-independent fashion. *J Allergy Clin Immunol.* (2013) 132:297–304.e3. doi: 10.1016/j.jaci.2013.03.037
137. Dhawan P, Christakos S. Novel regulation of 25-hydroxyvitamin D3 24-hydroxylase (24(OH)ase) transcription by glucocorticoids: cooperative effects of the glucocorticoid receptor, C/EBPβ, and the Vitamin D receptor in 24(OH)ase transcription. *J Cell Biochem.* (2010) 110:1314–23. doi: 10.1002/jcb.22645
138. Donaldson GC, Seemungal TAR, Bhowmik A, Wedzicha JA. Relationship between exacerbation frequency and lung function decline in chronic obstructive pulmonary disease. *Thorax.* (2002) 57:847–52. doi: 10.1136/thorax.57.10.847
139. Decramer M, Janssens W, Miravitlles M. Chronic obstructive pulmonary disease. *Lancet.* (2012) 379:1341–51. doi: 10.1016/S0140-6736(11)60968-9
140. Leung JM, Tiew PY, Mac Aogáin M, Budden KF, Yong VFL, Thomas SS, et al. The role of acute and chronic respiratory colonization and infections in the pathogenesis of COPD. *Respirology.* (2017) 22:634–50. doi: 10.1111/resp.13032
141. Wang Z, Bafadhel M, Haldar K, Spivak A, Mayhew D, Miller BE, et al. Lung microbiome dynamics in COPD exacerbations. *Eur Respir J.* (2016) 47:1082–92. doi: 10.1183/13993003.01406-2015
142. Bolcas PE, Brandt EB, Zhang Z, Myers JM, Ruff BP, Hershey GK. Vitamin D supplementation attenuates asthma development following traffic-related particulate matter exposure. *J Allergy Clin Immunol.* (2019) 143:386–94.e3. doi: 10.1016/j.jaci.2018.04.042
143. Wang H, Anthony D, Selemidis S, Vlahos R, Bozinovski S. Resolving viral-induced secondary bacterial infection in COPD: a concise review. *Front Immunol.* (2018) 9:2345. doi: 10.3389/fimmu.2018.02345
144. Stolz D, Papakonstantinou E, Grize L, Schilter D, Strobel W, Louis R, et al. Time-course of upper respiratory tract viral infection and COPD exacerbation. *Eur Respir J.* (2019) 54:1900407. doi: 10.1183/13993003.00407-2019
145. Schogler A, Muster RJ, Kieninger E, Casaulta C, Tapparel C, Jung A, et al. Vitamin D represses rhinovirus replication in cystic fibrosis cells by inducing LL-37. *Eur Respir J.* (2016) 47:520–30. doi: 10.1183/13993003.00665-2015
146. Sousa FH, Casanova V, Findlay F, Stevens C, Svoboda P, Pohl J, et al. Cathelicidins display conserved direct antiviral activity towards rhinovirus. *Peptides.* (2017) 95:76–83. doi: 10.1016/j.peptides.2017.07.013
147. Brockman-Schneider RA, Pickles RJ, Gern JE. Effects of vitamin D on airway epithelial cell morphology and rhinovirus replication. *PLoS ONE.* (2014) 9:e86755. doi: 10.1371/journal.pone.0086755
148. Gui B, Chen Q, Hu C, Zhu C, He G. Effects of calcitriol (1, 25-dihydroxy-vitamin D3) on the inflammatory response induced by H9N2 influenza virus infection in human lung A549 epithelial cells and in mice. *Virol J.* (2017) 14:10. doi: 10.1186/s12985-017-0683-y
149. Khare D, Godbole NM, Pawar SD, Mohan V, Pandey G, Gupta S, et al. Calcitriol [1, 25[OH]2 D3] pre- and post-treatment suppresses inflammatory response to influenza A (H1N1) infection in human lung A549 epithelial cells. *Eur J Nutr.* (2013) 52:1405–15. doi: 10.1007/s00394-012-0449-7
150. Sethi S, Murphy TF. Infection in the pathogenesis and course of chronic obstructive pulmonary disease. *N Engl J Med.* (2008) 359:2355–65. doi: 10.1056/NEJMra0800353
151. Sethi S, Evans N, Grant BJB, Murphy TF. New strains of bacteria and exacerbations of chronic obstructive pulmonary disease. *N Eng J Med.* (2002) 347:465–71. doi: 10.1056/NEJMoa012561
152. Wilkinson TMA, Aris E, Bourne S, Clarke SC, Peeters M, Pascal TG, et al. A prospective, observational cohort study of the seasonal dynamics of airway pathogens in the aetiology of exacerbations in COPD. *Thorax.* (2017) 72:919–27. doi: 10.1136/thoraxjnl-2016-209023
153. Yim S, Dhawan P, Ragunath C, Christakos S, Diamond G. Induction of cathelicidin in normal and CF bronchial epithelial cells by 1,25-dihydroxyvitamin D(3). *J Cystic Fibrosis.* (2007) 6:403–10. doi: 10.1016/j.jcf.2007.03.003
154. Dimitrov V, White JH. Species-specific regulation of innate immunity by vitamin D signaling. *J Steroid Biochem Mol Biol.* (2016) 164:246–53. doi: 10.1016/j.jsbmb.2015.09.016
155. Gombart AF, Borregaard N, Koeffler HP. Human cathelicidin antimicrobial peptide (CAMP) gene is a direct target of the vitamin D receptor and is strongly up-regulated in myeloid cells by 1,25-dihydroxyvitamin D3. *FASEB J.* (2005) 19:1067–77. doi: 10.1096/fj.04-3284com
156. Niederstrasser J, Herr C, Wolf L, Lehr CM, Beisswenger C, Bals R. Vitamin D deficiency does not result in a breach of host defense in murine models of pneumonia. *Infect Immun.* (2016) 84:3097–104. doi: 10.1128/IAI.00282-16
157. Lowry MB, Guo C, Zhang Y, Fantacone ML, Logan IE, Campbell Y, et al. A mouse model for vitamin D-induced human cathelicidin antimicrobial peptide gene expression. *J Steroid Biochem Mol Biol.* (2019) 198:105552. doi: 10.1016/j.jsbmb.2019.105552
158. Zuo W-L, Shenoy SA, Li S, O'Beirne SL, Strulovici-Barel Y, Leopold PL, et al. Ontogeny and biology of human small airway epithelial club cells. *Am J Respir Crit Care Med.* (2018) 198:1375–88. doi: 10.1164/rccm.201710-2107OC
159. Clark A, Mach N. Role of vitamin D in the hygiene hypothesis: the interplay between vitamin d, vitamin d receptors, gut microbiota, immune response. *Front Immunol.* (2016) 7:627. doi: 10.3389/fimmu.2016.00627
160. Salzman NH. Paneth cell defensins and the regulation of the microbiome: détente at mucosal surfaces. *Gut Microbes.* (2010) 1:401–6. doi: 10.4161/gmic.1.6.14076
161. Cullen TW, Schofield WB, Barry NA, Putnam EE, Rundell EA, Trent MS, et al. Gut microbiota. Antimicrobial peptide resistance mediates resilience of prominent gut commensals during inflammation. *Science.* (2015) 347:170–5. doi: 10.1126/science.1260580
162. Budden KF, Gellatly SL, Wood DLA, Cooper MA, Morrison M, Hugenholtz P, et al. Emerging pathogenic links between microbiota and the gut–lung axis. *Nat Rev Microbiol.* (2016) 15:55. doi: 10.1038/nrmicro.2016.142
163. Dang AT, Marsland BJ. Microbes, metabolites, and the gut-lung axis. *Mucosal Immunol.* (2019) 12:843–850. doi: 10.1038/s41385-019-0160-6
164. Waterhouse M, Hope B, Krause L, Morrison M, Protani MM, Zakrzewski M, et al. Vitamin D and the gut microbiome: a systematic review of *in vivo* studies. *Eur J Nutr.* (2019) 58:2895–910. doi: 10.1007/s00394-018-1842-7
165. Talsness CE, Penders J, E.Jansen HJM, Damoiseaux J, Thijs C, Mommers M. Influence of vitamin D on key bacterial taxa in infant microbiota in the KOALA birth cohort study. *PLoS ONE.* (2017) 12:e0188011. doi: 10.1371/journal.pone.0188011

166. Schaffler H, Herlemann DP, Klinitzke P, Berlin P, Kreikemeyer B, Jaster R, et al. Vitamin D administration leads to a shift of the intestinal bacterial composition in crohn's disease patients, but not in healthy controls. *J Dig Dis.* (2018) 19:225–34. doi: 10.1111/1751-2980.12591
167. Sullivan A, Hunt E, MacSharry J, Murphy DM. 'The microbiome and the pathophysiology of asthma'. *Respir Res.* (2016) 17:163. doi: 10.1186/s12931-016-0479-4
168. Mammen MJ, Sethi S. COPD and the microbiome. *Respirology.* (2016) 21:590–9. doi: 10.1111/resp.12732
169. Toivonen L, Hasegawa K, Ajami NJ, Celedon JC, Mansbach JM, Petrosino JF, et al. circulating 25-hydroxyvitamin D, nasopharyngeal microbiota, bronchiolitis severity. *Pediatr Allergy Immunol.* (2018) 29:877–80. doi: 10.1111/pai.12977
170. Kanhere M, He J, Chassaing B, Ziegler TR, Alvarez JA, Ivie EA, et al. Bolus weekly vitamin D3 supplementation impacts gut and airway microbiota in adults with cystic fibrosis: a double-blind, randomized, placebo-controlled clinical trial. *J Clin Endocrinol Metab.* (2018) 103:564–74. doi: 10.1210/jc.2017-01983
171. Zendedel A, Gholami M, Anbari K, Ghanadi K, Bachari EC, Azargon A. Effects of vitamin D Intake on FEV1 and COPD exacerbation: a randomized clinical trial study. *Glob J Health Sci.* (2015) 7:243–8. doi: 10.5539/gjhs.v7n4p243
172. Khan DM, Ullah A, Randhawa FA, Iqtadar S, Butt NF, Waheed K. Role of vitamin D in reducing number of acute exacerbations in chronic obstructive pulmonary disease (COPD) patients. *J Med Sci.* (2017) 33:610–4. doi: 10.12669/pjms.333.12397
173. Lehouck A, Mathieu C, Carremans C, Baeke F, Verhaegen J, Van Eldere J, et al. High doses of vitamin D to reduce exacerbations in chronic obstructive pulmonary disease: a randomized trial. *Ann Intern Med.* (2012) 156:105–14. doi: 10.7326/0003-4819-156-2-201201170-00004
174. Martineau AR, James WY, Hooper RL, Barnes NC, Jolliffe DA, Greiller CL, et al. Vitamin D3 supplementation in patients with chronic obstructive pulmonary disease (ViDiCO): a multicentre, double-blind, randomised controlled trial. *Lancet Respir Med.* (2015) 3:120–30. doi: 10.1016/S2213-2600(14)70255-3
175. Jolliffe DA, Greenberg L, Hooper RL, Mathyssen C, Rafiq R, de Jongh RT, et al. Vitamin D to prevent exacerbations of COPD: systematic review and meta-analysis of individual participant data from randomised controlled trials. *Thorax.* (2019) 74:337–45. doi: 10.1136/thoraxjnl-2018-212092
176. Rafiq R, Aleva FE, Schrumpf JA, Heijdra YF, Taube C, Daniels JMA, et al. Prevention of exacerbations in patients with COPD and vitamin D deficiency through vitamin D supplementation (PRECOVID): a study protocol. *BMC Pulm Med.* (2015) 15:106. doi: 10.1186/s12890-015-0101-4
177. Martineau AR, Jolliffe DA, Hooper RL, Greenberg L, Aloia JF, Bergman P, et al. Vitamin D supplementation to prevent acute respiratory tract infections: systematic review and meta-analysis of individual participant data. *BMJ.* (2017) 356:i6583. doi: 10.1136/bmj.i6583
178. Wang M, Liu M, Wang C, Xiao Y, An T, Zou M, et al. Association between vitamin D status and asthma control: a meta-analysis of randomized trials. *Respir Med.* (2019) 150:85–94. doi: 10.1016/j.rmed.2019.02.016
179. Ramos-Martínez E, López-Vancell MR, Fernández de Córdova-Aguirre JC, Rojas-Serrano J, Chavarría A, Velasco-Medina A, et al. Reduction of respiratory infections in asthma patients supplemented with vitamin D is related to increased serum IL-10 and IFNγ levels and cathelicidin expression. *Cytokine.* (2018) 108:239–46. doi: 10.1016/j.cyto.2018.01.001
180. Wani WA, Nazir M, Bhat JI, E.-u.-h. Malik, Ahmad QI, Charoo BA, et al. Vitamin D status correlates with the markers of cystic fibrosis-related pulmonary disease. *Pediatr Neonatol.* (2019) 60:210–215. doi: 10.1016/j.pedneo.2018.07.001
181. Tangpricha V, Lukemire J, Chen Y, Binongo JNG, Judd SE, Michalski ES, et al. Vitamin D for the immune system in cystic fibrosis (DISC): a double-blind, multicenter, randomized, placebo-controlled clinical trial. *Am J Clin Nutr.* (2019) 109:544–53. doi: 10.1093/ajcn/nqy291
182. Luo W, Hershberger PA, Trump DL, Johnson CS. 24-Hydroxylase in cancer: impact on vitamin D-based anticancer therapeutics. *J Steroid Biochem Mol Biol.* (2013) 136:252–7. doi: 10.1016/j.jsbmb.2012.09.031
183. Amatngalim GD, Broekman W, Daniel NM, van der Vlugt LEPM, van Schadewijk A, Taube C, et al. Cigarette smoke modulates repair and innate immunity following injury to airway epithelial cells. *PLoS ONE.* (2016) 11:e0166255. doi: 10.1371/journal.pone.0166255
184. Toshiyuki S, Kaori Y, Atsushi K, Keiko Y, Tai CC. CYP24A1 as a potential target for cancer therapy. *Anti-Cancer Agents Med Chem.* (2014) 14:97–108. doi: 10.2174/18715206113139990307
185. Lachapelle P, Li M, Douglass J, Stewart A. Safer approaches to therapeutic modulation of TGF-beta signaling for respiratory disease. *Pharmacol Ther.* (2018) 187:98–113. doi: 10.1016/j.pharmthera.2018.02.010

4

Role of Cystic Fibrosis Bronchial Epithelium in Neutrophil Chemotaxis

Giulio Cabrini[1,2,3*], *Alessandro Rimessi*[1,4], *Monica Borgatti*[1,2], *Ilaria Lampronti*[1,2], *Alessia Finotti*[1,2], *Paolo Pinton*[1,4] *and Roberto Gambari*[1,2*]

[1] Center for Innovative Therapies in Cystic Fibrosis, University of Ferrara, Ferrara, Italy, [2] Department of Life Sciences and Biotechnology, University of Ferrara, Ferrara, Italy, [3] Department of Neurosciences, Biomedicine and Movement, University of Verona, Verona, Italy, [4] Department of Medical Sciences, University of Ferrara, Ferrara, Italy

***Correspondence:**
Giulio Cabrini
giulio.cabrini@unife.it
Roberto Gambari
roberto.gambari@unife.it

A hallmark of cystic fibrosis (CF) chronic respiratory disease is an extensive neutrophil infiltrate in the mucosa filling the bronchial lumen, starting early in life for CF infants. The genetic defect of the CF Transmembrane conductance Regulator (CFTR) ion channel promotes dehydration of the airway surface liquid, alters mucus properties, and decreases mucociliary clearance, favoring the onset of recurrent and, ultimately, chronic bacterial infection. Neutrophil infiltrates are unable to clear bacterial infection and, as an adverse effect, contribute to mucosal tissue damage by releasing proteases and reactive oxygen species. Moreover, the rapid cellular turnover of lumenal neutrophils releases nucleic acids that further alter the mucus viscosity. A prominent role in the recruitment of neutrophil in bronchial mucosa is played by CF bronchial epithelial cells carrying the defective CFTR protein and are exposed to whole bacteria and bacterial products, making pharmacological approaches to regulate the exaggerated neutrophil chemotaxis in CF a relevant therapeutic target. Here we revise: (a) the major receptors, kinases, and transcription factors leading to the expression, and release of neutrophil chemokines in bronchial epithelial cells; (b) the role of intracellular calcium homeostasis and, in particular, the calcium crosstalk between endoplasmic reticulum and mitochondria; (c) the epigenetic regulation of the key chemokines; (d) the role of mutant CFTR protein as a co-regulator of chemokines together with the host-pathogen interactions; and (e) different pharmacological strategies to regulate the expression of chemokines in CF bronchial epithelial cells through novel drug discovery and drug repurposing.

Keywords: cystic fibrosis, epithelium, lung, chemotaxis, neutrophil, inflammation

LUNG PATHOLOGY IN CYSTIC FIBROSIS PATIENTS: AN EARLY EVENT ACCOMPANYING WHOLE LIFE

Autosomal recessive inheritance of mutations of the Cystic Fibrosis Transmembrane Conductance Regulator (*CFTR*) gene, encoding a chloride and bicarbonate transporting protein, is at the basis of the multiorgan Cystic Fibrosis (CF) disease (1–3). CF lung disease, characterized by chronic bacterial airway infection, neutrophilic inflammation, and dilation of bronchioles obstructed by mucus plugs, is presently the main limitation to the quality and expectancy of the life of CF patients. Although lung pathology and the mechanisms of the disease were prioritized for decades in CF research, what is between the *CFTR* gene defects and the overt clinical symptoms of the CF patients has still not been completely defined. Consensus has been reached that lung pathology begins in the early months of life for the majority of CF infants, often before the onset of clinical symptoms, as demonstrated by the presence of inflammatory cytokines in the bronchoalveolar lavage fluid of CF infants (4–6) and by the lung histopathology of CF infants who die within weeks or months after birth, showing bronchial lumena filled and plugged by neutrophils (7).

Different hypotheses have been proposed to link the chloride and bicarbonate transport defects of mutant CFTR protein and the onset of airway disease. Consensus on the mechanism can be summarized in that altered CFTR protein reduces the hydration, and possibly the pH, of the airway surface liquid (ASL), thus affecting the rate of the mucociliary clearance, the principal innate mechanism involved in the defense against microbial infection (8). ASL dehydration worsens the mucociliary clearance by reducing mucus fluidity in both ASL and in the submucosal glands of the airway mucosa. The precise mechanism(s) favoring the early recurrent infections with *Staphilococcus aureus* and *Haemophilus influenzae*, and the stable chronic bacterial infection with *Pseudomonas aeruginosa* (*P. aeruginosa*) that follows in at least 80% of CF teenagers, are not completely understood (9), as ALS dehydration and increased mucus viscosity are considered early predisposing events in CF lung pathophysiology (10, 11).

Hallmarks of the lung pathology of CF patients include defective mucociliary clearance and chronic bacterial infection (especially *P. aeruginosa*) associated with an exaggerated neutrophil dominated inflammation.

NEUTROPHILS IN CF AIRWAY INFLAMMATION: A DOUBLE-EDGED SWORD

Neutrophils are the predominant immune cells infiltrating the airway mucosa and filling the intralumenal space of bronchioles in CF patients (7). Although the recruitment of neutrophils in CF airways' begins early in life and becomes persistent, neutrophils are unable to solve CF bacterial infection. The inefficacy of neutrophils in clearing bacteria prompted a debate on the presence of a neutrophil dysfunction in CF airways, as has been extensively reviewed elsewhere (12, 13). Different *in vitro* and *in vivo* studies in human and mice models evidenced that defective CFTR expressed in CF neutrophils, which is essential for chloride transport into phagolysosome and production of HOCl, impairs bacterial killing, implicating a specific disadvantage in microbial clearance in CF airways (14–18). As an indirect confirmation of the role of CFTR in neutrophilic function, VX-770 CFTR potentiator and VRT-325 corrector partially restored the impaired bacterial killing function in neutrophils of patients bearing G551D-CFTR or F508del-CFTR mutations, respectively (19, 20).

Although defective in clearing the chronic respiratory infection of these patients, neutrophils in CF airways are exposed to bacteria and become a source of continuous release of proteases, mainly elastases, which further impair their killing ability upon cleavage of the CXCR1 chemokine receptor (21). The relevance of elastases released from neutrophils has become an intense field of investigation due to its multiple adverse effects in CF lung pathology. It has been directly correlated with the onset of bronchiectasis and the severity of lung disease. The imbalance between proteases and anti-proteases in the CF ASL has prompted researchers to consider neutrophil elastase as a relevant molecular target in this disease (22–31). Its role in CF lung tissue damage has been further increased by its effect on degradation of CFTR protein (32), which can potentially reduce the efficacy of novel CFTR modulators, and by the evidence that its expression is upregulated by the pro-inflammatory cytokine TNF-alpha (TNF-α) and the chemokine interleukin (IL)-8 (or CXCL8) in CF lung (33). Finally, it amplifies the autocrine circuitry of inflammation by potentiating the recruitment of elastase-producing neutrophils by inducing the release of the neutrophilic chemokine IL-8, acting with an autocrine mechanism on CXCR1 and with activation of TLR4 and MyD88-dependent signaling (34–36).

A second critical adverse effect of a huge amount of neutrophils is their contribution to increasing the pro-oxidant milieu of the CF ALS, as has been extensively reviewed elsewhere (37). Among the different sources of pro-oxidants in the CF airway milieu, neutrophils contribute by releasing reactive oxygen species (ROS) by mechanisms known as "frustrated phagocytosis" or as a result of continuous activation, being the neutrophil-derived ROS critical effectors of bronchial epithelial damage (38–41).

As a third critical adverse effect, the presence of a large amount of neutrophils in CF brochial lumena implies the release of abundant DNA on the surface of the mucosa, which further reduces the fluidity of the ASL and worsens the bronchial obstruction (42). For a long time, neutrophil-derived DNA was thought to be the result of the turnover of neutrophils ending in hypoxic necrosis and consequent DNA release (43). More recently, the free DNA in CF airways has been found to be derived from the Neutrophil Extracellular Traps (NETs) released by neutrophils instead of the results of hypoxic necrosis (44). NETs are part of the innate defense armamentarium that block bacteria, viruses, and parasites facilitating the phagocytosis by neutrophils. However, in the environment of CF lung infection and inflammation, the benefits of NETs seems to be overcome by the adverse effect of the release of DNA that further reduces ASL fluidity, which impairs the clearance of toxic enzymes, such as neutrophil elastase and myeloperoxidase, damaging the respiratory tissue. The balance between the pros and cons of NETs in CF lung disease is therefore critical (45, 46). A crucial issue in CF lung disease is that neutrophils in the bronchial lumena of CF patients are unable to clear the bacterial infection and are co-responsible, together with bacteria, for the tissue damage, since neutrophils release proteases and ROS and further affect the rheology of CF ASL with abundant DNA. A graphical summary is presented in **Figure 1**.

CHEMOKINES RECRUITING NEUTROPHILS AND THE ROLE OF BRONCHIAL EPITHELIAL CELLS

Elevated concentrations of cytokines have been found early in life in the bronchoalveolar lavage fluid of CF infants, even

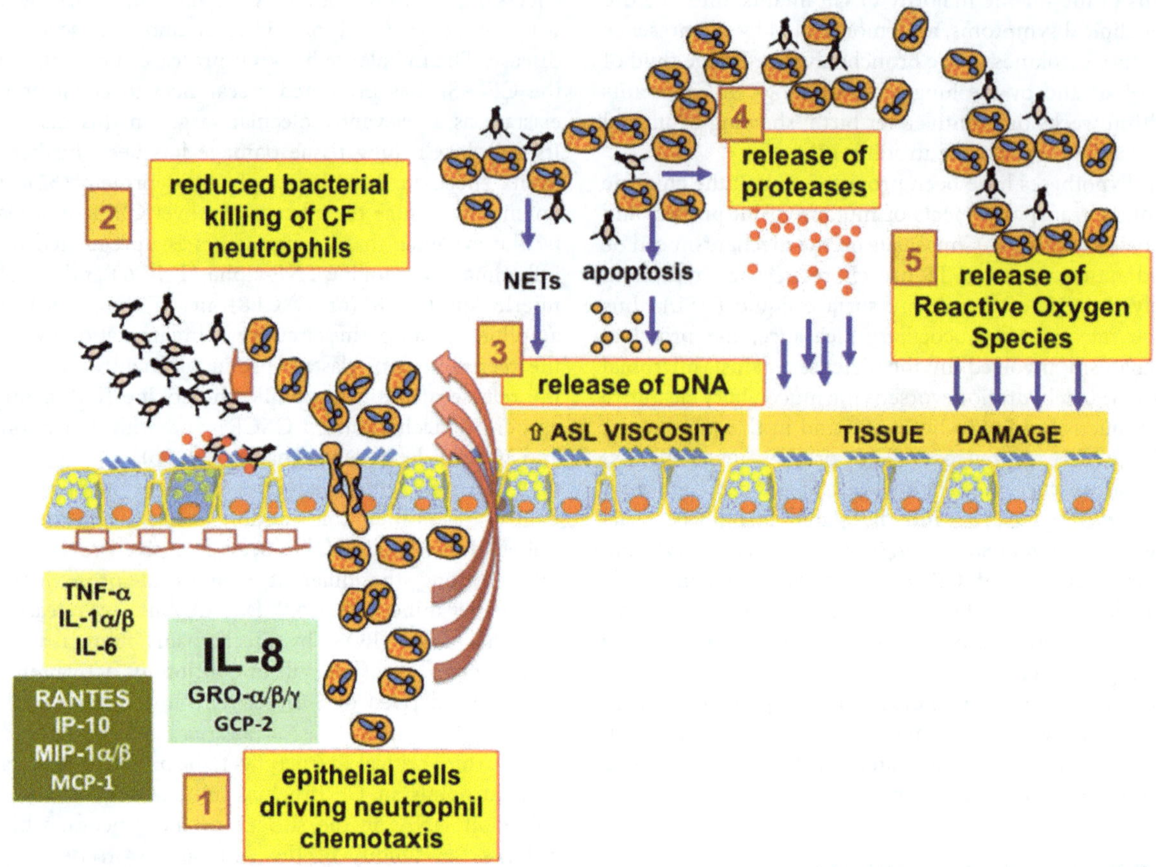

FIGURE 1 | CF bronchial epithelial cells and neutrophil chemotaxis. 1. epithelial cells driving neutrophil chemotaxis: bronchial epithelial cells drive the chemotaxis of neutrophils inside the lumen of bronchi and bronchioles of CF patients, mainly secreting the chemokine IL-8 (CXCL8) expressed upon interaction with bacteria with ASGM1R and TLR2/5 receptors exposed on the apical membrane. 2. reduced bacterial killing of CF neutrophils: CF neutrophils present different degrees of defective killing of the bacteria in the process of phagocytosis, being unable to clear completely the recurrent and, later on, chronic bacterial infection in the airways. 3. release of DNA: CF neutrophils are continuously stimulated in releasing Neutrophil Extracellular Traps. Despite the expected increase in efficiency of bacterial clearing, DNA from NETs increases the viscosity of the Airway Surface Liquid (ASL), further worsening the beat of cilia and the effectiveness of the CF mucociliary clearance. Moreover, CF neutrophils further release DNA as a consequence of apoptosis or necrosis due to the hypoxic environment resulting from mucus plugging of the conductive airways. 4. release of proteases: CF neutrophils exposed to bacteria or bacteria-derived components are prone to exocytosis of granules containing a wide armamentarium of proteases that are usually utilized by neutrophils to disrupt the tissues to allow their migration. In particular, an abundant amount of elastase has been found in CF lungs and its concentration has been related to CF lung disease progression and severity. 5. release of Reactive Oxygen Species: the unbalanced pro-oxidant milieu of the CF ASL due to excessive ROS derives mainly from "frustrated phagocytosis" of CF neutrophils and contributes together with proteases to a neutrophil-dependent airway tissue damage, a clear side effect dependent on the CFTR defect and worsened by an exaggerated neutrophil chemotaxis in CF bronchial lumen.

in the absence of an overt bacterial infection (4–6). Different mechanisms have been proposed to explain the early onset of sterile inflammation in CF lungs, including the role of airway surface mucus and hypoxia (47–49).

Among the soluble mediators of inflammation detected in CF bronchoalveolar lavage fluid, the most potent chemokines recruiting neutrophils have attracted particular interest, both in terms of pathophysiology and therapeutic perspectives, namely the complement system-derived C5a, the leukotriene B4 (LTB4), and the chemokine Interleukin(IL)-8.

C5a activated complement component receptor (C5aR) expressed on neutrophils was found to be critical in the defense against *P. aeruginosa* infection since knock-out mice deficient of C5aR were able to recruit neutrophils but succumbed to pneumonia because of the killing defect (50). Although it was earlier speculated that the C5aR decoy molecule C5L2 could be beneficial in reducing excessive inflammation in several lung diseases, including CF (51), it was later concluded that inactivation of C5aR by cleavage mediated by proteases released from CF neutrophils was at least partly responsible for the reduced killing and clearance of *P. aeruginosa* in CF lungs (52). Due to this critical role of C5aR in host defense, although elevated concentrations of C5a in CF airway fluids have been directly correlated with disease severity, very little effort has been invested in inhibiting the C5a-C5aR axis (53, 54).

LTB4 is released from neutrophils and macrophages in response to different stimuli, and in turn recruits and activates neutrophils (55). LTB4 has been found at elevated concentrations in different CF respiratory fluids (56–58). Because of its potent neutrophil chemotactic effect, novel drugs, or drug repositioning to inhibit either LTB4 or its receptor have been proposed in CF to reduce inflammatory-dependent tissue damage (59). Particularly relevant was the experience with BIIL 284 BS, a drug acting as an LTB4 receptor antagonist, which was tested in pre-clinical and clinical trials (60, 61). Unfortunately, the clinical trial resulted in major adverse events, as it was apparent that the drug, while effectively reducing the inflammatory response, was untowardly increasing *P. aeruginosa* bacterial load (61, 62), providing a first relevant alert on the delicate balance between the reduction of excessive inflammation by over-inhibiting neutrophil chemotaxis and the mandatory need of preserving a sufficient immune defense. To tackle the crucial issue of anticipating in pre-clinical assays the effect of potential anti-inflammatory molecules modulating neutrophil chemotaxis, an interesting CF *in vitro* model has been set-up, able to simulate closely the transepithelial neutrophil migration and the effect of candidate drugs (63). In spite of inhibiting the LTB4 receptor, such as in the previous unsuccessful experience with BIIL 284 BS (61, 62), acebilistat, a recent drug modulating LTB4 expression, has positively passed pre-clinical assays (63) and is now in clinical trials (64), keeping open the possibility of reducing excessive CF lung inflammation by modulating neutrophil chemotaxis targeting the leukotriene-LTB4 axis.

IL-8/CXCL8 is possibly the neutrophilic chemokine most extensively studied in CF lung pathophysiology. Different cells of the airway tract are known to contribute to the release IL-8; among these, bronchial epithelial cells have been highlighted as a relevant source. To dissect the specific contribution of bronchial epithelial cells in the expression of IL-8 and of several other soluble mediators of inflammation, different *in vitro* experimental models with immortalized cell lines or primary cell cultures have been tested and are currently utilized to investigate molecular mechanisms or novel anti-inflammatory molecules. Key pro-inflammatory challenges able to elicit inflammatory mediators in bronchial epithelial cells are different living bacteria (*S. aureus, P. aeruginosa*), heat-inactivated dead bacteria (Heat-Killed *P. aeruginosa*), flagella-defective or pili-defective recombinant strains of *P. aeruginosa*, single bacterial components (e.g., flagellin), *P. aeruginosa* clinical isolates and bacterial products from patients' airway specimens (e.g., Supernatant of Mucopurulent Material), different pro-inflammatory cytokines (e.g., TNF-α and IL-1), and oxidants such as hydrogen peroxide (65–72). Under these stimuli *in vitro*, bronchial epithelial cells upregulate the basal expression of many pro-inflammatory mediators, such as the cytokines (e.g., TNF-α, IL-1α/β, IL-6), chemokines attracting lympho-monocytes (e.g., IP-10, RANTES, MCP-1, MIP-1α/β), and, as anticipated, IL-8 and other chemokines attracting neutrophils (Gro α/β/γ, GCP-2) (67, 68, 70, 71, 73–81). Among these soluble mediators of inflammation, the neutrophilic chemokine IL-8 (CXCL8) is most strikingly expressed up to two orders of magnitude above the basal release (81). Wide consensus has been reached so far on the role of bronchial epithelial cells as relevant producers of the potent chemokine IL-8, which in turn forwards a strong recruiting soluble signal to neutrophils to reach the lumen of bronchi and bronchioles in the CF mucosa.

HOST-PATHOGEN INTERACTIONS AND INTRACELLULAR SIGNALING MODULATING IL-8/CXCL8 EXPRESSION

A growing series of evidence based on longitudinal clinical investigations of CF patients is building a strong consensus that the inflammatory process could be even more deleterious to CF lung structure and function than the bacterial infection by itself (83) Sterile inflammation in CF lungs has been evidenced based on the presence of elevated concentrations of cytokines in the bronchoalveolar lavage fluid of CF infants of a few months of age (4–6). Airway surface mucus plugging and hypoxia have been proposed to explain the onset of sterile inflammation in CF lungs (47–49). The possible direct contribution of intracellular CFTR protein defects has been proposed (as described later in paragraph 5), together with mechanisms more downstream than the CFTR-dependent ion transport alterations, such as mucus plugging (84). Although inflammation in the absence of detectable bacterial infection has been demonstrated as a likely initiating event, the whole inflammatory process in CF lung is undoubtedly amplified by the occurrence of polybacterial infection. Host-pathogen interactions between bacteria and bronchial epithelial cells in CF have been most extensively studied for *P. aeruginosa*, the pathogen that colonizes CF airways of almost all CF patients. *P. aeruginosa* in a planktonic state interacts through the pili with Asialo-GM1 receptor (AGM1R) on the apical membrane of airway epithelial cells (65). Flagellum-derived flagellin protein also binds to AGM1R, together with Toll-like receptors (TLR) 2 and 5 (85). Flagellin in particular has been found to elicit a strong intracellular pro-inflammatory signaling, as shown by the single purified protein and by recombinant lab strains of *P. aeruginosa*, in different converging studies led by Prince et al. (68, 72, 86, 87). MyD88-dependent signaling downstream TLR2 and TLR5, elicited by *P. aeruginosa*, activates Mitogen-Activated Protein (MAP) Kinases such as MAPK ERK1/2 and MAPK p38, together with ribosomal S6 kinase (RSK)1/2 and heat shock protein (HSP) 27, which are directly involved in inducing the expression of the neutrophilic chemokine IL-8 (88–90). Besides the activation of MyD88-dependent signaling, *P. aeruginosa* is known to also potentiate the expression of IL-8 by a nucleotide-purinergic receptors loop. Interaction of the bacteria with ASGM1R and TLR5 promotes sustained release of ATP as a classical "danger signal" from the apical membrane (85, 91), interacting with purinergic receptors P2Y2R (92). This activates an intracellular calcium signaling (see paragraph 6), in which phospholipase C beta 3 (PLCB3) plays a key role (78, 93).

For transcription factors (TFs) involved in chemokine expression, the promoter elements of IL-8 gene have been widely studied (89, 94, 95). The mapping of the transcription machinery of the IL-8 gene in human bronchial epithelial cells infected with *P. aeruginosa* was studied not only with the aim of understanding the molecular regulation of IL-8 transcription, but also to propose novel anti-inflammatory approaches and to identify potential pharmacological targets. This issue was addressed by investigating the role of TFs on the transcription of the IL-8 gene in human bronchial epithelial cells. Functional assays were based on the transfection of TF decoy oligodeoxynucleotides, designed to interfere with the interaction of the transcription factors nuclear factor-κB (NF-κB), activating protein (AP-1), CAAT/enhancer-binding protein β (C/EBPβ, also known as NF-IL-6), C/EBP homologous protein (CHOP), and cAMP response element binding protein (CREB) with the corresponding consensus sequences identified in the IL-8 promoter. The treatment of target cells with these decoy oligonucleotides reduced the *P. aeruginosa*-dependent transcription of IL-8, suggesting their participation in the transcriptional machinery (89, 94). These conclusions have been recently confirmed and reviewed (95). On the contrary, IL-8 gene expression is repressed by a combination of molecular events that includes: (a) deacetylation of histones, (b) octamer-1 (Oct-1) binding, and (c) active repression by NF-κB repressing factor (NRF). Histone deacetylase-1 (HDAC-1) activity is involved in IL-8 transcription inhibition, as demonstrated by the fact that HDAC1 inhibition derepresses the expression of IL-8, which involves the recruitment of CREB binding protein (CBP)/p300 to the IL-8 promoter, resulting in hyperacetylation of histones and chromatin remodeling, thus counteracting the repression (96, 97). In terms of Oct-1 activity, it has been demonstrated that Oct-1 (the IL-8 repressor) and CCAAT/enhancer-binding protein (C/EBP) (an IL-8 activator) bind to overlapping elements within the IL-8 promoter. The role of Oct-1 as a transcriptional repressor is sustained by experimental evidence that replacing the Oct-1 repressor with C/EBP induces transcription at the IL-8 promoter (98). Similarly, binding of NRF to a negative regulatory element (NRE) in the IL-8 gene promoter (which incompletely overlaps with the NF-κB response element) also represses IL-8 transcription (99). Interestingly, the transcription factors that have been suggested to regulate IL-8 are also involved in regulating the expression of other pro-inflammatory genes, such as GRO-γ, the intercellular adhesion molecule (ICAM)-1, and the cytokines IL-1β and IL-6 (94).

The possible application of transcription factor(s) targeting (for instance, using decoy oligonucleotides) might be a potential therapeutic intervention, especially in the case delivery issues are solved. In this respect, two recently reported studies have focused on nanomaterial-based delivery systems for overcoming limitations associated with clinical applications of decoy oligonucleotides targeting pro-inflammatory transcription factors (such as those targeting NF-kB) (100, 101).

THE EPIGENETIC REGULATION OF THE KEY CHEMOKINES

The epigenetic regulation of key chemokines in CF occurs at the level of: (a) histone acetyltransferase (HAT)/HDAC balance, (b) histone and DNA methylation, and (c) miRNA-dependent post-transcriptional regulation. It has been recently reported that the transcriptional regulation of IL-8 and other pro-inflammatory genes involves chromatin remodeling through histone acetylation. Interestingly, there is a possible regulatory loop between IL-8 gene transcription and CFTR. In fact, NF-κB facilitates histone acetylation of IL-8 and other pro-inflammatory gene promoters and the histone acetyltransferase (HAT)/HDAC balance is sensitive to CFTR function. This conclusion is supported by the observation that cells with a reduced or absent CFTR function have a decreased HDAC2 protein, resulting in hyperacetylation of the IL-8 promoter and increased IL-8 transcription. In agreement with (a), reduced HDAC2 and HDAC2 activity is observed in cells deficient in CFTR and (b) suppression of HDAC2 expression with HDAC2 shRNA (short hairpin RNA) resulted in enhanced IL-8 expression and promoter acetylation similar to CFTR-deficient cells (102). In conclusion, there is an intrinsic alteration in the HAT/HDAC balance in cells lacking CFTR function *in vitro* and in native CF tissue. This mechanism provides an explanation for the apparent dysregulation of inflammatory mediators seen in the CF airway, as reduced histone deacetylation would potentially influence many genes. IL-8 hypersecretion in CF airway epithelial cells is also caused by the abnormal epigenetic regulation of IL-8 gene involving histone methylation. Under basal conditions, CF cells had increased bromodomain (Brd)3 and Brd4 recruitment and enhanced NF-κB and C/EBPβ binding to the IL-8 promoter compared to non-CF cells due to trimethylation of histone H3 at lysine 4 (H3K4me3) and DNA hypomethylation at CpG6. IL-1β increased NF-κB, C/EBPβ, and Brd4 binding. Furthermore, inhibitors of bromodomain and extra-terminal domain family (BET) proteins reduced IL-8 production in CF cells, suggesting a therapeutic target for the BET pathway (103). Regarding microRNA (miRNA) involved in controlling IL-8 production in the CF lung, three recent studies have determined how miRNAs that are aberrantly expressed in the CF airways may post-transcriptionally regulate IL-8 expression. The first report was focused on miR-155, a miRNA that is highly expressed in CF lung. Bhattacharyya and Coll found that expression of miR-155 was elevated in CF IB3-1 lung epithelial cells in culture, compared with control IB3-1/S9 cells. In addition, clinical evidence indicated that miR-155 was also highly expressed in CF lung epithelial cells and circulating CF neutrophils from CF patients. High levels of miR-155 specifically reduced levels of SHIP1, thereby promoting PI3K/Akt activation and contributing to the pro-inflammatory expression of IL-8 in CF lung epithelial cells (104). The other two studies on this topic have investigated miRNAs that are decreased in the CF lung that directly target IL-8 mRNA. Fabbri et al. identified miR-93 as a miRNA that is decreased in IB3-1 and Cufi-1 cells infected with *P. aeruginosa*. The possible involvement of miR-93 in IL-8 gene regulation was validated using three luciferase vectors, including one carrying the complete 3'-UTR region of the IL-8 mRNA and one carrying the same region with a mutated miR-93 site. Specifically, the results obtained indicate that, in addition to NF-κB-dependent up-regulation of IL-8 gene transcription, IL-8 protein expression is post-transcriptionally regulated by interactions of the IL-8 mRNA with the inhibitory miR-93 (105). The involvement of microRNAs in IL-8 is also supported by the study of Oglesby et al. (106), who measured the expression and function of miRNAs decreased in the CF lung. MicroRNA miR-17 was identified as

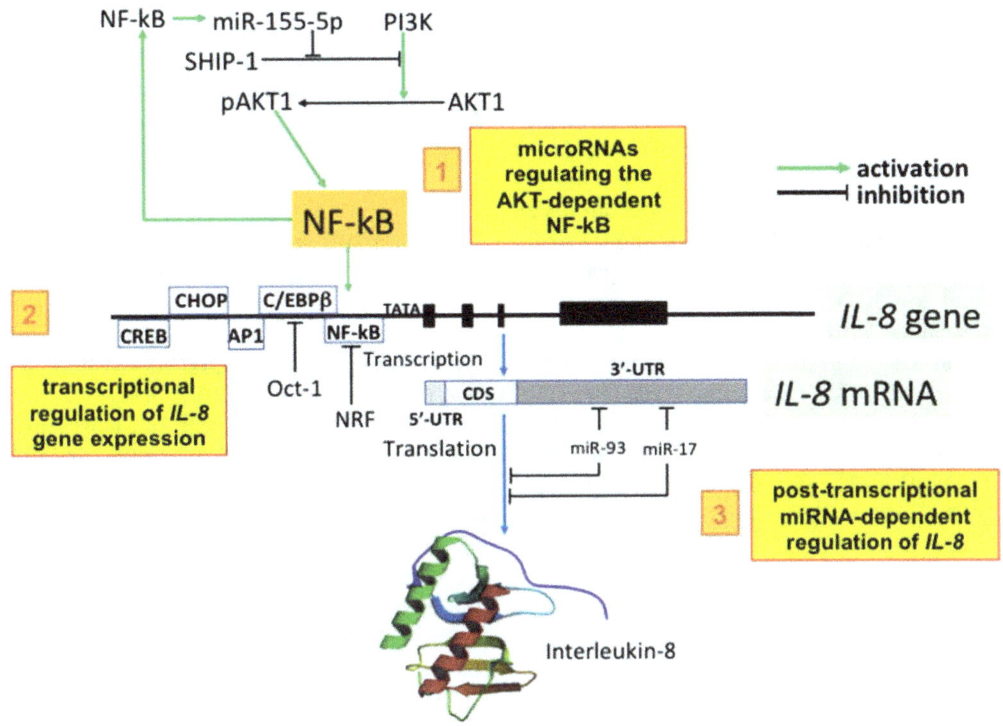

FIGURE 2 | Selected examples of the miRNA network regulating IL-8. 1. microRNAs regulating the AKT-dependent NF-kB: miR-155-5p expression is potentiated by NF-kB and is elevated in CF lung epithelial cells and circulating CF neutrophils biopsied from CF patients. High levels of miR-155 specifically reduce the levels of SHIP1, thereby promoting PI3K/Akt activation. Phospho-Akt levels are therefore elevated in CF lung epithelial cells and can be specifically lowered by either antagomir-155 or elevated expression of SHIP1. Elevated miR-155-5p contributes to the pro-inflammatory expression of IL-8 in CF lung epithelial cells by lowering SHIP1 expression and thereby activating the PI3K/Akt signaling pathway (104). 2. transcriptional regulation of *IL-8* gene expression: *IL-8* promoter is under the control of transcription factors enhancing *IL-8* mRNA production (examples are NF-κB, AP-1, C/EBPβ, CHOP, and CREB); furthermore, IL-8 gene expression is repressed by Oct-1 and by NF-κB repressing factor (NRF). All these transcription factors are regulated by microRNAs. 3. post-transcriptional miRNA-dependent regulation of IL-8: Fabbri et al. identified miR-93 as a miRNA that is decreased in cystic fibrosis IB3-1 and Cufi-1 cells infected with *P. aeruginosa*. The possible involvement of miR-93 in *IL-8* gene regulation was validated using luciferase vectors and the results obtained indicate that IL-8 protein expression is post-transcriptionally regulated by interactions of the *IL-8* mRNA with the inhibitory miR-93 (105). The involvement of microRNAs in IL-8 is also supported by the study of Oglesby et al. (106) who identified miR-17 as a miRNA regulating IL-8. Interestingly, its expression was decreased in adult CF bronchial brushings and bronchial epithelial cells chronically stimulated with *Pseudomonas*-conditioned medium (106). 5′-UTR, 3′-UTR: 5′ and 3′ untranslated region of the IL-8 mRNA; CDS, coding sequences.

a miRNA that regulates IL-8 and its expression was decreased in adult CF bronchial brushings and bronchial epithelial cells chronically stimulated with *Pseudomonas*-conditioned medium (106). Another microRNA involved in inflammation is miR-636, as recently demonstrated by Bardin et al. (107). By analyzing miRNAs in human primary air-liquid interface cell cultures, overexpression of miR-636 in CF patients compared to non-CF controls was shown. Functional studies demonstrated that miR-636 directly interacts with IL1R1 and RANK (two pro-inflammatory cytokine receptors), and IKBKB (which encodes IKKβ, a major protein in the NF-κB pathway). A summary of miRNA regulation is depicted in **Figure 2**.

CFTR PROTEIN DEFECTS COOPERATE TO PRO-INFLAMMATORY INTRACELLULAR SIGNALING

The origin of this abnormal inflammatory response in CF continues to be debated, with researchers unsure whether it is initiated by exogenous stimuli, such as persistent microbial infection, or by intrinsic deficiency of CFTR function, with alterations in signal transduction, or both. Dysregulation of the airway innate immune system is associated with CF, being both airway epithelial cells and immune cells susceptible to intrinsic CFTR-associated alterations in signal transduction.

No differences in TLRs expression have been observed between human CF and non-CF airway epithelial cell lines. However, increased expression of TLR2 and TLR5 on the apical membrane of the polarized human CF airway epithelial cells and in CFTR-knockout vs. WT mice were found (108, 109). These different cellular redistributions of TLRs render the CF airway epithelial cells more susceptible to host-pathogen interactions between bacterial constituents (pili and flagellin) and the receptors involved in the transduction of "danger signal" at apical membrane, favoring the release of cytokines (as described before in section host-pathogen interactions and intracellular signaling modulating IL-8/CXCL8 expression).

An intrinsic defect associated with CFTR deficiency is the susceptibility of CF airway cells to accumulate ROS, particularly during pathogen infection. Evidence shows increased oxidative stress in CF (37, 110–116). Although several studies suggest that the oxidative stress in CF is a direct consequence of mitochondrial dysfunction due to perturbed CFTR signaling, others suggest that the accumulation of ROS in CF depends on there being a reduced antioxidant capacity (113). Low mitochondrial reduced glutathione (mtGSH) levels were found in CF patient-derived tracheal cells and in CFTR-knockout mice (117, 118). Indeed, in CF patient-derived pancreatic and tracheal cells a reduction of protein expression of Cu/Zn-superoxide dismutase (SOD1) and Mn-SOD (SOD2) and a reduction in the activity of extracellular SOD (119) has been observed. The oxidative stress in CF lung may: (I) affect autophagy, compromising the expression of CFTR channel (120, 121); (II) induce mtDNA oxidation and damage, triggering inflammasome activation, and/or altering the OXPHOS activity, that in turn produces additional ROS (122, 123); and (III) destroy lung tissue, affecting the cell function and/or exacerbating the inflammatory response (37).

An inherent defective CFTR channel leads to transglutaminase (TG2) upregulation, resulting in defective autophagy with consequent accumulation of aggresomes and ROS (121). Lack of autophagy in macrophages and in airway epithelial cells result in a reduced bacterial clearance and in the accumulation of dysfunctional mitochondria, which in turn promotes secretion of pro-inflammatory cytokines, indicating that autophagy may regulate the inflammation responses by suppressing the secretion of immune mediators (124–126). In fact, the rescue of dysfunctional autophagy in CF, mediated by autophagy inducers such as MTOR inhibitor (rapamycin), TG2 inhibitor (cistamine), and/or modulators of Ca^{2+}-dependent signaling (KB-R7943), attenuated the hyperinflammation in CF lung, improving the CFTR transport to PM and reducing ROS production and cytokine release in macrophages and in primary CF airway cells *in vitro* and in CF mouse models *in vivo* (127–132).

The hyperinflammation of the CF airway is sustained by the accumulation of dysfunctional mitochondria, as an indirect consequence of perturbed CFTR signaling, responsible for ROS production and increased inflammasome-dependent IL-1β release. Mitochondrial defects associated with an abnormal oxidative stress and inflammatory response have been found in CF. The first evidence was shown in 1979, demonstrating that mitochondrial Ca^{2+} uptake and oxygen consumption were altered in mitochondria isolated from CF patient-derived fibroblast (133). In the same year, the mitochondrial NADH dehydrogenase (complex-1) was found altered in CF skin fibroblasts (134), while in 1981 a deficiency of 6-phosphate dehydrogenase in CF patients was found (135). Consistent with the first observations, in CF patient-derived tracheal cells a decreased mitochondrial NADH dehydrogenase activity and mitochondrial membrane potential ($\Delta\psi$) were measured, due to the down-regulation of the mt-ND4 gene that codifies for a subunit of the complex-1 essential for its assembly and activity (136). This alteration was rescued through the reintroduction of CFTR-wt, also indicating that mtGSH depletion in CF is responsible for the altered complex-1 activity (118). Recently, it has been observed that the CFTR corrector agent VX-809 and 4,6,4'-trimethylangelicin (TMA) treatment lead to partial restoration of the mitochondrial failure in CF airway cell lines, producing an improvement in complex-1 activity, $\Delta\psi$ generation, ANT-dependent ADP/ATP exchange, and membrane lipid peroxidation (137). These data indicate that the restoration of mitochondrial physiology is linked to the mitigation of the inflammatory response, suggesting that the mitochondrial defects found in CF airway cells contributes to the susceptibility of CF cells to bacterial infection, influencing the innate immune response.

Several pieces of evidence have shown how the hyperinflammation observed in CF lung is sustained by cell defects associated with CFTR deficiency intrinsic to epithelial, but also in inflammatory, cells. In CF patients, the differentiation of T lymphocytes to Th_{17} phenotype is increased (138), while monocyte-derived macrophages do not respond to IL-13/IL-4 and fail to polarize into M2 while the polarization to the M1 phenotype was unaffected (139). CF macrophages serve as a replicative niche for bacteria to avoid host defenses (140), present deficits in bacterial killing (141, 142), and produce excess cytokines (143). In synthesis, although the initiating event of CF lung inflammation between infection-derived exogenous and CFTR-related endogenous components remains a "chicken and egg" debate still without a final consensus, different converging evidence supports the hypothesis that CFTR-specific signal transduction alterations amplify the extent of the response.

In this context, analysis at a single-cell level might be very informative. For instance, Mould et al. (144) investigated inflammatory macrophage heterogeneity during acute lung inflammation in mice and performed single cell RNA sequencing of macrophages isolated from the airspaces during peak inflammation and resolution of inflammation. They found two transcriptionally distinct subdivisions of alveolar macrophages based on proliferative capacity and inflammatory programing. Of course, overcoming technical obstacles (due, for instance, to debris, and apoptotic cells) rendering difficult isolation of individual cells for single cell analyses is a key issue (145). Finally, on-a-chip devices are expected to bring key information at single-cell levels on hyperinflammation in pulmonary diseases, including CF (146–148). As far this key issue is concerned, starting from the notion that cell-to-cell variability in chemokine/cytokine secretion is largely unknown, Ramji et al. developed and validated a microfluidic device to integrate live-cell imaging of fluorescent reporter proteins with a single-cell assay of protein secretion (146). This device was used to image transcription factor dynamics in macrophages in response to LPS, followed by quantification of secretion of TNF, CCL2, CCL3, and CCL5.

INTRACELLULAR CALCIUM HOMEOSTASIS IN THE REGULATION OF THE EXPRESSION OF CHEMOKINES

Ca^{2+} homeostasis is a pivotal element in regulating the immunological and physical barriers of the airway epithelium in CF. Normally, the exposure to common respiratory bacterial pathogens, such as *P. aeruginosa*, originates in a cytosolic Ca^{2+} transient (about 100 nM) in airway epithelial cell lines necessary to initiate the inflammatory response, inducing the expression, and secretion of pro-inflammatory cytokines (149). A defective CFTR channel leads to the deregulation of Ca^{2+} homeostasis in CF cells, which is detrimental for lung inflammation. Ca^{2+} signaling dysregulations were observed in several human CF airway epithelial cell lines, where the intracellular Ca^{2+} concentration is increased compared to non-CF cells (150) due to: (I) intrinsic defects associated with CFTR deficiency, (II) chronic exposure to bacterial infection, and (III) persistent stimulation by pro-inflammatory mediators.

Intrinsic Defects Associated to CFTR Deficiency

In 1961, Donnell et al. published the first evidence of alterations of Ca^{2+} homeostasis in CF patients (151), which was then confirmed by Feigal et al., through direct measurement of the increased intracellular Ca^{2+} concentration in fibroblasts derived from CF patients (152, 153) and by Cabrini and De Togni as increased cytosolic Ca^{2+} concentration in CF neutrophils (154). In 1982, an increased mitochondrial Ca^{2+} uptake was observed in CF skin fibroblast, due to altered respiratory system activity (155). In 2009, Antigny et al. measured a decreased mitochondrial Ca^{2+} uptake in F508delCFTR airway epithelial cell lines as a consequence of depolarized and fragmented mitochondria (156). The debate is presently lessened because it has been demonstrated that a functional CFTR channel reduces the basal intracellular Ca^{2+} concentration in human airway epithelial cell lines and donor-derived primary airway epithelial cells, influencing the mitochondrial Ca^{2+} signals evoked by physiological and pathological stimuli (132). This abnormal intracellular Ca^{2+} increment in CF epithelial airway cells is in part justified by the reduced activity of Plasma Membrane (PM) Ca^{2+} ATPase (PMCA), which limits the Ca^{2+} efflux through the PM, and increased SERCA activity, which favors the endoplasmic reticulum (ER) Ca^{2+} accumulation (132). This increment in intracellular Ca^{2+} concentration in human epithelial airway cells is normalized by the administration of the corrector agent, VX809 (157). Several other pieces of evidence suggest that the increased intracellular Ca^{2+} concentration observed in CF airway cells depends on multifactorial aspects associated with defective CFTR, involving many Ca^{2+} channels expressed in the PM, including: (I) the Transient Receptor Potential Canonical channel 6 (TRPC6), normally expressed in human primary CF epithelial cells. Its Ca^{2+} influx capacity is enhanced in F508delCFTR and G551D-CFTR cells (158, 159); (II) the Store Operated Ca^{2+} Entry (SOCE) resulted in significantly increased CF airway cell lines and primary cells, due to an enhanced Orai1 channel insertion to PM, with consequent exacerbation of IL-8 secretion (160); and (III) the TRP channel TRPA1, expressed in bronchial columnar epithelial cells. Its direct activation by *P. aeruginosa* increases Ca^{2+} entry, mediating the release of cytokines such as IL-8, IL-1β, and TNF-α (81).

Chronic Exposure to Bacterial Infection and Persistent Stimulation by Pro-inflammatory Mediators

The chronic infection of CF airways amplifies the altered intracellular Ca^{2+} homeostasis of CF epithelial cells, predisposing the airway cells to a hyperinflammatory profile, which contributes to producing an excess of cytokines. Bacterial constituents and pro-inflammatory mediators cooperate, inducing an abnormal intracellular Ca^{2+} signaling in CF airway epithelia due to increased activation of apical G protein-coupled receptors (GPCRs) and a sustained ER Ca^{2+}-release (161). The higher intracellular Ca^{2+} concentration in CF cells contributes to a greater and more prolonged NF-κB activation with consequent effects on the expression and release of pro-inflammatory cytokines, such as IL-8 and IL-1β (82, 161). The persistent NF-κB activation in human CF airway cells is the consequence of the synergistic effects of bacterial components, such as flagellin, where flagellin interacting with asialoGM1 receptor favors the release of ATP from CF airway cell lines, which mediates purinergic receptors and activates downstream intracellular Ca^{2+} signaling that synergizes with the TLR5-dependent signaling to activate NF-κB (see section host-pathogen interactions and intracellular signaling modulating IL-8/CXCL8 expression) (92). The release of nucleotides from bronchial epithelial cells targeting P2Y2 purinergic receptors has been proposed to intervene on different aspects of CFTR regulation and lung pathophysiology (162–165). Bacterial constituents, pili and flagellin, interact with TLRs and TLR-associated glycolipid in airway cells (85, 166). In particular, TLR2 or asialoGM1 linked to TLR2 express both on the apical surface of airway cells and recognize bacterial constituents to induce the pro-inflammatory transcription of CXCL8 or MUC-2 gene via NF-κB activation, through the recruitment of PI3K and phospholipase C gamma (PLCγ), which in turn stimulate the release of Ca^{2+} through Inositol Triphosphate Receptors (IP3R) channels (167, 168). The generation of cytosolic Ca^{2+} transients activates classical Protein Kinase C (PKC) α and β isoforms, which through a phosphorylation cascade mediate the activation of NF-κB (169). In a similar molecular pathway, PLC beta 3 (PLCB3) also plays a relevant role in triggering cytosolic Ca^{2+} transients induced by *P. aeruginosa*, regulating the activation of PKCα and PKCβ to induce an NF-κB-dependent transcription of CXCL8 gene in human airway epithelial cell lines and in patient-derived primary cells (78). β-sitosterol (BSS) was used to inhibit the active form of PKCs involved in the transduction of *P. aeruginosa*-dependent pro-inflammatory Ca^{2+}-dependent signaling in CF patient-derived airway epithelial cells, leading to a significant reduction in expression of IL-8, growth-related oncogene (GRO)-α, and GRO-β (170). The role of PLCB3 in amplifying the expression and release of IL-8 during pathogen infection, through the regulation of intracellular Ca^{2+} transients, is associated with the severity and progression of CF lung disease. Single Nucleotide Polymorphisms (SNP) genetic study with the progression of CF lung disease severity, identify from a panel of 135 genes of immune response the association of c.2534C>T (p.S845L) variant of PLCB3 with a mild progression of pulmonary disease in CF (93). PLCB3-S845L results in a loss-of-function variant, where defective intracellular Ca^{2+} redistribution and PKCs' activation limited the IL-8, IL-1β, and MUC5 expression in CF patient-derived airway epithelial cells exposed to *P. aeruginosa* or CF patient-derived mucopurulent material. The IP3R-mediated ER Ca^{2+}-release is significantly augmented in CF epithelial cell lines (171), a consequence also of ER Ca^{2+} store expansion observed in CF cells (150). The ER expansion is not dependent on ER retention of misfolded CFTR, but reflects an airway epithelial response acquired following persistent bacterial infection, resulting in ER unfolded protein response (UPR) activation mediated by the IRE1/XBP-1 pathway and in a larger intracellular Ca^{2+} mobilization in response to abnormal GPCRs activation (172).

The sustained ER Ca^{2+}-release in CF airway cells conditions the mitochondria to a direct involvement in the pro-inflammatory response. CF airway cell lines and CF patient-derived airway primary cells are prone to *P. aeruginosa*-dependent mitochondrial perturbations, in which the mitochondrial Ca^{2+} uniporter (MCU) is a signal-integrating organelle that mediates mitochondrial ROS-dependent NLRP3 inflammasome activation and recruitment of both NLRP3 and NLRC4 inflammasome (132). The degree and quality of the inflammatory response in CF airway cells is also sustained by *P. aeruginosa*-dependent mitochondrial perturbations, initiated by flagellin, such as mitochondrial membrane potential loss, ROS production, and mitochondrial fragmentation (132). Rimessi et al. have characterized the role of mitochondria as drivers of the *P. aeruginosa*-triggered inflammatory exacerbation in CF airway cells, demonstrating that mitochondrial Ca^{2+} signaling plays a critical role in inflammasome NLRP3 recruitment and inflammasome-dependent IL-1β and IL-18 release in CF airway cell lines and in CF patient-derived airway primary cells (132). By modulating the MCU-dependent mitochondrial Ca^{2+}-uptake, genetically or mediating pharmacological inhibition with KB-R7943, it is possible to control the pathogen-dependent mitochondrial dysfunction preventing the integration of pro-inflammatory signals from mitochondria into CF patient-derived airway primary cells and *in vivo* mouse models (131, 132).

Although whether the Ca^{2+}-dependent activation of chloride channels in CF bronchial epithelial cells could partially vary the defects of CFTR ion transport is presently under scrutiny (173), the results recalled above support the concept that the up-regulation of intracellular Ca^{2+} signaling is a key amplifier of the inflammatory response and lung pathogenesis in CF, which opens the issue of new potential molecular therapeutic targets.

TARGETING NEUTROPHIL CHEMOTAXIS IN CF: NOVEL MOLECULES AND DRUG REPURPOSING

Preliminary observations in rat lung models (59) suggested the repurposing of ibuprofen, a non-steroideal anti-inflammatory drug used in conditions like osteoarthritis, rheumatoid arthritis, juvenile idiopathic arthritis, and acutely painful musculoskeletal conditions, to clinical use for CF patients (174, 175). Long-term application of this drug, as reported by a Cochrane analysis, has proved the concept that strategies to modulate lung inflammation can be beneficial for people with CF (176). As ibuprofen inhibits prostaglandin synthesis (177), a very broad anti-inflammatory mechanism that is not closely specific to the pathophysiology of CF lung inflammation, innovative approaches to target the adverse effects produced by the huge amount of neutrophils in the CF conductive airways have been recently tested. Some of these approaches have been launched upon the knowledge of the specificity of CF lung inflammation, whereas others were just pure empirical testing. The first attempts were focused on antagonizing neutrophil proteases elastase, one of the main deleterious effect of neutrophil inflammation in CF (28, 29, 178–186). Different elastase inhibitors have also been recently tested in clinical trial, with promising results in terms of safety and tolerability (187, 188), maintaining the high levels of interest in the rationale of targeting neutrophil elastase in CF lung inflammation (186).

Early signaling evoked by bacteria has been tested by inhibition of TLR2 or by inducing extracellular calcium entry through calcium ionophores (81, 189). More downstream the production of IL-8, different antagonists of its receptors that block its action on cell targets have been challenged (190–192). More recently, different molecular approaches targeting the intracellular signaling in bronchial epithelial cells have been developed. In consideration of the key role of NF-κB in the transcriptional regulation of IL-8 and other pro-inflammatory genes, several studies have been focused on pharmacological alteration of NF-κB activity. The transcription factor (TF) decoy strategy was applied by Bezzerri et al., using TF oligodeoxynucleotides (ODNs) to NF-κB able to inhibit transcription of IL-8 in bronchial cells (89). The TF decoy approach was based on the intracellular delivery of double-stranded ODNs causing inhibition of the binding of TF-related proteins (as determined *in vitro* using EMSA assays) to the different consensus sequences in the promoter of specific genes. When CF cells were transfected with double-stranded TF "decoy" ODNs, mimicking different NF-κB consensus sequences, partial inhibition of *P. aeruginosa*-dependent transcription of IL-8 was obtained. In addition, other NF-κB regulated genes were inhibited, such as GRO-gamma and IL-6. In order to demonstrate that TFD against NF-κB interferes with the NF-κB pathway, Finotti et al. demonstrated mediating chromatin immunoprecipitation (ChIP) treatment with TFD oligodeoxyribonucleotides of IB3-1 cells infected with *P. aeruginosa* leads to a decreased occupancy of the IL-8 gene promoter by NF-κB factors (193). Further studies were focused on the development of more stable therapeutic molecules and on the delivery strategy for TFD molecules. Among stable ODN analogs, peptide nucleic acids (PNAs)-based agents were found to be promising for CF. In this respect, PNA-DNA-PNA (PDP) chimeras are molecules of great interest from several points of view: (a) they can be complexed with liposomes and microspheres; (b) they are resistant to DNases, serum, and cytoplasmic extracts; and (c) they are potent decoy molecules (194, 195). By using electrophoretic mobility shift assay and RT-PCR analysis, it was demonstrated that: (a) the effects of PDP/PDP NF-κB decoy chimera on the accumulation of pro-inflammatory mRNAs in *P. aeruginosa*-infected IB3-1 cells in particular; (b) the PDP/PDP chimera is a strong inhibitor of IL-8 gene expression; and (c) the effect of PDP/PDP chimeras, unlike those of ODN-based decoys, are observed even in the absence of protection with lipofectamine (193–196). In another study, NF-κB decoys were employed with the hypothesis that they may limit lung inflammation in CF. In the study by De Stefano et al. (197), the effects of decoy ODN targeting NF-κB and delivered through biodegradable and respirable poly(D,L-lactide-co-glycolide) large porous particles (LPP) were determined on IL-6 and IL-8 mRNA expression in CF cells stimulated with lipopolysaccharide (LPS) from *P. aeruginosa*. The conclusion was that respirable biodegradable decoy ODN LPP may represent a promising strategy for inhibiting NF-κB transcriptional activity and related gene expression. This treatment, *in vivo*, was expected to reduce lung chronic inflammation in CF patients. Interestingly, De Stefano et al. (198) investigated the effects of NF-kB decoys delivered with inhalable nanoparticles in a rat model of lung inflammation induced by intratracheal aerosolization of LPS from *Pseudomonas aeruginosa*. A single intratracheal insufflation of the decoy ODNs reduced the bronchoalveolar neutrophil infiltration induced by LPS. This reduction was associated with decreased NF-κB/DNA binding activity, and decreased the content of IL-6, IL-8, and mucin-2 in lung homogenates.

In consideration of the involvement of microRNAs in the post-transcriptional regulation of IL-8 and other pro-inflammatory genes, both antagomiR and miRNA replacement approaches have been proposed (199–202). This confirmed that, in addition to relevance for the theoretical point of view, the studies on epigenetic regulation of chemokines (described in Chapter 5) might be important for the development of therapeutic protocols. For instance, transfection of CF cells with miR-93 (105) and miR-636 mimics (107) leads to an IL-8 decrease (105) and to a reduction of NF-κB activity, causing decreased secretion of IL-8 and IL-6 (200, 201). Another miRNA target to be considered is miR-199a-3p, whose expression is inversely correlated with increases in the expression of IKKβ and IL-8 (200). On the other hand, targeting miR-155 with antagomir might also be considered for IL-8 reduction (104). In fact, down-regulation of miR-155 was found to suppress the IL-8-associated pro-inflammatory phenotype in CF cells. In order to reduce the miR-155 levels in CF cells, antagomiR molecules against miR-155 were employed, modified with cholesterol to permit efficient entry into cells. Incubation of IB3-1 cells with antagomir-155 effectively down-regulated miR-155 expression, together with a sharp decrease in IL-8 mRNA and protein levels (104). On the other hand, as expected, miRNAs were also demonstrated to directly target the 3′UTR of IL-8 mRNA, such as miR-93 (105) and miR-17 (105). Therefore, modulating the expression of miRNAs that target IL-8 mRNA in CF bronchial epithelial cells is likely to represent a new therapeutic strategy for CF (199–201).

These studies have conclusively demonstrated that the pro-inflammatory status in CF is under the control of a complex network constituted by transcription factors and non-coding RNAs, responsible for transcriptional and post-transcriptional regulation of the expression of genes, such as IL-8, belonging to the pro-inflammatory CF network. These studies allowed the identification of novel targets for pharmacological interventions based on newly designed therapeutic approaches.

In addition to the development of new experimental approaches, recent efforts have been undertaken on drug repurposing, in order to bring new therapies based on drugs already used for other indications. This is expected to bring to the market several treatments at a lower risk, reduced cost, and less development time when compared to conventional drug development programs (202–204). One of the most interesting classes of molecules are psoralens, extensively studied as molecules to be employed in PUVA (Psoralen and Ultraviolet A)-therapy, a treatment extensively used in a variety of pathological conditions, including eczema, psoriasis, graft-vs.-host disease, vitiligo, mycosis fungoides, large-plaque parapsoriasis, and cutaneous T-cell lymphoma (205). It was in a study that found that 5-methoxypsoralen reduces *P. aeruginosa*-dependent IL-8 transcription in bronchial epithelial cell lines (206). When the analysis was extended to analogs of 5-methoxypsoralen (207, 208), a potent effect was observed with 4,6,4′-trimethyl-angelicin (TMA), which inhibited *P. aeruginosa*-dependent IL-8 transcription at a nanomolar concentration in IB3-1, CuFi-1, CFBE41o-, and Calu-3 bronchial epithelial cell lines. Analysis of phosphoproteins involved in pro-inflammatory transmembrane signaling evidenced that TMA reduces the phosphorylation of ribosomal S6 kinase-1 and AKT2/3, which were found to be involved in *P. aeruginosa*-dependent activation of IL-8 gene transcription (208). In addition, to understand whether the NF-κB pathway should be considered a target of TMA, chromatin immunoprecipitation was performed, demonstrating that TMA (100 nM) preincubated in whole living cells reduced the interaction of NF-κB with the promoter of IL-8 gene. These results suggest that TMA could inhibit IL-8 gene transcription mainly by intervening on driving the recruitment of activated transcription factors on the IL-8 gene promoter, as demonstrated in NF-κB (208). Recently, TMA was also shown to exhibit, in addition to anti-inflammatory activity, potentiation and correction of the CFTR. In conclusion, TMA is a triple-acting compound that reduces excessive IL-8 expression and potentiating/correcting CFTR function (209, 210). Another repurposed drug proposed for possible anti-inflammatory effects is azithromycin (AZM). IL-8 expression and DNA binding activity of two key pro-inflammatory transcription factors, NF-κB and AP-1, were investigated in CF and isogenic non-CF airway epithelial cell lines. AZM reduced both IL-8 mRNA and protein expression in CF cells reaching the levels of non-CF cells. In the presence of AZM reduction of NF-κB and AP-1, DNA binding was also observed (211). Regarding anti-inflammatory approaches, *in vitro* studies have tested the effects of genistein, fluvastatin, and corilagin, amongst others (212–214). The isoflavonoid genistein [5,7-Dihydroxy-3-(4-hydroxyphenyl)chromen-4-one] reduces IL-8 production in cultured CF bronchial gland cells by increasing cytosolic IκBα protein levels, thereby inhibiting NF-kB activation (212). The statin fluvastatin [(±)-(3R′,5S′,6E)-7-[3-(4-Fluorophenyl)-1-isopropylindol-2-yl]-3,5-dihydroxy-6-heptenoate] decreased IL-8 production in whole blood in response to *Pseudomonas* or

Aspergillus antigens, by preventing the prenylation of molecules, such as rho-A, ras, or rac, implicated in IL-8 signaling (213). Corilagin [beta-1-O-galloyl-3,6-(R)-hexahydroxydiphenoyl-d-glucose], a gallotannin identified in several plants, including *Phyllanthus urinaria*, binds to NF-κB, thus inhibiting NF-κB/DNA interactions and decreasing IL-8 gene expression in CF bronchial IB3-1 cells (214).

As for drug repurposing, corilagin, already shown to exhibit versatile medicinal activities, was found to be of potential use as a possible therapeutic molecule for CF. Interestingly, in addition of IL-8 inhibition, corilagin inhibits TNF-α-induced secretion of MCP-1 and RANTES (214).

The possible identification of repurposed drugs was also tackled by alternative approaches, such as connectivity mapping (ssCMap) to predict A20-inducing drugs and their anti-inflammatory action in CF. A20 is a NF-κB down-regulator that is expressed at low levels in CF and it is hypothesized to be a key target to normalize the inflammatory response (215). Publicly available gene array expression data, together with a statistically significant connections' map (sscMap), were employed. The objective was to predict drugs already licensed for therapeutic use in human pathologies to induce A20 mRNA and protein expression and thereby reduce inflammation. Ikarugamycin and quercetin have been identified as possible candidates for anti-inflammatory approaches, analyzing their effects on A20 and NF-κB(p65) expression (mRNA) as well as IL-8 pro-inflammatory cytokine release in the presence and absence of bacterial LPS in bronchial epithelial cells lines and in primary nasal epithelial cells from patients with CF and non-CF controls (215). Despite the very interesting results obtained from studies of drug repurposing in CF, the safety assessment in a new disease indication (CF in this case) is still an important concern in the regulatory process. While the safety assessment is based on drug label information, the drug repurposing approach may involve different formulations, changes in dosage that should be given great attention in the different patient populations considered.

CONCLUDING REMARKS AND PERSPECTIVES

The present review outlines different specific pathophysiological aspects of CF lung inflammation in which the bronchial epithelial cells represent a "crossroad of signaling" in this disease. Particular emphasis has been given to the role of bronchial epithelial cells in driving the process of neutrophil chemotaxis, with special regard to intracellular signaling, that could be considered a therapeutic target to reduce the lung tissue damage dependent on the byproducts released by hyper-activated neutrophils in the CF bronchial mucosa. To translate into therapy, a special focus was placed on innovative molecules or on drug repurposing to target pathways that are specific of the CF lung pathophysiology, instead of testing broad range anti-inflammatory molecules. As CF lung inflammation is a clearly secondary effect of altered CFTR protein defective ion transport, a question arises on whether in the era of CFTR modulators, with increasing efficacy in CFTR rescue, gating potentiation, and PM stabilization, anti-inflammatory drugs maintain a specific therapeutic rationale. It has already been shown that rescue of F508del CFTR in CF in experimental model systems can partly reduce the release of pro-inflammatory mediators, including IL-8 (216–218). However, the CFTR correctors and potentiators are not available for all the classes of CFTR molecular defects, leaving a significant fraction of CF patients without this treatment option. The clinical response has been shown to be variable within patients with the same class of mutations; the advanced inflammatory disease in adolescent and adult CF patients is unlikely to be completely halted using only CFTR correctors and potentiators, leaving the development of novel anti-inflammatory drugs a rational unmet need for CF treatment (219, 220).

AUTHOR CONTRIBUTIONS

GC, AR, PP, and RG initiated the concept and wrote the manuscript together with MB, IL, and AF. All authors contributed to the article and approved the submitted version.

ACKNOWLEDGMENTS

We are grateful to Mirko Pinotti, Marco Cipolli, Adriana Chilin, Marco Prosdocimi, Maria Cristina Dechecchi, Anna Tamanini, Valentino Bezzerri, Paola Prandini, Lisa Provezza, Alessandra Santangelo, Silvia Munari, and Simone Patergnani for helpful discussions. PP is grateful to Camilla degli Scrovegni for continuous support.

REFERENCES

1. Riordan JR, Rommens JM, Kerem B, Alon N, Rozmahel R, Grzelczak Z, et al. Identification of the cystic fibrosis gene: cloning and characterization of complementary DNA. *Science.* (1989) 245:1066–73. doi: 10.1126/science.2475911
2. Rommens JM, Iannuzzi MC, Kerem B, Drumm ML, Melmer G, Dean M, et al. Identification of the cystic fibrosis gene: chromosome walking and jumping. *Science.* (1989) 245:1059–65. doi: 10.1126/science.2772657
3. Kerem B, Rommens JM, Buchanan JA, Markiewicz D, Cox TK, Chakravarti A, et al. Identification of the cystic fibrosis gene: genetic analysis. *Science.* (1989) 245:1073–80. doi: 10.1126/science.2570460
4. Khan TZ, Wagener JS, Bost T, Martinez J, Accurso FJ, Riches DW. Early pulmonary inflammation in infants with cystic fibrosis. *Am J Respir Crit Care Med.* (1995) 151:1075–82. doi: 10.1164/ajrccm.151.4.7697234
5. Noah TL, Black HR, Cheng PW, Wood RE, Leigh MW. Nasal and bronchoalveolar lavage fluid cytokines in early cystic fibrosis. *J Infect Dis.* (1997) 175:638–47. doi: 10.1093/infdis/175.3.638
6. Armstrong DS, Grimwood K, Carlin JB, Carzino R, Gutièrrez JP, Hull J, et al. Lower airway inflammation in infants and young children with cystic fibrosis. *Am J Respir Crit Care Med.* (1997) 156:1197–204. doi: 10.1164/ajrccm.156.4.96-11058
7. Stoltz DA, Meyerholz DK, Welsh MJ. Origins of cystic fibrosis lung disease. *N Engl J Med.* (2015) 372:351–62. doi: 10.1056/NEJMra1300109

8. Boucher RC. Evidence for airway surface dehydration as the initiating event in CF airway disease. *J Intern Med.* (2007) 261:5–16. doi: 10.1111/j.1365-2796.2006.01744.x
9. Tingpej P, Smith L, Rose B, Zhu H, Conibear T, Al Nassafi K, et al. Phenotypic characterization of clonal and non-clonal *Pseudomonas aeruginosa* strains isolated from lungs of adults with cystic fibrosis. *J Clin Microbiol.* (2007) 45:1697–704. doi: 10.1128/JCM.02364-06
10. Boucher RC. Airway surface dehydration in cystic fibrosis: pathogenesis and therapy. *Annu Rev Med.* (2007) 58:157–70. doi: 10.1146/annurev.med.58.071905.105316
11. Derichs N, Jin BJ, Song Y, Finkbeiner WE, Verkman AS. Hyperviscous airway periciliary and mucous liquid layers in cystic fibrosis measured by confocal fluorescence photobleaching. *FASEB J.* (2011) 25:2325–32. doi: 10.1096/fj.10-179549
12. Hayes E, Pohl K, McElvaney NG, Reeves EP. The cystic fibrosis neutrophil: a specialized yet potentially defective cell. *Arch Immunol Ther Exp.* (2011) 59:97–112. doi: 10.1007/s00005-011-0113-6
13. Laval J, Ralhan A, Hartl D. Neutrophils in cystic fibrosis. *Biol Chem.* (2016) 397:485–96. doi: 10.1515/hsz-2015-0271
14. Painter RG, Valentine VG, Lanson NA Jr, Leidal K, Zhang Q, Lombard G, et al. CFTR Expression in human neutrophils and the phagolysosomal chlorination defect in cystic fibrosis. *Biochemistry.* (2006) 45:10260–9. doi: 10.1021/bi060490t
15. Painter RG, Bonvillain RW, Valentine VG, Lombard GA, LaPlace SG, Nauseef WM, et al. The role of chloride anion and CFTR in killing of *Pseudomonas aeruginosa* by normal and CF neutrophils. *J Leukoc Biol.* (2008) 83:1345–53. doi: 10.1189/jlb.0907658
16. Painter RG, Marrero L, Lombard GA, Valentine VG, Nauseef WM, Wang G. CFTR-mediated halide transport in phagosomes of human neutrophils. *J Leukoc Biol.* (2010) 87:933–42. doi: 10.1189/jlb.1009655
17. Bonfield TL, Hodges CA, Cotton CU, Drumm ML. Absence of the cystic fibrosis transmembrane regulator (Cftr) from myeloid-derived cells slows resolution of inflammation and infection. *J Leukoc Biol.* (2012) 92:1111–22. doi: 10.1189/jlb.0412188
18. Ng HP, Zhou Y, Song K, Hodges CA, Drumm ML, Wang G. Neutrophil-mediated phagocytic host defense defect in myeloid Cftr-inactivated mice. *PLoS ONE.* (2014) 9:e106813. doi: 10.1371/journal.pone.0106813
19. Zhou Y, Song K, Painter RG, Aiken M, Reiser J, Stanton BA, et al. Cystic fibrosis transmembrane conductance regulator recruitment to phagosomes in neutrophils. *J Innate Immun.* (2013) 5:219–30. doi: 10.1159/000346568
20. Pohl K, Hayes E, Keenan J, Henry M, Meleady P, Molloy K, et al. A neutrophil intrinsic impairment affecting Rab27a and degranulation in cystic fibrosis is corrected by CFTR potentiator therapy. *Blood.* (2014) 124:999–1009. doi: 10.1182/blood-2014-02-555268
21. Hartl D, Latzin P, Hordijk P, Marcos V, Rudolph C, Woischnik M, et al. Cleavage of CXCR1 on neutrophils disables bacterial killing in cystic fibrosis lung disease. *Nat Med.* (2007) 13:1423–30. doi: 10.1038/nm1690
22. Döring G. Polymorphonuclear leukocyte elastase: its effects on the pathogenesis of *Pseudomonas aeruginosa* infection in cystic fibrosis. *Antibiot Chemother.* (1989) 42:169–76. doi: 10.1159/000417617
23. Nadel JA. Protease actions on airway secretions. Relevance to cystic fibrosis. *Ann N Y Acad Sci.* (1991) 624:286–96. doi: 10.1111/j.1749-6632.1991.tb17027.x
24. Birrer P, McElvaney NG, Rüdeberg A, Sommer CW, Liechti-Gallati S, Kraemer R, et al. Protease-antiprotease imbalance in the lungs of children with cystic fibrosis. *Am J Respir Crit Care Med.* (1994) 150:207–13. doi: 10.1164/ajrccm.150.1.7912987
25. Döring G. The role of neutrophil elastase in chronic inflammation. *Am J Respir Crit Care Med.* (1994) 150:S114–7. doi: 10.1164/ajrccm/150.6_Pt_2.S114
26. Suter S. The role of bacterial proteases in the pathogenesis of cystic fibrosis. *Am J Respir Crit Care Med.* (1994) 150:S118–22. doi: 10.1164/ajrccm/150.6_Pt_2.S118
27. Venaille TJ, Ryan G, Robinson BW. Epithelial cell damage is induced by neutrophil-derived, not pseudomonas-derived, proteases in cystic fibrosis sputum. *Respir Med.* (1998) 92:233–40. doi: 10.1016/S0954-6111(98)90101-9
28. Kelly E, Greene CM, McElvaney NG. Targeting neutrophil elastase in cystic fibrosis. *Expert Opin Ther Targets.* (2008) 12:145–57. doi: 10.1517/14728222.12.2.145
29. Griese M, Kappler M, Gaggar A, Hartl D. Inhibition of airway proteases in cystic fibrosis lung disease. *Eur Respir J.* (2008) 32:783–95. doi: 10.1183/09031936.00146807
30. Dittrich AS, Kühbandner I, Gehrig S, Rickert-Zacharias V, Twigg M, Wege S, et al. Elastase activity on sputum neutrophils correlates with severity of lung disease in cystic fibrosis. *Eur Respir J.* (2018) 51:1701910. doi: 10.1183/13993003.01910-2017
31. McKelvey MC, Weldon S, McAuley DF, Mall MA, Taggart CC. Targeting proteases in cystic fibrosis lung disease: paradigms, progress, and potential. *Am J Respir Crit Care Med.* (2019). 201:141–7. doi: 10.1164/rccm.201906-1190PP
32. Le Gars M, Descamps D, Roussel D, Saussereau E, Guillot L, Ruffin M, et al. Neutrophil elastase degrades cystic fibrosis transmembrane conductance regulator via calpains and disables channel function *in vitro* and *in vivo*. *Am J Respir Crit Care Med.* (2013) 187:170–9. doi: 10.1164/rccm.201205-0875OC
33. Taggart C, Coakley RJ, Greally P, Canny G, O'Neill SJ, McElvaney NG. Increased elastase release by CF neutrophils is mediated by tumor necrosis factor-alpha and interleukin-8. *Am J Physiol Lung Cell Mol Physiol.* (2000) 278:L33–41. doi: 10.1152/ajplung.2000.278.1.L33
34. Nakamura H, Yoshimura K, McElvaney NG, Crystal RG. Neutrophil elastase in respiratory epithelial lining fluid of individuals with cystic fibrosis induces interleukin-8 gene expression in a human bronchial epithelial cell line. *J Clin Invest.* (1992) 89:1478–84. doi: 10.1172/JCI115738
35. Walsh DE, Greene CM, Carroll TP, Taggart CC, Gallagher PM, O'Neill SJ, et al. Interleukin-8 up-regulation by neutrophil elastase is mediated by MyD88/IRAK/TRAF-6 in human bronchial epithelium. *J Biol Chem.* (2001) 276:35494–9. doi: 10.1074/jbc.M103543200
36. Devaney JM, Greene CM, Taggart CC, Carroll TP, O'Neill SJ, McElvaney NG. Neutrophil elastase up-regulates interleukin-8 via toll-like receptor 4. *FEBS Lett.* (2003) 544:129–32. doi: 10.1016/S0014-5793(03)00482-4
37. Galli F, Battistoni A, Gambari R, Pompella A, Bragonzi A, Pilolli F, et al. Oxidative stress and antioxidant therapy in cystic fibrosis. *Biochim Biophys Acta.* (2012) 1822:690–713. doi: 10.1016/j.bbadis.2011.12.012
38. Cantin AM, North SL, Fells GA, Hubbard RC, Crystal RG. Oxidant-mediated epithelial cell injury in idiopathic pulmonary fibrosis. *J Clin Invest.* (1987) 79:1665–73. doi: 10.1172/JCI113005
39. Cantin A, Woods DE. Protection by antibiotics against myeloperoxidase-dependent cytotoxicity to lung epithelial cells *in vitro*. *J Clin Invest.* (1993) 91:38–45. doi: 10.1172/JCI116196
40. Witko-Sarsat V, Delacourt C, Rabier D, Bardet J, Nguyen AT, Descamps-Latscha B. Neutrophil-derived long-lived oxidants in cystic fibrosis sputum. *Am J Respir Crit Care Med.* (1995) 152:1910–6. doi: 10.1164/ajrccm.152.6.8520754
41. Worlitzsch D, Herberth G, Ulrich M, Döring G. Catalase, myeloperoxidase and hydrogen peroxide in cystic fibrosis. *Eur Respir J.* (1998) 11:377–83. doi: 10.1183/09031936.98.11020377
42. Marcos V, Zhou-Suckow Z, Önder Yildirim A, Bohla A, Hector A, Vitkov L, et al. Free DNA in cystic fibrosis airway fluids correlates with airflow obstruction. *Mediators Inflamm.* (2015) 2015:408935. doi: 10.1155/2015/408935
43. Lethem MI, James SL, Marriott C, Burke JF. The origin of DNA associated with mucus glycoproteins in cystic fibrosis sputum. *Eur Respir J.* (1990) 3:19–23.
44. Marcos V, Zhou Z, Yildirim AO, Bohla A, Hector A, Vitkov L, et al. CXCR2 mediates NADPH oxidase-independent neutrophil extracellular trap formation in cystic fibrosis airway inflammation. *Nat Med.* (2010) 16:1018–23. doi: 10.1038/nm.2209
45. Cheng OZ, Palaniyar N. NET balancing: a problem in inflammatory lung diseases. *Front Immunol.* (2013) 4:1. doi: 10.3389/fimmu.2013.00001
46. Porto BN, Stein RT. Neutrophil extracellular traps in pulmonary diseases: too much of a good thing? *Front Immunol.* (2016) 7:311. doi: 10.3389/fimmu.2016.00311

47. Schultz A, Stick S. Early pulmonary inflammation and lung damage in children with cystic fibrosis. *Respirology.* (2015) 20:569–78. doi: 10.1111/resp.12521
48. Montgomery ST, Mall MA, Kicic A, Stick SM, AREST CF. Hypoxia and sterile inflammation in cystic fibrosis airways: mechanisms and potential therapies. *Eur Respir J.* (2017) 49:1600903. doi: 10.1183/13993003.00903-2016
49. Esther CR Jr, Muhlebach MS, Ehre C, Hill DB, Wolfgang MC, Kesimer M, et al. Mucus accumulation in the lungs precedes structural changes and infection in children with cystic fibrosis. *Sci Transl Med.* (2019) 11:eaav3488. doi: 10.1126/scitranslmed.aav3488
50. Höpken UE, Lu B, Gerard NP, Gerard C. The C5a chemoattractant receptor mediates mucosal defence to infection. *Nature.* (1996) 383:86–9. doi: 10.1038/383086a0
51. Gerard NP, Lu B, Liu P, Craig S, Fujiwara Y, Okinaga S, et al. An anti- inflammatory function for the complement anaphylatoxin C5a-binding protein, C5L2. *J Biol Chem.* (2005) 280:39677–80. doi: 10.1074/jbc.C500287200
52. van den Berg CW, Tambourgi DV, Clark HW, Hoong SJ, Spiller OB, McGreal EP. Mechanism of neutrophil dysfunction: neutrophil serine proteases cleave and inactivate the C5a receptor. *J Immunol.* (2014) 192:1787–95. doi: 10.4049/jimmunol.1301920
53. Sass LA, Hair PS, Perkins AM, Shah TA, Krishna NK, Cunnion KM. Complement effectors of inflammation in cystic fibrosis lung fluid correlate with clinical measures of disease. *PLoS ONE.* (2015) 10:e0144723. doi: 10.1371/journal.pone.0144723
54. Hair PS, Sass LA, Vazifedan T, Shah TA, Krishna NK, Cunnion KM. Complement effectors, C5a and C3a, in cystic fibrosis lung fluid correlate with disease severity. *PLoS ONE.* (2017) 12:e0173257. doi: 10.1371/journal.pone.0173257
55. Ford-Hutchinson AW, Bray MA, Doig MV, Shipley ME, Smith MJ. Leukotriene B, a potent chemokinetic and aggregating substance released from polymorphonuclear leukocytes. *Nature.* (1980) 286:264–5. doi: 10.1038/286264a0
56. Sampson AP, Spencer DA, Green CP, Piper PJ, Price JF. Leukotrienes in the sputum and urine of cystic fibrosis children. *Br J Clin Pharmacol.* (1990) 30:861–9. doi: 10.1111/j.1365-2125.1990.tb05452.x
57. Konstan MW, Walenga RW, Hilliard KA, Hilliard JB. Leukotriene B4 markedly elevated in the epithelial lining fluid of patients with cystic fibrosis. *Am Rev Respir Dis.* (1993) 148:896–901. doi: 10.1164/ajrccm/148.4_Pt_1.896
58. Carpagnano GE, Barnes PJ, Geddes DM, Hodson ME, Kharitonov SA. Increased leukotriene B4 and interleukin-6 in exhaled breath condensate in cystic fibrosis. *Am J Respir Crit Care Med.* (2003) 167:1109–12. doi: 10.1164/rccm.200203-179OC
59. Konstan MW, Vargo KM, Davis PB. Ibuprofen attenuates the inflammator response to Pseudomonas aeruginosa in a rat model of chronic pulmonary infection. Implications for antiinflammatory therapy in cystic fibrosis. *Am Rev Respir Dis.* (1990) 141:186–92. doi: 10.1164/ajrccm/141.1.186
60. Konstan MW, Davis PB. Pharmacological approaches for the discovery and development of new anti-inflammatory agents for the treatment of cystic fibrosis. *Adv Drug Deliv Rev.* (2002) 54:1409–23. doi: 10.1016/S0169-409X(02)00146-1
61. Konstan MW, Döring G, Heltshe SL, Lands LC, Hilliard KA, Koker P, et al. A randomized double blind, placebo controlled phase 2 trial of BIIL 284BS (an LTB4 receptor antagonist) for the treatment of lung disease in children and adults with cystic fibrosis. *J Cyst Fibros.* (2014) 13:148–55. doi: 10.1016/j.jcf.2013.12.009
62. Döring G, Bragonzi A, Paroni M, Aktürk FF, Cigana C, Schmidt A, et al. BIIL 284 reduces neutrophil numbers but increases P. aeruginosa bacteremia and inflammation in mouse lungs. *J Cyst Fibros.* (2014) 13:156–63. doi: 10.1016/j.jcf.2013.10.007
63. Forrest OA, Ingersoll SA, Preininger MK, Laval J, Limoli DH, Brown MR, et al. Frontline Science: pathological conditioning of human neutrophils recruited to the airway milieu in cystic fibrosis. *J Leukoc Biol.* (2018) 104:665–75. doi: 10.1002/JLB.5HI1117-454RR
64. Elborn JS, Ahuja S, Springman E, Mershon J, Grosswald R, Rowe SM. EMPIRE-CF: a phase II randomized placebo-controlled trial of once-daily, oral acebilustat in adult patients with cystic fibrosis–study design and patient demographics. *Contemp Clin Trials.* (2018) 72:86–94. doi: 10.1016/j.cct.2018.07.014
65. Saiman L, Prince A. *Pseudomonas aeruginosa* pili bind to asialoGM1 which is increased on the surface of cystic fibrosis epithelial cells. *J Clin Invest.* (1993) 92:1875–80. doi: 10.1172/JCI116779
66. Imundo L, Barasch J, Prince A, Al-Awqati Q. Cystic fibrosis epithelial cells have a receptor for pathogenic bacteria on their apical surface. *Proc Natl Acad Sci USA.* (1995) 92:3019–23. doi: 10.1073/pnas.92.7.3019
67. DiMango E, Zar HJ, Bryan R, Prince A. Diverse *Pseudomonas aeruginosa* gene products stimulate respiratory epithelial cells to produce interleukin-8. *J Clin Invest.* (1995) 96:2204–10. doi: 10.1172/JCI118275
68. Feldman M, Bryan R, Rajan S, Scheffler L, Brunnert S, Tang H, et al. Role of flagella in pathogenesis of *Pseudomonas aeruginosa* pulmonary infection. *Infect Immun.* (1998) 66:43–51. doi: 10.1128/IAI.66.1.43-51.1998
69. DiMango E, Ratner AJ, Bryan R, Tabibi S, Prince A. Activation of NF-kappaB by adherent *Pseudomonas aeruginosa* in normal and cystic fibrosis respiratory epithelial cells. *J Clin Invest.* (1998) 101:2598–605. doi: 10.1172/JCI2865
70. Bryan R, Prince A. Bacterial-epithelial interactions. *Mol Med.* (2002) 70:465–78. doi: 10.1385/1-59259-187-6:465
71. Rastogi D, Ratner AJ, Prince A. Host-bacterial interactions in the initiation of inflammation. *Paediatr Respir Rev.* (2001) 2:245–52. doi: 10.1053/prrv.2001.0147
72. Parker D, Prince A. Epithelial uptake of flagella initiates pro-inflammatory signaling. *PLoS ONE.* (2013) 8:e59932. doi: 10.1371/journal.pone.0059932
73. Massion PP, Inoue H, Richman-Eisenstat J, Grunberger D, Jorens PG, Housset B, et al. Novel *Pseudomonas* product stimulates interleukin-8 production in airway epithelial cells *in vitro*. *J Clin Invest.* (1994) 93:26–32. doi: 10.1172/JCI116954
74. Jorens PG, Richman-Eisenstat JB, Housset BP, Massion PP, Ueki I, Nadel JA. *Pseudomonas*-induced neutrophil recruitment in the dog airway *in vivo* is mediated in part by IL-8 and inhibited by a leumedin. *Eur Respir J.* (1994) 7:1925–31.
75. Moura JA, Cristina de Assis M, Ventura GC, Saliba AM, Gonzaga L Jr, Si-Tahar M, et al. Differential interaction of bacterial species from the *Burkholderia cepacia* complex with human airway epithelial cells. *Microbes Infect.* (2008) 10:52–9. doi: 10.1016/j.micinf.2007.10.002
76. Zhao X, Town JR, Li F, Zhang X, Cockcroft DW, Gordon JR. ELR-CXC chemokine receptor antagonism targets inflammatory responses at multiple levels. *J Immunol.* (2009) 182:3213–22. doi: 10.4049/jimmunol.0800551
77. Kaza SK, McClean S, Callaghan M. IL-8 released from human lung epithelial cells induced by cystic fibrosis pathogens *Burkholderia cepacia* complex affects the growth and intracellular survival of bacteria. *Int J Med Microbiol.* (2011) 301:26–33. doi: 10.1016/j.ijmm.2010.06.005
78. Bezzerri V, d'Adamo P, Rimessi A, Lanzara C, Crovella S, Nicolis E, et al. Phospholipase C-β3 is a key modulator of IL-8 expression in cystic fibrosis bronchial epithelial cells. *J Immunol.* (2011) 186:4946–58. doi: 10.4049/jimmunol.1003535
79. Dechecchi MC, Nicolis E, Mazzi P, Cioffi F, Bezzerri V, Lampronti I, et al. Modulators of sphingolipid metabolism reduce lung inflammation. *Am J Respir Cell Mol Biol.* (2011) 45:825–33. doi: 10.1165/rcmb.2010-0457OC
80. Mizunoe S, Shuto T, Suzuki S, Matsumoto C, Watanabe K, Ueno-Shuto K, et al. Synergism between interleukin (IL)-17 and Toll-like receptor 2 and 4 signals to induce IL-8 expression in cystic fibrosis airway epithelial cells. *J Pharmacol Sci.* (2012) 118:512–20. doi: 10.1254/jphs.11240FP
81. Prandini P, De Logu F, Fusi C, Provezza L, Nassini R, Montagner G, et al. Transient receptor potential ankyrin 1 channels modulate inflammatory response in respiratory cells from patients with cystic fibrosis. *Am J Respir Cell Mol Biol.* (2016) 55:645–56. doi: 10.1165/rcmb.2016-0089OC
82. Ribeiro CM, Paradiso AM, Schwab U, Perez-Vilar J, Jones L, O'neal W, et al. Chronic airway infection/inflammation induces a Ca2+i-dependent hyperinflammatory response in human cystic fibrosis airway epithelia. *J Biol Chem.* (2005) 280:17798–806. doi: 10.1074/jbc.M410618200
83. Rosenow T, Mok LC, Turkovic L, Berry LJ, Sly PD, Ranganathan S, et al. The cumulative effect of inflammation and infection on structural lung disease in early cystic fibrosis. *Eur Respir J.* (2019) 54:1801771. doi: 10.1183/13993003.01771-2018
84. Balázs A, Mall MA. Mucus obstruction and inflammation in early cystic fibrosis lung disease: emerging role of the IL-1 signaling pathway. *Pediatr Pulmonol.* (2019) 54(suppl.3):S5–12. doi: 10.1002/ppul.24462

85. Adamo R, Sokol S, Soong G, Gomez MI, Prince A. Pseudomonas aeruginosa flagella activate airway epithelial cells through asialoGM1 and toll-like receptor 2 as well as toll-like receptor 5. *Am J Respir Cell Mol Biol.* (2004) 30:627–34. doi: 10.1165/rcmb.2003-0260OC
86. Sadikot RT, Blackwell TS, Christman JW, Prince AS. Pathogen-host interactions in *Pseudomonas aeruginosa* pneumonia. *Am J Respir Crit Care Med.* (2005) 171:1209–23. doi: 10.1164/rccm.200408-1044SO
87. Prince A. Flagellar activation of epithelial signaling. *Am J Respir Cell Mol Biol.* (2006) 34:548–51. doi: 10.1165/rcmb.2006-0022SF
88. Ratner AJ, Bryan R, Weber A, Nguyen S, Barnes D, Pitt A, et al. Cystic fibrosis pathogens activate Ca2+-dependent mitogen-activated protein kinase signaling pathways in airway epithelial cells. *J Biol Chem.* (2001) 276:19267–75. doi: 10.1074/jbc.M007703200
89. Bezzerri V, Borgatti M, Finotti A, Tamanini A, Gambari R, Cabrini G. Mapping the transcriptional machinery of the IL-8 gene in human bronchial epithelial cells. *J Immunol.* (2011) 187:6069–81. doi: 10.4049/jimmunol.1100821
90. Illek B, Fu Z, Schwarzer C, Banzon T, Jalickee S, Miller SS, et al. Flagellin-stimulated Cl- secretion and innate immune responses in airway epithelia: role for p38. *Am J Physiol Lung Cell Mol Physiol.* (2008) 295:L531–42. doi: 10.1152/ajplung.90292.2008
91. McNamara N, Khong A, McKemy D, Caterina M, Boyer J, Julius D, et al. ATP transduces signals from ASGM1, a glycolipid that functions as a bacterial receptor. *Proc Natl Acad Sci USA.* (2001) 98:9086–91. doi: 10.1073/pnas.161290898
92. McNamara N, Gallup M, Sucher A, Maltseva I, McKemy D, Basbaum C. AsialoGM1 and TLR5 cooperate in flagellin-induced nucleotide signaling to activate Erk1/2. *Am J Respir Cell Mol Biol.* (2006) 34:653–60. doi: 10.1165/rcmb.2005-0441OC
93. Rimessi A, Bezzerri V, Salvatori F, Tamanini A, Nigro F, Dechecchi MC, et al. PLCB3 loss of function reduces *Pseudomonas aeruginosa*-dependent IL-8 release in cystic fibrosis. *Am J Respir Cell Mol Biol.* (2018) 59:428–36. doi: 10.1165/rcmb.2017-0267OC
94. Bezzerri V, Borgatti M, Nicolis E, Lampronti I, Dechecchi MC, Mancini I, et al. Transcription factor oligodeoxynucleotides to NF-kappaB inhibit transcription of IL-8 in bronchial cells. *Am J Respir Cell Mol Biol.* (2008) 39:86–96. doi: 10.1165/rcmb.2007-0176OC
95. Jundi K, Greene CM. Transcription of interleukin-8: how altered regulation can affect cystic fibrosis lung disease. *Biomolecules.* (2015) 5:1386–98. doi: 10.3390/biom5031386
96. Ashburner BP, Westerheide SD, Baldwin AS Jr. The p65 (RelA) subunit of NF-κB interacts with the histone deacetylase (HDAC) corepressors HDAC1 and HDAC2 to negatively regulate gene expression. *Mol Cell Biol.* (2001) 21:7065–77. doi: 10.1128/MCB.21.20.7065-7077.2001
97. Vanden Berghe W, de Bosscher K, Boone E, Plaisance S, Haegeman G. The nuclear factor-κB engages CBP/p300 and histone acetyltransferase activity for transcriptional activation of the interleukin-6 gene promoter. *J Biol Chem.* (1999) 274:32091–8. doi: 10.1074/jbc.274.45.32091
98. Wu GD, Lai EJ, Huang N, Wen X. Oct-1 and CCAAT/enhancer-binding protein (C/EBP) bind to overlapping elements within the interleukin-8 promoter. The role of Oct-1 as a transcriptional repressor. *J Biol Chem.* (1997) 272:2396–403. doi: 10.1074/jbc.272.4.2396
99. Nourbakhsh M, Kalble S, Dorrie A, Hauser H, Resch K, Kracht M. The NF-κB repressing factor is involved in basal repression and interleukin (IL)-1-induced activation of IL-8 transcription by binding to a conserved NF-κB-flanking sequence element. *Biol Chem.* (2001) 276:4501–8. doi: 10.1074/jbc.M007532200
100. Farahmand L, Darvishi B, Majidzadeh AK. Suppression of chronic inflammation with engineered nanomaterials delivering nuclear factor κB transcription factor decoy oligodeoxynucleotides. *Drug Deliv.* (2017) 24:1249–61. doi: 10.1080/10717544.2017.1370511
101. Wardwell PR, Bader RA. Immunomodulation of cystic fibrosis epithelial cells via NF-κB decoy oligonucleotide-coated polysaccharide nanoparticles. *J Biomed Mater Res A.* (2015) 103:1622–31. doi: 10.1002/jbm.a.35296
102. Bartling TR, Drumm ML. Loss of CFTR results in reduction of histone deacetylase 2 in airway epithelial cells. *Am J Physiol Lung Cell Mol Physiol.* (2009) 297:L35–43. doi: 10.1152/ajplung.90399.2008
103. Poghosyan A, Patel JK, Clifford RL, Knox AJ. Epigenetic dysregulation of interleukin 8 (CXCL8) hypersecretion in cystic fibrosis airway epithelial cells. *Biochem Biophys Res Commun.* (2016) 476:431–7. doi: 10.1016/j.bbrc.2016.05.140
104. Bhattacharyya S, Kumar P, Tsuchiya M, Bhattacharyya A, Biswas R. Regulation of miR-155 biogenesis in cystic fibrosis lung epithelial cells: antagonistic role of two mRNA-destabilizing proteins, KSRP and TTP. *Biochem Biophys Res Commun.* (2013) 433:484–8. doi: 10.1016/j.bbrc.2013.03.025
105. Fabbri E, Borgatti M, Montagner G, Bianchi N, Finotti A, Lampronti I, et al. Expression of microRNA-93 and Interleukin-8 during *Pseudomonas aeruginosa*-mediated induction of proinflammatory responses. *Am J Respir Cell Mol Biol.* (2014) 50:1144–55. doi: 10.1165/rcmb.2013-0160OC
106. Oglesby IK, Vencken SF, Agrawal R, Gaughan K, Molloy K, Higgins G, et al. miR-17 overexpression in cystic fibrosis airway epithelial cells decreases interleukin-8 production. *Eur Respir J.* (2015) 46:1350–60. doi: 10.1183/09031936.00163414
107. Bardin P, Foussignière T, Rousselet N, Rebeyrol C, Porter JC, Corvol H, et al. miR-636: a newly-identified actor for the regulation of pulmonary inflammation in cystic fibrosis. *Front Immunol.* (2019) 10:2643. doi: 10.3389/fimmu.2019.02643
108. Muir A, Soong G, Sokol S, Reddy B, Gomez MI, Van Heeckeren A, et al. Toll-like receptors in normal and cystic fibrosis airway epithelial cells. *Am J Respir Cell Mol Biol.* (2004) 30:777–83. doi: 10.1165/rcmb.2003-0329OC
109. Greene CM, Carroll TP, Smith SG, Taggart CC, Devaney J, Griffin S, et al. TLR-induced inflammation in cystic fibrosis and non-cystic fibrosis airway epithelial cells. *J Immunol.* (2005) 174:1638–46. doi: 10.4049/jimmunol.174.3.1638
110. Brown RK, Kelly FJ. Evidence for increased oxidative damage in patients with cystic fibrosis. *Pediatr Res.* (1994) 36:487–93. doi: 10.1203/00006450-199410000-00013
111. Boncoeur E, Criq VS, Bonvin E, Roque T, Henrion-Caude A, Gruenert DC, et al. Oxidative stress induces extracellular signal-regulated kinase 1/2 mitogen-activated protein kinase in cystic fibrosis lung epithelial cells: potential mechanism for excessive IL-8 expression. *Int J Biochem Cell Biol.* (2008) 40:432–46. doi: 10.1016/j.biocel.2007.08.013
112. Livnat G, Bentur L, Kuzmisnsky E, Nagler RM. Salivary profile and oxidative stress in children and adolescents with cystic fibrosis. *J Oral Pathol Med.* (2010) 39:16–21. doi: 10.1111/j.1600-0714.2009.00813.x
113. Dickerhof N, Pearson JF, Hoskin TS, Berry LJ, Turner R, Sly PD, et al. Oxidative stress in early cystic fibrosis lung disease is exacerbated by airway glutathione deficiency. *Free Radic Biol Med.* (2017) 113:236–43. doi: 10.1016/j.freeradbiomed.2017.09.028
114. Tucker MA, Fox BM, Seigler N, Rodriguez-Miguelez P, Looney J, Thomas J, et al. Endothelial dysfunction in cystic fibrosis: role of oxidative stress. *Oxid Med Cell Longev.* (2019) 2019:1629638. doi: 10.1155/2019/1629638
115. Favia M, de Bari L, Bobba A, Atlante A. An intriguing involvement of mitochondria in cystic fibrosis. *J Clin Med.* (2019) 8:1890. doi: 10.3390/jcm8111890
116. Scholte BJ, Horati H, Veltman M, Vreeken RJ, Garratt LW, Tiddens HAWM, et al. Oxidative stress and abnormal bioactive lipids in early cystic fibrosis lung disease. *J Cyst Fibros.* (2019) 18:781–9. doi: 10.1016/j.jcf.2019.04.011
117. Velsor LW, Kariya C, Kachadourian R, Day BJ. Mitochondrial oxidative stress in the lungs of cystic fibrosis transmembrane conductance regulator protein mutant mice. *Am J Respir Cell Mol Biol.* (2006) 35:579–86. doi: 10.1165/rcmb.2005-0473OC
118. Kelly-Aubert M, Trudel S, Fritsch J, Nguyen-Khoa T, Baudouin-Legros M, Moriceau S, et al. GSH monoethyl ester rescues mitochondrial defects in cystic fibrosis models. *Hum Mol Genet.* (2011) 20:2745–59. doi: 10.1093/hmg/ddr173
119. Rottner M, Tual-Chalot S, Mostefai HA, Andriantsitohaina R, Freyssinet JM, Martínez MC. Increased oxidative stress induces apoptosis in human cystic fibrosis cells. *PLoS ONE.* (2011) 6:e24880. doi: 10.1371/journal.pone.0024880
120. Cantin AM, Bilodeau G, Ouellet C, Liao J, Hanrahan JW. Oxidant stress suppresses CFTR expression. *Am J Physiol Cell Physiol.* (2006) 290:C262–70. doi: 10.1152/ajpcell.00070.2005
121. Luciani A, Villella VR, Esposito S, Brunetti-Pierri N, Medina D, Settembre C, et al. Defective CFTR induces aggresome formation and lung inflammation

in cystic fibrosis through ROS-mediated autophagy inhibition. *Nat Cell Biol.* (2010) 12:863–75. doi: 10.1038/ncb2090
122. Rimessi A, Previati M, Nigro F, Wieckowski MR, Pinton P. Mitochondrial reactive oxygen species and inflammation: molecular mechanisms, diseases and promising therapies. *Int J Biochem Cell Biol.* (2016) 81:281–93. doi: 10.1016/j.biocel.2016.06.015
123. Escames G, López LC, García JA, García-Corzo L, Ortiz F, Acuña-Castroviejo D. Mitochondrial DNA and inflammatory diseases. *Hum Genet.* (2012) 131:161–73. doi: 10.1007/s00439-011-1057-y
124. Nakahira K, Haspel JA, Rathinam VA, Lee SJ, Dolinay T, Lam HC, et al. Autophagy proteins regulate innate immune responses by inhibiting the release of mitochondrial DNA mediated by the NALP3 inflammasome. *Nat Immunol.* (2011) 12:222–30. doi: 10.1038/ni.1980
125. Junkins RD, Shen A, Rosen K, McCormick C, Lin TJ. Autophagy enhances bacterial clearance during *P. aeruginosa* lung infection. *PLoS ONE.* (2013) 8:e72263. doi: 10.1371/journal.pone.0072263
126. Maiuri L, Kroemer G. Autophagy delays progression of the two most frequent human monogenetic lethal diseases: cystic fibrosis and Wilson disease. *Aging.* (2018) 10:3657–61. doi: 10.18632/aging.101736
127. Abdulrahman BA, Khweek AA, Akhter A, Caution K, Kotrange S, Abdelaziz DH, et al. Autophagy stimulation by rapamycin suppresses lung inflammation and infection by *Burkholderia cenocepacia* in a model of cystic fibrosis. *Autophagy.* (2011) 7:1359–70. doi: 10.4161/auto.7.11.17660
128. Rubinsztein DC, Codogno P, Levine B. Autophagy modulation as a potential therapeutic target for diverse diseases. *Nat Rev Drug Discov.* (2012) 11:709–30. doi: 10.1038/nrd3802
129. De Stefano D, Villella VR, Esposito S, Tosco A, Sepe A, De Gregorio F, et al. Restoration of CFTR function in patients with cystic fibrosis carrying the F508del-CFTR mutation. *Autophagy.* (2014) 10:2053–74. doi: 10.4161/15548627.2014.973737
130. Villella VR, Esposito S, Ferrari E, Monzani R, Tosco A, Rossin F, et al. Autophagy suppresses the pathogenic immune response to dietary antigens in cystic fibrosis. *Cell Death Dis.* (2019) 10:258. doi: 10.1038/s41419-019-1500-x
131. Rimessi A, Pozzato C, Carparelli L, Rossi A, Ranucci S, De Fino I, et al. Pharmacological modulation of Mitochondrial Calcium Uniporter controls lung inflammation in cystic fibrosis. *Sci Adv.* (2020) 16:aax9093. doi: 10.1126/sciadv.aax9093
132. Rimessi A, Bezzerri V, Patergnani S, Marchi S, Cabrini G, Pinton P. Mitochondrial Ca2+-dependent NLRP3 activation exacerbates the *Pseudomonas aeruginosa*-driven inflammatory response in cystic fibrosis. *Nat Commun.* (2015) 6:6201. doi: 10.1038/ncomms7201
133. Feigal RJ, Shapiro BL. Mitochondrial calcium uptake and oxygen consumption in cystic fibrosis. *Nature.* (1979) 278:276–7. doi: 10.1038/278276a0
134. Shapiro BL, Feigal RJ, Lam LF. Mitrochondrial NADH dehydrogenase in cystic fibrosis. *Proc Natl Acad Sci USA.* (1979) 76:2979–83. doi: 10.1073/pnas.76.6.2979
135. Congdon PJ, Littlewood JM, Aggarwal RK, Shapiro H. Glucose 6-phosphate dehydrogenase deficiency and cystic fibrosis. *Postgrad Med J.* (1981) 57:453–4. doi: 10.1136/pgmj.57.669.453
136. Valdivieso AG, Marcucci F, Taminelli G, Guerrico AG, Alvarez S, Teiber ML, et al. The expression of the mitochondrial gene MT-ND4 is downregulated in cystic fibrosis. *Biochem Biophys Res Commun.* (2007) 356:805–9. doi: 10.1016/j.bbrc.2007.03.057
137. Atlante A, Favia M, Bobba A, Guerra L, Casavola V, Reshkin SJ. Characterization of mitochondrial function in cells with impaired cystic fibrosis transmembrane conductance regulator (CFTR) function. *J Bioenerg Biomembr.* (2016) 48:197–210. doi: 10.1007/s10863-016-9663-y
138. Kushwah R, Gagnon S, Sweezey NB. Intrinsic predisposition of naïve cystic fibrosis T cells to differentiate towards a Th17 phenotype. *Respir Res.* (2013) 14:138. doi: 10.1186/1465-9921-14-138
139. Tarique AA, Sly PD, Holt PG, Bosco A, Ware RS, Logan J, et al. CFTR-dependent defect in alternatively-activated macrophages in cystic fibrosis. *J Cyst Fibros.* (2017) 16:475–82. doi: 10.1016/j.jcf.2017.03.011
140. Assani K, Tazi MF, Amer AO, Kopp BT. IFN-γ stimulates autophagy-mediated clearance of *Burkholderia cenocepacia* in human cystic fibrosis macrophages. *PLoS ONE.* (2014) 9:e96681. doi: 10.1371/journal.pone.0096681
141. Assani K, Shrestha CL, Robledo-Avila F, Rajaram MV, Partida-Sanchez S, Schlesinger LS, et al. Human cystic fibrosis macrophages have defective calcium-dependent protein kinase C activation of the NADPH oxidase, an effect augmented by *Burkholderia cenocepacia. J Immunol.* (2017) 198:1985–94. doi: 10.4049/jimmunol.1502609
142. Lamothe J, Valvano MA. *Burkholderia cenocepacia*-induced delay of acidification and phagolysosomal fusion in cystic fibrosis transmembrane conductance regulator (CFTR)-defective macrophages. *Microbiology.* (2008) 154:3825–34. doi: 10.1099/mic.0.2008/023200-0
143. Kopp BT, Abdulrahman BA, Khweek AA, Kumar SB, Akhter A, Montione R, et al. Exaggerated inflammatory responses mediated by *Burkholderia cenocepacia* in human macrophages derived from Cystic fibrosis patients. *Biochem Biophys Res Commun.* (2012) 424:221–7. doi: 10.1016/j.bbrc.2012.06.066
144. Mould KJ, Jackson ND, Henson PM, Seibold M, Janssen WJ. Single cell RNA sequencing identifies unique inflammatory airspace macrophage subsets. *JCI Insight.* (2019) 4:126556. doi: 10.1172/jci.insight.126556
145. Hisert KB, Liles WC, Manicone AM. A flow cytometric method for isolating cystic fibrosis airway macrophages from expectorated sputum. *Am J Respir Cell Mol Biol.* (2019) 61:42–50. doi: 10.1165/rcmb.2018-0236MA
146. Ramji R, Alexander AF, Muñoz-Rojas AR, Kellman LN, Miller-Jensen K. Microfluidic platform enables live-cell imaging of signaling and transcription combined with multiplexed secretion measurements in the same single cells. *Integr Biol.* (2019) 11:142–53. doi: 10.1093/intbio/zyz013
147. Irimia D, Wang X. Inflammation-on-a-chip: probing the immune system *ex vivo. Trends Biotechnol.* (2018) 36:923–37. doi: 10.1016/j.tibtech.2018.03.011
148. Kongsuphol P, Liu Y, Ramadan Q. On-chip immune cell activation and subsequent time-resolved magnetic bead-based cytokine detection. *Biomed Microdevices.* (2016) 18:93. doi: 10.1007/s10544-016-0117-4
149. Fu Z, Bettega K, Carroll S, Buchholz KR, Machen TE. Role of Ca2+ in responses of airway epithelia to *Pseudomonas aeruginosa*, flagellin, ATP, and thapsigargin. *Am J Physiol Lung Cell Mol Physiol.* (2007) 292:L353–64. doi: 10.1152/ajplung.00042.2006
150. Ribeiro CM. The role of intracellular calcium signals in inflammatory responses of polarised cystic fibrosis human airway epithelia. *Drugs R D.* (2006) 7:17–31. doi: 10.2165/00126839-200607010-00002
151. Donnell GN, Cleland RS. Intestinal atresia or stenosis in the newborn associated with fibrocystic disease of the pancreas. *Calif Med.* (1961) 94:165–70.
152. Feigal RJ, Shapiro BL. Altered intracellular calcium in fibroblasts from patients with cystic fibrosis and heterozygotes. *Pediatr Res.* (1979) 13:764–8. doi: 10.1203/00006450-197906000-00009
153. Shapiro BL, Lam LF. Intracellular calcium in cystic fibrosis heterozygotes. *Life Sci.* (1987) 40:2361–6. doi: 10.1016/0024-3205(87)90510-8
154. Cabrini G, De Togni P. Increased cytosolic calcium in cystic fibrosis neutrophils. Effect on stimulus-secretion coupling. *Life Sci.* (1985) 36:1561–7. doi: 10.1016/0024-3205(85)90380-7
155. Feigal RJ, Tomczyk MS, Shapiro BL. The calcium abnormality in cystic fibrosis mitochondria: relative role of respiration and ATP hydrolysis. *Life Sci.* (1982) 30:93–8. doi: 10.1016/0024-3205(82)90640-3
156. Antigny F, Girardin N, Raveau D, Frieden M, Becq F, Vandebrouck C. Dysfunction of mitochondria Ca2+ uptake in cystic fibrosis airway epithelial cells. *Mitochondrion.* (2009) 9:232–41. doi: 10.1016/j.mito.2009.02.003
157. Philippe R, Antigny F, Buscaglia P, Norez C, Becq F, Frieden M, et al. SERCA and PMCA pumps contribute to the deregulation of Ca2+ homeostasis in human CF epithelial cells. *Biochim Biophys Acta.* (2015) 1853:892–903. doi: 10.1016/j.bbamcr.2015.01.010
158. Antigny F, Norez C, Dannhoffer L, Bertrand J, Raveau D, Corbi P, et al. Transient receptor potential canonical channel 6 links Ca2+ mishandling to cystic fibrosis transmembrane conductance regulator channel dysfunction in cystic fibrosis. *Am J Respir Cell Mol Biol.* (2011) 44:83–90. doi: 10.1165/rcmb.2009-0347OC
159. Vachel L, Norez C, Becq F, Vandebrouck C. Effect of VX-770 (ivacaftor) and OAG on Ca2+ influx and CFTR activity in G551D and F508del-CFTR expressing cells. *J Cyst Fibros.* (2013) 12:584–91. doi: 10.1016/j.jcf.2013.05.008

160. Balghi H, Robert R, Rappaz B, Zhang X, Wohlhuter-Haddad A, Evagelidis A, et al. Enhanced Ca2+ entry due to Orai1 plasma membrane insertion increases IL-8 secretion by cystic fibrosis airways. *FASEB J.* (2011) 25:4274–91. doi: 10.1096/fj.11-187682
161. Tabary O, Boncoeur E, de Martin R, Pepperkok R, Clément A, Schultz C, et al. Calcium-dependent regulation of NF-(kappa)B activation in cystic fibrosis airway epithelial cells. *Cell Signal.* (2006) 18:652–60. doi: 10.1016/j.cellsig.2005.06.004
162. Lazarowski ER, Boucher RC. Purinergic receptors in airway epithelia. *Curr Opin Pharmacol.* (2009) 9:262–7. doi: 10.1016/j.coph.2009.02.004
163. Huang P, Gilmore E, Kultgen P, Barnes P, Milgram S, Stutts MJ. Local regulation of cystic fibrosis transmembrane regulator and epithelial sodium channel in airway epithelium. *Proc Am Thorac Soc.* (2004) 1:33–7. doi: 10.1513/pats.2306012
164. Faria D, Schreiber R, Kunzelmann K. CFTR is activated through stimulation of purinergic P2Y2 receptors. *Pflugers Arch.* (2009) 457:1373–80. doi: 10.1007/s00424-008-0606-2
165. Billet A, Hanrahan JW. The secret life of CFTR as a calcium-activated chloride channel. *J Physiol.* (2013) 591:5273–8. doi: 10.1113/jphysiol.2013.261909
166. Triantafilou M, Morath S, Mackie A, Hartung T, Triantafilou K. Lateral diffusion of Toll-like receptors reveals that they are transiently confined within lipid rafts on the plasma membrane. *J Cell Sci.* (2004) 117:4007–14. doi: 10.1242/jcs.01270
167. Chun J, Prince A. Activation of Ca2+-dependent signaling by TLR2. *J Immunol.* (2006) 177:1330–7. doi: 10.4049/jimmunol.177.2.1330
168. Dohrman A, Miyata S, Gallup M, Li JD, Chapelin C, Coste A, et al. Mucin gene (MUC 2 and MUC 5AC) upregulation by Gram-positive and Gram-negative bacteria. *Biochim Biophys Acta.* (1998) 1406:251–9. doi: 10.1016/S0925-4439(98)00010-6
169. Asehnoune K, Strassheim D, Mitra S, Yeol Kim J, Abraham E. Involvement of PKCalpha/beta in TLR4 and TLR2 dependent activation of NF-kappaB. *Cell Signal.* (2005) 17:385–94. doi: 10.1016/j.cellsig.2004.08.005
170. Lampronti I, Dechecchi MC, Rimessi A, Bezzerri V, Nicolis E, Guerrini A, et al. β-sitosterol reduces the expression of chemotactic cytokine genes in cystic fibrosis bronchial epithelial cells. *Front Pharmacol.* (2017) 8:236. doi: 10.3389/fphar.2017.00236
171. Martins JR, Kongsuphol P, Sammels E, Dahimène S, Aldehni F, Clarke LA, et al. F508del-CFTR increases intracellular Ca(2+) signaling that causes enhanced calcium-dependent Cl(-) conductance in cystic fibrosis. *Biochim Biophys Acta.* (2011) 1812:1385–92. doi: 10.1016/j.bbadis.2011.08.008
172. Ribeiro CM, Lubamba BA. Role of IRE1α/XBP-1 in cystic fibrosis airway inflammation. *Int J Mol Sci.* (2017) 18:E118. doi: 10.3390/ijms18010118
173. Kunzelmann K, Kongsuphol P, Chootip K, Toledo C, Martins JR, Almaca J, et al. Role of the Ca2+ -activated Cl- channels bestrophin and anoctamin in epithelial cells. *Biol Chem.* (2011) 392:125–34. doi: 10.1515/bc.2011.010
174. Konstan MW, Hoppel CL, Chai BL, Davis PB. Ibuprofen in children with cystic fibrosis: pharmacokinetics and adverse effects. *J Pediatr.* (1991) 118:956–64. doi: 10.1016/S0022-3476(05)82218-8
175. Konstan MW, Byard PJ, Hoppel CL, Davis PB. Effect of high-dose ibuprofen in patients with cystic fibrosis. *N Engl J Med.* (1995) 332:848–54. doi: 10.1056/NEJM199503303321303
176. Lands LC, Stanojevic S. Oral non-steroidal anti-inflammatory drug therapy for lung disease in cystic fibrosis. *Cochrane Database Syst Rev.* (2019) 9:CD001505. doi: 10.1002/14651858.CD001505.pub5
177. Kantor TG. Ibuprofen. *Ann Intern Med.* (1979) 91:877–82. doi: 10.7326/0003-4819-91-6-877
178. McElvaney NG, Nakamura H, Birrer P, Hébert CA, Wong WL, Alphonso M, et al. Modulation of airway inflammation in cystic fibrosis. *In vivo* suppression of interleukin-8 levels on the respiratory epithelial surface by aerosolization of recombinant secretory leukoprotease inhibitor. *J Clin Invest.* (1992) 90:1296–301. doi: 10.1172/JCI115994
179. Allen ED. Opportunities for the use of aerosolized alpha 1-antitrypsin for the treatment of cystic fibrosis. *Chest.* (1996) 110:256S–60S. doi: 10.1378/chest.110.6_Supplement.256S
180. Vogelmeier C, Gillissen A, Buhl R. Use of secretory leukoprotease inhibitor to augment lung antineutrophil elastase activity. *Chest.* (1996) 110(6 suppl.):261S–6S. doi: 10.1378/chest.110.6_Supplement.261S
181. Bingle L, Tetley TD. Secretory leukoprotease inhibitor: partnering alpha 1-proteinase inhibitor to combat pulmonary inflammation. *Thorax.* (1996) 51:1273–4. doi: 10.1136/thx.51.12.1273
182. Tremblay GM, Janelle MF, Bourbonnais Y. Anti-inflammatory activity of neutrophil elastase inhibitors. *Curr Opin Investig Drugs.* (2003) 4:556–65.
183. Roghanian A, Sallenave JM. Neutrophil elastase (NE) and NE inhibitors: canonical and non-canonical functions in lung chronic inflammatory diseases (cystic fibrosis and chronic obstructive pulmonary disease). *J Aerosol Med Pulm Drug Deliv.* (2008) 21:125–44. doi: 10.1089/jamp.2007.0653
184. Zani ML, Tanga A, Saidi A, Serrano H, Dallet-Choisy S, Baranger K, et al. SLPI and trappin-2 as therapeutic agents to target airway serine proteases in inflammatory lung diseases: current and future directions. *Biochem Soc Trans.* (2011) 39:1441–6. doi: 10.1042/BST0391441
185. Dunlevy FK, Martin SL, de Courcey F, Elborn JS, Ennis M. Anti-inflammatory effects of DX-890, a human neutrophil elastase inhibitor. *J Cyst Fibros.* (2012) 11:300–4. doi: 10.1016/j.jcf.2012.02.003
186. McElvaney NG. Alpha-1 antitrypsin therapy in cystic fibrosis and the lung disease associated with alpha-1 antitrypsin deficiency. *Ann Am Thorac Soc.* (2016) 13(suppl.2):S191–6. doi: 10.1513/AnnalsATS.201504-245KV
187. Keir HR, Fong CJ, Crichton ML, Barth P, Chevalier E, Brady G, et al. Personalised anti- inflammatory therapy for bronchiectasis and cystic fibrosis: selecting patients for controlled trials of neutrophil elastase inhibition. *ERJ Open Res.* (2019) 5:00252-2018. doi: 10.1183/23120541.00252-2018
188. Watz H, Nagelschmitz J, Kirsten A, Pedersen F, van der Mey D, Schwers S, et al. Safety and efficacy of the human neutrophil elastase inhibitor BAY 85-8501 for the treatment of non-cystic fibrosis bronchiectasis: a randomized controlled trial. *Pulm Pharmacol Ther.* (2019) 56:86–93. doi: 10.1016/j.pupt.2019.03.009
189. Greene CM, Ramsay H, Wells RJ, O'Neill SJ, McElvaney NG. Inhibition of Toll-like receptor 2-mediated interleukin-8 production in Cystic Fibrosis airway epithelial cells via the alpha7-nicotinic acetylcholine receptor. *Mediators Inflamm.* (2010) 2010:423241. doi: 10.1155/2010/423241
190. Ha H, Debnath B, Odde S, Bensman T, Ho H, Beringer PM, et al. Discovery of novel CXCR2 inhibitors using ligand-based pharmacophore models. *J Chem Inf Model.* (2015) 55:1720–38. doi: 10.1021/acs.jcim.5b00181
191. Leaker BR, Barnes PJ, O'Connor B. Inhibition of LPS-induced airway neutrophilic inflammation in healthy volunteers with an oral CXCR2 antagonist. *Respir Res.* (2013) 14:137. doi: 10.1186/1465-9921-14-137
192. Jackson PL, Noerager BD, Jablonsky MJ, Hardison MT, Cox BD, Patterson JC, et al. A CXCL8 receptor antagonist based on the structure of N-acetyl-proline-glycine-proline. *Eur J Pharmacol.* (2011) 668:435–42. doi: 10.1016/j.ejphar.2011.02.045
193. Finotti A, Borgatti M, Bezzerri V, Nicolis E, Lampronti I, Dechecchi M, et al. Effects of decoy molecules targeting NF-kappaB transcription factors in Cystic fibrosis IB3-1 cells: recruitment of NF-kappaB to the IL-8 gene promoter and transcription of the IL-8 gene. *Artif DNA PNA XNA.* (2012) 3:97–296. doi: 10.4161/adna.21061
194. Romanelli A, Pedone C, Saviano M, Bianchi N, Borgatti M, Mischiati C, et al. Molecular interactions with nuclear factor kappaB (NF-kappaB) transcription factors of a PNA-DNA chimera mimicking NF-kappaB binding sites. *Eur J Biochem.* (2001) 268:6066–75. doi: 10.1046/j.0014-2956.2001.02549.x
195. Borgatti M, Lampronti I, Romanelli A, Pedone C, Saviano M, Bianchi N, et al. Transcription factor decoy molecules based on a peptide nucleic acid (PNA)-DNA chimera mimicking Sp1 binding sites. *J Biol Chem.* (2003) 278:7500–9. doi: 10.1074/jbc.M206780200
196. Borgatti M, Finotti A, Romanelli A, Saviano M, Bianchi N, Lampronti I, et al. Peptide nucleic acids (PNA)-DNA chimeras targeting transcription factors as a tool to modify gene expression. *Curr Drug Targets.* (2004) 5:735–44. doi: 10.2174/1389450043345155
197. De Stefano D, Ungaro F, Giovino C, Polimeno A, Quaglia F, Carnuccio R. Sustained inhibition of IL-6 and IL-8 expression by decoy ODN to NF-κB delivered through respirable large porous particles in LPS-stimulated cystic fibrosis bronchial cells. *J Gene Med.* (2011) 13:200–8. doi: 10.1002/jgm.1546
198. De Stefano D, Coletta C, Bianca Rd, Falcone L, d'Angelo I, Ungaro F, et al. A decoy oligonucleotide to NF-κB delivered through inhalable particles

prevents LPS-induced rat airway inflammation. *Am J Respir Cell Mol Biol.* (2013) 49:288–95. doi: 10.1165/rcmb.2012-0473OC

199. Bardin P, Sonneville F, Corvol H, Tabary O. Emerging microRNA therapeutic approaches for cystic fibrosis. *Front Pharmacol.* (2018) 9:1113. doi: 10.3389/fphar.2018.01113
200. Bardin P, Marchal-Duval E, Sonneville F, Blouquit-Laye S, Rousselet N, Le Rouzic P, et al. Small RNA and transcriptome sequencing reveal the role of miR-199a-3p in inflammatory processes in cystic fibrosis airways. *J Pathol.* (2018) 245:410–20. doi: 10.1002/path.5095
201. Luly FR, Lévêque M, Licursi V, Cimino G, Martin-Chouly C, Théret N, et al. MiR-146a is over-expressed and controls IL-6 production in cystic fibrosis macrophages. *Sci Rep.* (2019) 9:16259. doi: 10.1038/s41598-019-52770-w
202. Tambuyzer E, Vandendriessche B, Austin CP, Brooks PJ, Larsson K, Miller Needleman KI, et al. Therapies for rare diseases: therapeutic modalities, progress and challenges ahead. *Nat Rev Drug Discov.* (2019) 19:93–111. doi: 10.1038/s41573-019-0049-9
203. Liu Z, Borlak J, Tong W. Deciphering miRNA transcription factor feed-forward loops to identify drug repurposing candidates for cystic fibrosis. *Genome Med.* (2014) 6:94. doi: 10.1186/s13073-014-0094-2
204. Newman SP. Delivering drugs to the lungs: the history of repurposing in the treatment of respiratory diseases. *Adv Drug Deliv Rev.* (2018) 133:5–18. doi: 10.1016/j.addr.2018.04.010
205. Marka A, Carter JB., Phototherapy for cutaneous T-cell lymphoma. *Dermatol Clin.* (2020) 38:127–35. doi: 10.1016/j.det.2019.08.013
206. Nicolis E, Lampronti I, Dechecchi MC, Borgatti M, Tamanini A, Bezzerri V, et al. Modulation of expression of IL-8 gene in bronchial epithelial cells by 5-methoxypsoralen. *Int Immunopharmacol.* (2009) 9:1411–22. doi: 10.1016/j.intimp.2009.08.013
207. Borgatti M, Chilin A, Piccagli L, Lampronti I, Bianchi N, Mancini I, et al. Development of a novel furocoumarin derivative inhibiting NF-κB dependent biological functions: design, synthesis and biological effects. *Eur J Med Chem.* (2011) 46:4870–7. doi: 10.1016/j.ejmech.2011.07.032
208. Tamanini A, Borgatti M, Finotti A, Piccagli L, Bezzerri V, Favia M, et al. Trimethylangelicin reduces IL-8 transcription and potentiates CFTR function. *Am J Physiol Lung Cell Mol Physiol.* (2011) 300:L380–90. doi: 10.1152/ajplung.00129.2010
209. Favia M, Mancini MT, Bezzerri V, Guerra L, Laselva O, Abbattiscianni AC, et al. Trimethylangelicin promotes the functional rescue of mutant F508del CFTR protein in cystic fibrosis airway cells. *Am J Physiol Lung Cell Mol Physiol.* (2014) 307:L48–61. doi: 10.1152/ajplung.00305.2013
210. Laselva O, Marzaro G, Vaccarin C, Lampronti I, Tamanini A, Lippi G, et al. Molecular mechanism of action of trimethylangelicin derivatives as CFTR modulators. *Front Pharmacol.* (2018) 9:719. doi: 10.3389/fphar.2018.00719
211. Cigana C, Nicolis E, Pasetto M, Assael BM, Melotti P. Anti-inflammatory effects of azithromycin in cystic fibrosis airway epithelial cells. *Biochem Biophys Res Commun.* (2006) 350:977–82. doi: 10.1016/j.bbrc.2006.09.132
212. Tabary O, Escotte S, Couetil JP, Hubert D, Dusser D, Puchelle E, et al. Genistein inhibits constitutive and inducible NF-κB activation and decreases IL-8 production by human cystic fibrosis bronchial gland cells. *Am J Pathol.* (1999) 155:473–81. doi: 10.1016/S0002-9440(10)65143-7
213. Jouneau S, Bonizec M, Belleguic C, Desrues B, Brinchault G, Galaine J, et al. Anti-inflammatory effect of fluvastatin on IL-8 production induced by Pseudomonas aeruginosa and *Aspergillus fumigatus* antigens in cystic fibrosis. *PLoS ONE.* (2011) 6:e22655. doi: 10.1371/journal.pone.0022655
214. Gambari R, Borgatti M, Lampronti I, Fabbri E, Brognara E, Bianchi N, et al. Corilagin is a potent inhibitor of NF-κB activity and downregulates TNF-α induced expression of IL-8 gene in cystic fibrosis IB3-1 cells. *Int Immunopharmacol.* (2012) 13:308–15. doi: 10.1016/j.intimp.2012.04.010
215. Malcomson B, Wilson H, Veglia E, Thillaiyampalam G, Barsden R, Donegan S, et al. Connectivity mapping (ssCMap) to predict A20-inducing drugs and their antiinflammatory action in cystic fibrosis. *Proc Natl Acad Sci USA.* (2016) 113:E3725–34. doi: 10.1073/pnas.1520289113
216. Veit G, Bossard F, Goepp J, Verkman AS, Galietta LJ, Hanrahan JW, et al. Proinflammatory cytokine secretion is suppressed by TMEM16A or CFTR channel activity in human cystic fibrosis bronchial epithelia. *Mol Biol Cell.* (2012) 23:4188–202. doi: 10.1091/mbc.e12-06-0424
217. Ruffin M, Roussel L, Maillé É, Rousseau S, Brochiero E. Vx-809/Vx-770 treatment reduces inflammatory response to Pseudomonas aeruginosa in primary differentiated cystic fibrosis bronchial epithelial cells. *Am J Physiol Lung Cell Mol Physiol.* (2018) 314:L635–41. doi: 10.1152/ajplung.00198.2017
218. Zeng M, Szymczak M, Ahuja M, Zheng C, Yin H, Swaim W, et al. Restoration of CFTR activity in ducts rescues acinar cell function and reduces inflammation in pancreatic and salivary glands of mice. *Gastroenterology.* (2017) 153:1148–59. doi: 10.1053/j.gastro.2017.06.011
219. Roesch EA, Nichols DP, Chmiel JF. Inflammation in cystic fibrosis: an update. *Pediatr Pulmonol.* (2018) 53:S30–50. doi: 10.1002/ppul.24129
220. Perrem L, Ratjen F. Anti-inflammatories and mucociliary clearance therapies in the age of CFTR modulators. *Pediatr Pulmonol.* (2019) 54(suppl.3):S46–55. doi: 10.1002/ppul.24364

5

Influenza A Virus Pre-Infection Exacerbates *Pseudomonas aeruginosa*-Mediated Lung Damage through Increased MMP-9 Expression, Decreased Elafin Production and Tissue Resilience

Berengère Villeret [1]***, Brigitte Solhonne*** [1]***, Marjolène Straube*** [1]***, Flora Lemaire*** [1]***,***
Aurélie Cazes [1,2]***, Ignacio Garcia-Verdugo*** [1] ***and Jean-Michel Sallenave*** [1*]

[1] Inserm, UMR1152, Laboratoire d'Excellence Inflamex, Département Hospitalo-Universtaire FIRE (Fibrosis, Inflammation and Remodeling), Université de Paris, Paris, France, [2] Assistance Publique-Hôpitaux de Paris (APHP), Hôpital Bichat, Service de Pneumologie A, Paris, France

***Correspondence:**
Jean-Michel Sallenave
jean-michel.sallenave@inserm.fr

Individuals with impaired immune responses, such as ventilated and cystic fibrosis patients are often infected with *Pseudomonas aeruginosa* (*P.a*) bacteria, and a co-infection with the *Influenza* virus (IAV) is often present. It has been known for many years that infection with IAV predisposes the host to secondary bacterial infections (such as *Streptococcus pneumoniae* or *Staphylococcus aureus*), and there is an abundance of mechanistic studies, including those studying the role of desensitization of TLR signaling, type I IFN- mediated impairment of neutrophil chemokines and antimicrobial production, attenuation of IL1β production etc., showing this. However, little is known about the mechanistic events underlying the potential deleterious synergy between *Influenza* and *P.a* co-infections. We demonstrate here *in vitro* in epithelial cells and *in vivo* in three independent models (two involving mice given IAV +/– *P.a*, and one involving mice given IAV +/– IL-1β) that IAV promotes secondary *P.a*-mediated lung disease or augmented IL-1β-mediated inflammation. We show that IAV-*P.a*-mediated deleterious responses includes increased matrix metalloprotease (MMP) activity, and MMP-9 in particular, and that the use of the MMP inhibitor improves lung resilience. Furthermore, we show that IAV post-transcriptionally inhibits the antimicrobial/anti-protease molecule elafin/trappin-2, which we have shown previously to be anti-inflammatory and to protect the host against maladaptive neutrophilic inflammation in *P.a* infections. Our work highlights the capacity of IAV to promote further *P.a*-mediated lung damage, not necessarily through its interference with host resistance to the bacterium, but by down-regulating tissue resilience to lung inflammation instead. Our study therefore suggests that restoring tissue resilience in clinical settings where IAV/*P.a* co-exists could prove a fruitful strategy.

Keywords: *Pseudomonas aeruginosa*, *influenza* virus, elafin, metalloprotease, lung tissue resilience

INTRODUCTION

Individuals with impaired immune responses, such as cystic fibrosis (1–5) and ventilated patients (6, 7) demonstrate frequent respiratory viral infections with a variety of viruses, including the *Influenza A* virus (IAV). For example, clinical studies have shown correlations between viral infections with pulmonary exacerbations (1–3, 5), with the former often predisposing the host to secondary bacterial infections (8–11). Specifically, in a CF population study spanning over 6 years, which recruited in excess of 31,000 individuals and which reported an excess of 91,000 pulmonary exacerbations, the latter were associated with IAV activity (mostly of the H3N2 serotype) in both children and adults, with a *Pseudomonas aeruginosa* (*P.a*) prevalence of 48 and 82%, respectively. By contrast, an RSV association was only observed in adults (12). Surprisingly however, despite their simultaneous occurrence in such situations as acute nosocomial infections or chronic exacerbations in cystic fibrosis (see above) and COPD/emphysema, none of these studies have extensively tackled the interaction between *Influenza* and *Pseudomonas aeruginosa* (*P.a*). Indeed, mechanistic studies dealing with IAV and bacteria have mainly concerned *Staphylococcus aureus* and *Streptococcus pneumoniae*, for the latter, and a variety of mechanisms (often potentially contradictory) have been put forward to explain the deleterious consequences of such interactions.

These include, not exhaustively however, IAV-mediated desensitization of TLR signaling (13), type I interferon-mediated impairment of neutrophil chemokines or function (14–17), down-regulation of antimicrobial production (18–20), attenuation of IL1β production or IL1β-mediated alveolar macrophage activity (21, 22), exaggerated inflammatory responses (23, 24), or loss of lung repair potential (25, 26).

Mechanistically, we demonstrated here *in vitro* and *in vivo* in three independent models (two involving mice given IAV +/− *P.a*, and one involving mice given IAV +/− IL-1β) that IAV pre-treatment promoted secondary PAO1-mediated lung disease or augmented IL-1β-mediated inflammation, by enhancing deleterious inflammatory responses. These included increased matrix metalloprotease (MMP) activity, particularly MMP-9. Importantly, we showed that the MMP inhibitor batimastat improved lung resilience, and interestingly, this was not associated with an increase in bacterial clearance. Furthermore, we showed that IAV post-transcriptionally inhibited the antimicrobial/anti-protease molecule elafin/trappin-2, which we have shown previously to be anti-inflammatory in a variety of settings (27–29) and protects the host against maladaptive neutrophilic inflammation in *P.a* (27, 28, 30) infections, as well as against Plasmodium-mediated lung damage (29).

Altogether, out work highlights the capacity of IAV to promote further PAO1-mediated lung damage, not through its interference with host resistance to the bacterium (16, 19), but through down-regulating tissue resilience to lung inflammation instead. Our study therefore suggests that restoring tissue resilience in clinical settings where IAV/*P.a* co-exist could be a fruitful strategy.

MATERIALS AND METHODS

Materials

Phosphoramidon and batimastat were obtained from Sigma-Aldrich. Recombinant human and murine interleukin 1β were purchased from R&D Systems. Tace II metalloprotease substrate was obtained from Enzolife Science. Neutrophil elastase (NE) was obtained from Elastin products.

PAO1 and *Influenza A* Preparation

PAO1 WT (obtained from the ATCC; 15692), was grown overnight in Luria Broth (LB) medium (1% Bactotryptone, 0.5% Bacto Yeast Extract, 0.5% NaCl) under agitation. On the next day, an aliquot of PAO1 culture was grown over 3–4 h in an exponential phase and the OD was checked (600 nm). Bacteria were then centrifuged (4,000 rpm for 15 min) and pellets resuspended at the desired multiplicity of infection (moi) or colony forming units (cfu) in PBS.

The virus strain A/Scotland/20/74 (H3N2) was routinely amplified in MDCK cells (ATCC CCL-34), as described before Barbier et al. (31) and Villeret et al. (32). From the supernatants of infected cells, the *influenza* virus was purified by centrifugation in sucrose gradient, quantified by the virus plaque assay (32), aliquoted, and kept at −80°C until use.

When needed, purified samples were inactivated by heating at 95°C for 10 min in a block heater. Inability of heat-inactivated *influenza* virus (IAV*) to replicate was then confirmed by viral gene M2 q-PCR analysis (see below).

Adenovirus Constructs

The replication-deficient adenovirus (Ad) Ad-MCMV-elafin is described in Sallenave et al. (33).

Cells, Cell Cultures, and Protocols

NCI-H292 cells (ATCC reference number CRL-1848), a human pulmonary mucoepidermoid carcinoma cell line, BEAS-2B cells (ATCC CRL-9609), a SV-40 transformed bronchial epithelial cell line, and A549 (ATCC CCL-185) a cell line from a lung adenocarcinoma, were cultured in RPMI (NCI-H292) or F12/K Nutrient mixture (BEAS-2B and A549) medium supplemented with Glutamax, antibiotics, and 10% de-complemented fetal calf serum (all reagents from Gibco). Cells were incubated at 37°C in a water-jacketed CO_2 incubator. Cells were infected in serum-free medium with either IAV or PAO1. Alternatively, they were stimulated with either h-IL-1β, 5′ triphosphate double stranded RNA (5′ ppp dsRNA at 1.2 μg/ml) (Invivogen), complexed to lipofectamine 2000 (Invitrogen), with polyinosinic-polycytidylic acid (poly IC at 10 μg/ml) (Invivogen), or with combinations thereof.

Cell viability was assessed by measuring Lactate dehydrogenase (LDH) activity in cell lysates and supernatants, using the CytoTox 96 Nonradioactive Cytotoxicity assay (Promega).

Cells were washed twice with ice-cold PBS and lysed in TrisHCl 50 mM, NaCl 150 mM, NP40 1%, Glycerol 3%, EDTA 2 mM, and EGTA 2 mM buffer. After centrifugation (14,000 rpm, 15 min, 4°C) pellets were discarded. Cell supernatants and lysates were then recovered and stored at −80°C until further analysis.

In vivo Experiments

Procedures involving mice were approved by our Ethical Committee (Paris-Nord/No 121) and by the French ministry of Research (agreement numbers 4537.03 and 02012). Eight-week-old male C57Bl/6 mice and human elafin/trappin-2 transgenic mice (hereafter called eTg mice) were obtained from Janvier (Le Genest-Saint-Isle, France) and generated by our group (34), respectively. Mice were anesthetized using an intramuscular injection of ketamine 500 and xylazine 2% in 0.9% NaCl (20:10:70). Either the *Influenza A* virus (IAV), PAO1 bacteria, or m-IL-1ß recombinant protein were given intra-nasally (i.n) or through the oro-pharyngeal route, in a final volume of 40 µl instilled through a fine polypropylene tubing. Mice were then monitored for survival or were humanely killed (overdose of 100 µl intra-peritoneally-injected pentobarbital) for mechanistic studies. For the latter, bronchoalveolar lavages (BALs) fluid was obtained by cannulating the trachea and instilling 2 × 1 ml of PBS. Typically, a volume of 1.7 ml of BALF was retrieved and centrifuged at 2,000 rpm for 10 min. Supernatants were used for protein, cytokine/chemokine (ELISA), protease activity, and hemoglobin, as a surrogate for lung damage (absorbance reading at 405 nm) measurements. BAL cell pellets were used to perform cytospins for cell differential analysis (Diff-Quick, Dade Diagnostika GmbH, Unterschleissheim, Germany).

Lung tissues were used for RNA quantification, for assessment of bacterial count, after plating extracts on agarose plates, or for histological studies.

Cytokines/Chemokines/Antimicrobials Measurement

The concentration of mediators in cell cultures supernatants/lysates or murine BALs were quantified by sandwich ELISA kits following the manufacturer's indications (R&D Bio-Techne, Minneapolis, MN) or used in our in house ELISA (33).

BAL Protease Activities

BAL metalloprotease, trypsin-like, and neutrophil-elastase activities were measured using fluorogenic substrates, as

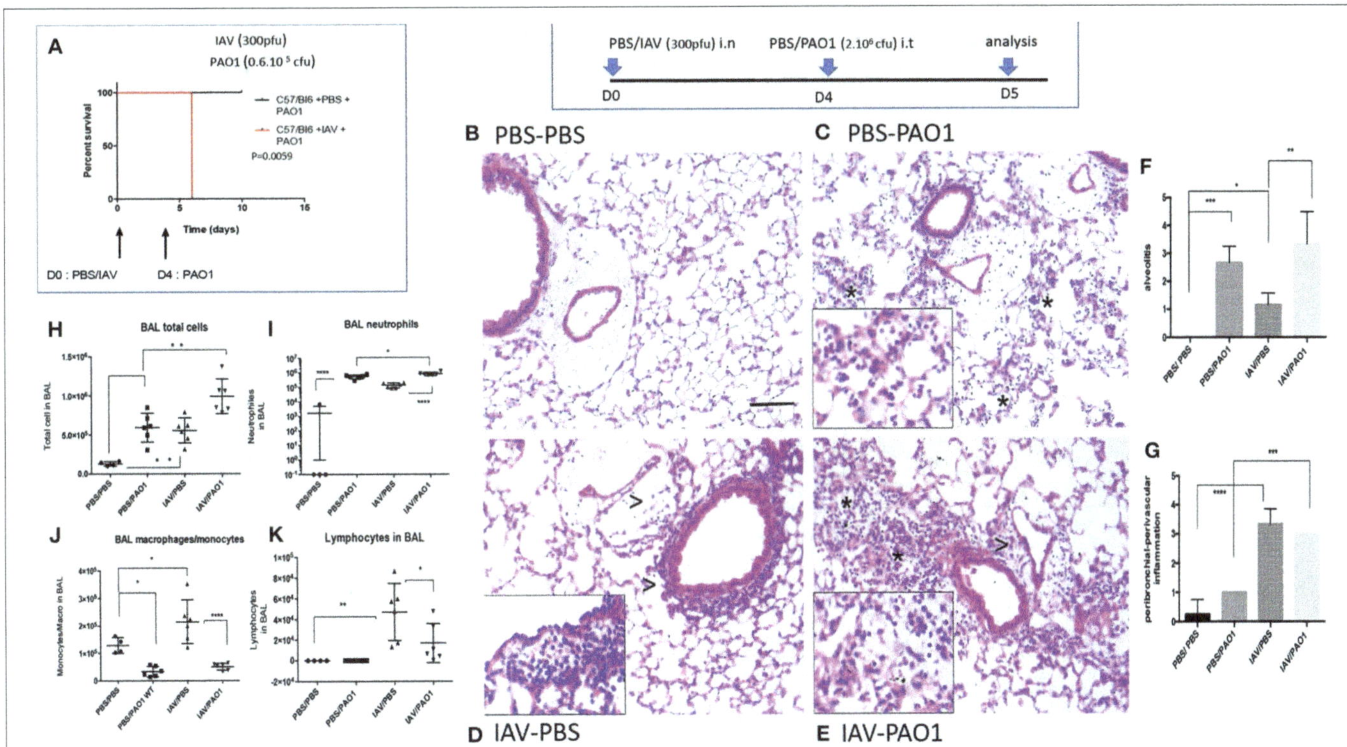

FIGURE 1 | IAV lung pre-infection sensitizes WT C57Bl/6 mice to further PAO1-mediated inflammation. **(A)** Survival experiment: C57Bl/6 WT mice were instilled i.n with either PBS or IAV (300 pfu) (two cohorts of six animals for each treatment). Four days later, mice were further instilled i.t with PAO1 ($0.6.10^6$ cfu), and mice survival was assessed, using Kaplan-Meier curves. Statistical tests were performed with the GraphPad Prism 6 package, using the Log-rank (Mantel-Cox) test, $p = 0.0059$. **(B–K)** Mechanistic experiment: at D0, C57Bl/6 WT mice were instilled i.n with either PBS or IAV (300 pfu). Four days later, mice were further instilled i.t with either PBS or PAO1 (2.10^6 cfu). At day 5, mice were sacrificed, and a bronchoalveolar lavage (BAL) was performed for cytospin cellular quantification **(H–K)**. Lungs were also obtained, inflated, cut and used for histological observation **(B–E)** and inflammation scoring **(F–G)**. NB: The three animals used for histology for the PBS/PAO1 and IAV/PAO1 groups all scored similarly, respectively 1 ($n = 3$) and 3 ($n = 3$). There are therefore no error bars. **(B–E)** (PBS/PBS; PBS/PAO1; IAV/PBS; IAV/PAO1, respectively): inflammatory lesions of treated lungs. Representative images of each condition on H&E slides at x20 original magnification. Scale bar: 200 µm. Stars indicate neutrophilic alveolar influx; arrow heads indicate perivascular and peribronchial mononuclear cell inflammation. Inserts are x40 magnification of cellular influx (mostly neutrophils in PBS-PAO1, mononuclear cells in IAV-PBS and a mix in IAV-PAO1). Results are shown as means ± SD. Statistical significance: ANOVA, multiple comparison, Tukey's test, with each point representing an individual mouse, *$p < 0.05$; **$p < 0.01$; ***$p < 0.001$; ****$p < 0.0001$.

described in Barbier et al. (31) Bastaert et al. (35), and Le Gars et al. (36), respectively. Alternatively, BAL MMP activity was measured by zymography (30).

RNA Preparation

Cell monolayers were directly lysed in RNA lysis buffer. RNA isolation was performed using the PureLink® RNA Mini Kit (12183018A, Ambion, Life technologies), following the manufacturer's instructions. For lung RNA assessment, frozen lungs were homogenized in RNA lysis buffer provided by the Pure Link RNA extraction kit (Life Technologies), using lysing matrix D tubes and the FastPrep-24 5G mixer (MP Biomedical) at 4°C (two cycles of 40s, level 5). Briefly, lysates were mixed with 70% ethanol and loaded onto a silica-membrane column. After different washings, total RNA was eluted in DNAse-RNAse-free water and stored at −80°C until use.

DNase treatment was performed prior to Reverse transcription polymerase chain reaction (RT-PCR) using RNAse-free DNAse I (Roche) at 37°C for 10 min. DNAse was then inactivated by increasing the temperature to 70°C for 10 min. Complementary DNA (cDNA) was synthesized from total RNA (500 ng) using M-MLV Reverse Transcriptase (Promega) as per the supplier's protocol (1 h at 37°C followed by 1 min at 70°C).

Real-time PCR was done in a 7500 Fast Real-Time PCR System (Applied Biosystems). Reactions were performed in a total volume of 15 μl using 2x Fast SYBR® Green Master Mix (Life Technologies), 2 μl of diluted cDNA, 2 μmol forward primer, and 2 μmol reverse primer in a 96-well plate. PCR was run with the standard program: 95°C 10 min, 40 times of cycling 95°C 15 s and 60°C 1 min in a 96-well plate. Triplicate Ct values were obtained, and results were expressed as dCT = CT gene of interest-CT HPRT/18S (with low and high values representing high and low levels of the gene of interest, respectively). Alternatively, the results were expressed using the comparative Ct (ΔΔCt) calculation and the following formula: Fold change (RQ) = $2^{-(\Delta\Delta CT)}$, using "control cells" as calibrator (arbitrary unit =1).

The primers used were the following: M2 viral protein: (Fw: aagaccaatcctgtcacctct; Rw: caaagcgtctacgctgcagtc); CCL-5: (Fw: cagtcgtctttgtcacccgaa; Rw: tcccaagctaggacaagagca); IL-8 (Fw: agagacagcagagcacacaa; Rw: ttagcactccttggcaaaac); IL-6 (Fw: tcaatgaggagacttgcctg; Rw: tgtactcatctgcacagcctc); HPRT (Fw: ttgctttccttggtcaggca; Rw: atccaacacttcgtggggtc); 18s rRNA (Fw: cttagagggacaagtggcg; Rw: acgctgagccagtcagtgta).

Histology

Perfused and fixed lungs (4% PFA in PBS, overnight at 4°C) were embedded in paraffin and sectioned in slides (4 μm), stained

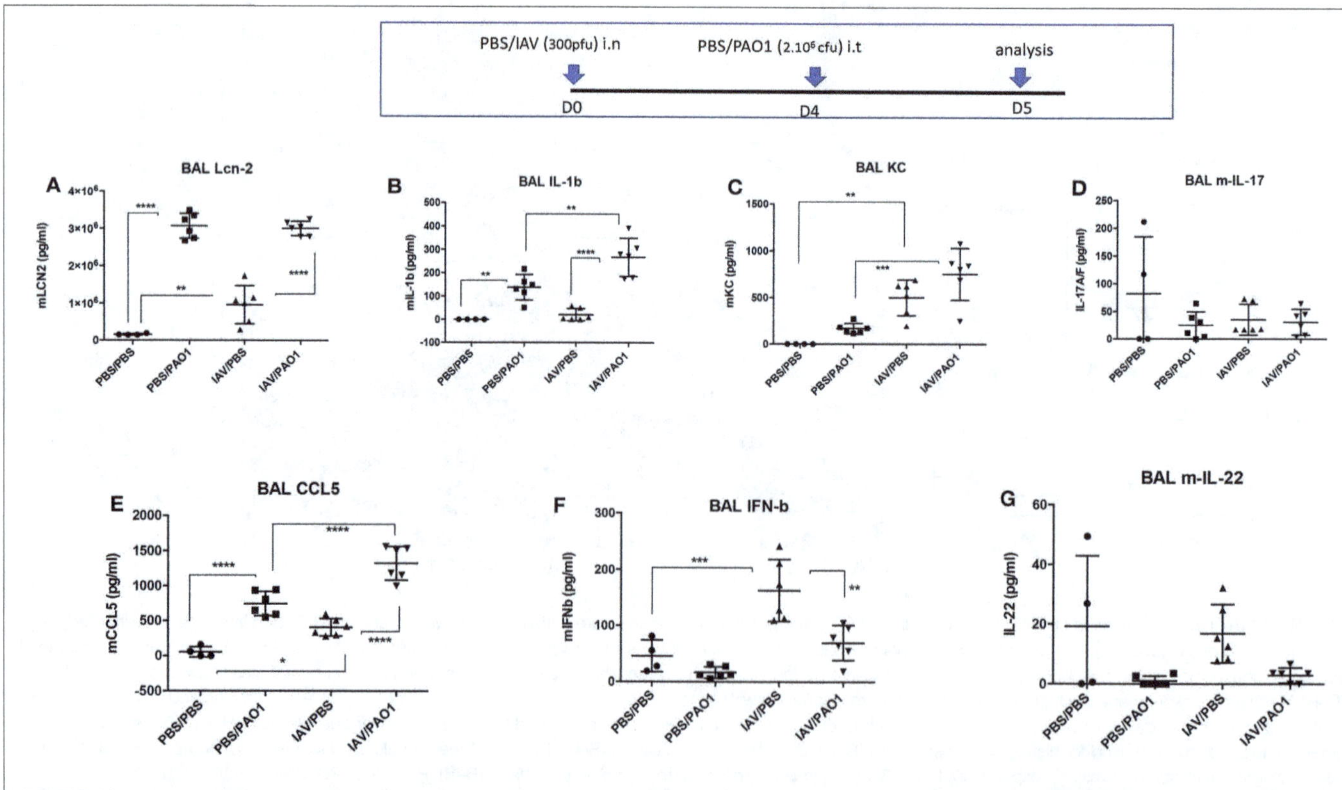

FIGURE 2 | IAV lung pre-infection sensitizes WT C57Bl/6 mice to further PAO1-mediated cytokine production. BAL supernatants (see **Figure 1** legend) were further used for assessment of cytokines and mediators. Each symbol represent an individual mouse. Statistical significance: ANOVA, multiple comparison, Tukey's test, with each point representing an individual mouse, *p < 0.05; **p < 0.01; ***p < 0.001; ****p < 0.0001. **(A)** Lcn-2 levels, **(B)** IL-1b levels, **(C)** KC levels, **(D)** IL-17 levels, **(E)** CCL5 levels, **(F)** IFN-b levels, **(G)** IL-22 levels.

with Hematoxylin-eosin. Inflammation was scored with a semi-quantitative scale (0: no inflammation to 4: severe inflammation with exudate) both in alveolar and in peribronchial/interstitial lung compartments.

Statistical Analysis

Data were expressed as means ± standard errors of the mean (SEM) unless otherwise stated. One-way ANOVA was used to determine statistically significant differences among groups followed by Tukey's multiple test for comparisons. Survival curves in murine model experiments were plotted using Kaplan-Meier curves and statistical tests were performed using the Log-rank (Mantel-Cox) test. All analyses were performed with Prism version 7, GraphPad.

RESULTS

IAV Pre-Infection Exacerbates *P. aeruginosa* Inflammation in C57Bl/6 Murine Lungs

In survival experiments, neither IAV (not shown) nor PAO1 alone (**Figure 1A**), induced any fatalities of C57Bl/6 mice, at the doses used. In contrast, IAV pre-treatment followed by PAO1 infection induced the death of all animals (**Figure 1A**).

In mechanistic experiments, C57Bl/6 mice infected with IAV (**Figures 1D,F,G**) or PAO1 (**Figures 1C,F,G**) exhibited increased lung tissue inflammation, compared to PBS mock-treated animals (**Figures 1B,F,G**). Neutrophils were the overwhelming cell type present after "PAO1 alone" infection, mainly in the alveoli (**Figures 1C,F**). By contrast, lymphocytes and monocytes (even though neutrophils were also present) were predominant in "IAV-alone"-infected animals and were mostly located in perivascular/peribronchial areas (**Figures 1D,G**).

Sequential IAV and PAO1 infections gave rise to increased neutrophilia, compared to "PAO1 alone" treatment (**Figures 1E–G**), especially in the peribronchial/perivascular areas, even though, notably, neither IL-17 nor IL-22 levels were increased over controls (**Figures 2D–G**).

This tissue inflammation was mirrored in BALs (**Figures 1H–K**), showing increased cytokine and inflammatory mediators in infected animals (IL-1β, KC, CCL-5, Lcn2, **Figures 2A–C,E,F**). IL-1β levels were only significantly increased following "PAO1-alone" and after "IAV+PAO1" infections (**Figure 2B**). With the notable exception of IFN-β, which was reduced, when compared to IAV alone (**Figure 2F**), and IL-17 and IL-22, which were not increased (**Figures 2D,G**), all inflammatory parameters

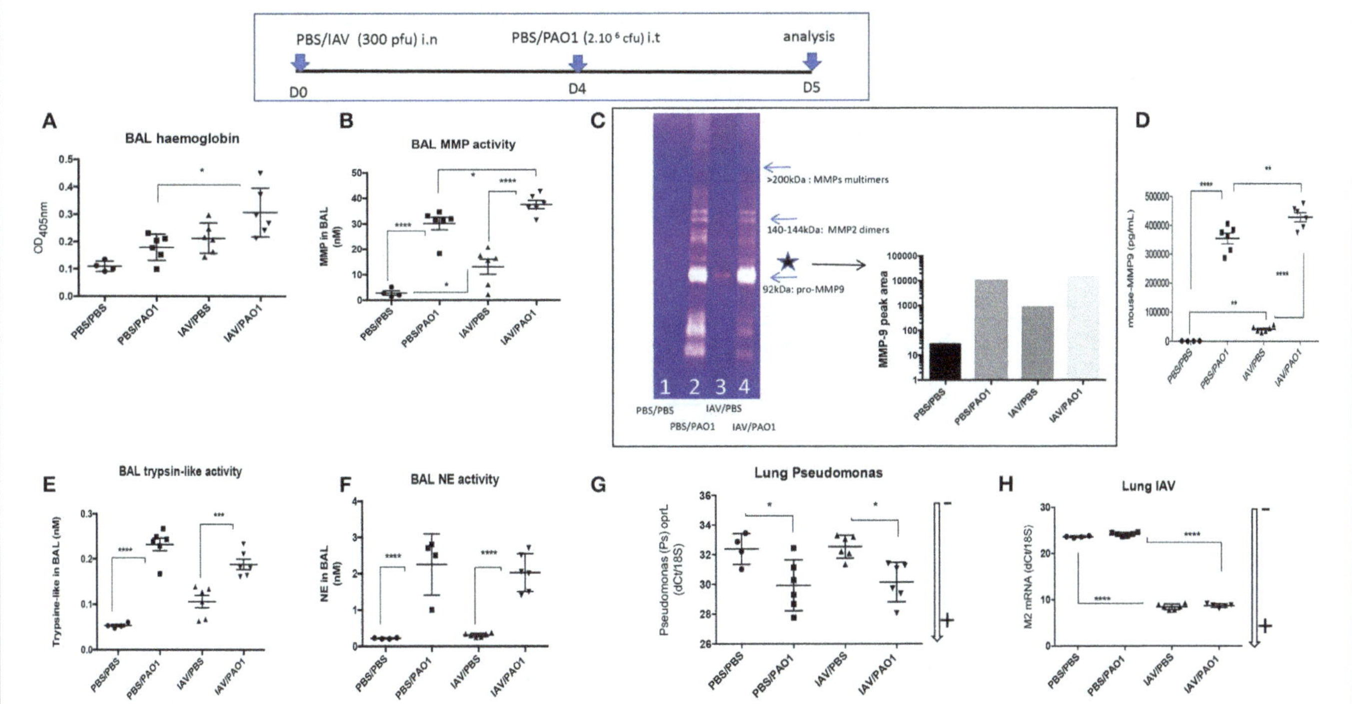

FIGURE 3 | IAV lung pre-infection sensitizes WT C57Bl/6 mice to further PAO1-mediated metalloprotease activity and lung injury. BAL supernatants (see **Figure 1** legend) was further used for hemoglobin content (absorbance at 405 nm, **A**) and protease activity **(B–H)**. **(B)** BAL metalloprotease bioactivity was assessed with the synthetic substrate 5-FAM-Ser-Pro-Leu-Ala-Gln-Ala-ValArg-Ser-Ser-Ser-Arg-Lys(5-TAMRA)-NH2 (35). **(C)** BAL metalloprotease bioactivity was also assessed by zymography. BALs from individual mice within the same experimental group (1: PBS/PBS; 2: PBS/PAO1; 3: IAV/PBS; 4: IAV/PAO1) were pooled and Pro-MMP-9 (*, left panel) intensity was assessed by densitometry (right panel). **(D)** BAL MMP-9 levels were measured by ELISA. **(E)** BAL trypsin-like activity was assessed with the synthetic substrate Boc-Phe-Ser-Arg-7-amido-4-méthylcoumarin (37). **(F)** BAL NE bioactivity was assessed with the synthetic substrate MeOSuc-Ala-Ala-Pro-Val-AMC (27). Lung extracts were also used for RNA preparation and RT-PCR analysis of M2 and oprL genes [as read-outs for IAV and PAO1 loads, respectively **(G–H)**]. Low and high RNA content is marked with an arrow indicating low (–) or high (+) level of expression. Results are shown as means ± SD. Statistical significance: ANOVA, multiple comparison, Tukey's test, with each point representing an individual mouse, $^{*}p < 0.05$; $^{**}p < 0.01$; $^{***}p < 0.001$; $^{****}p < 0.0001$.

were increased in IAV + PAO1-treated animals, compared to IAV alone. Compared to "PAO1" alone, IL-1β, KC and CCL-5 were significantly increased in the "IAV + PAO1" treatment.

Inflammation resulted in lung injury, demonstrated by increased BAL hemoglobin levels, and again IAV pre-treatment potentiated the latter (**Figure 3A**). Potentially explaining this, BALF metalloprotease activity (MMP), as measured with a synthetic substrate, was increased in IAV-alone- and PAO1-alone-treated mice (**Figure 3B**). This activity was again potentiated, when IAV preceded PAO1 treatment. Using zymography, we further showed that MMP-9 was present and was clearly the most abundant MMP in BAL of IAV-infected animals (*, 3C), which was confirmed by ELISA (3D). Importantly, and specifically, IAV/PAO1 induced more MMP-9 than PAO1 alone (3D).

Other protease activities were also present in BAL, albeit at much lower concentrations: trypsin-like activity was mostly increased in PAO1-alone and IAV+PAO1 arms of the experiment (**Figure 3E**), compared to MMP levels.

NE BALF activity was also increased in PAO1-alone and in IAV+PAO1-treated mice, but very poorly in "IAV-alone" mice (**Figure 3F**).

Notably, neither IAV nor PAO1 influenced each other's infection, using M2 and oprL genes as a read-out for IAV and PAO1 loads, respectively (**Figures 3G,H**), suggesting that dysregulated direct antimicrobial activity was not a major player here.

Epithelial Cell Modeling of IAV/PAO1/IL-1b Stimulations

Because epithelial cells are the main IAV targets, the interactions studied above *in vivo* were then modeled *in vitro* in these cells. After a comparative study in NCI-H292, BEAS-2B, and A549 lung cells, we found (not shown) that A549 cells were most responsive to IAV-, IAV PAMPs-, PAO1-, and IL-1ß-mediated infection/stimulation, and these cells were therefore further studied below:

(a) IAV differentially regulate inflammatory/anti-viral and antimicrobial mediators in A549 cells.

We either infected A549 cells with IAV (moi 1) or stimulated them with either poly IC, 5′ ppp ds RNA, synthetic ligands for TLR-3, RIG-I and MDA-5, respectively, or with IL-1ß, a sterile inflammatory stimulus. We then measured the RNA and protein levels of a variety of mediators (cytokines, antimicrobial/anti-inflammatory molecules), all relevant to the *in vivo* model described in **Figures 1–3**.

At the RNA level (**Figure 4**: NB: ΔdCT values are inversely proportional to RNA levels, and arrows indicate gene expression +/−), we showed that IL-8 was clearly induced by IAV and IL-1ß (ΔdCT of −4 and −7.5 respectively, **Figure 4B**), but modestly by

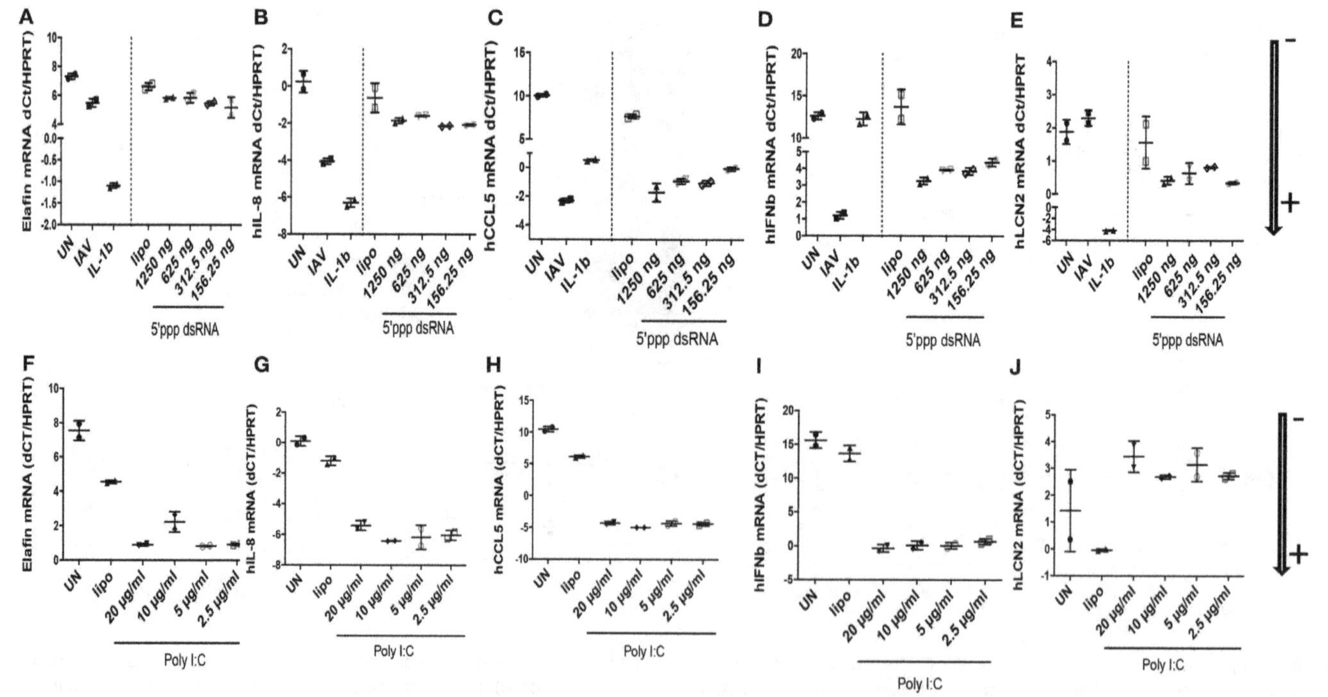

FIGURE 4 | IAV-, polyIC-, 5′ppp dsRNA-, and IL-1β- mediated induction of elafin, IL-8, CCL5, IFN- β, Lcn-2 RNA in A549 cells. At D0, A549 cells (24 wells plates, 70% confluence) were either left unstimulated (UN), infected with IAV (moi 1), or stimulated with either IL-1β (10 ng/ml), lipofectamine control (CLT lipo), 5′ ppp dsRNA (Invitrogen) or poly IC (Invitrogen), at various concentrations during 4 h at 37°C in OPTI-MEM medium. Cells were then washed, medium replenished, and 16 h later, cell lysates were recovered for further analysis of RNA **(A–J)**, respectively, for elafin, IL-8, CCL5, IFN- β, Lcn-2. q-PCR analysis was performed, and results expressed as dCT (CT gene of interest-CT HPRT), with low and high values representing high and low levels of the gene of interest, respectively (marked with an arrow indicating low (−) or high (+) level of expression). Two independent experiments (individual symbols) were performed. Results are shown as means ± SD.

5′ ppp dsRNA (ΔdCT of −1.0, **Figure 4B**) and at intermediate levels by poly-IC (ΔdCT of −4, **Figure 4G**). By contrast, CCL-5 RNA was robustly induced by all stimuli (ΔdCT of respectively −12, −10, −9.5, and −10, **Figures 4C,H**). Lcn-2 RNA was also strongly up-regulated by IL-1ß (ΔdCT of −7, **Figure 4E**), modestly by 5′ ppp dsRNA (**Figure 4E**) and even inhibited by poly IC (**Figure 4J**).

IFN-ß RNA stood alone since it was not induced by IL-1ß (**Figure 4D**), but was, as expected, strongly up-regulated by IAV, 5′ ppp dsRNA, and polyIC (ΔdCT of −11.5, −8, and −15, respectively, **Figures 4D,I**). When elafin, an antimicrobial molecule with anti-inflammatory/anti-NF-kb activity (27–30) was considered, IL-1ß was again clearly the greatest inducer of elafin mRNA (ΔdCT of −8, **Figure 4A**), with polyIC and IAV being strong and intermediate inducers (ΔdCT of −6.5 and −2, **Figures 4A,F**), respectively.

When protein levels were studied (**Figure 5**), we observed that IAV had important post-transcriptional regulatory activities: IAV clearly up-regulated IL-8, CCL-5, IFN-ß proteins (**Figures 5B–D**, respectively), in keeping with increased RNA levels, while having no effect on elafin and Lcn2 proteins (**Figures 5A,E**, respectively). Poly IC and 5′ ppp dsRNA effects were even more contrasted: poly IC slightly down-regulated the accumulation of IL-8 (**Figure 5G**) and drastically down-regulated that of elafin and Lcn-2 (**Figures 5F,J**) proteins, while very robustly inducing that of CCL-5 (**Figure 5H**) and IFN-ß (**Figure 5I**). Similarly, 5′ ppp dsRNA also sharply induced CCL-5 and IFN-ß protein accumulation (**Figures 5C,D**, respectively), in keeping with its effect on RNA, but had virtually no effect on elafin (**Figure 5A**), IL-8 (**Figure 5B**), or Lcn2 (**Figure 5E**) protein accumulation. These results demonstrated that IAV had specific down-regulatory post transcriptional activity on elafin and Lcn-2, and that its effect is mimicked by its nucleic acid analogs, either polyIC or 5′ppp dsRNA, suggesting an intra-cellular mode of action:

(b) IAV, but not PAO1, post-transcriptionally down-regulates elafin expression in A549 cells.

We then demonstrated in further *in vitro* independent experiments that the post-transcriptional regulation observed in **Figures 4, 5**, in which IAV induced RNA, but not protein levels of elafin, was indeed "IAV-specific," since PAO1 up-regulated both RNA and protein levels of elafin and IL-8 instead (see **Figures S1G,H,J,K** and the **Supplementary Materials**).

(c) IAV exacerbates IL-1ß- and PAO1-mediated inflammatory responses and down-regulates elafin and Lcn-2 accumulation in A549 cells.

Having shown *in vivo* that IAV could exacerbate PAO1 responses (**Figures 1–3**) and that, studied individually, IAV alone (but not PAO1) could inhibit *in vitro* elafin and Lcn-2 protein production specifically (**Figure 5** and **Figure S1**), we set up a "multi-hit inflammatory model" in A549 cells, where combinations of "mixes" were studied together (**Figures 6, 7**), similarly to the *in*

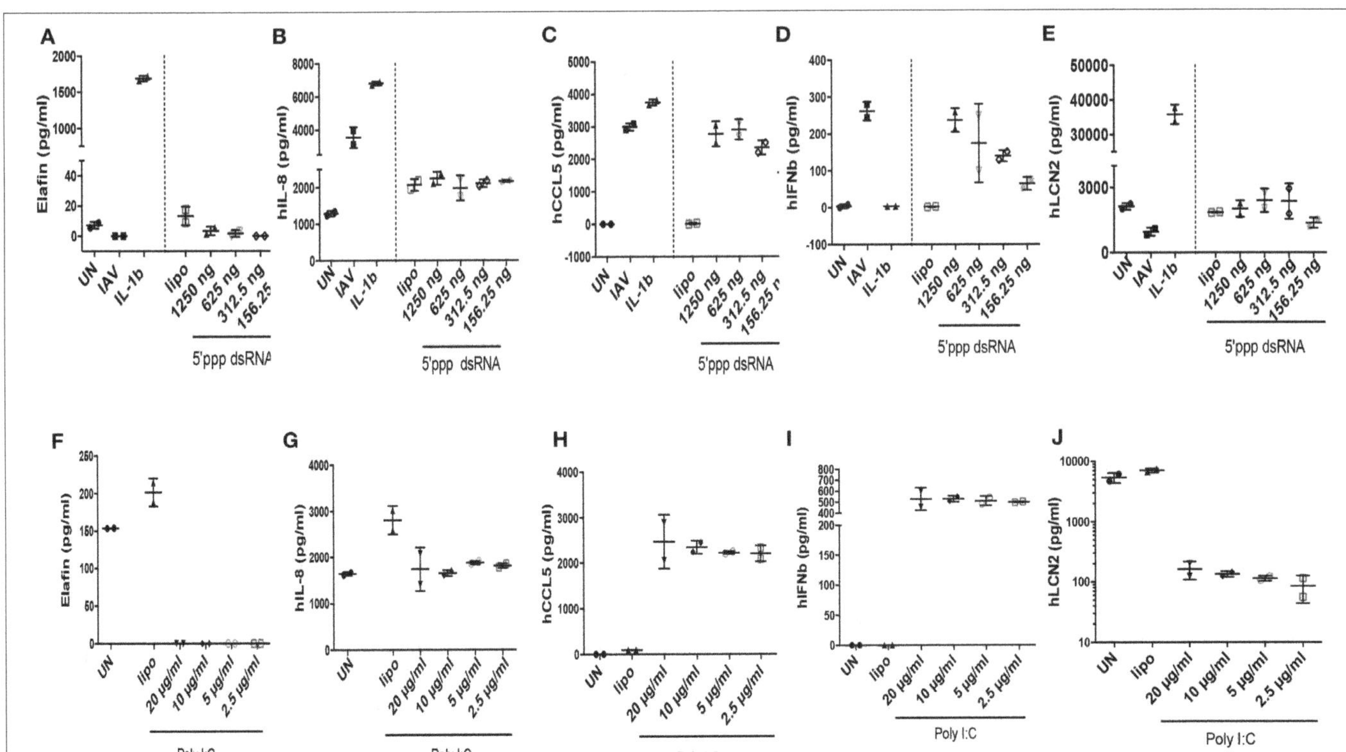

FIGURE 5 | IAV-, polyIC-, 5′ppp dsRNA- and IL-1β- mediated induction of elafin, IL-8, CCL5, IFN- β, Lcn-2 protein in A549 cells. The supernatants obtained from the experiments depicted in **Figure 4** were recovered and used for protein measurement (ELISA) of elafin, IL-8, CCL5, IFN- β, Lcn-2 **(A–J)**.

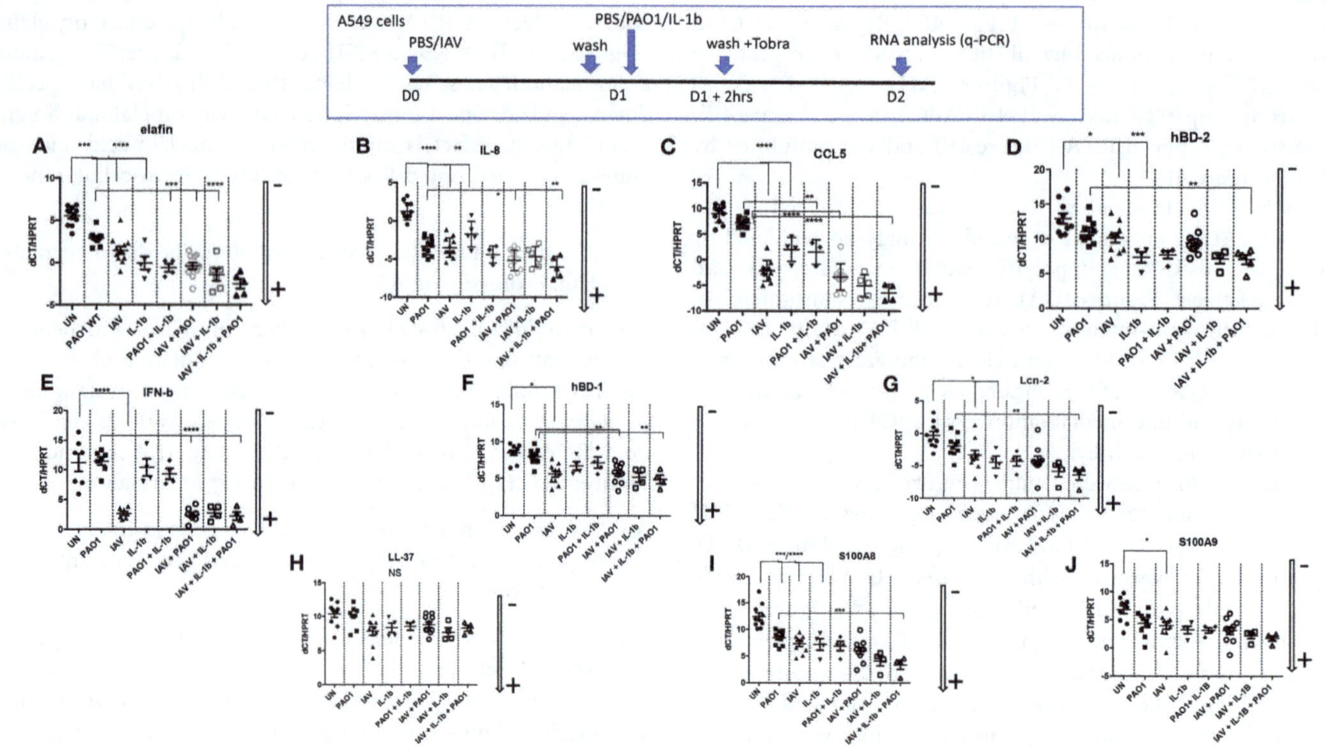

FIGURE 6 | Epithelial cell regulation of cytokines/chemokines and antimicrobials transcription in IAV/PAO1/IL-1β co-infection models. At D0, A549 cells (24 wells plates) were either uninfected or infected with IAV (moi 1) in serum-free medium for 1 h. After washing, and o/n incubation, cells were either replenished with fresh medium and left untreated (UN), or treated with either PAO1 alone (moi 1), IL-1β alone (10 ng/ml), or IL-1β + PAO1 (at the same doses). After a further 2 h, cells were washed with F12K medium containing tobramycin (40 μg/ml), to remove PAO1 load, and left for 24 h in medium. At the end of the incubation, at D2, supernatants and cell lysates were recovered, and cytokines/chemokines/antimicrobials were assessed for RNA (this figure) and protein levels (ELISAs, **Figure 7**). For RNA analysis, gene expression is marked with an arrow indicating low (–) or high (+) level of expression (see **Figure 4** for the full explanation). Results are shown as means ± SD. Statistical significance: ANOVA, multiple comparison, Tukey's test, with each point representing an individual mouse, $^*p < 0.05$; $^{**}p < 0.01$; $^{***}p < 0.001$; $^{****}p < 0.0001$. **(A)** Elafin RNA, **(B)** IL-8 RNA, **(C)** CCL5 RNA, (D) hBD-2 RNA, **(E)** IFN-b RNA, **(F)** hBD-1 RNA, **(G)** Lcn-2 RNA, **(H)** LL-37 RNA, **(I)** S100 A8 RNA, **(J)** S100A9 RNA.

vivo protocol. In addition to IAV and PAO1, IL-1ß was added in this model, as an important "first wave" cytokine up-regulated *in vivo* (**Figure 2**).

Echoing these *in vivo* data, we showed that all these agents up-regulated the transcription of many inflammatory/antimicrobial molecules in A549 cells, as evidenced by a reduction in dCT levels (**Figure 6**). Notably, compared to "PAO1 alone," pre-infection with IAV followed by PAO1 infection further increased IL-8 (**Figure 6B**), CCL-5 (**Figure 6C**), hBD-1 (**Figure 6F**), and elafin (**Figure 6A**) mRNA levels.

IFN-ß inductions stood out as notable exceptions (**Figure 6E**), where only IAV-containing "mixes" were effective agonists, and LL-37 (**Figure 6H**), whose expression was relatively stable, in keeping with the described relative constitutiveness of this antimicrobial.

When protein levels were assessed in supernatants (**Figure 7**), IAV again demonstrated post-transcriptional regulation on elafin and Lcn-2; indeed, there was a trend for decreased elafin and Lcn-2 production in IAV + PAO1 treatments, compared to PAO1 alone, and IAV had a clear down-regulating effect on these mediators when "IAV+ IL-1β" and "IAV+ PAO1 + IL-1β" were compared to "IL-1β" and "IAV+ PAO1," respectively (**Figures 7A,B**). Again, this regulatory effect was specific since, as demonstrated above, IAV clearly up-regulated IL-8 and CCL-5 proteins, compared to untreated cells, and did either not change for IL-8 (**Figure 7C**) or even increased for CCL-5 (**Figure 7D**) protein production, when cells were infected with IAV and further treated with PAO1 and/or IL-1β.

To assess whether the IAV regulatory effect was acting intra- or extra-cellularly, the levels of the same mediators were measured in A549 lysates (instead of in supernatants). We found that, mirroring the effects observed in A549 supernatants, IAV again down-regulated the IL-1β-mediated intracellular accumulation of elafin and Lcn2 (**Figures 8A,B**), but not those of IL-8 and CCL-5 (**Figures 8C,D**).

In addition, we also studied the IAV regulation of an exogenously added Adenovirus-h-elafin construct in A549 cells (**Figures 8E–G**) and found that IAV also down-regulated elafin accumulation in both supernatants and lysates (**Figures 8E,F**).

Importantly, this IAV-mediated down-regulation was not due to an interference of IAV with Ad infection, since IAV

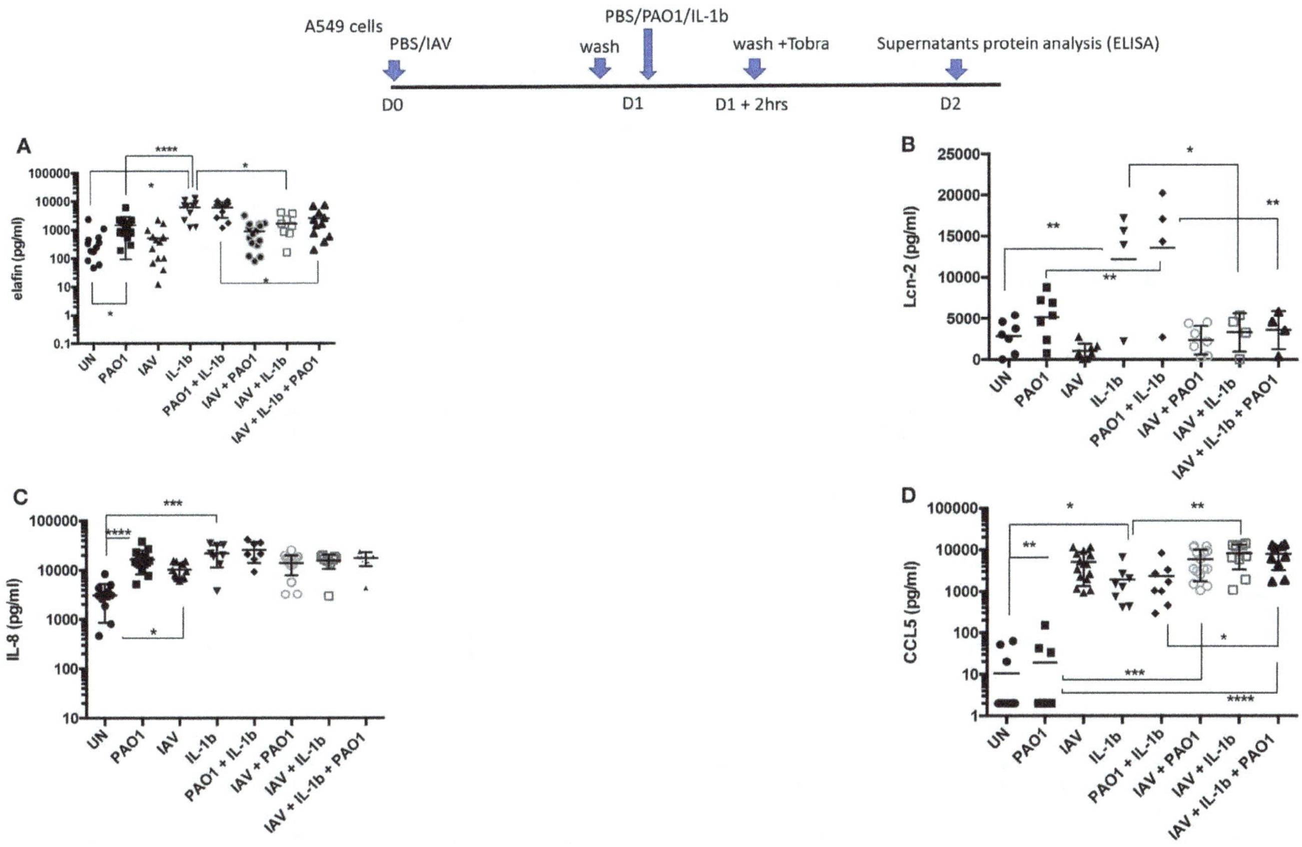

FIGURE 7 | Cytokines/chemokines and antimicrobials protein production in IAV/PAO1 and IAV/ IL-1β co-infection models. Elafin, IL-8, CCL5, and Lcn-2 protein content was assessed by ELISA in the supernatants from the experiment described in **Figure 6**. Results are shown as means ± SD. Statistical significance: ANOVA, multiple comparison, Tukey's test, with each point representing an individual mouse, *$p < 0.05$; **$p < 0.01$; ***$p < 0.001$; ****$p < 0.0001$. **(A)** Elafin levels, **(B)** Lcn-2 levels, **(C)** IL-8 levels, **(D)** CCL5 levels.

+ Ad-h-elafin- RNA levels were even higher than in the Ad-elafin "alone" condition, as demonstrated with lower dCT levels; showing that the Ad vector efficiently delivered its genetic cargo (**Figure 8G**).

IAV Pre-Infection Down-Regulate Elafin Expression *in vivo* and Exacerbates *P. aeruginosa* Inflammation in Elafin-Over-Expressing Mice

Having demonstrated *in vitro* that IAV specifically inhibited elafin and Lcn-2 protein production in lung epithelial cells, two important antimicrobial/anti-inflammatory molecules (27–30, 38), we then tested whether this regulatory effect was also observed *in vivo*. Because C57Bl/6 WT mice are "natural KO" for elafin (34), this was tested in h-elafin over-expressers, using the Ad-h-elafin over-expressing system (33). Since elafin expression was only required in our protocol as a "read out target" for IAV, Ad-h-elafin was only given 16 h (at the same time as either PBS or PAO1) before animals were culled for analysis. Expectedly, given its anti-inflammatory nature as demonstrated previously (27–30), the PBS/Ad-elafin/PBS "Control" arm of the experiment did not induce any inflammation "per se," as assessed by a "typical" percentage of macrophages and neutrophils recovered in BALs, 99 and 1%, respectively, **Figures S2B–D**. Importantly, although IAV did not decrease either basal or PAO1-induced lung elafin RNA levels (**Figure 9A**), it drastically reduced elafin protein accumulation in BALs, akin to that observed *in vitro* (**Figure 9B**). In contrast, IAV up-regulated both Lcn-2 RNA and protein levels (**Figures 9C,D**) and did not significantly affect PAO1-mediated Lcn-2 protein up-regulation (**Figure 9D**), contrary to that observed *in vitro* in epithelial cells.

Irrespectively, infection of Ad-h-elafin-treated mice with either IAV or PAO1 exhibited increased inflammation, as assessed by BAL total inflammatory cells, neutrophilia (**Figures S2A–F**), increase in cytokine and antimicrobials levels (**Figures S2G–N**), protease activity (**Figures 9E–G,J**), and tissue injury (**Figure 9L**). This confirmed what was observed in WT C57Bl/6 mice (**Figures 1–3**), i.e., the exacerbated effect of IAV on PAO1 infection and the key involvement of metalloproteases, including MMP-9 (**Figures 9G,J**). Importantly again, as also demonstrated in WT C57Bl/6 mice (**Figure 3G**), neither IAV nor PAO1 influenced each other's infection (**Figures 9H,I**),

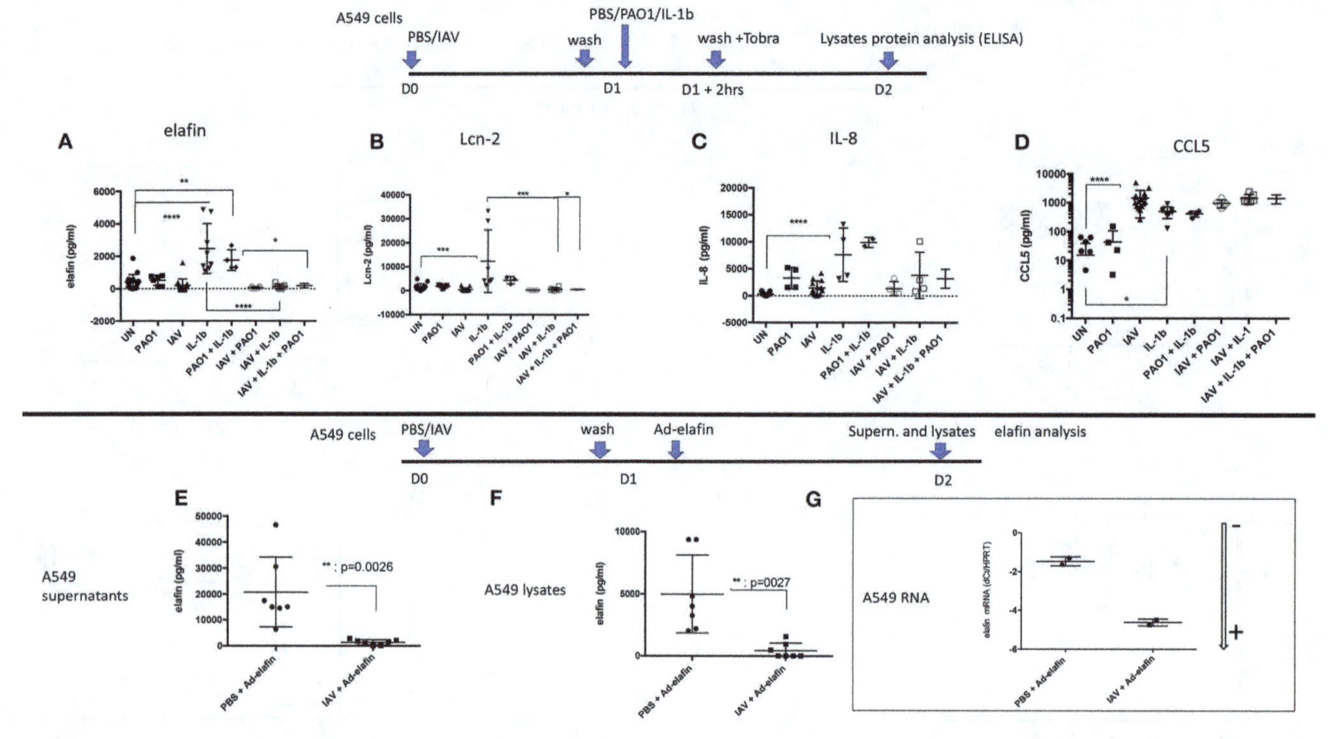

FIGURE 8 | IAV-mediated post-transcriptional regulation occurs intra-cellularly and in an Adenovirus-elafin reporter system in A549 cells. Top panel: A549 cells were treated as explained in the **Figure 6** legend. Cell lysates were recovered and protein levels for elafin, Lcn-2, IL-8, CCL-5 (**A–D**, respectively) were measured by ELISA. Bottom panel: A549 cells were mock-infected or infected with IAV (moi =1), as explained above. After 16 h, cells were further infected with replication-deficient Adenovirus-h-elafin (33). After a further 24 h, A549 supernatants and lysates were recovered and elafin protein levels measured by ELISA (**E,F** respectively). In a subset experiment, cell lysates were recovered for q-PCR assessment of elafin RNA content. The latter is marked with an arrow indicating low (–) or high (+) level of expression **(G)** (see **Figure 4** for full explanation). Results are shown as means ± SD. Statistical significance (except for **G**): ANOVA, multiple comparison, Tukey's test, with each point representing an individual mouse, *$p < 0.05$; **$p < 0.01$; ***$p < 0.001$; ****$p < 0.0001$).

reinforcing that dysregulated direct antimicrobial activity was not the major cause of IAV-induced inflammatory exacerbations. This was further strengthened by the use of the MMP inhibitor batimastat (see below, **Figure 10**). The latter was chosen because it does not inhibit LasB (39), quantitatively the most abundant PAO1 metalloprotease (30, 35), therefore allowing us to specifically address the effect of IAV on host (and not PAO1) metalloproteases. Importantly, because host proteases are known to be important for IAV replication (40, 41), and in order not to affect that cycle, batimastat was given "therapeutically" at D4 at the peak of IAV replication, at the same time as PAO1, and not "prophylactically" at the time of IAV infection (D0).

We showed that batimastat delayed the lethality of mice co-infected with IAV and PAO1 (**Figure 10A**), and down-regulated gelatinolytic activity, including MMP-9 expression, as shown by zymography (**Figure 10B**), and ELISA (**Figure 10C**). In addition, batimastat treatment down-regulated neutrophilic inflammation (**Figures 10D–G**) and tissue injury (**Figure 10L**), confirming that MMPs are indeed instrumental in the IAV-subversion of lung tissue resilience.

Interestingly, the beneficial effect of batimastat did not extend to rescuing elafin protein levels (**Figure 10I**), and even down-regulated Lcn-2 accumulation (**Figure 10J**), suggesting that proteolytic digestion of elafin by MMPs was not at play here, neither *in vivo* nor *in vitro* (not shown). Interestingly, batimastat was strikingly associated with a sharp increase in PAO1 load in lungs (**Figures 10M,O**), assessed by two independent methods, and in spleen (**Figure 10N**), demonstrating bacterial translocation into the periphery, and suggesting again a clear dissociation increase between tissue resilience and resistance to PAO1. In contrast, batimastat did not influence IAV load (**Figure 10P**). Some of the above results are described in more detail in the **Supplementary Material** (**Supplementary Material Results** and **Figure S2**).

DISCUSSION

Bacterial superinfections are an established risk of primary viral infections (e.g., rhinovirus, *Influenza* virus). Among the many potential mechanisms advocated, previous studies have suggested that IAV might promote further bacterial outgrowth by down-regulating neutrophilic function (14–17) or antimicrobial molecules (18–20). Notably, most

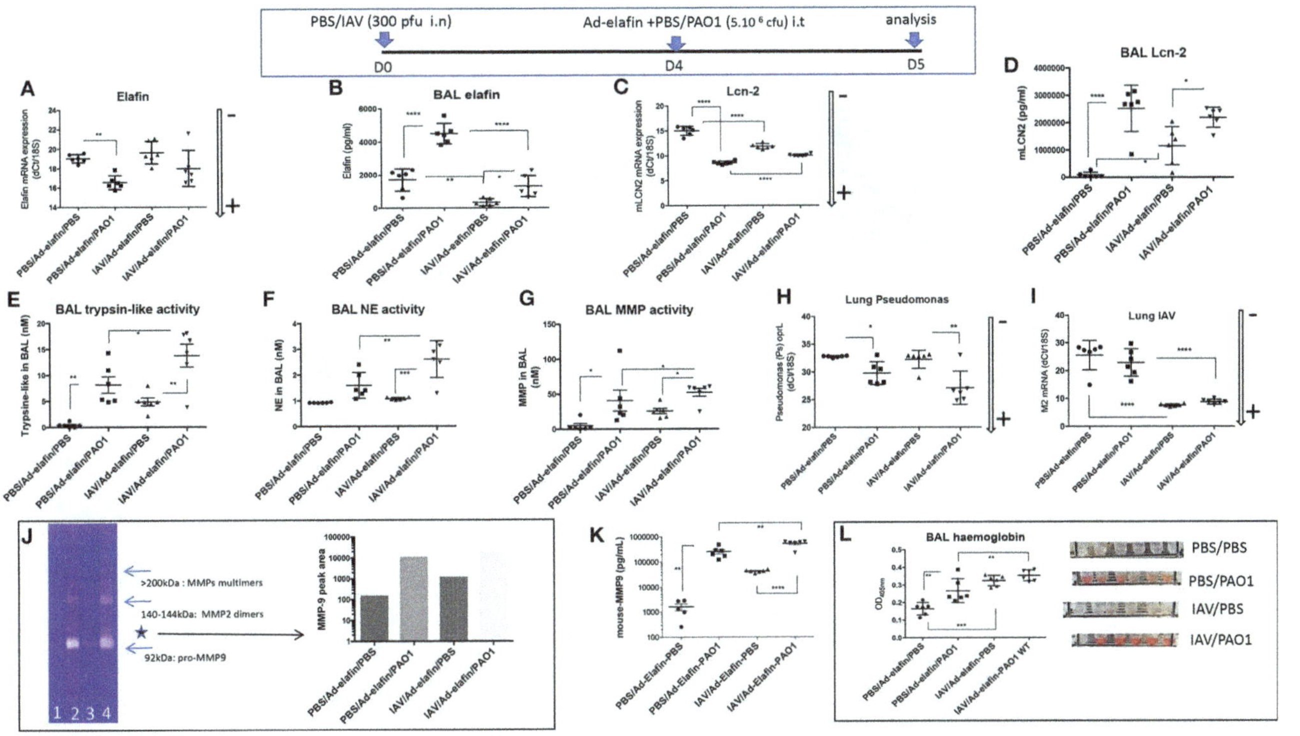

FIGURE 9 | IAV lung pre-infection sensitizes elafin over-expressing mice to further PAO1-mediated inflammation, metalloprotease activity, and lung injury. At D0, C57Bl/6 WT mice were instilled i.n with either PBS or IAV (300 pfu). Four days later, mice were further instilled i.t with Ad-elafin (3.10^6 pfu) plus either PBS or PAO1 (5.10^6 cfu). At day 5, mice were sacrificed, and a bronchoalveolar lavage (BAL) was performed. Lungs were also obtained, and RNA prepared for q-PCR assessment of elafin and Lcn-2 **(A,C)**. BAL was also used for elafin and Lcn-2 protein measurements **(B,D)**, and protease activity **(E–G)**, using synthetic substrates, or zymography **(J)**, as explained in the **Figure 3** legend. **(E)** BAL trypsin-like activity; **(F)** BAL NE bioactivity; **(G)** BAL MMP bioactivity; **(H)** Lung PAO1 load was assessed by q-PCR by measuring oprL expression; **(I)** Lung IAV load was similarly measured by q-PCR (M2 gene). As for other Figures, gene expression is marked with an arrow indicating low (–) or high (+) level of expression. **(J)** MMP bio activity was assessed by zymography: BALs from individual mice within the same experimental group (1: PBS/PBS; 2: PBS/PAO1; 3: IAV/PBS; 4: IAV/PAO1) were pooled and Pro-MMP-9 (*, left panel) intensity was assessed by densitometry (right panel). **(K)** BAL MMP-9 levels were measured by ELISA. **(L)** Hemoglobin levels were measured by absorbance at 413 nm. Results are shown as means ± SD. Statistical significance: ANOVA, multiple comparison, Tukey's test, with each point representing an individual mouse, $^*p < 0.05$; $^{**}p < 0.01$; $^{***}p < 0.001$; $^{****}p < 0.0001$.

authors have modeled their studies using *S. aureus* or *S. pneumoniae* as the secondary bacterial "hit," and despite its obvious clinical importance, no studies have, to our knowledge, comprehensively investigated mechanisms linking *Influenza* (IAV) and *P. aeruginosa* infections (16, 19). Using the latter combination, with the H3N2 and PAO1 strains, respectively, we show here in a variety of *in vitro* and *in vivo* models, that IAV dramatically down-regulates, at the post-transcriptional level, the antimicrobial/anti-inflammatory elafin/trappin-2 *in vitro* (**Figures 4–8** and **Figure S1**) and *in vivo* in PAO1- (**Figures 9**, **10** and **Figure S2**) and IL-1β-mediated models of inflammation (**Figures S3, S4** and **Supplementary Material Results**). Unfortunately, our attempts to determine whether other antimicrobial molecules might also be inhibited by IAV were thwarted by the previously reported unreliability of current available ELISA kits for antimicrobial molecules (not shown). An important exception was Lcn-2, which we also showed to be inhibited by IAV *in vitro* in epithelial cells (**Figures 4, 5, 7**), but not, unlike elafin, *in vivo* in mice lungs (**Figures 9**, **10** and **Figure S3**). Although the exact mechanism still remains obscure, IAV likely down-regulates, at least *in vitro*, an epithelial intra-cellular/cytosolic event, since elafin and Lcn2 intra-cellular protein levels were also drastically reduced (**Figure 8**).

Relatedly, in a previous study, Robinson et al. also showed that pre-infecting C57Bl/6 mice with PR8 H1N1 IAV down-regulated the antimicrobials Lcn2, RegIIIγ, and S100A8 mRNA levels upon further *S. aureus* infection, but the effect on protein levels was not reported, again likely because of the paucity of reliable ELISA kits (18). Relevantly, Mallia et al. showed that rhinovirus induced neutrophil elastase in COPD patients and suggests that the ensuing down-regulation of secretory leukocyte protease inhibitor and elafin is causative in triggering exacerbations in these patients (20). Relatedly, although no bacterial data were reported, in a transcriptomic study enrolling 1,610 individuals, 142 of which were followed for evaluation of acute viral respiratory illness, the elafin gene (PI3) was found to be the top downregulated gene in the acute phase of the *Influenza* infection, but not in the rhinovirus or other infection groups (42).

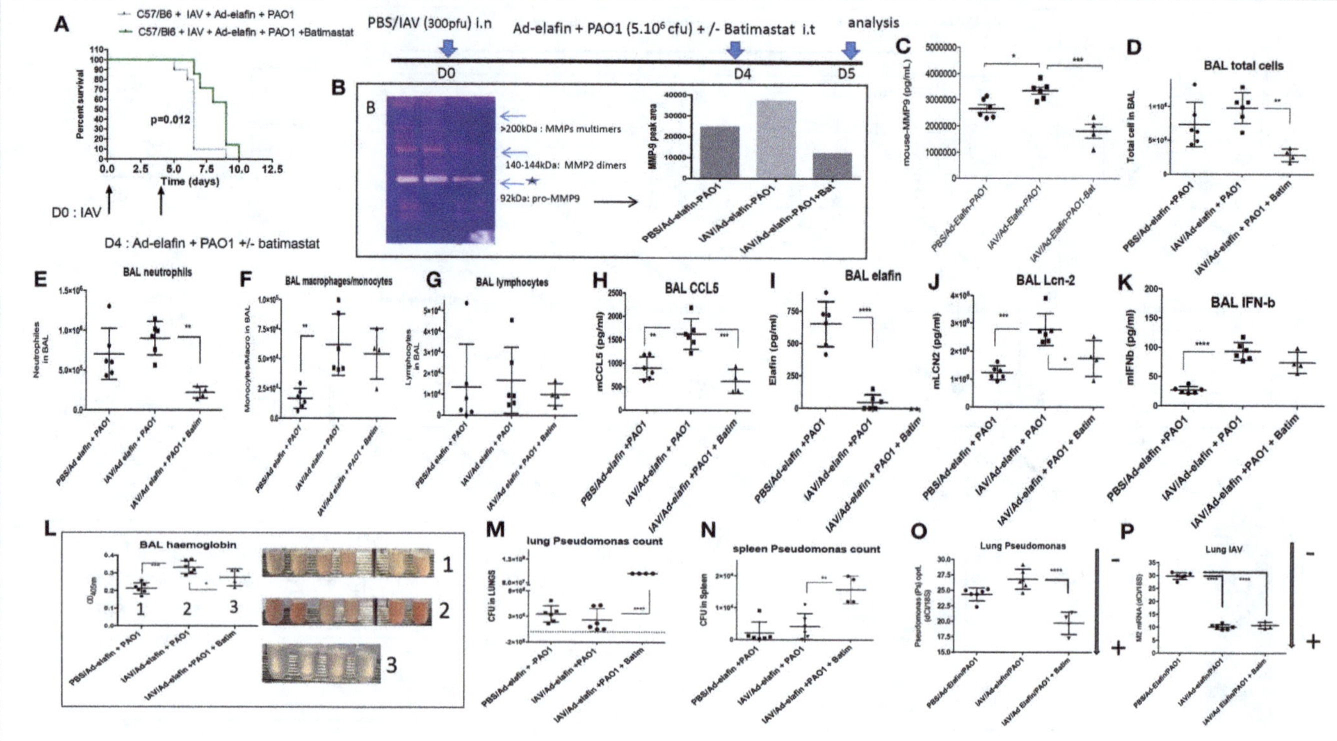

FIGURE 10 | The metalloprotease batimastat delays lethality in IAV + PAO1 infection and reduces inflammation and lung injury. **(A)** Survival experiment: C57/Bl6 mice were instilled i.n with IAV (300 pfu). Four days later, mice were further instilled i.t with Ad-elafin (3.10^6 pfu) and PAO1 (1.10^5 cfu) +/− the metalloprotease inhibitor batimastat (200 μgs). Survival was then followed and analyzed using Kaplan-Meier curves. Statistical tests were performed with the GraphPad Prism 6 package, using the Log-rank (Mantel-Cox) test. **(B–N)** Mechanistic experiments: C57Bl/6 WT mice were instilled i.n with either PBS or IAV (300 pfu). Four days later, mice were further instilled i.t with Ad-elafin (3.10^6 pfu) and PAO1 (5.10^6 cfu) +/− batimastat (200 μgs). At day 5, mice were sacrificed, and a bronchoalveolar lavage (BAL) was performed. BAL fluid supernatant was used for MMP measurements (zymography, **B**, and MMP-9 ELISA, **C**), cystospin cellular quantification **(D–G)**, ELISA assessment of a variety of mediators **(H–K)**, hemoglobin measurements **(L)**. Lungs and spleens were also harvested and used to measure PAO1 load (cfu counts on agarose plates, **M** and **N**, respectively). NB: in **(M)**, bacteria numbers were too high to be counted with the required precision. The value was therefore set at the maximum countable, considering the dilution used, i.e., 10^8 bacteria. PAO1 and IAV load were also independently assessed by measuring by q-PCR oprL and M2 gene expression, **O** and **P** respectively. Gene expression is marked, as above, with an arrow indicating low (−) or high (+) level of expression. Results are shown as means ± SD. Statistical significance: ANOVA, multiple comparison, Tukey's test, with each point representing an individual mouse, $^*p < 0.05$; $^{**}p < 0.01$; $^{***}p < 0.001$; $^{****}p < 0.0001$.

Regardless of the mechanisms, a reduction in some antimicrobial molecule levels, like elafin in our study, is certainly a plausible mechanism to explain further sensitivity to bacterial infections. However, although it has long been assumed that these molecules only have a direct bacteriostatic/bactericidal activity on microbes, it is now apparent that they have more complex and pleiotropic activities (43). Specifically, we have previously demonstrated that a 5 day local over-expression of elafin protected mice lungs against maladaptive neutrophilic inflammation in *P.a* infections (27, 28, 30), and also against Plasmodium-induced inflammation, through the induction of anti-inflammatory pathways (29). Importantly, the focus of the present study was not to "re-demonstrate" the protective effect of elafin against *P.a* (see above, 27), since elafin expression was short-lived in our Ad-elafin *in vivo* protocol (16 h), but allowed us, as discussed above, to demonstrate for the first time that it is down-regulated by IAV.

Equally as important, and indeed the initial focus of our study, was the demonstration that IAV pre-infection exacerbated further PAO1-mediated inflammatory responses, regardless of elafin presence (Ad-elafin protocol, **Figure 9** and **Figure S2**), or of its absence (in C57Bl/6 WT mice, **Figures 1–3**). Indeed, in the context of IAV+ PAO1 infection, increased lung inflammatory cell influx, particularly neutrophils, which were activated, as evidenced by increased NE bioactivity, was associated with enhanced inflammatory markers, e.g., IL-1β, KC, and with an increase in protease (mainly MMP) activity, and with tissue injury.

Strengthening previously reported data that IAV can induce metalloproteases in the lung and other organs (44–48), we further demonstrated that induced MMP activity (including that of MMP-9) by IAV pre-infection was indeed likely an important factor in sensitization of mice to further PAO1-mediated lung damage, since the MMP inhibitor batimastat significantly delayed lethality (**Figure 10A**) and diminished inflammatory responses (**Figures 10D–G**) and tissue damage (**Figure 10L**).

Although the cellular source of MMPs was not investigated here, neutrophils are known to secrete MMP-2 and 9 and they were likely a significant source (48). Interestingly, there was very little NE bio-activity in BALs from "IAV-alone"-infected animals, suggesting that either MMPs are more readily secreted than NE post-IAV, or that "IAV-alone" induced the secretion of elastase inhibitors capable of blocking NE activity.

Importantly, in contrast to previous IAV/bacteria associations studied in the past, e.g., IAV/*S.aureus*; IAV/*S. pneumoniae*, IAV pre-treatment did not condition the host to further PAO1 infection by restraining the IL-1β-IL-17 pathway (21, 22), and/or neutrophilic responses to bacteria (14–17). Although these differences may partly be explained by differences in the strains of *Influenza* used (H3N2 Scotland here), we believe that *P.a* may clearly respond differentially from other bacteria. This combination sets the scene for a furthered deleterious protease (MMP mainly) response and a down-regulation of elafin, a key anti-inflammatory molecule, resulting in increased tissue injury, where neutrophils probably play a major role (37, 49, 50).

In conclusion, as demonstrated by the fact that bacterial growth and dissemination does not equate with decreased survival (**Figure 10**), our data strengthen the concept (26, 51) that improvement of tissue resilience by inhibiting host proteases [(27–30), this study] and up-regulating antimicrobials/anti-inflammatory molecules inhibited by IAV, such as elafin (27–30) is not necessarily associated with bacterial clearance (specifically *P.a* in our study). Indeed, the MMP inhibitor batimastat even promoted bacterial dissemination, suggesting that MMPs might have anti-bacterial activities. This may have to be carefully considered in clinical situations where IAV/*P.a* co-infections are found (VAP, cystic fibrosis...).

AUTHOR CONTRIBUTIONS

BV, BS, MS, and FL performed experiments. AC performed histological analysis. IG-V helped in the design of the experiments and critically appraised drafts of the document. J-MS designed experiments, analyzed data, and wrote the manuscript.

ACKNOWLEDGMENTS

We wish to thank Dr. S. Kheir for his help with some of the *in vivo* experiments and Mr. O. Thibaudeau, from the histology platform (INSERM U1152, Bichat Hospital) for his help with tissue processing.

REFERENCES

1. Wat D, Doull I. Respiratory virus infections in cystic fibrosis. *Paediatr Respir Rev.* (2003) 4:172–7. doi: 10.1016/S1526-0542(03)00059-9
2. Collinson J, Nicholson KG, Cancio E, Ashman J, Ireland DC, Hammersley V, et al. Effects of upper respiratory tract infections in patients with cystic fibrosis. *Thorax.* (1996) 51:1115–22. doi: 10.1136/thx.51.11.1115
3. Smyth AR, Smyth RL, Tong CY, Hart CA, Heaf DP. Effect of respiratory virus infections including rhinovirus on clinical status in cystic fibrosis. *Arch Dis Child.* (1995) 73:117–20. doi: 10.1136/adc.73.2.117
4. Armstrong D, Grimwood K, Carlin JB, Carzino R, Hull J, Olinsky A, et al. Severe viral respiratory infections in infants with cystic fibrosis. *Pediatr Pulmonol.* (1998) 26:371–9. doi: 10.1002/(sici)1099-0496(199812)26:6<371::aid-ppul1>3.0.co;2-n
5. Hiatt PW, Grace SC, Kozinetz CA, Raboudi SH, Treece DG, Taber LH, et al. Effects of viral lower respiratory tract infection on lung function in infants with cystic fibrosis. *Pediatrics.* (1999) 103:619–26. doi: 10.1542/peds.103.3.619
6. Iregui MG, Kollef MH. Ventilator-associated pneumonia complicating the acute respiratory distress syndrome. *Semin Respir Crit Care Med.* (2001) 22:317–26. doi: 10.1055/s-2001-15788
7. Nguyen C, Kaku S, Tutera D, Kuschner WG, Barr J. Viral respiratory infections of adults in the intensive care unit. *J Intensive Care Med.* (2016) 31:427–41. doi: 10.1177/0885066615585944
8. Cawcutt K, Kalil AC. Pneumonia with bacterial and viral co-infection. *Curr Opin Crit Care.* (2017) 23:385–90. doi: 10.1097/MCC.0000000000000435
9. Muscedere J, Ofner M, Kumar A, Long J, Lamontagne F, Cook D, et al. The occurrence and impact of bacterial organisms complicating critical care illness associated with 2009 influenza A(H1N1) infection. *Chest.* (2013) 144:39–47. doi: 10.1378/chest.12-1861
10. Scheiblauer H, Reinacher M, Tashiro M, Rott R. Interactions between bacteria and influenza A virus in the development of influenza pneumonia. *J Infect Dis.* (1992) 166:783–91. doi: 10.1093/infdis/166.4.783
11. Kiedrowski MR, Bomberger JM. Viral-bacterial co-infections in the cystic fibrosis respiratory tract. *Front Immunol.* (2018) 9:3067. doi: 10.3389/fimmu.2018.03067
12. Somayaji R, Goss CH, Khan U, Neradilek M, Neuzil KM, Ortiz JR. Cystic fibrosis pulmonary exacerbations attributable to respiratory syncytial virus and influenza: a population-based study. *Clin Infect Dis.* (2017) 64:1760–7. doi: 10.1093/cid/cix203
13. Didierlaurent A, Goulding J, Patel S, Snelgrove R, Low L, Bebien M, et al. Sustained desensitization to bacterial Toll-like receptor ligands after resolution of respiratory influenza infection. *J Exp Med.* (2008) 205:323–9. doi: 10.1084/jem.20070891
14. Jochems SP, Marcon F, Carniel BF, Holloway M, Mitsi E, Smith E, et al. Inflammation induced by influenza virus impairs human innate immune control of pneumococcus. *Nat Immunol.* (2018) 19:1299–308. doi: 10.1038/s41590-018-0231-y
15. Kudva A, Scheller EV, Robinson KM, Crowe CR, Choi SM, Slight SR, et al. IFN-beta -mediated down-regulation of IL17/neutrophilic responses/antimicrobial responses. *J Immunol.* (2011) 186:1666–74. doi: 10.4049/jimmunol.1002194
16. Ishikawa H, Fukui T, Ino S, Sasaki H, Awano N, Kohda C, et al. Influenza virus infection causes neutrophil dysfunction through reduced G-CSF production and an increased risk of secondary bacterial infection in the lung. *Virology.* (2016) 499:23–9. doi: 10.1016/j.virol.2016.08.025
17. Shahangian A, Chow EK, Tian X, Kang JR, Ghaffari A, Liu SY, et al. Type I IFNs mediate development of postinfluenza bacterial pneumonia in mice. *J Clin Invest.* (2009) 119:1910–20. doi: 10.1172/JCI35412

18. Robinson KM, McHugh KJ, Mandalapu S, Clay ME, Lee B, Scheller EV, et al. Influenza A virus exacerbates *Staphylococcus aureus* pneumonia in mice by attenuating antimicrobial peptide production. *J Infect Dis.* (2014) 209:865–75. doi: 10.1093/infdis/jit527
19. Lee B, Robinson KM, McHugh KJ, Scheller EV, Mandalapu S, Chen C, et al. Influenza-induced type I interferon enhances susceptibility to gram-negative and gram-positive bacterial pneumonia in mice. *Am J Physiol Lung Cell Mol Physiol.* (2015) 309:L158–67. doi: 10.1152/ajplung.00338.2014
20. Mallia P, Footitt J, Sotero R, Jepson A, Contoli M, Trujillo-Torralbo MB, et al. Rhinovirus infection induces degradation of antimicrobial peptides and secondary bacterial infection in chronic obstructive pulmonary disease. *Am J Respir Crit Care Med.* (2012) 186:1117–24. doi: 10.1164/rccm.201205-0806OC
21. Bansal S, Yajjala VK, Bauer C, Sun K. IL-1 signaling prevents alveolar macrophage depletion during influenza and *Streptococcus pneumoniae* coinfection. *J Immunol.* (2018) 200:1425–33. doi: 10.4049/jimmunol.1700210
22. Robinson KM, Choi SM, McHugh KJ, Mandalapu S, Enelow RI, Kolls JK, et al. Influenza A exacerbates *Staphylococcus aureus* pneumonia by attenuating IL-1β production in mice. *J Immunol.* (2013) 191:5153–9. doi: 10.4049/jimmunol.1301237
23. Ivanov S, Renneson J, Fontaine J, Barthelemy A, Paget C, Fernandez EM, et al. Interleukin-22 reduces lung inflammation during influenza A virus infection and protects against secondary bacterial infection. *J Virol.* (2013) 87:6911–24. doi: 10.1128/JVI.02943-12
24. Lee KM, Morris-Love J, Cabral DJ, Belenky P, Opal SM, Jamieson AM. Coinfection with Influenza A virus and *Klebsiella oxytoca*: an underrecognized impact on host resistance and tolerance to pulmonary infections. *Front Immunol.* (2018) 9:2377. doi: 10.3389/fimmu.2018.02377
25. Kash JC, Walters KA, Davis AS, Sandouk A, Schwartzman LM, Jagger BW, et al. Lethal synergism of 2009 pandemic H1N1 influenza virus and *Streptococcus pneumoniae* coinfection is associated with loss of murine lung repair responses. *MBio.* (2011) 2:e00172–11. doi: 10.1128/mBio.00172-11
26. Morgan DJ, Casulli J, Chew C, Connolly E, Lui S, Brand OJ, et al. Innate immune cell suppression and the link with secondary lung bacterial pneumonia. *Front Immunol.* (2018) 9:2943. doi: 10.3389/fimmu.2018.02943
27. Simpson AJ, Wallace WA, Marsden ME, Govan JR, Porteous DJ, Haslett C, et al. Adenoviral augmentation of elafin protects the lung against acute injury mediated by activated neutrophils and bacterial infection. *J Immunol.* (2001) 167:1778–86. doi: 10.4049/jimmunol.167.3.1778
28. Henriksen PA, Hitt M, Xing Z, Wang J, Haslett C, Riemersma RA, et al. Adenoviral gene delivery of elafin and secretory leukocyte protease inhibitor attenuates NF-kappa B-dependent inflammatory responses of human endothelial cells and macrophages to atherogenic stimuli. *J Immunol.* (2004) 172:4535–44. doi: 10.4049/jimmunol.172.7.4535
29. Roussilhon C, Bang G, Bastaert F, Solhonne B, Garcia-Verdugo I, Peronet R, et al. The antimicrobial molecule trappin-2/elafin has anti-parasitic properties and is protective *in vivo* in a murine model of cerebral malaria. *Sci Rep.* (2017) 7:42243. doi: 10.1038/srep42243
30. Saint-Criq V, Villeret B, Bastaert F, Kheir S, Hatton A, Cazes A, et al. *Pseudomonas aeruginosa* LasB protease impairs innate immunity in mice and humans by targeting a lung epithelial cystic fibrosis transmembrane regulator-IL-6-antimicrobial-repair pathway. *Thorax.* (2018) 73:49–61. doi: 10.1136/thoraxjnl-2017-210298
31. Barbier D, Garcia-Verdugo I, Pothlichet J, Khazen R, Descamps D, Rousseau K, et al. Influenza A induces the major secreted airway mucin MUC5AC in a protease-EGFR-extracellular regulated kinase-Sp1-dependent pathway. *Am J Respir Cell Mol Biol.* (2012) 47:149–57. doi: 10.1165/rcmb.2011-0405OC
32. Villeret B, Dieu A, Straube M, Solhonne B, Miklavc P, Hamadi S, et al. Silver nanoparticles impair retinoic acid-inducible gene I-mediated mitochondrial antiviral immunity by blocking the autophagic flux in lung epithelial cells. *ACS Nano.* (2018) 12:1188–202. doi: 10.1021/acsnano.7b06934
33. Sallenave JM, Xing Z, Simpson AJ, Graham FL, Gauldie J. Adenovirus-mediated expression of an elastase-specific inhibitor (elafin): a comparison of different promoters. *Gene Ther.* (1998) 5:352–60. doi: 10.1038/sj.gt.3300610
34. Sallenave JM, Cunningham GA, James RM, McLachlan G, Haslett C. Regulation of pulmonary and systemic bacterial lipopolysaccharide responses in transgenic mice expressing human elafin. *Infect Immun.* (2003) 71:3766–74. doi: 10.1128/IAI.71.7.3766-3774.2003
35. Bastaert F, Kheir S, Saint-Criq V, Villeret B, My-Chan Dang P, El-Benna J, et al. *Pseudomonas aeruginosa* LasB subverts alveolar macrophage activity by interfering with bacterial killing through downregulation of innate immune defense, reactive oxygen species generation, and complement activation. *Front Immunol.* (2018) 9:1675. doi: 10.3389/fimmu.2018.01675
36. Le Gars M, Descamps D, Roussel D, Saussereau E, Guillot L, Ruffin M, et al. Neutrophil elastase degrades cystic fibrosis transmembrane conductance regulator via calpains and disables channel function *in vitro* and *in vivo*. *Am J Respir Crit Care Med.* (2013) 187:170–9. doi: 10.1164/rccm.201205-0875OC
37. Sallenave JM, Donnelly SC, Grant IS, Robertson C, Gauldie J, Haslett C. Secretory leukocyte proteinase inhibitor is preferentially increased in patients with acute respiratory distress syndrome. *Eur Respir J.* (1999) 13:1029–36. doi: 10.1183/09031936.99.13510299
38. Guglani L, Gopal R, Rangel-Moreno J, Junecko BF, Lin Y, Berger T, et al. Lipocalin 2 regulates inflammation during pulmonary mycobacterial infections. *PLoS ONE.* (2012) 7:e50052. doi: 10.1371/journal.pone.0050052
39. Sandri A, Ortombina A, Boschi F, Cremonini E, Boaretti M, Sorio C, et al. Inhibition of *Pseudomonas aeruginosa* secreted virulence factors reduces lung inflammation in CF mice. *Virulence.* (2018) 9:1008–18. doi: 10.1080/21505594.2018.1489198
40. Kido H, Okumura Y, Takahashi E, Pan HY, Wang S, Yao D, et al. Role of host cellular proteases in the pathogenesis of influenza and influenza-induced multiple organ failure. *Biochim Biophys Acta.* (2012) 1824:186–94. doi: 10.1016/j.bbapap.2011.07.001
41. Kido H, Okumura Y, Takahashi E, Pan HY, Wang S, Chida J, et al. Host envelope glycoprotein processing proteases are indispensable for entry into human cells by seasonal and highly pathogenic avian influenza viruses. *J Mol Genet Med.* (2008) 3:167–75.
42. Zhai Y, Franco LM, Atmar RL, Quarles JM, Arden N, Bucasas KL, et al. Host transcriptional response to influenza and other acute respiratory viral infections–a prospective cohort study. *PLoS Pathog.* (2015) 11:e1004869. doi: 10.1371/journal.ppat.1004869
43. Leiva-Juárez MM, Kolls JK, Evans SE. Lung epithelial cells: therapeutically inducible effectors of antimicrobial defense. *Mucosal Immunol.* (2018) 11:21–34. doi: 10.1038/mi.2017.71
44. Yeo SJ, Kim SJ, Kim JH, Lee HJ, Kook YH. Influenza A virus infection modulates the expression of type IV collagenase in epithelial cells. *Arch Virol.* (1999) 144:1361–70. doi: 10.1007/s007050050592
45. Wang S, Quang Le T, Chida J, Cisse Y, Yano M, Kido H. Mechanisms of matrix metalloproteinase-9 upregulation and tissue destruction in various organs in influenza A virus infection. *J Med Invest.* (2010) 57:26–34. doi: 10.2152/jmi.57.26
46. Lee YH, Lai CL, Hsieh SH, Shieh CC, Huang LM, Wu-Hsieh BA. Influenza A virus induction of oxidative stress and MMP-9 is associated with severe lung pathology in a mouse model. *Virus Res.* (2013) 178:411–22. doi: 10.1016/j.virusres.2013.09.011
47. Talmi-Frank D, Altboum Z, Solomonov I, Udi Y, Jaitin DA, Klepfish M, et al. Extracellular matrix proteolysis by MT1-MMP contributes to influenza-related tissue damage and mortality. *Cell Host Microbe.* (2016) 20:458–70. doi: 10.1016/j.chom.2016.09.005
48. Bradley LM, Douglass MF, Chatterjee D, Akira S, Baaten BJ. Matrix metalloprotease 9 mediates neutrophil migration into the airways in response to influenza virus-induced toll-like receptor signaling. *PLoS Pathog.* (2012) 8:e1002641. doi: 10.1371/journal.ppat.1002641
49. Sallenave JM, Shulmann J, Crossley J, Jordana M, Gauldie J. Regulation of secretory leukocyte proteinase inhibitor (SLPI) and elastase-specific inhibitor (ESI/elafin) in human airway epithelial cells by cytokines and neutrophilic enzymes. *Am J Respir Cell Mol Biol.* (1994) 11:733–41. doi: 10.1165/ajrcmb.11.6.7946401
50. Wilkinson TS, Conway Morris A, Kefala K, O'Kane CM, Moore NR, Booth NA, et al. Ventilator-associated pneumonia is characterized by excessive release of neutrophil proteases in the lung. *Chest.* (2012) 142:1425–32. doi: 10.1378/chest.11-3273

6

Mechanisms of Virus-Induced Airway Immunity Dysfunction in the Pathogenesis of COPD Disease, Progression and Exacerbation

Hong Guo-Parke[1], Dermot Linden[1], Sinéad Weldon[1], Joseph C. Kidney[2†] and Clifford C. Taggart[1†]*

[1] Airway Innate Immunity Research Group, Wellcome Wolfson Institute for Experimental Medicine, School of Medicine, Dentistry & Biomedical Sciences, Queens University Belfast, Belfast, United Kingdom, [2] Department of Respiratory Medicine Mater Hospital Belfast, Belfast, United Kingdom

***Correspondence:**
Clifford C. Taggart
c.taggart@qub.ac.uk

[†] These authors share senior authorship

Chronic obstructive pulmonary disease (COPD) is the integrated form of chronic obstructive bronchitis and pulmonary emphysema, characterized by persistent small airway inflammation and progressive irreversible airflow limitation. COPD is characterized by acute pulmonary exacerbations and associated accelerated lung function decline, hospitalization, readmission and an increased risk of mortality, leading to huge social-economic burdens. Recent evidence suggests ~50% of COPD acute exacerbations are connected with a range of respiratory viral infections. Nevertheless, respiratory viral infections have been linked to the severity and frequency of exacerbations and virus-induced secondary bacterial infections often result in a synergistic decline of lung function and longer hospitalization. Here, we review current advances in understanding the cellular and molecular mechanisms underlying the pathogenesis of COPD and the increased susceptibility to virus-induced exacerbations and associated immune dysfunction in patients with COPD. The multiple immune regulators and inflammatory signaling pathways known to be involved in host-virus responses are discussed. As respiratory viruses primarily target airway epithelial cells, virus-induced inflammatory responses in airway epithelium are of particular focus. Targeting virus-induced inflammatory pathways in airway epithelial cells such as Toll like receptors (TLRs), interferons, inflammasomes, or direct blockade of virus entry and replication may represent attractive future therapeutic targets with improved efficacy. Elucidation of the cellular and molecular mechanisms of virus infections in COPD pathogenesis will undoubtedly facilitate the development of these potential novel therapies that may attenuate the relentless progression of this heterogeneous and complex disease and reduce morbidity and mortality.

Keywords: chronic obstructive pulmonary disease, virus, inflammation, infection, lung damage, acute pulmonary exacerbation

INTRODUCTION

Chronic obstructive pulmonary disease (COPD) is the umbrella term for chronic obstructive bronchitis and pulmonary emphysema, and is characterized by persistent small airway inflammation and progressive irreversible airflow limitation (1–5). COPD is associated with acute pulmonary exacerbations, accelerated lung function decline and increased risk of mortality (6, 7). As a common global epidemic, COPD affects 10% of the population and is the third leading cause of death worldwide (3). Viral and bacterial infections are key elements in the pathogenesis of exacerbations (5–9). Recent evidence suggests respiratory viral infections cause ~50% of COPD acute exacerbations (5, 6, 10). Secondary bacterial infections often ensue with pronounced illness (6).

However, the underlying mechanisms of how viruses subvert host immune defense systems in COPD exacerbations are not completely understood. Herein, we review current advances in understanding the cellular and molecular mechanisms associated with the increased susceptibility to virus infections. As respiratory viruses preferentially infect airway epithelial cells, we focus on virus-induced inflammatory responses in airway epithelium. Understanding these pathogenic pathways may facilitate the development of potential novel therapies to attenuate the relentless progression of the disease.

COPD PATHOGENESIS

Cigarette smoking is the predominant etiologic factor in the development of COPD (3–5). Other risk factors include host genetic factors, which is most evident in alpha-1 antitrypsin (AAT) deficiency (11–13). Recently, childhood respiratory viral infections have been postulated as an independent risk factor associated with COPD later in life (14). Other environmental factors such as pollutant and occupational exposure to dusts or fumes, particularly organic dusts are strongly associated with COPD (4, 13, 15, 16). Social deprivation is also a factor in the development of COPD (6, 17, 18).

Cigarette smoke and other inhale noxious gases induce an abnormal inflammatory response, that is further amplified by protease and oxidative stress, which are central to COPD pathogenesis (8, 11). Persistent small airway inflammation and the resulting destruction of the lung architecture leads to emphysema and loss of lung elastic recoil, chronic bronchitis induced mucus hypersecretion and airflow obstruction, as well as peribronchial fibrosis (11, 19, 20). Excessive neutrophilic infiltration and associated proteolytic enzymes including neutrophil elastase are hallmark features of smoke-induced inflammation (19, 21–25). Consequently, the protease/antiprotease imbalance contributes to the pathogenesis of emphysema due to the increased breakdown of elastin and loss of elastic recoil in the lung parenchyma (19, 21–24). Diminished activity of protein phosphatase 2A (PP2A), a regulator of the inflammatory response in the airways, has been demonstrated in COPD and upregulation of PP2A activity can ameliorate inflammation in a cigarette smoke model of COPD by reducing activity of the cysteine protease, cathepsin S (26). Recent research has proposed a role for formylated peptides and formyl peptide receptor (FPR) receptor signaling in the initiation and progression of lung disease in current and former smokers (27, 28). These peptides are present in tobacco leaves and are actively secreted by bacteria or passively released from dead and dying host cells after tissue injury (29). FPR1 and FPR2 activation may play a role in neutrophil migration, degranulation, reactive oxygen species (ROS) production, and phagocytosis (29, 30). A novel cross-talk mechanism was identified in neutrophils, by which signals generated by the purinergic receptor for ATP ($P2Y_2$) reactivate ligand-bound inactive FPRs, which resume signaling (31). Furthermore, a role for purinergic receptors in the pathophysiology of COPD has been demonstrated in human and experimental models (32–35), however, further work is needed to elucidate its role in the immune dysfunction associated with COPD (36). Excessive production of ROS results in an oxidant-antioxidant imbalance leading to oxidative stress and is a major predisposing feature in the development of the disease (37–41). Therefore, a vicious cycle is created in which inflammation drives a protease-antiprotease and oxidant-antioxidant imbalance, as well as multiple intracellular cell signaling mechanisms, which potentiate inflammation, goblet cell hyperplasia and mucus hypersecretion (8, 40).

Chronic low-grade respiratory syncytial virus (RSV) infection has also been implicated in COPD pathogenesis (42–45). However, the detection of RSV infection in stable COPD remains controversial (46, 47). Hogg and colleagues showed that the E1A region of the adenovirus may contribute to COPD pathogenesis by enhancing soluble ICAM-1 expression and inflammatory cells infiltration (48). In contrast, another study failed to demonstrate the persistent presence of adenovirus V or E1A (49). Polosukhin at al. detected Epstein Barr Virus (EBV) positive cells in COPD lung tissue sections by immunochemistry staining (50). Consistent with this finding, we have demonstrated that EBV DNA is frequently present in COPD sputum compared with unaffected smokers (51). Latent viral infections and cigarette smoke may synergistically contribute to the chronic inflammation in COPD (52). COPD is a heterogeneous disease with a complex etiology, however, acute and chronic lower respiratory tract infections occur with increased frequency in patients with COPD. Whatever the cause, it is clear that a defective host response plays an important role and improving our understanding of the mechanisms involved is essential to improving prevention and treatment strategies.

AIRWAY EPITHELIUM DYSFUNCTION IN COPD

Normal airway epithelial cells play a pivotal role in innate immune defense. They act as a barrier to pathogens and noxious stimuli and produce mediators and enzymes to orchestrate and maintain proper functioning of the innate and adaptive immune responses (24, 53, 54). As illustrated in **Figure 1**, the COPD airway epithelium responds to cigarette smoke by secreting inflammatory mediators and recruiting immune cells to the site of damage to orchestrate the inflammatory response. A robust infiltration of macrophages and $CD8^+$ T cells, and to a lesser extent $CD4^+$ T cells, in the airway mucosa as well as elevated neutrophils in the airway lumen are the hallmark features of COPD inflammation, the degree of which correlates to disease severity (46, 55). Increased levels of epithelial-derived CXCL9 (MIG), CXCL10 (IP-10), and CXCL11 (I-TAC) and their receptor CXCR3 has been demonstrated to contribute, in part, to the mechanism of $CD8^+$ cellular accumulation (40, 53, 54). $CD8^+$ T cells release IP-10, TNF-α, IFN-γ, perforins, and granzyme, and have been associated with alveolar epithelial cell apoptosis (19, 37, 56, 57). As COPD progresses, elevated numbers of dendritic cells and B lymphocytes also appear in the airways and alveolar walls. $CD8^+$ T cells and B cells organize into lymphoid follicles and may contribute to increased "immune surveillance" in COPD (19, 37, 39). The airway epithelium also releases a cascade of secondary mediators including cytokines, lipid mediators, growth factors, proteases, antiproteases and ROS to escalate COPD inflammation (53, 54, 58). Cigarette smoke and other irritants also activate epithelial cells and macrophages to release neutrophil and macrophage chemoattractants, such as LTB4, IL-8, and related CXC chemokines (MCP-1, GRO-α and GM-CSF), which contribute to the development of emphysema (39, 46, 59, 60).

The mechanism of neutrophilic inflammation has been linked to CD11b/CD18 on neutrophils binding to ICAM-1 on bronchial epithelium, which is up-regulated in COPD (54, 61–63). Neutrophils migrate to the respiratory tract and release serine proteases, matrix metalloproteinases (MMPs) and oxidants (24, 40, 46). Neutrophil serine proteases are associated with emphysema, mucus hypersecretion, increased risk of exacerbation and accelerated forced expiratory volume in 1 s (FEV_1) decline (64–66). Subsequently, these proteases degrade extracellular matrix components leading to the destruction of the alveolar wall, epithelial barrier dysfunction, reduction in mucociliary clearance, mucus hypersecretion and goblet cell metaplasia through activation of the epidermal growth factor receptor (EGFR) (37, 59, 64). Moreover, alveolar epithelial cells also secrete transforming growth factor-β (TGF-β) which may contribute to small airway fibrosis and emphysema (67).

MOLECULAR MECHANISMS ASSOCIATED WITH VIRAL-INDUCED COPD EXACERBATIONS

Viral-Induced COPD Exacerbations

Acute exacerbations of COPD are characterized by a sudden decline in lung function, hospitalization and high mortality (7, 9, 46). The complicated interaction between the host and viral or bacterial infections or co-infection, as well as environmental factors, precipitate the onset of exacerbations. These factors amplify the inflammatory burden in the small airway, overpowering host anti-inflammatory mechanisms leading to profound airway obstruction in COPD (46, 68–70). Severe virus-associated exacerbations also induce elevated levels of $CD8^+$ T cells, neutrophils, eosinophils, TNF-α and IL-6 in the sputum of COPD patients (68–70).

Exacerbations often occur seasonally accompanied by common cold-like symptoms implicating respiratory viral infections rather than hitherto suspected bacterial infection (43, 44). Respiratory virus infection, including human rhinovirus (HRV), influenza virus (IAV), coronavirus, RSV, human parainfluenza, metapneumovirus (hMPV) and adenovirus initiate nearly 50% of COPD exacerbations often with more severe symptoms (69–73). Viruses have developed a myriad of aversion strategies to subvert and manipulate host immune responses and these have been recently reviewed elsewhere (74, 75). Most respiratory viruses target airway epithelial cells leading to epithelial barrier destruction, microvascular dilatation, oedema and immune cell infiltration (58, 70–72). These viruses are associated with small airway secondary bacterial infection, thus magnifying the inflammatory response in COPD leading to a synergistic deterioration in lung function and prolonged hospitalization (42, 44, 71).

As detailed below, recent research has focused on immune regulators and inflammatory signaling pathways orchestrating the underlying mechanisms of increased susceptibility to virus-associated exacerbation and the exaggerated inflammatory response in COPD airways and potential therapeutic inventions.

T Cell Exhaustion

Although accumulated $CD8^+$ T cells are present in greater numbers in severe COPD, a diminished $CD8^+$ T cell antiviral response, worsened airflow limitation and respiratory symptoms have been reported in IAV and HRV-induced COPD exacerbations (68, 71, 76, 77). As a result, $CD8^+$ cells potentially amplify airway epithelium destruction and promote tissue injury through mechanisms including direct cytotoxic effects, pro-inflammatory signaling and recruitment of other immune cells, leading to increased susceptibility to virus infections of airway epithelium (42–44, 69).

In COPD, prolonged receptor–ligand interaction during T cell activation may be linked to T cell exhaustion. McKendry and colleagues investigated increased $CD8^+$ activation through the programmed cell death protein (PD)-1 exhaustion pathway as a potential mechanism of viral-induced COPD exacerbations (76). Dysregulation of T-cell cytotoxicity was associated with elevated levels of PD-1, which further increased following influenza infection in COPD patients (76). In contrast, infection-induced expression of the ligand PD-L1 on COPD macrophages was diminished, with a concomitant increase in IFN-γ release. These synergistic effects may cause excessive T-cell inflammation in response to virus infection.

The NF-κB Pathway

The NF-κB pathway is consistently activated in COPD macrophages and airway epithelium, in particular, during bacterial or viral infections (78). Upon pathogen stimulation, the canonical pathway is mainly triggered by Toll like receptors (TLRs) and pro-inflammatory cytokines such as TNFα and IL-1 leading to the activation of the RelA containing NF-κB complexes. This initiates the translocation of RelA (p65)/p50 to the nucleus, where it induces the transcriptional response of pro-inflammatory and cell survival genes (78–80). The alternative

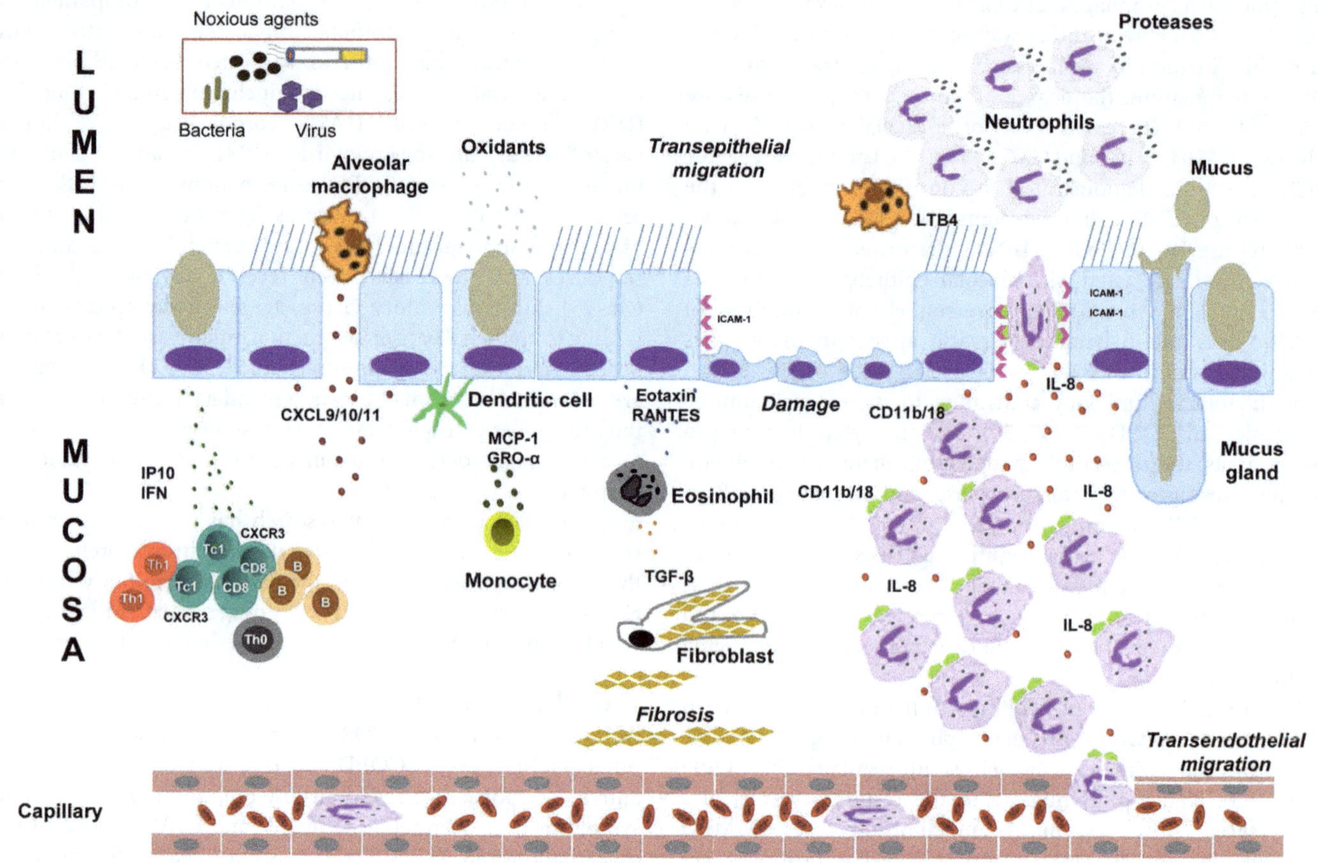

FIGURE 1 | Mechanisms of airway immunity dysfunction in COPD. Cigarette smoke and noxious agents activate epithelial cells and macrophages to release chemotactic factors such as CXCL9 (MIG), CXCL10 (IP10), and CXCL11 (I-TAC), which increase CD8+ T cells, dendritic cells, B lymphocytes and eosinophil infiltration into the airway mucosa. These inflammatory cells together with macrophages and epithelial cells initiate an inflammatory cascade that triggers the release of inflammatory mediators such as TNF-α, IFN-γ, proteases (such as MMPs), inflammatory cytokines and chemokines (IL-1, IL-6, IL-8) and growth factors. These inflammatory mediators sustain the airway mucosal inflammatory process in COPD, which cause elastin degradation and emphysema. Epithelial cells and macrophages also release TGF-β, which stimulates fibroblast proliferation resulting in small airway fibrosis. During exacerbation, the inflammatory burden in the small airways over-powers host anti-inflammatory mechanisms leading to profound alveolar damage and inflammation. Cigarette smoke and other irritants activate epithelial cells and macrophages to release neutrophil chemoattractants, such as LTB4, IL-8, TNFα, CXC chemokines (MCP-1, GRO-α, and GM-CSF). CXC chemokines also act as chemoattractants for monocytes. Cigarette smoke causes increased level of ROS produced in the airways is reflected by increased markers of oxidative stress. Oxidative stress is involved in several events in the pathogenesis of COPD including oxidative inactivation of anti-proteases and surfactants, mucus hypersecretion, alveolar epithelial injury, remodeling of extracellular matrix and apoptosis. Neutrophils bind to ICAM-1, the level of which has been found to upregulated in bronchial epithelial cells in COPD. Neutrophils then migrate to the respiratory tract under the control of IL8/LTB4 chemotactic gradient. These cells then release proteases that break down connective tissue in the lung parenchyma, resulting in emphysema. Neutrophil elastase release in airway induces epithelial barrier dysfunction, mucus hypersecretion and reduces mucociliary clearance. GM-CSF, Granulocyte-macrophage colony-stimulating factor: GRO-α, Growth-regulated oncogene-α; ICAM-1, epithelial intercellular adhesion molecule-1; LTB4, leukotriene B4; IL, interleukin; IP10, CXCL10, interferon g-induced protein 10; I-TAC, CXCL11, interferon-inducible T-cell α chemoattractant; MCP-1, monocyte chemoattractant protein-1; MIG, CXCL9, monokine induced by g interferon; MMPs, matrix metalloproteinases; RANTES, regulated on activation, normal T cell expressed and secreted; ROS: reactive oxygen species; TGF, transforming growth factor; TNF-α, Tumor necrosis factor-α; IFN, interferon.

non-canonical NF-κB pathway signals through a subset of receptors to activate the kinase NIK and IKKα complexes and downstream NF-κB2 p100 leading to the p52/RelB nucleus translocation and lymphoid organogenesis and B cell activation (78, 79).

Persistent or prolonged activation of NF-κB may contribute to COPD pathogenesis by switching on the transcriptional response of pro-inflammatory cytokines, chemokines, cell adhesion molecules (CAMs), proteases, and inhibitors of apoptosis to amplify inflammation. Therefore, strategies, which block the activation of NF-κB, offer attractive therapeutic options to regulate COPD inflammation. Several IKK-β inhibitors have been identified to inhibit p65 nuclear translocation and exert anti-inflammatory effects (81, 82). Lung-targeted overexpression of RelB has also been demonstrated to protect against cigarette smoke–induced inflammation by reducing inflammatory mediator production (83). In COPD airway epithelium, influenza virus infection increased microRNA-125a/b, which directly inhibits A20 and mitochondrial antiviral-signaling protein (MAVS) to promote inflammation and impair antiviral responses in COPD (84). Thus, miR-125a/b may provide a potential therapeutic target for both inflammation and antiviral responses in COPD.

TLR Sensing and EGFR Signaling

Figure 2 illustrates key virus innate recognition signaling pathways in COPD airway epithelium. Briefly, ssRNAs of HRV, RSV, and IAV are recognized by TLR3 in the endosomes which consequently activate IRF-3 via the Toll/IL-1 receptor domain-containing adaptor (TRIF), leading to the induction of IFN-β and IFN-λ1. Other endosomal TLRs (TLR7/8 and TLR7/9) recognize the dsRNAs of IAV and adenovirus through MyD88-dependent pathway to activate NF-κB and IRF-7 to secrete pro-inflammatory mediators and IFNs, respectively. TLR4 expressed on the cell surface senses RSV and IAV, signaling through both the MyD88 and TRIF pathways to activate NF-κB and IRF-7. The airway epithelium may recognize EBV by endosomal TLRs and TLR2 at the cell surface to activate downstream pathways (85, 86). As a risk factor for RSV-induced COPD exacerbations, TLR3 activation has been found to correlate with lung function deterioration during exacerbations highlighting TLR3 blockade as a therapeutic target (87). However, Silkoff et al. showed that TLR3 inhibition was inefficient in attenuating HRV-induced experimental asthma exacerbation (88).

Many TLRs recognize pathogen-associated molecular patterns (PAMPs) to activate airway epithelial EGFR signaling cascades. Aberrant EGFR signaling promotes progressive lung fibrosis and mucus hypersecretion; characteristic features of COPD, asthma and cystic fibrosis pathogenesis (24, 89). The EGFR cascade consists of multiple receptors and extracellular ligands that function via receptor auto-phosphorylation and cytoplasmic protein binding of four downstream complexes including the mitogen-activated protein kinases/extracellular signal–regulated kinases (MEK/ERK), phosphatidylinositol 3-kinases/protein kinase B (PKB) (PI3K/AKT), Just Another Kinase/signal transducer and activator of transcription (JAK/STAT) and mammalian target of rapamycin (mTOR) pathways (89). In a murine COPD model, EGFR activation through PI3K inhibited ciliated cell apoptosis and allowed IL-13 to stimulate the trans-differentiation of ciliated to goblet cell metaplasia (90). HRV infection induced the phosphorylation of PKD, a downstream kinase of PI3K. PKD inhibitors have been reported to effectively block HRV, poliovirus (PV) and foot-and-mouth disease virus (FMDV) replication at an early stage of infection, highlighting the potential of PKD inhibition in anti-HRV therapy in COPD (91). Chronic inflammation can also induce ICAM-1 and its ligand fibrinogen has been shown to promote EGFR-dependent mucin production in the airways of subjects with mucus hypersecretion (92).

EGF and the EGFR ligand, TGF-α, have been reported to directly enhance TNF-α-induced IL-8 secretion in airway inflammation (93). Ganesan et al. found that abnormal EGFR activation contributed to enhanced IL-8 expression in COPD airways via the NF-κB regulator, FoxO3A (94). Interestingly, TLR3 also induced EGFR activation and EGFR ligands (TGF-α and amphiregulin), which in turn promote EGFR-ERK signaling and mucin production through an autocrine/paracrine loop (95). Collectively, TLR antiviral defense mechanisms integrate with the EGFR mediated epithelial proliferation/repair pathways and may play an important role in viral-induced airway remodeling and airway disease exacerbations (93, 95, 96).

Viral infection *per se* also activates EGFR and EGFR signaling to ERK1/2, while STATs control the severity of HRV mediated airway inflammation. *In vitro*, HRV induced goblet cell hyperplasia was demonstrated to function through NF-κB-dependent MMP-mediated TGF-α release, leading to EGFR activation and mucus secretion (97). Interestingly, virus-induced EGFR activation suppressed interferon regulatory factor 1 (IRF1)-dependent IFN-λ airway epithelial antiviral signaling (98, 99). Inhibiting virus-mediated EGFR signaling augmented IRF1, IFN-λ secretion and viral clearance, indicating EGFR pathways as potential therapeutic targets in viral-induced COPD exacerbations (99).

Cytoplasmic-Sensing Pathways

As shown in **Figure 2**, the airway epithelium also detects viral invasion through cytoplasmic pathogen recognition receptors. DNA and RNA viruses release their genomes into cytoplasm, which are detected by the host through cytoplasmic retinoic acid-inducible gene I/melanoma differentiation-associated protein 5-mitochondrial antiviral-signaling protein (RIG-I/MDA5–MAVS) RNA-sensing and the cyclic GMP–AMP synthase- signaling effector stimulator of interferon genes (cGAS–STING) DNA-sensing pathways, respectively (100). Upon ss/dsRNA binding, the RNA helicases, RIG-I and MDA5, interact with the adaptor protein MAVS on the mitochondrial outer membrane to activate the downstream signaling of type I interferon antiviral responses (100, 101). In contrast, the cGAS receptor senses retroviral replication products, dsDNA and RNA/DNA hybrids, to induce the synthesis of cGAMP which binds and activates STING (100). Interferon γ-inducible protein 16 (IFI16), a novel DNA sensor, has been found to recruit STING to activate type I IFN signaling through an unknown molecular mechanism (102). STING and MAVS also stimulate downstream multiple kinase signaling cascades resulting in IRF3 phosphorylation and NF-κB nuclear translocation (101, 102).

The primary consequence of these virus-sensing pathways is the induction of type I/type III IFNs and IFN stimulated genes as well as the production of inflammatory cytokines and chemokines. Attenuation of the IFN response following virus infection could result in uncontrolled viral replication and an escalated inflammatory response, a potential mechanism of virus-induced exacerbations in COPD. IFNα/β deficiency has been demonstrated in bronchial biopsies of asthmatic patients with rhinovirus-induced exacerbations and smoking-induced COPD (103). Farazuddin et al. have demonstrated that quercetin, a potent antioxidant and anti-inflammatory agent with antiviral properties, effectively mitigates rhinovirus-induced COPD exacerbation in a mouse model (104). Elevated ICAM-1 expression on the surface of airway epithelium has been directly linked to the mechanism of increased susceptibility of HRV-induced acute exacerbation. As the receptor of the major group of HRV and a ligand of lymphocyte function-associated antigen 1 (LFA-1) on neutrophils, ICAM-1 over-expression has been

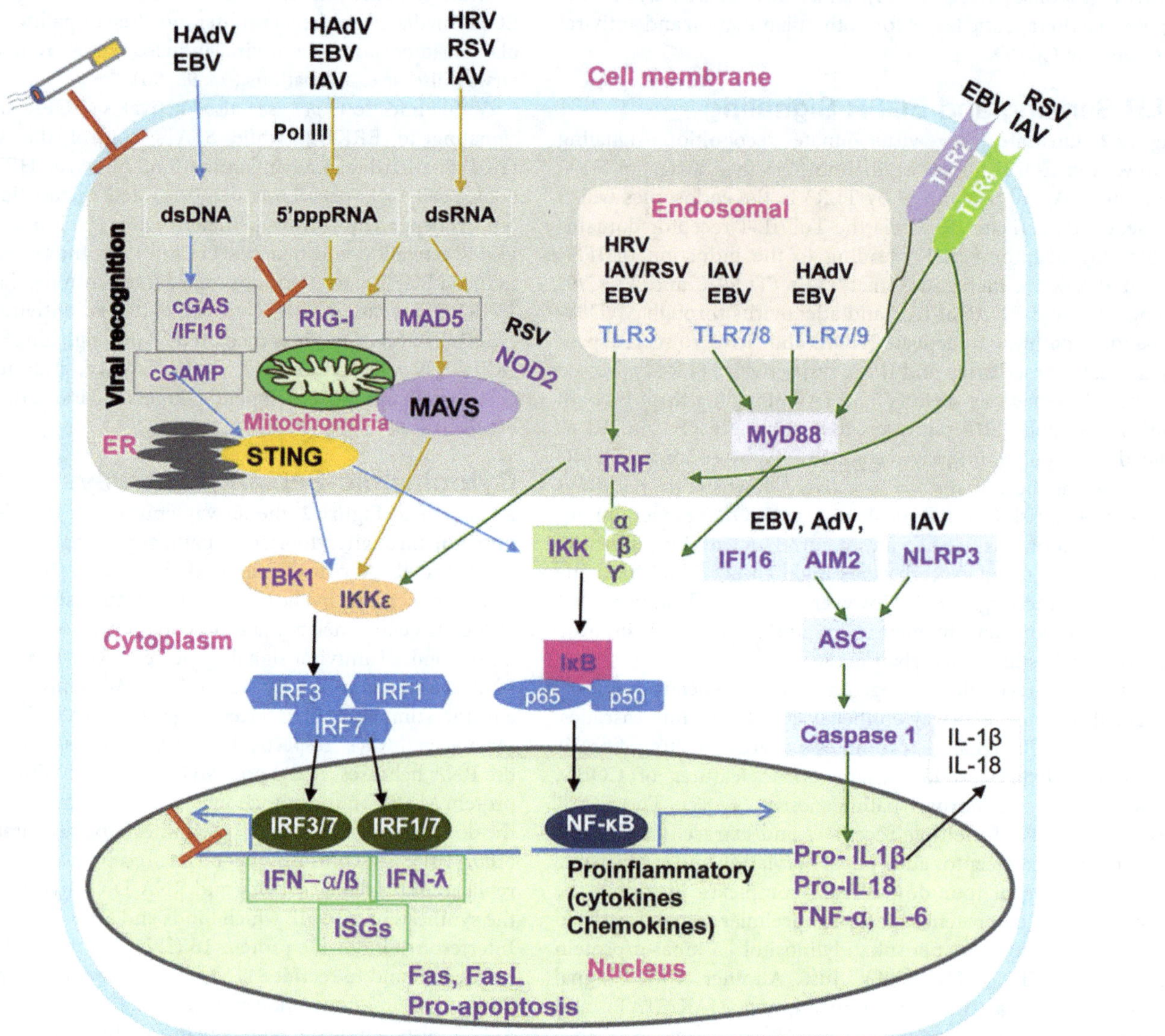

FIGURE 2 | Intracellular Viral Sensing Pathways. DNA and RNA viruses release their genomes in the cytoplasm, where host innate sensors for nucleic acids reside. Upon ss/dsRNA binding, RIG-I engages the adaptor protein MAVS on the mitochondrial outer membrane. The cGAS receptor recognizes dsDNA and the RNA:DNA hybrids generated during retroviral replication and catalyzes the synthesis of cGAMP, which is the primary agonist of the adaptor protein STING. Another sensor, IFI16 can recruit STING in response to cytoplasmic DNA through a molecular mechanism yet to be described. Both STING and MAVS stimulate downstream signaling cascades that involve multiple kinases and finally lead to IRF3 phosphorylation and nuclear translocation. The primary consequence of these virus sensing pathways is the induction of type I IFN and IFN stimulated genes. cGAS, cyclic GMP-AMP synthase; cGAMP, 2′3′guanosine-adenosine monophosphate; IFI16, interferon-g inducible protein 16; IKK, IkB kinase; IRF3, interferon regulatory factor 3; MAVS, mitochondrial antiviral-signaling protein; RIG-I, retinoic acid inducible gene-I; ss/dsRNA, single-stranded/double-stranded RNA; vRNA/DNA, viral RNA/DNA; STING, stimulator of interferon genes; TANK, TRAF-associated NF-kB activator; TBK1, TANK binding kinase 1.

shown on epithelial cells in smokers and patients with COPD (63, 105, 106). Blocking ICAM-1 may also represent as a potential therapeutic option in HRV-induced exacerbations.

Direct Targeting of Viral Binding, Entry, and Replication

Strategies that directly prevent virus binding, entry and replication may provide attractive alternatives in the treatment of COPD exacerbations (107). Capsid binders represent attractive potential inhibitors of HRV entry, however, they are strain-specific and have shown no effect on improving lung function and exacerbation in clinical trials to date (106). Mousnier and colleagues demonstrated that a dual inhibitor of human N-myristoyltransferases NMT1 and NMT2 can inhibit host-cell N-myristoylation and completely prevent rhinoviral replication, highlighting the therapeutic potential of targeting myristoylation in blocking rhinovirus infection in COPD (108). Short palate, lung, nasal epithelium clone 1 (SPLUNC1), a multifunctional host defense protein, was demonstrated to inhibit IAV binding and entry into airway epithelial cells, indicating an antiviral role for this protein in the airways (109). Therefore, in the COPD lung, SPLUNC1 degradation by proteases such as neutrophil elastase and/or inactivation by cigarette smoke may increase susceptibility to viral as well as bacterial infections, in addition to airway dehydration (110, 111). Recent research suggests that, in addition to modulating neutrophil chemotaxis, FPR2 signaling may be an important player in viral replication and IAV pathogenesis (30, 112, 113).

Inflammasome

The inflammasome is a multiprotein pro-inflammatory complex and serves as an important link between the innate and adaptive immune responses. Inflammasomes that are activated by IAV RNA, EBV and adenoviral DNA include the nucleotide binding and oligomerization domain (NOD)-like receptor family pyrin domain-containing 3 (NLRP3) protein, absent in melanoma 2 (AIM2) protein and IFI16 protein (114). The inflammasome complexes assemble after recognition of PAMPs or danger-associated molecular patterns (DAMPs) induced by virus-killed cells or tissue damage and interact with apoptosis-associated speck like protein containing a caspase recruitment domain (ASC) via caspase activation and recruitment domains (CARD)-CARD/caspase-1 pathway (115–117). Activation of the inflammasome complex results in the autocatalytic cleavage of caspase-1 and ultimately leads to the production of pro-inflammatory cytokines including IL-1β, IL-18 and pro-IL-33 (116, 117). Upon maturation, these cytokines mediate inflammatory responses by activating lymphocytes and facilitating their infiltration to the site of primary infection and by inducing IFNs and other pro-inflammatory cytokines secretions (116).

CONCLUDING REMARKS

COPD is a heterogeneous and complex disease resulting from the deregulation of multiple immune regulators and inflammatory signaling pathways. Significant progress has been made to elucidate the causative mechanism of COPD pathophysiology including viral infection in disease development, severity and exacerbations. Targeting virus-induced inflammatory pathways such as T cell exhaustion, NF-κB, TLRs, EGFR, interferons and the inflammasome provide attractive future therapeutic options. Understanding the cellular and molecular mechanisms of virus-induced COPD pathogenesis could potentially limit pathogen-mediated disease exacerbations and minimize viral-associated inflammation, tissue destruction and pulmonary function deterioration.

AUTHOR CONTRIBUTIONS

All authors listed have made a substantial, direct and intellectual contribution to the work, and approved it for publication.

REFERENCES

1. Buist AS, McBurnie MA, Vollmer WM, Gillespie S, Burney P, Mannino DM, et al. International variation in the prevalence of COPD (the BOLD study): a population-based prevalence study. *Lancet.* (2007) 370:741–50. doi: 10.1016/S0140-6736(07)61377-4
2. Mirza S, Clay RD, Koslow MA, Scanlon PD. COPD guidelines: a review of the 2018. GOLD Report. *Mayo Clin Proc.* (2018) 93:1488–502. doi: 10.1016/j.mayocp.2018.05.026
3. Barnes PJ. Chronic obstructive pulmonary disease: a growing but neglected global epidemic. *PLoS Med.* (2007) 4:e112. doi: 10.1371/journal.pmed.0040112
4. Salvi S. Tobacco smoking and environmental risk factors for chronic obstructive pulmonary disease. *Clin Chest Med.* (2014) 35:17–27. doi: 10.1016/j.ccm.2013.09.011
5. Bauer CMT, Morissette MC, Stämpfli MR. The influence of cigarette smoking on viral infections. *Chest.* (2013) 143:196–206. doi: 10.1378/chest.12-0930
6. Mohan A, Chandra S, Agarwal D, Guleria R, Broor S, Gaur B, et al. Prevalence of viral infection detected by PCR and RT-PCR in patients with acute exacerbation of COPD: a systematic review. *Respirology.* (2010) 15:536–42. doi: 10.1111/j.1440-1843.2010.01722.x
7. Merinopoulou E, Raluy-Callado M, Ramagopalan S, MacLachlan S, Khalid JM. COPD exacerbations by disease severity in England. *Int J Chron Obstruct Pulmon Dis.* (2016) 11:697–709. doi: 10.2147/COPD.S100250
8. Sethi S, Murphy TF. Infection in the pathogenesis and course of chronic obstructive pulmonary disease. *N Engl J Med.* (2008) 359:2355–65. doi: 10.1056/NEJMra0800353
9. Ko FW, Chan KP, Hui DS, Goddard JR, Shaw JG, Reid DW, et al. Acute exacerbation of COPD. *Respirology.* (2016) 21:1152–65. doi: 10.1111/resp.12780
10. Linden D, Guo-Parke H, Coyle P V., Fairley D, McAuley DF, Taggart CC, et al. Respiratory viral infection: a potential "missing link" in the pathogenesis of COPD. *Eur Respir Rev.* (2019) 28:180063. doi: 10.1183/16000617.0063-2018
11. Calverley PMA, Walker P. Chronic obstructive pulmonary disease. *Lancet.* (2003) 362:1053–61. doi: 10.1016/S0140-6736(03)14416-9
12. Pauwels RA, Rabe KF. Burden and clinical features of chronic obstructive pulmonary disease (COPD). *Lancet.* (2004) 364:613–20. doi: 10.1016/S0140-6736(04)16855-4
13. Mannino DM, Buist AS. Global burden of COPD: risk factors, prevalence, and future trends. *Lancet.* (2007) 370:765–73. doi: 10.1016/S0140-6736(07)61380-4
14. Marsico S, Caccuri F, Mazzuca P, Apostoli P, Roversi S, Lorenzin G, et al. Human lung epithelial cells support human metapneumovirus persistence by overcoming apoptosis. *Pathog Dis.* (2018) 76:fty013. doi: 10.1093/femspd/fty013
15. Marsh S, Aldington S, Shirtcliffe P, Weatherall M, Beasley R. Smoking and COPD: what really are the risks? *Eur Respir J.* (2006) 28:883–4. doi: 10.1183/09031936.06.00074806
16. Lundbäck B, Lindberg A, Lindström M, Rönmark E, Jonsson AC, Jönsson E, et al. Obstructive lung disease in northern Sweden studies. Not 15 but 50% of smokers develop COPD?–Report from the obstructive lung disease in northern Sweden studies. *Respir Med.* (2003) 97:115–22. doi: 10.1053/rmed.2003.1446

17. GBD 2015 Chronic Respiratory Disease Collaborators. Global, regional, and national deaths, prevalence, disability-adjusted life years, and years lived with disability for chronic obstructive pulmonary disease and asthma, 1990-2015: a systematic analysis for the global burden of disease study 2015. *Lancet Respir Med.* (2017) 5:691–706. doi: 10.1016/S2213-2600(17)30293-X
18. Rycroft CE, Heyes A, Lanza L, Becker K. Epidemiology of chronic obstructive pulmonary disease: a literature review. *Int J Chron Obstruct Pulmon Dis.* (2012) 7:457–94. doi: 10.2147/COPD.S32330
19. Hogg JC, Chu F, Utokaparch S, Woods R, Elliott WM, Buzatu L, et al. The nature of small-airway obstruction in chronic obstructive pulmonary disease. *N Engl J Med.* (2004) 350:2645–53. doi: 10.1056/NEJMoa032158
20. Kim V, Criner GJ. Chronic bronchitis and chronic obstructive pulmonary disease. *Am J Respir Crit Care Med.* (2013) 187:228–37. doi: 10.1164/rccm.201210-1843CI
21. Navratilova Z, Kolek V, Petrek M. Matrix metalloproteinases and their inhibitors in chronic obstructive pulmonary disease. *Arch Immunol Ther Exp.* (2016) 64:177–93. doi: 10.1007/s00005-015-0375-5
22. Owen CA. Roles for proteinases in the pathogenesis of chronic obstructive pulmonary disease. *Int J Chron Obstruct Pulmon Dis.* (2008) 3:253–68. doi: 10.2147/COPD.S2089
23. Shapiro SD. Proteolysis in the lung. *Eur Respir J.* (2003) 22:30s–2. doi: 10.1183/09031936.03.00000903a
24. Bagdonas E, Raudoniute J, Bruzauskaite I, Aldonyte R. Novel aspects of pathogenesis and regeneration mechanisms in COPD. *Int J Chron Obstruct Pulmon Dis.* (2015) 10:995–1013. doi: 10.2147/COPD.S82518
25. Hoenderdos K, Condliffe A. The neutrophil in chronic obstructive pulmonary disease. Too Little, Too Late or Too Much, Too Soon? *Am J Respir Cell Mol Biol.* (2013) 48:531–9. doi: 10.1165/rcmb.2012-0492TR
26. Doherty DF, Nath S, Poon J, Foronjy RF, Ohlmeyer M, Dabo AJ, et al. Protein phosphatase 2a reduces cigarette smoke-induced cathepsin s and loss of lung function. *Am J Respir Crit Care Med.* (2019) 200:51–62. doi: 10.1164/rccm.201808-1518OC
27. Cardini S, Dalli J, Fineschi S, Perretti M, Lungarella G, Lucattelli M. Genetic ablation of the fpr1 gene confers protection from smoking-induced lung emphysema in mice. *Am J Respir Cell Mol Biol.* (2012) 47:332–9. doi: 10.1165/rcmb.2012-0036OC
28. De Cunto G, Bartalesi B, Cavarra E, Balzano E, Lungarella G, Lucattelli M. Ongoing lung inflammation and disease progression in mice after smoking cessation: beneficial effects of formyl-peptide receptor blockade. *Am J Pathol.* (2018) 188:2195–206. doi: 10.1016/j.ajpath.2018.06.010
29. Dorward DA, Lucas CD, Chapman GB, Haslett C, Dhaliwal K, Rossi AG. The role of formylated peptides and formyl peptide receptor 1 in governing neutrophil function during acute inflammation. *Am J Pathol.* (2015) 185:1172–84. doi: 10.1016/j.ajpath.2015.01.020
30. Bozinovski S, Anthony D, Anderson GP, Irving LB, Levy BD, Vlahos R. Treating neutrophilic inflammation in COPD by targeting ALX/FPR2 resolution pathways. *Pharmacol Ther.* (2013) 140:280–9. doi: 10.1016/j.pharmthera.2013.07.007
31. Önnheim K, Christenson K, Gabl M, Burbiel JC, Müller CE, Oprea TI, et al. A novel receptor cross-talk between the ATP receptor P2Y2 and formyl peptide receptors reactivates desensitized neutrophils to produce superoxide. *Exp Cell Res.* (2014) 323:209–17. doi: 10.1016/j.yexcr.2014.01.023
32. Lommatzsch M, Cicko S, Müller T, Lucattelli M, Bratke K, Stoll P, et al. Extracellular adenosine triphosphate and chronic obstructive pulmonary disease. *Am J Respir Crit Care Med.* (2010) 181:928–34. doi: 10.1164/rccm.200910-1506OC
33. Lazar Z, Müllner N, Lucattelli M, Ayata CK, Cicko S, Yegutkin GG, et al. NTPDase1/CD39 and aberrant purinergic signalling in the pathogenesis of COPD. *Eur Respir J.* (2016) 47:254–63. doi: 10.1183/13993003.02144-2014
34. Cicko S, Lucattelli M, Müller T, Lommatzsch M, De Cunto G, Cardini S, et al. Purinergic receptor inhibition prevents the development of smoke-induced lung injury and emphysema. *J Immunol.* (2010) 185:688–97. doi: 10.4049/jimmunol.0904042
35. Lucattelli M, Cicko S, Müller T, Lommatzsch M, De Cunto G, Cardini S, et al. P2X7 receptor signaling in the pathogenesis of smoke-induced lung inflammation and emphysema. *Am J Respir Cell Mol Biol.* (2011) 44:423–9. doi: 10.1165/rcmb.2010-0038OC
36. Antonioli L, Blandizzi C, Pacher P, Haskó G. The purinergic system as a pharmacological target for the treatment of immune-mediated inflammatory diseases. *Pharmacol Rev.* (2019) 71:345–82. doi: 10.1124/pr.117.014878
37. Barnes PJ. Cellular and molecular mechanisms of asthma and COPD. *Clin Sci.* (2017) 131:1541–58. doi: 10.1042/CS20160487
38. Eapen MS, Myers S, Walters EH, Sohal SS. Airway inflammation in chronic obstructive pulmonary disease (COPD): a true paradox. *Expert Rev Respir Med.* (2017) 11:827–39. doi: 10.1080/17476348.2017.1360769
39. Barnes PJ, Shapiro SD, Pauwels RA. Chronic obstructive pulmonary disease: molecular and cellular mechanisms. *Eur Respir J.* (2003) 22:672–88. doi: 10.1183/09031936.03.00040703
40. MacNee W. Pathogenesis of chronic obstructive pulmonary disease. *Proc Am Thorac Soc.* (2005) 2:258–66. doi: 10.1513/pats.200504-045SR
41. McGuinness A, Sapey E. Oxidative stress in COPD: sources, markers, and potential mechanisms. *J Clin Med.* (2017) 6:21. doi: 10.3390/jcm6020021
42. Sikkel MB, Quint JK, Mallia P, Wedzicha JA, Johnston SL. Respiratory syncytial virus persistence in chronic obstructive pulmonary disease. *Pediatr Infect Dis J.* (2008) 27:S63–70. doi: 10.1097/INF.0b013e3181684d67
43. Seemungal T, Harper-Owen R, Bhowmik A, Moric I, Sanderson G, Message S, et al. Respiratory viruses, symptoms, and inflammatory markers in acute exacerbations and stable chronic obstructive pulmonary disease. *Am J Respir Crit Care Med.* (2001) 164:1618–23. doi: 10.1164/ajrccm.164.9.2105011
44. Singanayagam A, Joshi P V, Mallia P, Johnston SL. Viruses exacerbating chronic pulmonary disease: the role of immune modulation. *BMC Med.* (2012) 10:27. doi: 10.1186/1741-7015-10-27
45. Wilkinson TMA, Donaldson GC, Johnston SL, Openshaw PJM, Wedzicha JA. Respiratory syncytial virus, airway inflammation, and FEV1 decline in patients with chronic obstructive pulmonary disease. *Am J Respir Crit Care Med.* (2006) 173:871–6. doi: 10.1164/rccm.200509-1489OC
46. Papi A, Bellettato CM, Braccioni F, Romagnoli M, Casolari P, Caramori G, et al. Infections and airway inflammation in chronic obstructive pulmonary disease severe exacerbations. *Am J Respir Crit Care Med.* (2006) 173:1114–21. doi: 10.1164/rccm.200506-859OC
47. Falsey AR, Formica MA, Hennessey PA, Criddle MM, Sullender WM, Walsh EE. Detection of respiratory syncytial virus in adults with chronic obstructive pulmonary disease. *Am J Respir Crit Care Med.* (2006) 173:639–43. doi: 10.1164/rccm.200510-1681OC
48. Matsuse T, Hayashi S, Kuwano K, Keunecke H, Jefferies WA, Hogg JC. Latent adenoviral infection in the pathogenesis of chronic airways obstruction. *Am Rev Respir Dis.* (1992) 146:177–84. doi: 10.1164/ajrccm/146.1.177
49. McManus TE, Marley A-M, Baxter N, Christie SN, Elborn JS, Heaney LG, et al. Acute and latent adenovirus in COPD. *Respir Med.* (2007) 101:2084–90. doi: 10.1016/j.rmed.2007.05.015
50. Polosukhin VV, Cates JM, Lawson WE, Zaynagetdinov R, Milstone AP, Massion PP, et al. Bronchial secretory immunoglobulin a deficiency correlates with airway inflammation and progression of chronic obstructive pulmonary disease. *Am J Respir Crit Care Med.* (2011) 184:317–27. doi: 10.1164/rccm.201010-1629OC
51. McManus TE, Marley A-M, Baxter N, Christie SN, Elborn JS, O'Neill HJ, et al. High levels of epstein-barr virus in COPD. *Eur Respir J.* (2008) 31:1221–6. doi: 10.1183/09031936.00107507
52. Foronjy RF, Dabo AJ, Taggart CC, Weldon S, Geraghty P. Respiratory syncytial virus infections enhance cigarette smoke induced COPD in Mice. *PLoS ONE.* (2014) 9:e90567. doi: 10.1371/journal.pone.0090567
53. Gao W, Li L, Wang Y, Zhang S, Adcock IM, Barnes PJ, et al. Bronchial epithelial cells: the key effector cells in the pathogenesis of chronic obstructive pulmonary disease? *Respirology.* (2015) 20:722–9. doi: 10.1111/resp.12542
54. Vareille M, Kieninger E, Edwards MR, Regamey N. The airway epithelium: soldier in the fight against respiratory viruses. *Clin Microbiol Rev.* (2011) 24:210–29. doi: 10.1128/CMR.00014-10
55. O'Shaughnessy TC, Ansari TW, Barnes NC, Jeffery PK. Inflammation in bronchial biopsies of subjects with chronic bronchitis: inverse relationship of CD8+ T lymphocytes with FEV1. *Am J Respir Crit Care Med.* (1997) 155:852–7. doi: 10.1164/ajrccm.155.3.9117016
56. Kim W-D, Chi H-S, Choe K-H, Oh Y-M, Lee S-D, Kim K-R, et al. A possible role for CD8 + and non-CD8 + cell granzyme B in early small

airway wall remodelling in centrilobular emphysema. *Respirology.* (2013) 18:688–96. doi: 10.1111/resp.12069

57. Majo J, Ghezzo H, Cosio MG. Lymphocyte population and apoptosis in the lungs of smokers and their relation to emphysema. *Eur Respir J.* (2001) 17:946–53. doi: 10.1183/09031936.01.17509460
58. Aghapour M, Raee P, Moghaddam SJ, Hiemstra PS, Heijink IH. Airway epithelial barrier dysfunction in chronic obstructive pulmonary disease: role of cigarette smoke exposure. *Am J Respir Cell Mol Biol.* (2018) 58:157–69. doi: 10.1165/rcmb.2017-0200TR
59. Barnes PJ. Inflammatory mechanisms in patients with chronic obstructive pulmonary disease. *J Allergy Clin Immunol.* (2016) 138:16–27. doi: 10.1016/j.jaci.2016.05.011
60. Wang Y, Xu J, Meng Y, Adcock IM, Yao X. Role of inflammatory cells in airway remodeling in COPD. *Int J Chron Obstruct Pulmon Dis.* (2018) 13:3341–8. doi: 10.2147/COPD.S176122
61. Lopez-Campos JL, Calero C, Arellano-Orden E, Marquez-Martín E, Cejudo-Ramos P, Ortega Ruiz F, et al. Increased levels of soluble ICAM-1 in chronic obstructive pulmonary disease and resistant smokers are related to active smoking. *Biomark Med.* (2012) 6:805–11. doi: 10.2217/bmm.12.64
62. Kidney JC, Proud D. Neutrophil transmigration across human airway epithelial monolayers: mechanisms and dependence on electrical resistance. *Am J Respir Cell Mol Biol.* (2000) 23:389–95. doi: 10.1165/ajrcmb.23.3.4068
63. Shukla SD, Mahmood MQ, Weston S, Latham R, Muller HK, Sohal SS, et al. The main rhinovirus respiratory tract adhesion site (ICAM-1) is upregulated in smokers and patients with chronic airflow limitation (CAL). *Respir Res.* (2017) 18:6. doi: 10.1186/s12931-016-0483-8
64. Dey T, Kalita J, Weldon S, Taggart CC. Proteases and their inhibitors in chronic obstructive pulmonary disease. *J Clin Med.* (2018) 7:244. doi: 10.3390/jcm7090244
65. Sommerhoff CP, Nadel JA, Basbaum CB, Caughey GH. Neutrophil elastase and cathepsin G stimulate secretion from cultured bovine airway gland serous cells. *J Clin Invest.* (1990) 85:682–9. doi: 10.1172/JCI114492
66. Weiss SJ. Tissue destruction by neutrophils. *N Engl J Med.* (1989) 320:365–76. doi: 10.1056/NEJM198902093200606
67. Aschner Y, Downey GP. Transforming growth factor-β: master regulator of the respiratory system in health and disease. *Am J Respir Cell Mol Biol.* (2016) 54:647–55. doi: 10.1165/rcmb.2015-0391TR
68. Kurai D, Saraya T, Ishii H, Takizawa H. Virus-induced exacerbations in asthma and COPD. *Front Microbiol.* (2013) 4:293. doi: 10.3389/fmicb.2013.00293
69. Frickmann H, Jungblut S, Hirche TO, Groß U, Kuhns M, Zautner AE. The influence of virus infections on the course of COPD. *Eur J Microbiol Immunol.* (2012) 2:176–85. doi: 10.1556/EuJMI.2.2012.3.2
70. Allie SR, Randall TD. Pulmonary immunity to viruses. *Clin Sci.* (2017) 131:1737–62. doi: 10.1042/CS20160259
71. Schneider D, Ganesan S, Comstock AT, Meldrum CA, Mahidhara R, Goldsmith AM, et al. Increased cytokine response of rhinovirus-infected airway epithelial cells in chronic obstructive pulmonary disease. *Am J Respir Crit Care Med.* (2010) 182:332–40. doi: 10.1164/rccm.200911-1673OC
72. Potena A, Caramori G, Casolari P, Contoli M, Johnston SL, Papi A. Pathophysiology of viral-induced exacerbations of COPD. *Int J Chron Obstruct Pulmon Dis.* (2007) 2:477–83.
73. Jafarinejad H, Moghoofei M, Mostafaei S, Salimian J, Azimzadeh Jamalkandi S, Ahmadi A. Worldwide prevalence of viral infection in AECOPD patients: a meta-analysis. *Microb Pathog.* (2017) 113:190–6. doi: 10.1016/j.micpath.2017.10.021
74. Christiaansen A, Varga SM, Spencer J V. Viral manipulation of the host immune response. *Curr Opin Immunol.* (2015) 36:54–60. doi: 10.1016/j.coi.2015.06.012
75. Moreno-Altamirano MMB, Kolstoe SE, Sánchez-García FJ. Virus control of cell metabolism for replication and evasion of host immune responses. *Front Cell Infect Microbiol.* (2019) 9:95. doi: 10.3389/fcimb.2019.00095
76. McKendry RT, Spalluto CM, Burke H, Nicholas B, Cellura D, Al-Shamkhani A, et al. Dysregulation of antiviral function of cd8(+) t cells in the chronic obstructive pulmonary disease lung. Role of the PD-1-PD-L1 Axis. *Am J Respir Crit Care Med.* (2016) 193:642–51. doi: 10.1164/rccm.201504-0782OC
77. Singanayagam A, Loo S-L, Calderazzo MA, Finney LJ, Trujillo Torralbo M-B, Bakhsoliani E, et al. Anti-viral immunity is impaired in COPD patients with frequent exacerbations. *Am J Physiol Lung Cell Mol Physiol.* (2019) 317:L893–903. doi: 10.1101/632372
78. Schuliga M. NF-kappaB signaling in chronic inflammatory airway disease. *Biomolecules.* (2015) 5:1266–83. doi: 10.3390/biom5031266
79. Lawrence T. The nuclear factor NF- B pathway in inflammation. *Cold Spring Harb Perspect Biol.* (2009) 1:a001651. doi: 10.1101/cshperspect.a001651
80. Zhou L, Liu Y, Chen X, Wang S, Liu H, Zhang T, et al. Over-expression of nuclear factor-κB family genes and inflammatory molecules is related to chronic obstructive pulmonary disease. *Int J Chron Obstruct Pulmon Dis.* (2018) 13:2131–8. doi: 10.2147/COPD.S164151
81. Gagliardo R, Chanez P, Profita M, Bonanno A, Albano GD, Montalbano AM, et al. IκB kinase-driven nuclear factor-κB activation in patients with asthma and chronic obstructive pulmonary disease. *J Allergy Clin Immunol.* (2011) 128:635–45.e1-2. doi: 10.1016/j.jaci.2011.03.045
82. Banerjee A, Koziol-White C, Panettieri R. p38 MAPK inhibitors, IKK2 inhibitors, and TNFα inhibitors in COPD. *Curr Opin Pharmacol.* (2012) 12:287–92. doi: 10.1016/j.coph.2012.01.016
83. McMillan DH, Baglole CJ, Thatcher TH, Maggirwar S, Sime PJ, Phipps RP. Lung-targeted overexpression of the NF-κB member RelB inhibits cigarette smoke-induced inflammation. *Am J Pathol.* (2011) 179:125–33. doi: 10.1016/j.ajpath.2011.03.030
84. Hsu AC-Y, Dua K, Starkey MR, Haw T-J, Nair PM, Nichol K, et al. MicroRNA-125a and -b inhibit A20 and MAVS to promote inflammation and impair antiviral response in COPD. *JCI Insight.* (2017) 2:e90443. doi: 10.1172/jci.insight.90443
85. Shehab M, Sherri N, Hussein H, Salloum N, Rahal EA. Endosomal toll-like receptors mediate enhancement of interleukin-17a production triggered by Epstein-Barr virus DNA in mice. *J Virol.* (2019) 93:e00987-19. doi: 10.1128/JVI.00987-19
86. West JA, Gregory SM, Damania B. Toll-like receptor sensing of human herpesvirus infection. *Front Cell Infect Microbiol.* (2012) 2:122. doi: 10.3389/fcimb.2012.00122
87. Liu D, Chen Q, Zhu H, Gong L, Huang Y, Li S, et al. Association of respiratory syncytial virus toll-like receptor 3-mediated immune response with COPD exacerbation frequency. *Inflammation.* (2018) 41:654–66. doi: 10.1007/s10753-017-0720-4
88. Silkoff PE, Flavin S, Gordon R, Loza MJ, Sterk PJ, Lutter R, et al. Toll-like receptor 3 blockade in rhinovirus-induced experimental asthma exacerbations: a randomized controlled study. *J Allergy Clin Immunol.* (2018) 141:1220–30. doi: 10.1016/j.jaci.2017.06.027
89. Vallath S, Hynds RE, Succony L, Janes SM, Giangreco A. Targeting EGFR signalling in chronic lung disease: therapeutic challenges and opportunities. *Eur Respir J.* (2014) 44:513–22. doi: 10.1183/09031936.00146413
90. Tyner JW, Kim EY, Ide K, Pelletier MR, Roswit WT, Morton JD, et al. Blocking airway mucous cell metaplasia by inhibiting EGFR antiapoptosis and IL-13 transdifferentiation signals. *J Clin Invest.* (2006) 116:309–21. doi: 10.1172/JCI25167
91. Guedán A, Swieboda D, Charles M, Toussaint M, Johnston SL, Asfor A, et al. Investigation of the role of protein kinase D in human rhinovirus replication. *J Virol.* (2017) 91:e00217-17. doi: 10.1128/JVI.00217-17
92. Kim S, Nadel JA. Fibrinogen binding to ICAM-1 promotes EGFR-dependent mucin production in human airway epithelial cells. *Am J Physiol Lung Cell Mol Physiol.* (2009) 297:L174–83. doi: 10.1152/ajplung.00032.2009
93. Subauste MC, Proud D. Effects of tumor necrosis factor-α, epidermal growth factor and transforming growth factor-α on interleukin-8 production by, and human rhinovirus replication in, bronchial epithelial cells. *Int Immunopharmacol.* (2001) 1:1229–34. doi: 10.1016/S1567-5769(01)00063-7
94. Ganesan S, Unger BL, Comstock AT, Angel KA, Mancuso P, Martinez FJ, et al. Aberrantly activated EGFR contributes to enhanced IL-8 expression in COPD airways epithelial cells via regulation of nuclear FoxO3A. *Thorax.* (2013) 68:131–41. doi: 10.1136/thoraxjnl-2012-201719
95. Zhu L, Lee P-K, Lee W-M, Zhao Y, Yu D, Chen Y. Rhinovirus-induced major airway mucin production involves a novel TLR3-EGFR-dependent pathway. *Am J Respir Cell Mol Biol.* (2009) 40:610–9. doi: 10.1165/rcmb.2008-0223OC
96. Hewson CA, Haas JJ, Bartlett NW, Message SD, Laza-Stanca V, Kebadze T, et al. Rhinovirus induces MUC5AC in a human infection model and

in vitro via NF-κB and EGFR pathways. *Eur Respir J.* (2010) 36:1425–35. doi: 10.1183/09031936.00026910
97. Stolarczyk M, Scholte BJ. The EGFR-ADAM17 axis in chronic obstructive pulmonary disease and cystic fibrosis lung pathology. *Mediators Inflamm.* (2018) 2018:1067134. doi: 10.1155/2018/1067134
98. Ueki IF, Min-Oo G, Kalinowski A, Ballon-Landa E, Lanier LL, Nadel JA, et al. Respiratory virus-induced EGFR activation suppresses IRF1-dependent interferon λ and antiviral defense in airway epithelium. *J Exp Med.* (2013) 210:1929–36. doi: 10.1084/jem.20121401
99. Kalinowski A, Galen BT, Ueki IF, Sun Y, Mulenos A, Osafo-Addo A, et al. Respiratory syncytial virus activates epidermal growth factor receptor to suppress interferon regulatory factor 1-dependent interferon-lambda and antiviral defense in airway epithelium. *Mucosal Immunol.* (2018) 11:958–67. doi: 10.1038/mi.2017.120
100. Abe T, Marutani Y, Shoji I. Cytosolic DNA-sensing immune response and viral infection. *Microbiol Immunol.* (2019) 63:51–64. doi: 10.1111/1348-0421.12669
101. Chan YK, Gack MU. Viral evasion of intracellular DNA and RNA sensing. *Nat Rev Microbiol.* (2016) 14:360–73. doi: 10.1038/nrmicro.2016.45
102. Orzalli MH, Broekema NM, Diner BA, Hancks DC, Elde NC, Cristea IM, et al. cGAS-mediated stabilization of IFI16 promotes innate signaling during herpes simplex virus infection. *Proc Natl Acad Sci USA.* (2015) 112:E1773–81. doi: 10.1073/pnas.1424637112
103. Zhu J, Message SD, Mallia P, Kebadze T, Contoli M, Ward CK, et al. Bronchial mucosal IFN-α/β and pattern recognition receptor expression in patients with experimental rhinovirus-induced asthma exacerbations. *J Allergy Clin Immunol.* (2019) 143:114–25.e4. doi: 10.1016/j.jaci.2018.04.003
104. Farazuddin M, Mishra R, Jing Y, Srivastava V, Comstock AT, Sajjan US. Quercetin prevents rhinovirus-induced progression of lung disease in mice with COPD phenotype. *PLoS ONE.* (2018) 13:e0199612. doi: 10.1371/journal.pone.0199612
105. Traub S, Nikonova A, Carruthers A, Dunmore R, Vousden KA, Gogsadze L, et al. An anti-human ICAM-1 antibody inhibits rhinovirus-induced exacerbations of lung inflammation. *PLoS Pathog.* (2013) 9:e1003520. doi: 10.1371/journal.ppat.1003520
106. Mirabelli C, Scheers E, Neyts J. Novel therapeutic approaches to simultaneously target rhinovirus infection and asthma/COPD pathogenesis. *F1000Res.* (2017) 6:1860. doi: 10.12688/f1000research.11978.1
107. Beigel JH, Nam HH, Adams PL, Krafft A, Ince WL, El-Kamary SS, et al. Advances in respiratory virus therapeutics - a meeting report from the 6th isirv antiviral group conference. *Antiviral Res.* (2019) 167:45–67. doi: 10.1016/j.antiviral.2019.04.006
108. Mousnier A, Bell AS, Swieboda DP, Morales-Sanfrutos J, Pérez-Dorado I, Brannigan JA, et al. Fragment-derived inhibitors of human N-myristoyltransferase block capsid assembly and replication of the common cold virus. *Nat Chem.* (2018) 10:599–606. doi: 10.1038/s41557-018-0039-2
109. Schaefer N, Li X, Seibold MA, Jarjour NN, Denlinger LC, Castro M, et al. The effect of BPIFA1/SPLUNC1 genetic variation on its expression and function in asthmatic airway epithelium. *JCI Insight.* (2019) 4:e127237. doi: 10.1172/jci.insight.127237
110. Jiang D, Wenzel SE, Wu Q, Bowler RP, Schnell C, Chu HW. Human neutrophil elastase degrades SPLUNC1 and impairs airway epithelial defense against bacteria. *PLoS ONE.* (2013) 8:e64689. doi: 10.1371/journal.pone.0064689
111. Seys LJM, Verhamme FM, Dupont LL, Desauter E, Duerr J, Seyhan Agircan A, et al. Airway surface dehydration aggravates cigarette smoke-induced hallmarks of COPD in mice. *PLoS ONE.* (2015) 10:e0129897. doi: 10.1371/journal.pone.0129897
112. Tcherniuk S, Cenac N, Comte M, Frouard J, Errazuriz-Cerda E, Galabov A, et al. Formyl peptide receptor 2 plays a deleterious role during influenza a virus infections. *J Infect Dis.* (2016) 214:237–47. doi: 10.1093/infdis/jiw127
113. Ampomah PB, Moraes LA, Lukman HM, Lim LHK. Formyl peptide receptor 2 is regulated by RNA mimics and viruses through an IFN-b-STAT3-dependent pathway. *FASEB J.* (2018) 32:1468–78. doi: 10.1096/fj.201700584RR
114. Lupfer C, Malik A, Kanneganti T-D. Inflammasome control of viral infection. *Curr Opin Virol.* (2015) 12:38–46. doi: 10.1016/j.coviro.2015.02.007
115. Chen I-Y, Ichinohe T. Response of host inflammasomes to viral infection. *Trends Microbiol.* (2015) 23:55–63. doi: 10.1016/j.tim.2014.09.007
116. Colarusso C, Terlizzi M, Molino A, Pinto A, Sorrentino R. Role of the inflammasome in chronic obstructive pulmonary disease (COPD). *Oncotarget.* (2017) 8:81813–24. doi: 10.18632/oncotarget.17850
117. Hikichi M, Mizumura K, Maruoka S, Gon Y. Pathogenesis of chronic obstructive pulmonary disease (COPD) induced by cigarette smoke. *J Thorac Dis.* (2019) 11:S2129–40. doi: 10.21037/jtd.2019.10.43

7

Epigenetic Regulation of Airway Epithelium Immune Functions in Asthma

Bilal Alashkar Alhamwe[1,2,3], *Sarah Miethe*[1,4], *Elke Pogge von Strandmann*[3], *Daniel P. Potaczek*[1,5†] *and Holger Garn*[1,4*†]

[1] Institute of Laboratory Medicine, Philipps-University Marburg, Member of the German Center for Lung Research (DZL), Universities of Giessen and Marburg Lung Center, Marburg, Germany, [2] College of Pharmacy, International University for Science and Technology (IUST), Daraa, Syria, [3] Center for Tumor Biology and Immunology, Institute of Tumor Immunology, Philipps University Marburg, Marburg, Germany, [4] Translational Inflammation Research Division & Core Facility for Single Cell Multiomics, Philipps University Marburg, Marburg, Germany, [5] John Paul II Hospital, Kraków, Poland

***Correspondence:**
Holger Garn
garn@staff.uni-marburg.de

† These authors have contributed equally to this work

Asthma is a chronic inflammatory disease of the respiratory tract characterized by recurrent breathing problems resulting from airway obstruction and hyperresponsiveness. Human airway epithelium plays an important role in the initiation and control of the immune responses to different types of environmental factors contributing to asthma pathogenesis. Using pattern recognition receptors airway epithelium senses external stimuli, such as allergens, microbes, or pollutants, and subsequently secretes endogenous danger signaling molecules alarming and activating dendritic cells. Hence, airway epithelial cells not only mediate innate immune responses but also bridge them with adaptive immune responses involving T and B cells that play a crucial role in the pathogenesis of asthma. The effects of environmental factors on the development of asthma are mediated, at least in part, by epigenetic mechanisms. Those comprise classical epigenetics including DNA methylation and histone modifications affecting transcription, as well as microRNAs influencing translation. The common feature of such mechanisms is that they regulate gene expression without affecting the nucleotide sequence of the genomic DNA. Epigenetic mechanisms play a pivotal role in the regulation of different cell populations involved in asthma pathogenesis, with the remarkable example of T cells. Recently, however, there is increasing evidence that epigenetic mechanisms are also crucial for the regulation of airway epithelial cells, especially in the context of epigenetic transfer of environmental effects contributing to asthma pathogenesis. In this review, we summarize the accumulating evidence for this very important aspect of airway epithelial cell pathobiology.

Keywords: airway, allergy, asthma, epigenetic, epithelium, histone, methylation, microRNA (miRNA)

INTRODUCTION

Asthma is a chronic inflammatory disease of the airways, in which airway obstruction and hyperresponsiveness underlie recurrent breathing problems, with symptoms being especially pronounced during disease exacerbations (1, 2). Respiratory tract epithelium plays an important role in asthma by initiating and controlling immune responses to different types of pathogenic environmental factors, including allergens, viruses, pollutants, and others. The biology of the airway epithelium in health and its pathobiology in asthma are regulated by epigenetic mechanisms forming the intercellular homeostatic system responding to internal as well as external changing conditions on the level of transcriptional and posttranscriptional regulation of gene expression (3, 4).

AIRWAY EPITHELIUM AND ASTHMA

The airway epithelium is the first structure of the body getting into contact with inhaled air with all its containing environmental components. Initially, it was thought to just constitute a mechanical barrier to enable the bidirectional transfer of air to and from the gas-exchanging alveolar structures. Over the last years, it turned out, however, that the airway epithelium in general and the bronchial epithelium as a major part of it in particular represent a much more complex tissue fulfilling a variety of additional functions such as retrograde transport of inhaled particles, establishment of a biochemical barrier system, and initiation and regulation of innate and adaptive immune mechanisms by release of various cytokines and chemokines. By this, it represents an integrative part of the innate immune system, the coordinated activity of which is essential for maintaining the local tissue and even systemic body integrity (5). To exert these diverse functions, the bronchial epithelium is composed of multiple structurally and/or functionally differing cell types, such as ciliated cells (mucociliary transport), goblet cells (mucus secretion), tuft and M cells (luminal signal sampling and antigen presentation), ionocytes (water regulation), and club cells (mucus and surfactant protein production) (6). All these cell types develop from local stem cell precursors, called basal cells (7). It is quite obvious that the continuous development of the different cell types from such precursors, as well as their concerted action under healthy conditions, requires a high level of control and regulation (8). In asthma, the underlying control mechanisms are disturbed by both external (environmental factors such as allergens, pollen, bacteria, viruses) and internal (i.e., cytokines, chemokines, low-molecular-weight mediators produced by innate and adaptive immune cells) influences, resulting in dysregulated activities of the bronchial epithelium (9). This includes hypersecretion of mucus, release of epithelial-derived cytokines called alarmins [e.g., interleukin 25 (IL-25), IL-33, thymic stromal lymphopoietin], chemokines, and antimicrobial peptides, as well as uncontrolled proliferation and differentiation processes, altogether leading to functional [e.g., airway hyperresponsiveness(AHR)] and structural (e.g., airway remodeling) changes that represent characteristic features of asthma pathology (10). Not unexpectedly, because of the close relation to environmental influences and their changes, epigenetic regulation processes are crucially involved in the appropriate development, maintenance, and functionality of the different components of the airway epithelium (11). Chronic inflammatory processes such as in asthma are expected to interfere with these well-balanced epigenetic mechanisms in the epithelium of the airways. This may happen at the level of the aforementioned finally differentiated cell types and by changing related gene expression patterns that influence their functional behavior. It is also conceivable that epigenetic changes occur already at the level of the basal cells, which would then be inherited to all kinds of cells developing from the affected precursors with multiple functional consequences (12). It needs to be considered that these mechanisms may either lead to further perpetuation of the disease process or, alternatively, represent repair activities initiated to get the complex system back to steady state, that is, healthy conditions.

EPIGENETIC MECHANISMS

Epigenetics comprises molecular mechanisms of inheritable but reversible phenotypic changes that lead to modified gene expression without alterations at the level of the DNA sequence (13). In the human genome, 80% of the DNA is packed into nucleosomes, and the rest forms linkers between nucleosomes. The nucleosomes are further packed into dense three-dimensional structures called chromosomes (14). The core components of the nucleosome are histone proteins, which are accessible to different types of posttranslational modifications (PTMs), including acetylation, methylation, phosphorylation, sumoylation, and ubiquitination. Posttranslational modifications, especially if occurring at important regulatory genomic regions such as enhancers or promoters, are able to change the accessibility of the DNA to the transcriptional machinery, which is associated with active, poised, or silenced status of transcriptional activity. For example, histone acetylations, the changes introduced by histone acetyltransferases (HATs) and removed by histone deacetylases (HDACs), are usually associated with transcriptional activation of the gene (15, 16). DNA methylation, in which a methyl group is enzymatically added to the cytosine ring of DNA, is another type of the epigenetic modification. While the methylation reaction is catalyzed by DNA methyltransferases, ten-eleven translocation (TET) methylcytosine dioxygenase family proteins mediate DNA demethylation. DNA methylation is typically associated with gene repression (3, 17). In addition to the classical epigenetic modifications mentioned above, different types of the non-coding RNAs such as microRNAs (miRNAs) and others, for instance, piwi-interacting RNAs or small nucleolar RNAs, are involved in the epigenetic regulation of gene expression. Briefly, miRNAs exert their silencing effects through the binding to the mature mRNA molecules in the cytosol that leads to mRNA degradation or reduction in the translational efficiency of the ribosomes (18, 19) (**Figure 1**).

DNA METHYLATION

DNA methylation is probably the best studied epigenetic modification in general but also in relation to asthma. Although studies conducted so far on the involvement of DNA methylation in asthma have mostly used already available DNA samples and/or DNA extracted from easily available tissues, also

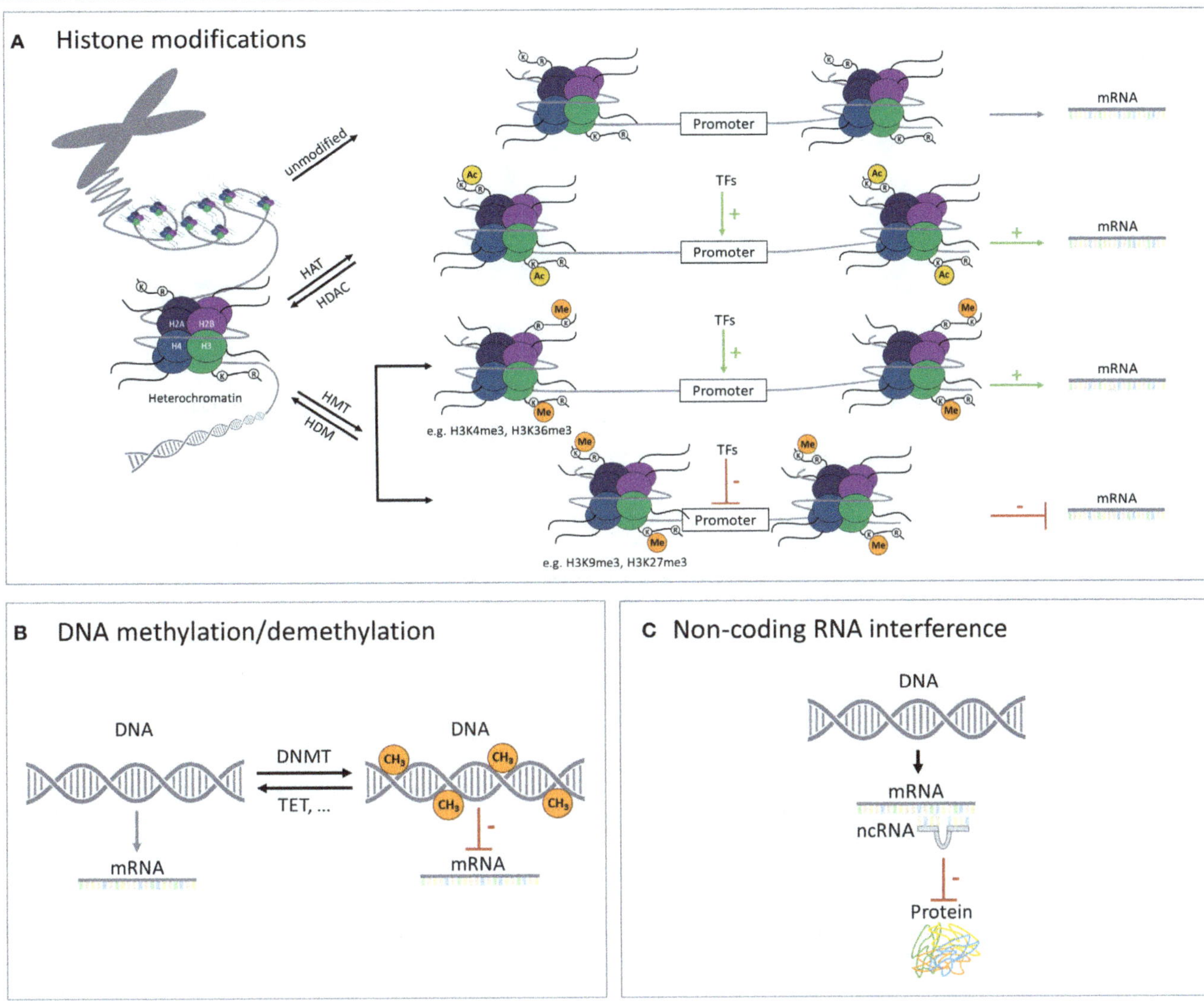

FIGURE 1 | Schematic illustration of major epigenetic modifications. **(A)** Modification of histones such as histone acetylation/deacetylation via histone acetyltransferases (HATs)/histone deacetylases (HDAC) and methylation/demethylation via histone methyltransferases (HMT)/histone demethylases (HDM) can either activate or repress the target gene transcription. Histone acetylation is typically associated with higher expression of the gene. Histone methylation can be related to either higher or lower transcriptional activity, depending on the amino acid residue modified and the number of methyl groups added. **(B)** DNA methylation or demethylation of genomic DNA through DNA methyltransferases (DNMT) or ten-eleven translocation (TET) enzymes and others, respectively. Higher level of DNA methylation is typically associated with lower transcriptional activity of the respective gene. **(C)** MicroRNAs (miRNAs) and further small non-coding RNAs can interfere with gene expression through base pairing with messenger RNAs and thus inhibiting their translation into the encoded protein.

lower airway epithelial cells (AECs) have been investigated (**Figure 2**). Stefanowicz et al. (20) performed a comparative DNA methylation analysis of 807 genes in bronchial AECs and peripheral blood mononuclear cells (PBMCs) obtained from atopics, atopic asthmatics, non-atopic asthmatics, or healthy controls. They identified signature sets of CpG sites differentially methylated between AECs and PBMCs, which were either independent of the disease phenotype or specific to healthy controls, atopics, or asthmatics. Although no differences in the DNA methylation status were found between disease phenotypes in PBMCs, they were observed between asthmatics and atopics in AECs (20). Kim et al. (21) comparatively analyzed genome-wide DNA methylation levels in bronchial mucosa tissues obtained from atopic and non-atopic asthmatics and healthy controls. Although the methylation levels were similar between asthmatics and controls, a set of loci has been identified with significant differences in DNA methylation between atopic and non-atopic asthmatics (21). Clifford et al. (22) investigated in turn the effects of experimental respiratory tract exposure to allergen, diesel exhaust, or both as a coexposure, always observing only minimal resulting changes in the bronchial epithelial DNA methylome of the participating individuals. They found, however, that if any of the two insults occurs in advance of the other (crossover exposure with a 4-week interval), the initial

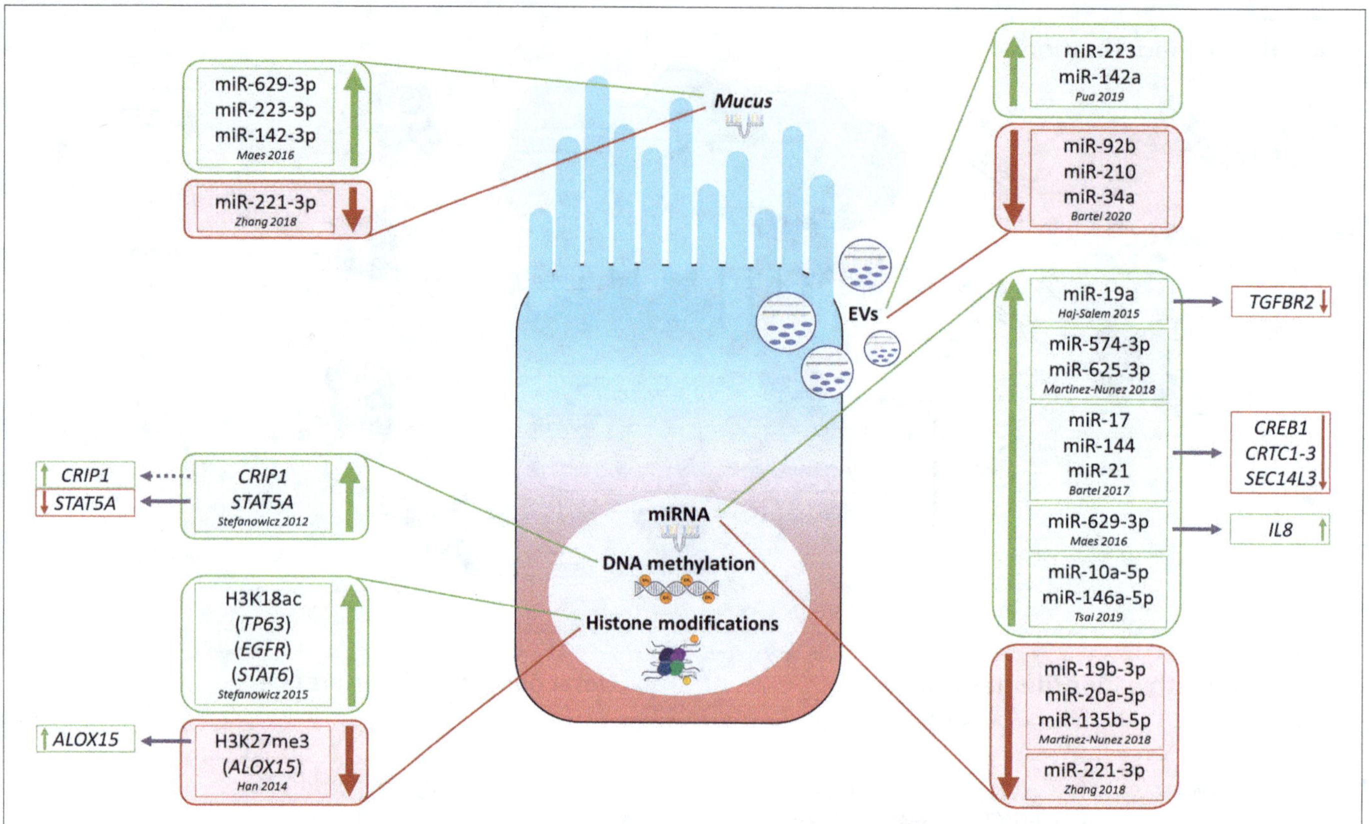

FIGURE 2 | Overview of currently known key epigenetic modifications observed in lower airway epithelial cells from asthma/allergic airway inflammation conditions and—if known—associated functional consequences. The green color always indicates upregulation of the respective modification in asthmatics vs. healthy while red color identifies opposite regulation. EVs, extracellular vesicles; miRNA, microRNA; H3K18ac, histone H3K18 acetylation; H3K27me3, histone H3K27me3 trimethylation.

one primes the bronchial epithelial DNA methylome for the second, resulting in cumulative epigenetic changes with potential biological relevance (22).

In most cases, however, DNA methylation studies conducted in airway tissue in the context of asthma have not been performed in bronchial or lung ACEs but rather in nasal epithelial cells (NECs) due to easier accessibility (23–28). Cardenas et al. (23) conducted an epigenome-wide study on DNA methylation using nasal swabs collected in a large group of early teenagers deriving from a birth cohort. They identified multiple DNA methylation loci associated with asthma, allergies, and related clinical or laboratory parameters (23). In another cohort of adolescents, Forno et al. (24) performed in turn an epigenome-wide analysis of DNA methylation in nasal epithelium. The major findings of this study, replicated in two independent cohorts, comprised the identification of specific DNA methylation profiles associated with atopy and atopic asthma and a nasal methylation panel that could classify children by atopy or atopic asthma (24). Reese et al. (25) sought to identify differential DNA methylation related to pediatric asthma in blood from newborns and school-aged children. Interestingly, they were able to replicate in eosinophils or nasal respiratory epithelium most of the asthma-related differential methylation signatures initially detected in blood (25). Brugha et al. (29) comparatively analyzed DNA methylation in airway and surrogate tissues. They found that the methylation profile in nasal epithelium was most representative of that in the airway epithelium, whereas the profile in buccal cells was moderately and that in blood was least similar (29). In our view, these results clearly suggest that DNA methylation studies performed in the context of asthma as an airway disease should preferentially be conducted using AECs or NECs. Although beyond the scope of this review, we would like to mention that, in our view, sorted specific white blood cell populations would be highly valuable to study systemic adaptive immunity DNA methylation patterns underlying asthma. However, how well those signatures correspond to local lung DNA methylation patterns would need to be assessed in separate studies. Back to NECs, Xiao et al. (27) showed that nasal DNA methylation at the promoter of the vanin 1 gene (*VNN1*) might be a clinically useful biomarker of corticosteroid treatment response in asthmatic children. Another study from the same group demonstrated in turn that DNA methylation at the TET methylcytosine dioxygenase 1 gene (*TET1*) contributes to traffic-related air pollution and asthma (26).

Finally, allelic differences in DNA methylation and thus gene expression in AECs can mediate the effects of certain genetic variants known to be associated with susceptibility to childhood asthma, such as those in chromosome 17q21 (30, 31).

HISTONE MODIFICATIONS

In addition to DNA methylation, also histone modifications participate in epithelial (patho-) mechanisms related to asthma (**Figure 2**). Stefanowicz et al. (32) compared global and gene-specific alveolar epithelial cells histone acetylation and methylation status between asthmatics and healthy subjects. Generally, they observed higher global H3K18ac and H3K9me3 levels in asthmatic subjects. In more detail, they found in asthmatics a higher association of H3K18ac (but not H3K9me3) around the transcription start sites of *TP63* (tumor protein p63, ΔNp63 isoform), *EGFR* (epidermal growth factor receptor), and *STAT6* (signal transducer and activator of transcription 6) genes. Finally, they detected a non-significant increase in protein expression of those three genes in AECs treated with trichostatin A, an HDAC inhibitor (HDACi) (32). In another work, the same group comparatively analyzed the expression of 82 epigenetic modifying enzymes in AECs and bronchial fibroblasts obtained from asthmatics and healthy controls (33). Thirty-nine enzymes were differentially expressed between AECs and bronchial fibroblasts, 24 of which passed the correction for multiple testing. Six histone modifiers turned out to be differentially expressed in AECs between asthmatics and non-asthmatics, however, mostly not significantly when corrected for multiple testing (33).

Beneficial effects of HDACi have been observed in murine models of allergic airway inflammation (AAI) mimicking features of human allergic asthma (34, 35). Application of HDACi in an ovalbumin (OVA)-based model reduced airway inflammation, remodeling, and AHR. In addition, HDACi treatment was associated with lower expression of transforming growth factor β1 (TGF-β1) in AECs and diminished synthesis of contractile proteins by airway smooth muscle cells (34). HDACi treatment in mice subjected to a house dust mite (HDM)–based model was in turn able to prevent them from developing AHR and AAI. Moreover, HDACi restored the integrity of the *ex vivo*–cultured NECs isolated from AR patients (35). Significantly lower H3K27me3 levels at the promoter of the arachidonate 15-lipoxygenase (ALOX15) gene (*ALOX15*) were observed in human lung epithelial A549 cells after the treatment with IL-4, which coincided with higher *ALOX15* mRNA levels (36).

Targeting histone modification—related mechanisms turned out to be effective also in a cockroach allergen extract–induced mouse model of mixed granulocytic (eosinophilic and neutrophilic), T_H2/T_H17-driven asthma (37). Specifically, whereas a bromo- and extraterminal (BET) inhibitor was already alone able to abolish T_H17-driven neutrophilic inflammation, in combination with dexamethasone it completely blocked both T_H2- and T_H17-driven immune responses in the lung, which was associated with reductions in lung eosinophilia and neutrophilia, and mucin secretion. Furthermore, BET inhibition improved cockroach allergen extract- or IL-17A–induced increase in markers of glucocorticoid insensitivity [i.e., decrease in HDAC2 expression (38)] in murine or human AECs, respectively (37). In another study, *Hdac2*$^{+/-}$ mice subjected to an HDM-induced AAI model demonstrated stronger inflammatory infiltration as well as higher expression of type 2 cytokines and IL-17A in the lung tissue compared to wild-type animals. Additional IL-17A depletion was able to reverse these HDAC2 impairment-induced effects (39). In turn, HDM and IL-17A synergistically reduced HDAC2 expression in human bronchial epithelial cells (BECs) *in vitro*. Besides, silencing the HDAC2-encoding gene further enhanced HDM- and/or IL-17A–induced inflammatory cytokines in human BECs, whereas HDAC2 overexpression or knockdown of the gene encoding IL-17A was able to reduce the release of such inflammatory cytokines (39). Taken together, original findings by Zijlstra et al. (38), who first discovered IL-17A–induced steroid resistance mediated by a reduction of HDAC2 activity, have thus been corroborated and expanded.

MICRORNA

Several recent studies have highlighted the importance of miRNAs in the regulation of epithelial pathobiology in asthma (**Figure 2**). Bartel et al. (40) combined different approaches such as *in vivo* studies in mice with OVA- or HDM-induced AAI, *ex vivo*/*in vitro* experiments including luciferase reporter assay and stimulation–expression analyses, miRNA/mRNA microarrays, and *in silico* approaches. This composed strategy enabled the authors to identify the transcription factor cAMP-responsive element binding protein (*Creb1*) and its transcriptional coactivators (*Crtc1-3*) as targets for miR-17, miR-144, and miR-21, all three deregulated in lungs of mice with AAI. Moreover, they observed downregulation of Sec14-like 3 (*Sec14l3*), a putative target of Creb1, in both AAI models and in primary normal human BECs upon IL-13 treatment suggesting that miRNA-regulated Crtc1-3 and Sec14l3 play a role in early epithelial responses to type 2 stimuli (40). Microarray analysis of miRNA expression in bronchoscopy-isolated human BECs showed in turn an upregulation of miR-19a in samples obtained from severe asthmatic subjects compared to those from mild asthmatics and healthy controls (41). Furthermore, luciferase reporter assay- and Western blot–based functional studies demonstrated miR-19a to enhance proliferation of BECs in severe asthma through targeting TGF-β receptor 2 gene (*TGFBR2*) mRNA (41). Using subcellular fractionation and RNA sequencing (Frac-seq) in human primary BECs from healthy controls and severe asthmatics, Martinez-Nunez et al. (42) assessed paired genome-wide expression of miRNAs along with cytoplasmic (total) and polyribosome-bound (translational) mRNA levels. They identified a hub of six dysregulated miRNAs, displaying preference for polyribosome-bound mRNAs, which accounted for ~90% of whole miRNA targeting. Interestingly, transfection of such miRNAs into BECs obtained from healthy subjects turned them into cells mimicking features of those obtained from severe asthmatics (42).

Recently, extracellular vesicles (EVs) transferring miRNAs between cells have been identified as a novel mechanism of intercellular communication (3, 43, 44). Of note, the composition of the extracellular miRNA pool in the lung of mice was very similar to that of the airway epithelium, and ~80% of the detected EVs were of epithelial origin (45). However, following the induction of AAI, the presence of miRNAs preferentially expressed by immune cells, such as miR-223 and miR-142a, and hematopoietic cell–derived EVs increased also substantially, indicating an importance of the extracellular miRNA pool for the development of local allergic inflammatory processes (45). Gupta et al. (46) focused on EVs secreted by two kinds of human airway cell cultures, that is, primary tracheobronchial cells and a cultured AEC line (Calu-3). Their data suggest that cellular information can be transferred between AECs via miRNA-containing EVs, which may thereby contribute to epithelial biology and remodeling (46). Another study profiled the expression of miRNAs in EVs secreted from the apical and basal sides by normal human BECs treated with IL-13 in order to induce an asthma-like response (47). Significant candidates were then confirmed in EVs isolated from nasal lavages obtained from children with mild to moderate or severe asthma and healthy control subjects. Interestingly, levels of miR-92b, miR-210, and miR-34a turned out to correlate with lung function measures (47).

Two studies investigated miRNAs in asthmatic sputum (48, 49). In two independent cohorts, Maes et al. (48) found a significant upregulation of miR-629-3p, miR-223-3p, and miR-142-3p in sputum of severe asthmatics compared to healthy controls, with the highest levels in patients with neutrophilic asthma. Of those three miRNAs associated with sputum neutrophilia and airway obstruction, miR-629-3p was expressed in BECs. Interestingly, transfection of human BECs with a miR-629-3p mimic induced expression of IL-8, the sputum levels of which were significantly increased and positively correlated with sputum neutrophilia in severe asthmatics (48). Zhang et al. (49) found in turn that epithelial, sputum, and plasma miR-221-3p levels were significantly lower in asthmatics compared to healthy controls. In addition, levels of epithelial and sputum miR-221-3p inversely correlated with airway eosinophilia (49).

Finally, Tsai et al. (50) sought to find the common miRNA-related effects in BECs obtained from subjects with asthma and chronic obstructive pulmonary disease (COPD). First detected with next-generation sequencing, the upregulation of miR-10a-5p and miR-146a-5p in BECs obtained from both asthma and COPD patients was subsequently confirmed by quantitative polymerase chain reaction. Moreover, compared to healthy controls, also serum miR-146a-5p levels were higher in asthma and COPD subjects (50). Further research will establish whether miRNAs mediating intercellular communication can be used for clinical applications as biomarkers or therapeutic targets.

SPECIAL ASPECTS

Airborne viruses, for instance, human rhinoviruses (HRVs), stimulate asthma exacerbations. In addition, repeated early life infections with such viruses can lead to the development of a persistent asthma phenotype, especially in children with atopic susceptibility (3, 51). Interestingly, some studies suggest that the effects of respiratory viral infections are at least partly mediated by epigenetic changes in airway epithelial cells. It has been demonstrated that *ex vivo* experimental HRV infection of NECs obtained from asthmatic children significantly changes patterns of DNA methylation and mRNA expression (52). Moreover, HRV infection in young children has been associated with changes in the airway secretory miRNome, characterized by a highly specific additional appearance of miR-155 in nasal secretion EVs (53). In turn, BECs obtained from asthmatics have been shown to be characterized by dysregulated miR-22 expression after experimental *ex vivo* infection with influenza A virus (IAV) (54). Other epigenetic modifications, specifically histone methylations, also seem to be involved in the regulation of epithelial antiviral responses (55).

Dysregulated epithelial–mesenchymal transition (EMT) is the process driven mostly by TGF-β1, which strongly contributes to the establishment of the persistent asthma phenotype, that is, to disease chronification (56). Epigenetic mechanisms seem to play an important role in EMT. It has been demonstrated in mouse models mimicking allergic asthma that miR-448-5p can inhibit TGF-β1–induced EMT and pulmonary fibrosis (57). Applying an epigenome-wide approach in a human study, McErlean et al. (58) identified in turn multiple loci showing differential H3K27ac enrichment in asthma, which clustered at genes associated with type 2–driven asthma and EMT.

CONCLUSIONS AND PERSPECTIVES

Epigenetic mechanisms play a very important role in the epithelial pathobiology of asthma. While histone modifications seem to be especially interesting as possible therapeutic targets, DNA methylation and miRNAs, also from the easily accessible nasal epithelium, show a substantial diagnostic potential. Although the data gathered by now (for overview, see also **Supplementary Table 1**) already strongly suggest a usefulness of epigenetics in the asthma management, further studies, especially those considering the complex interplay of different epigenetic mechanisms and those focusing on a single-cell type or investigations on the single cell level, are needed.

AUTHOR CONTRIBUTIONS

BA: draft writing and figure drafts. SM: draft writing and final figures. ES: editing and reviewing. DP: conceptualization, draft writing, and reviewing. HG: conceptualization, coordination, draft writing, and reviewing. All authors contributed to the article and approved the submitted version.

REFERENCES

1. Miethe S, Guarino M, Alhamdan F, Simon H-U, Renz H, Dufour J-F, et al. Effects of obesity on asthma: immunometabolic links. *Polish Arch Internal Med.* (2018) 128:469–77. doi: 10.20452/pamw.4304
2. Koczulla AR, Vogelmeier CF, Garn H, Renz H. New concepts in asthma: clinical phenotypes and pathophysiological mechanisms. *Drug Discov Today.* (2017) 22:388–96. doi: 10.1016/j.drudis.2016.11.008
3. Potaczek DP, Harb H, Michel S, Alhamwe BA, Renz H, Tost J. Epigenetics and allergy: from basic mechanisms to clinical applications. *Epigenomics.* (2017) 9:539–71. doi: 10.2217/epi-2016-0162
4. Pepper AN, Renz H, Casale TB, Garn H. Biologic therapy and novel molecular targets of severe asthma. *J Allergy Clin Immunol Pract.* (2017) 5:909–16. doi: 10.1016/j.jaip.2017.04.038
5. Potaczek DP, Miethe S, Schindler V, Alhamdan F, Garn H. Role of airway epithelial cells in the development of different asthma phenotypes. *Cell Signal.* (2020) 69:109523. doi: 10.1016/j.cellsig.2019.109523
6. Plasschaert LW, Žilionis R, Choo-Wing R, Savova V, Knehr J, Roma G, et al. A single-cell atlas of the airway epithelium reveals the CFTR-rich pulmonary ionocyte. *Nature.* (2018) 560:377–81. doi: 10.1038/s41586-018-0394-6
7. Watson JK, Rulands S, Wilkinson AC, Wuidart A, Ousset M, van Keymeulen A, et al. Clonal dynamics reveal two distinct populations of basal cells in slow-turnover airway epithelium. *Cell Rep.* (2015) 12:90–101. doi: 10.1016/j.celrep.2015.06.011
8. Loxham M, Davies DE. Phenotypic and genetic aspects of epithelial barrier function in asthmatic patients. *J Allergy Clin Immunol.* (2017) 139:1736–51. doi: 10.1016/j.jaci.2017.04.005
9. Holgate ST. The sentinel role of the airway epithelium in asthma pathogenesis. *Immunol Rev.* (2011) 242:205–19. doi: 10.1111/j.1600-065X.2011.01030.x
10. Lloyd CM, Saglani S. Epithelial cytokines and pulmonary allergic inflammation. *Curr Opin Immunol.* (2015) 34:52–8. doi: 10.1016/j.coi.2015.02.001
11. Wawrzyniak P, Wawrzyniak M, Wanke K, Sokolowska M, Bendelja K, Rückert B, et al. Regulation of bronchial epithelial barrier integrity by type 2 cytokines and histone deacetylases in asthmatic patients. *J Allergy Clin Immunol.* (2017) 139:93–103. doi: 10.1016/j.jaci.2016.03.050
12. Ordovas-Montanes J, Dwyer DF, Nyquist SK, Buchheit KM, Vukovic M, Deb C, et al. Allergic inflammatory memory in human respiratory epithelial progenitor cells. *Nature.* (2018) 560:649–54. doi: 10.1038/s41586-018-0449-8
13. Lacal I, Ventura R. Epigenetic inheritance: concepts, mechanisms and perspectives. *Front Mol Neurosci.* (2018) 11:292. doi: 10.3389/fnmol.2018.00292
14. Alberts B, Johnson A, Lewis J, Raff M, Roberts K, Walter P. *Molecular Biology of the Cell: Chromosomal DNA and Its Packaging in the Chromatin Fiber.* 4th ed. New York, NY: Garland Science (2002).
15. Harb H, Alashkar Alhamwe B, Garn H, Renz H, Potaczek DP. Recent developments in epigenetics of pediatric asthma. *Curr Opin Pediatr.* (2016) 28:754–63. doi: 10.1097/MOP.0000000000000424
16. Alaskhar Alhamwe B, Khalaila R, Wolf J, Bülow V, von Harb H, Alhamdan F, et al. Histone modifications and their role in epigenetics of atopy and allergic diseases. *Allergy Asthma Clin Immunol.* (2018) 14:39. doi: 10.1186/s13223-018-0259-4
17. Alashkar Alhamwe B, Alhamdan F, Ruhl A, Potaczek DP, Renz H. The role of epigenetics in allergy and asthma development. *Curr Opin Allergy Clin Immunol.* (2020) 20:48–55. doi: 10.1097/ACI.0000000000000598
18. Hu G, Niu F, Humburg BA, Liao K, Bendi S, Callen S, et al. Molecular mechanisms of long noncoding RNAs and their role in disease pathogenesis. *Oncotarget.* (2018) 9:18648–63. doi: 10.18632/oncotarget.24307
19. Karlsson O, Baccarelli AA. Environmental health and long non-coding RNAs. *Curr Environ Health Rep.* (2016) 3:178–87. doi: 10.1007/s40572-016-0092-1
20. Stefanowicz D, Hackett T-L, Garmaroudi FS, Günther OP, Neumann S, Sutanto EN, et al. DNA methylation profiles of airway epithelial cells and PBMCs from healthy, atopic and asthmatic children. *PLoS ONE.* (2012) 7:e44213. doi: 10.1371/journal.pone.0044213
21. Kim Y-J, Park S-W, Kim T-H, Park J-S, Cheong HS, Shin HD, et al. Genome-wide methylation profiling of the bronchial mucosa of asthmatics: relationship to atopy. *BMC Med Genet.* (2013) 14:39. doi: 10.1186/1471-2350-14-39
22. Clifford RL, Jones MJ, MacIsaac JL, McEwen LM, Goodman SJ, Mostafavi S, et al. Inhalation of diesel exhaust and allergen alters human bronchial epithelium DNA methylation. *J Allergy Clin Immunol.* (2017) 139:112–21. doi: 10.1016/j.jaci.2016.03.046
23. Cardenas A, Sordillo JE, Rifas-Shiman SL, Chung W, Liang L, Coull BA, et al. The nasal methylome as a biomarker of asthma and airway inflammation in children. *Nat Commun.* (2019) 10:3095. doi: 10.1038/s41467-019-11058-3
24. Forno E, Wang T, Qi C, Yan Q, Xu C-J, Boutaoui N, et al. DNA methylation in nasal epithelium, atopy, and atopic asthma in children: a genome-wide study. *Lancet Respir Med.* (2019) 7:336–46. doi: 10.1016/S2213-2600(18)30466-1
25. Reese SE, Xu C-J, den Dekker HT, Lee MK, Sikdar S, Ruiz-Arenas C, et al. Epigenome-wide meta-analysis of DNA methylation and childhood asthma. *J Allergy Clin Immunol.* (2019) 143:2062–74. doi: 10.1016/j.jaci.2018.11.043
26. Somineni HK, Zhang X, Biagini Myers JM, Kovacic MB, Ulm A, Jurcak N, et al. Ten-eleven translocation 1 (TET1) methylation is associated with childhood asthma and traffic-related air pollution. *J Allergy Clin Immunol.* (2016) 137:797–805.e5. doi: 10.1016/j.jaci.2015.10.021
27. Xiao C, Biagini Myers JM, Ji H, Metz K, Martin LJ, Lindsey M, et al. Vanin-1 expression and methylation discriminate pediatric asthma corticosteroid treatment response. *J Allergy Clin Immunol.* (2015) 136:923–31.e3. doi: 10.1016/j.jaci.2015.01.045
28. Zhang X, Biagini Myers JM, Burleson JD, Ulm A, Bryan KS, Chen X, et al. Nasal DNA methylation is associated with childhood asthma. *Epigenomics.* (2018) 10:629–41. doi: 10.2217/epi-2017-0127
29. Brugha R, Lowe R, Henderson AJ, Holloway JW, Rakyan V, Wozniak E, et al. DNA methylation profiles between airway epithelium and proxy tissues in children. *Acta Paediatr.* (2017) 106:2011–6. doi: 10.1111/apa.14027
30. Moussette S, Al Tuwaijri A, Kohan-Ghadr H-R, Elzein S, Farias R, Bérubé J, et al. Role of DNA methylation in expression control of the IKZF3-GSDMA region in human epithelial cells. *PLoS ONE.* (2017) 12:e0172707. doi: 10.1371/journal.pone.0172707
31. Toncheva AA, Potaczek DP, Schedel M, Gersting SW, Michel S, Krajnov N, et al. Childhood asthma is associated with mutations and gene expression differences of ORMDL genes that can interact. *Allergy.* (2015) 70:1288–99. doi: 10.1111/all.12652
32. Stefanowicz D, Lee JY, Lee K, Shaheen F, Koo H-K, Booth S, et al. Elevated H3K18 acetylation in airway epithelial cells of asthmatic subjects. *Respir Res.* (2015) 16:95. doi: 10.1186/s12931-015-0254-y
33. Stefanowicz D, Ullah J, Lee K, Shaheen F, Olumese E, Fishbane N, et al. Epigenetic modifying enzyme expression in asthmatic airway epithelial cells and fibroblasts. *BMC Pulm Med.* (2017) 17:24. doi: 10.1186/s12890-017-0371-0
34. Ren Y, Su X, Kong L, Li M, Zhao X, Yu N, et al. Therapeutic effects of histone deacetylase inhibitors in a murine asthma model. *Inflamm Res.* (2016) 65:995–1008. doi: 10.1007/s00011-016-0984-4
35. Steelant B, Wawrzyniak P, Martens K, Jonckheere A-C, Pugin B, Schrijvers R, et al. Blocking histone deacetylase activity as a novel target for epithelial barrier defects in patients with allergic rhinitis. *J Allergy Clin Immunol.* (2019) 144:1242–53.e7. doi: 10.1016/j.jaci.2019.04.027
36. Han H, Xu D, Liu C, Claesson H-E, Björkholm M, Sjöberg J. Interleukin-4-mediated 15-lipoxygenase-1 trans-activation requires UTX recruitment and H3K27me3 demethylation at the promoter in A549 cells. *PLoS ONE.* (2014) 9:e85085. doi: 10.1371/journal.pone.0085085
37. Nadeem A, Ahmad SF, Al-Harbi NO, Siddiqui N, Ibrahim KE, Attia SM. Inhibition of BET bromodomains restores corticosteroid responsiveness in a mixed granulocytic mouse model of asthma. *Biochem Pharmacol.* (2018) 154:222–33. doi: 10.1016/j.bcp.2018.05.011
38. Zijlstra GJ, Hacken NHT, ten Hoffmann RF, van Oosterhout AJM, Heijink IH. Interleukin-17A induces glucocorticoid insensitivity in human bronchial epithelial cells. *Eur Respir J.* (2012) 39:439–45. doi: 10.1183/09031936.00017911
39. Lai T, Wu M, Zhang C, Che L, Xu F, Wang Y, et al. HDAC2 attenuates airway inflammation by suppressing IL-17A production in HDM-challenged mice. *Am J Physiol Lung Cell Mol Physiol.* (2019) 316:L269–79. doi: 10.1152/ajplung.00143.2018
40. Bartel S, Schulz N, Alessandrini F, Schamberger AC, Pagel P, Theis FJ, et al. Pulmonary microRNA profiles identify involvement of Creb1 and Sec14l3

in bronchial epithelial changes in allergic asthma. *Sci Rep.* (2017) 7:46026. doi: 10.1038/srep46026

41. Haj-Salem I, Fakhfakh R, Bérubé J-C, Jacques E, Plante S, Simard MJ, et al. MicroRNA-19a enhances proliferation of bronchial epithelial cells by targeting TGFβR2 gene in severe asthma. *Allergy.* (2015) 70:212–9. doi: 10.1111/all.12551
42. Martinez-Nunez RT, Rupani H, Platé M, Niranjan M, Chambers RC, Howarth PH, et al. Genome-wide posttranscriptional dysregulation by MicroRNAs in human asthma as revealed by Frac-seq. *J Immunol.* (2018) 201:251–63. doi: 10.4049/jimmunol.1701798
43. Tost J. A translational perspective on epigenetics in allergic diseases. *J Allergy Clin Immunol.* (2018) 142:715–26. doi: 10.1016/j.jaci.2018.07.009
44. Guiot J, Struman I, Louis E, Louis R, Malaise M, Njock M-S. Exosomal miRNAs in lung diseases: from biologic function to therapeutic targets. *J Clin Med.* (2019) 8:1345. doi: 10.3390/jcm8091345
45. Pua HH, Happ HC, Gray CJ, Mar DJ, Chiou N-T, Hesse LE, et al. Increased hematopoietic extracellular RNAs and vesicles in the lung during allergic airway responses. *Cell Rep.* (2019) 26:933–44.e4. doi: 10.1016/j.celrep.2019.01.002
46. Gupta R, Radicioni G, Abdelwahab S, Dang H, Carpenter J, Chua M, et al. Intercellular communication between airway epithelial cells is mediated by exosome-like vesicles. *Am J Respir Cell Mol Biol.* (2019) 60:209–20. doi: 10.1165/rcmb.2018-0156OC
47. Bartel S, La Grutta S, Cilluffo G, Perconti G, Bongiovanni A, Giallongo A, et al. Human airway epithelial extracellular vesicle miRNA signature is altered upon asthma development. *Allergy.* (2020) 75:346–56. doi: 10.1111/all.14008
48. Maes T, Cobos FA, Schleich F, Sorbello V, Henket M, Preter K, et al. Asthma inflammatory phenotypes show differential microRNA expression in sputum. *J Allergy Clin Immunol.* (2016) 137:1433–46. doi: 10.1016/j.jaci.2016.02.018
49. Zhang K, Liang Y, Feng Y, Wu W, Zhang H, He J, et al. Decreased epithelial and sputum miR-221-3p associates with airway eosinophilic inflammation and CXCL17 expression in asthma. *Am J Physiol Lung Cell Mol Physiol.* (2018) 315:L253–L264. doi: 10.1152/ajplung.00567.2017
50. Tsai M-J, Tsai Y-C, Chang W-A, Lin Y-S, Tsai P-H, Sheu C-C, et al. Deducting microRNA-mediated changes common in bronchial epithelial cells of asthma and chronic obstructive pulmonary disease-a next-generation sequencing-guided bioinformatic approach. *Int J Mol Sci.* (2019) 20:553. doi: 10.3390/ijms20030553
51. Potaczek DP, Unger SD, Zhang N, Taka S, Michel S, Akdag N, et al. Development and characterization of DNAzyme candidates demonstrating significant efficiency against human rhinoviruses. *J Allergy Clin Immunol.* (2019) 143:1403–15. doi: 10.1016/j.jaci.2018.07.026
52. Pech M, Weckmann M, König IR, Franke A, Heinsen F-A, Oliver B, et al. Rhinovirus infections change DNA methylation and mRNA expression in children with asthma. *PLoS ONE.* (2018) 13:e0205275. doi: 10.1371/journal.pone.0205275
53. Gutierrez MJ, Gomez JL, Perez GF, Pancham K, Val S, Pillai DK, et al. Airway secretory microRNAome changes during rhinovirus infection in early childhood. *PLoS ONE.* (2016) 11:e0162244. doi: 10.1371/journal.pone.0162244
54. Moheimani F, Koops J, Williams T, Reid AT, Hansbro PM, Wark PA, et al. Influenza A virus infection dysregulates the expression of microRNA-22 and its targets; CD147 and HDAC4, in epithelium of asthmatics. *Respir Res.* (2018) 19:145. doi: 10.1186/s12931-018-0851-7
55. Spalluto CM, Singhania A, Cellura D, Woelk CH, Sanchez-Elsner T, Staples KJ, et al. IFN-γ influences epithelial antiviral responses via histone methylation of the RIG-I promoter. *Am J Respir Cell Mol Biol.* (2017) 57:428–38. doi: 10.1165/rcmb.2016-0392OC
56. Rout-Pitt N, Farrow N, Parsons D, Donnelley M. Epithelial mesenchymal transition (EMT): a universal process in lung diseases with implications for cystic fibrosis pathophysiology. *Respir Res.* (2018) 19:136. doi: 10.1186/s12931-018-0834-8
57. Yang Z-C, Qu Z-H, Yi M-J, Shan Y-C, Ran N, Xu L, et al. MiR-448-5p inhibits TGF-β1-induced epithelial-mesenchymal transition and pulmonary fibrosis by targeting Six1 in asthma. *J Cell Physiol.* (2019) 234:8804–14. doi: 10.1002/jcp.27540
58. McErlean P, Kelly A, Dhariwal J, Kirtland M, Watson J, Ranz I, et al. Genome-wide profiling of an enhancer-associated histone modification reveals the influence of asthma on the epigenome of the airway epithelium. *bioRxiv.* (2018) 6. doi: 10.1101/282889

8

Impaired Airway Epithelial Barrier Integrity in Response to *Stenotrophomonas maltophilia* Proteases, Novel Insights using Cystic Fibrosis Bronchial Epithelial Cell Secretomics

Kevin Molloy[1], Gerard Cagney[2], Eugene T. Dillon[2], Kieran Wynne[2], Catherine M. Greene[3] and Noel G. McElvaney[1]*

[1] Department of Medicine, Royal College of Surgeons in Ireland, Beaumont Hospital, Dublin, Ireland, [2] School of Biomolecular and Biomedical Science, University College Dublin, Dublin, Ireland, [3] Department of Clinical Microbiology, Royal College of Surgeons in Ireland, Beaumont Hospital, Dublin, Ireland

***Correspondence:**
Catherine M. Greene
cmgreene@rcsi.ie

Stenotrophomonas maltophilia is a Gram-negative opportunistic pathogen that can chronically colonize the lungs of people with cystic fibrosis (CF) and is associated with lethal pulmonary hemorrhage in immunocompromised patients. Its secreted virulence factors include the extracellular serine proteases StmPR1, StmPR2, and StmPR3. To explore the impact of secreted virulence determinants on pulmonary mucosal defenses in CF, we examined the secretome of human CFBE41o- bronchial epithelial cells in response to treatment with *S. maltophilia* K279a cell culture supernatant (CS) using a liquid-chromatography-tandem mass spectrometry (LC-MS/MS) based label-free quantitative (LFQ) shotgun proteomics approach for global profiling of the cell secretome. Secretome analysis identified upregulated pathways mainly relating to biological adhesion and epithelial cell signaling in infection, whereas no specific pathways relating to the immune response were enriched. Further exploration of the potentially harmful effects of K279a CS on CF bronchial epithelial cells, demonstrated that K279a CS caused CFBE41o- cell condensation and detachment, reversible by the serine protease inhibitor PMSF. K279a CS also decreased trans-epithelial electrical resistance in CFBE41o- cell monolayers suggestive of disruption of tight junction complexes (TJC). This finding was corroborated by an observed increase in fluorescein isothiocyanate (FITC) dextran permeability and by demonstrating PMSF-sensitive degradation of the tight junction proteins ZO-1 and occludin, but not JAM-A or claudin-1. These observations demonstrating destruction of the CFBE41o- TJC provide a novel insight regarding the virulence of *S. maltophilia* and may explain the possible injurious effects of this bacterium on the CF bronchial epithelium and the pathogenic mechanism leading to lethal pulmonary hemorrhage.

Keywords: *Stenotrophomonas maltophilia*, cystic fibrosis, extracellular proteases, secretomics, tight junction, epithelial barrier dysfunction

INTRODUCTION

Culture supernatant (CS) from bacteria, most notably *Pseudomonas aeruginosa,* has been used extensively to study host-pathogen interactions in the cystic fibrosis (CF) lung. Studies have explored its effects on TLR-induced inflammation (1), pro-inflammatory cytokine production (2, 3), innate immunity proteins (4–6) and degradation of extracellular matrix components (5, 7, 8), amongst others. However, there is a paucity of information regarding the effects of the important emerging CF pathogen, *Stenotrophomonas maltophilia* on airway epithelial cells *in vitro.* Given that the pathogenesis of *S. maltophilia* is complex and multifactorial, high-throughput technologies such as proteomics can help decipher differences in protein expression in composite circumstances such as host-pathogen interactions. Secretome analysis is a promising area of research permitting novel insights into the pathogenesis of different infections. Proteins secreted by a pathogen are present at the interface between the pathogen and the host cells and can thus regulate or mediate the host responses and cause disease (9).

The cell secretome is a collection of proteins that have been shed and proteins secreted by cells into the extracellular space and are important for maintaining cell-cell communication and proliferation. Examples of secretory proteins include extracellular matrix proteins, digestive enzymes, cytokines, chemokines, and growth factors (10). Identification of proteins released by cells into culture supernatants *in vitro* may help to better understand pathological conditions and mechanisms *in vivo*. For example, using high-throughput subcellular proteomics Lietzen et al. showed a robust secretion of different danger-associated molecular patterns in human macrophages in response to influenza A, and that the P2X7 receptor and Src tyrosine kinase activity are essential for inflammasome activation (11). Secretome analysis of A549 cells infected with *Mycoplasma pneumoniae* revealed higher levels of IL-33 mimicking *in vivo* conditions whereby higher than normal IL-33 levels are evident in plasma and bronchoalveolar lavage fluid from patients with *M. pneumonia*-associated pneumonia (12). Analysis of the *in vitro* proteome response of a human bronchial epithelial cell line to *Aspergillus fumigatus* demonstrated previously unknown aspects of bronchial epithelial cell behavior in response to infection including both cellular defense mechanisms and immune reactions (13).

Airway epithelial cells provide the first line of defense following exposure to inhaled infectious agents. Virulence factors such as secreted proteases expressed by *S. maltophilia* are likely to be important mediators of the pathogenic interaction between *S. maltophilia* and these cells. Indeed *S. maltophilia* has been shown to preferentially adhere along intercellular junctions, raising the possibility that tight junction dysfunction may be an important pathogenic mechanism of this bacterium (14). *S. maltophilia* has also been shown to induce morphological changes in fibroblast monolayers resulting in the cell layer partially condensing, formation of cell-free areas, and detachment from the culture plate (15). StmPR1 is likely a causative factor leading to the clinical observation of lethal pulmonary hemorrhage in those who are immunocompromised (16). Moreover, purified StmPr1 induces cell rounding and detachment of A549 cells by targeting cell integrin-extracellular matrix connections (matrilysis) as well as adherence and tight junction proteins for degradation (17, 18).

In this study, using K279a as the reference clinical strain for *S. maltophilia* infection, we provide an insight into host-pathogen interaction using a liquid-chromatography-tandem mass spectrometry (LC-MS/MS) based label-free quantitative shotgun proteomics approach for global profiling of the K279a CS treated human CFBE41o- (cystic fibrosis airway epithelial cell line) cell secretome. Using data from this secretomic analysis we examine the effects of K279a CS on epithelial barrier integrity and degradation of components of CFBE41o- cell tight junctions.

MATERIALS AND METHODS

Reference Bacterial Strain

K279a was used as the reference clinical strain for this work (19). K279a was cultivated by scraping the surface of the frozen bacterial stock (−80°C) with a sterile 10 μL inoculating loop, placed in Luria-Bertani broth (LBB) and incubated overnight at 37°C on an orbital shaker at 200 rpm prior to use. Working stocks were maintained on agar plates at 4°C for up to 2 weeks. Cultures were regularly examined for purity using MALDI-TOF mass spectrometry (MS) analysis.

Preparation of K279a Culture Supernatant (CS)

We have previously shown that Dulbecco's modified essential medium (DMEM) low glucose (5.6 mM) medium (Invitrogen) is the optimal growth medium for inducing K279a protease activity (20). To prepare a stock solution of K279a CS, 10 μL of an overnight K279a culture was inoculated in 6 x 15 mls of DMEM low glucose (5.6 mM) medium and grown for 48 h at 37°C on an orbital shaker. K279a CS was passed sequentially through 0.45-μm and 0.2-μm filters millex filters (Millipore Corporation, Bedford, MA). Culture supernatant (90 mls) was then concentrated using 5-kDa nominal-weight limit (NMWL) cut-off Amicon® Ultra-15 filter devices (Millipore Corporation, Bedford, MA). All concentrates were centrifuged at 4,000 × g and subsequently diafiltered by centrifugation with sterile DPBS to remove any low molecular weight contaminants including glucose and amino acids present in DMEM. An equivalent volume of DMEM was used as a negative control and for correction during protein quantification using the BCA (bicinchoninic acid) assay.

Measurement of K279a CS Protease Activity

Protease activity was measured using the SensoLyte Red Protease Fluorometric Assay Kit (AnaSpec) as previously described (20). Prior to treatment of CFBE41o- airway epithelial cells, protease activity based on the known concentration of protein in K279a CS was adjusted based on a standard curve of K279a CS protease activity (measured in RFU/min).

CFBE41o- Cell Culture

CFBE41o–, an SV40-transformed human ΔF508 homozygote bronchial epithelial cell line was maintained in 75 cm^2 flasks at 37°C humidified CO_2 incubator in minimal essential medium (MEM) supplemented with 10% fetal calf serum (FCS), 1% L-glutamine, 1% penicillin/streptomycin (Invitrogen). The cell line was originally obtained as a gift from D. Gruenert (California Pacific Medical Center Research Institute, San Francisco). Prior to treatment, cells were washed twice with sterile DPBS to remove excess FCS and were placed in serum free medium for 6 h. Immediately prior to treatment with K279a CS, cells were placed in fresh serum-free media.

Romanowsky Stain of CFBE41o- Cells

To visualize morphological effects CFB41o- cells were untreated (control) or treated with K279a CS for 16 h at 37°C. Cells were stained using the Hema–Rapid staining set GURR® (VWR, UK), air dried and then fixed in methanol for 5 s following by staining with reagent one and reagent two for 3 and 6 s, respectively. Images were captured using an Olympus CKX41 and processed using CELL B by Soft Imaging System (Olympus, Tokyo, Japan).

LDH CFBE41o- Cell Viability Assay

LDH assays were performed using the CytoTox 96® Non-Radioactive Cytotoxicity Assay (Promega, USA) according to the manufacturer's instructions. Absorbance was measured 490 nm on a microplate reader (Victor™ X3 Multilabel Plate Reader, PerkinElmer, Massachusetts, USA).

CFBE41o- Cell Secretome In-Solution Digestion (ISD) and Mass Spectrometry

CFBE41o- cells were grown to 90% confluence, washed twice with warm DPBS and then either left untreated (control) or treated with K279a CS (protease activity: 500 RFU/min) for16 h. Supernatants were harvested, centrifuged at 4,500 × g for 10 min at 4°C and concentrated using Amicon-Ultra centrifugal filters (3-kDa NMWL) and protein concentration was determined by the BCA assay. Samples concentrations were adjusted to contain 20 μg of protein in 50 μL of 50 mM NH_4HCO_3 buffer for in solution digestion. Concentrated secretome samples were stored at −80° until processing for in solution digestion and mass spectrometry as described in the **Supplementary Methods**.

Bioinformatic Data Analysis

Methods by which proteomic analysis, cellular localization of identified proteins, gene ontology analysis, prediction of disease related proteins using candidate gene prioritization and CFBE41o- cell secretome and sub-network analysis are described in the **Supplementary Material**.

Tight Junction Studies

Monolayer Culture and TEER Measurement

CFBE41o- cells were seeded at 5 × 10^5 cells/cm^2 onto clear permeable filter inserts (Millipore Corporation, Bedford, MA, 6.5 mm diameter, 0.4 μm pore size), grown for 7 days prior to experiments, and medium was changed on alternate days. Prior to treatment, cells were washed with DPBS and the media replaced with serum free DMEM and allowed to equilibrate for 2 days prior to treatment. Tight junction integrity was assessed by measuring the TEER with an EVOM epithelial voltmeter in a Chopstick Electrode Set for EVOM (World Precision Instruments, Sarasota, FL, USA). The TEER of the background filter inserts was 20 Ω × cm^2.

Fluorescein Isothiocyanate (FITC) Dextran Permeability Assay

Inserts were gently washed twice with 200 μL of Hanks' Balanced Salt Solution (HBSS), pre-warmed to 37°C then transferred using sterile tweezers, to a fresh 24 well plate. FITC-labeled dextran (10 kDa) was added (200 μL) to the upper chamber at a concentration of 0.5 mg/ml and 1 ml of pre-warmed HBSS added to the lower chamber. Cells were incubated for 1 h at 37°C. FITC dextran permeability was then measured by transferring 100 uL from each of the basal chambers to a black 96-well-plate and read using a microplate reader (Victor™ X3 Multilabel Plate Reader, PerkinElmer, Massachusetts, USA) at excitation 485 nm and emission 535 nm.

Western Blotting

CFBE41o- cells were washed in ice cold DBPS and lysed for 15 min in 100 μL of RIPA buffer [50 mM Tris-Cl (pH 7.6), 1 mM EDTA (pH), 0.5 mM EGTA, 1% Triton X-100, 0.1% sodium deoxycholate, 0.1% SDS and 140 mM NaCl] in the presence of a protease inhibitor cocktail (Calbiochem, 539132), centrifuged at 14,000 × g for 5 min at 4°C and then heated to 95°C for 5 min prior to the addition of reducing sample buffer. Fifty microgram CFBE41o- lysate was separated using SDS-PAGE, transferred to PVDF using a semi-dry Novex XCell SureLock blotting system (ThermoFisher) and membranes were blocked (3% w/v Marvel skimmed milk, 1% bovine serum albumin in 0.1% PBS-Tween) then incubated with the respective primary antibodies for ZO-1 (1:500, rabbit polyclonal, ThermoFisher Scientific, #61-7300), Occludin (1:500, rabbit polyclonal, ThermoFisher Scientific, #71-1500), JAM-A (1:500, rabbit polyclonal, ThermoFisher Scientific, #36-1700), or Claudin-1 (1:500, rabbit polyclonal, ThermoFisher Scientific, #71-7800) overnight. β-actin was used a loading control (1:10,000 mouse monoclonal, Merck Millipore, #MAB1501). Visualization of immunoreactive protein bands was achieved using secondary antibodies to rabbit (Anti-rabbit IgG, HRP-linked antibody, 1:2,000, Cell Signaling, #7074S) or mouse (Anti-mouse IgG, HRP-linked antibody, 1:2,000, Cell Signaling, #7076S) and Immobilon Western chemiluminescent HRP substrate (Millipore) and the Syngene G:Box Chemi XL gel documentation system. Densitometry was performed using the GeneSnap Syngene program (Synoptics).

Statistical Analysis

All statistical analyses were performed using GraphPad Prism 5.0 software package (San Diego, CA). All experiments were performed in triplicate and results are expressed as the mean ± SEM and were compared by Student's *t*-test (two-tailed) or analysis of variance where appropriate followed by Tukey *post-hoc* test for multiple comparisons where appropriate. Differences were considered significant at $p \leq 0.05$.

RESULTS

Morphological Effects of K279a CS on CFBE41o- Cells

There are many example reports using bacterial CS to study the behavior of virulence factors *in vitro* (3, 21–23). As a first step toward assessing the role, if any, of secreted proteases in the pathogenesis of *S. maltophilia* pulmonary infection, we examined the effect of differing concentrations of K279a CS (5 and 10% v/v) on CFBE41o- cell monolayers compared with untreated control cells (**Figure 1A**). Monolayers incubated with K279a CS displayed morphological changes including cell condensation, rounding and detachment after incubation for 16 h, the effects of which were most pronounced in those treated with 10% v/v K279a CS (**Figures 1B,C**). To determine whether extracellular serine protease(s) were responsible for these effects, K279a proteases were inhibited using 1 mM PMSF. The destructive effect of K279a CS was prevented by incubation with PMSF, which has been shown to be a potent inhibitor of K279a protease activity (**Figure 1D**).

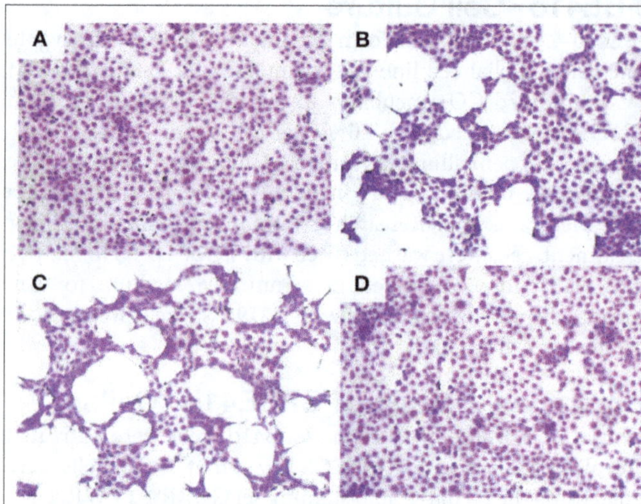

FIGURE 1 | Romanowsky stain (Hema-Gurr) of untreated and treated CFBE41o- cells with K279a CS in the absence and presence of PMSF. Wells were seeded with CFBE41o- cells (3 × 10^5 cells/ml) in MEM supplemented with 10% FCS and grown to 90% confluence in 24 well-tissue culture plates. The following day, medium was removed and washed twice with pre-warmed (37°C) DPBS to fully remove FCS. Cells were then placed in fresh serum free medium for 6 h prior to treatment. CFBE41o- cells were untreated (control, **A**) or incubated with 5% **(B)** or 10% v/v of K279a CS which was untreated **(C)** or treated with 1 mM PMSF **(D)** for 16 h. The following day the cell CS was removed and the remaining cells were stained using the Hema-Rapid staining set GURR® for hematology (VWR, UK). Cells were air dried and then fixed in methanol for 5 s following by staining with reagent one and reagent two for 3 and 6 s, respectively. Representative images were captured using an Olympus CKX41 and processed using CELL B by Soft Imaging System (Olympus, Tokyo, Japan).

Label-Free Quantitative (LFQ) Shotgun Proteomic Analysis of CFBE41o- Secretome Following Treatment With K279a CS

To further elucidate the potential pathological changes occurring in cystic fibrosis airway epithelial cells following *S. maltophilia* infection, we used label-free quantitative (LFQ) shotgun proteomic analysis of the CFBE41o- secretome following treatment with K279a CS. We compared the relative abundance of proteins between two experimental conditions, CFBE41o- cells left untreated (control) and those treated with K279a CS (with protease activity of 500 RFU/min). Cells were treated for 16 h in the presence or absence of K279a CS followed by collection of cell secreted proteins (24). A schematic representation of the experimental design is outlined in **Supplementary Figure 1**.

LDH cytotoxicity assay showed that treatment with K279a CS did not significantly affect CFBE41o- cell integrity within 16 h. Cells treated with K279a CS with the highest protease activity (5 × 10^3 RFU/min) released 40% greater LDH compared to control and the effect was prevented by PMSF. However, this was not statistically significant after correcting for multiple comparisons (**Supplementary Figure 2**).

Based on the LC-MS/MS data, 1290 proteins were identified, of which 972 ± 91 and 424.3 ± 9 were in the control group and the treatment group, respectively. A total of 376 proteins were included in the final analysis following filtration for proteins found in at least two out of three replicates in at least one group (**Figure 2A**). Among them, proteins were quantified on the basis of two or more peptides, with mean sequence coverage of 45.5 ± 17% (**Figure 2B**). Overall 271 statistically significant proteins were differentially expressed (Benjamini Hochberg false discovery rate <0.05) between treatment and control. Hierarchical clustering was also performed separately on the two groups (i.e., treated and untreated control), to determine proteins which were either up-regulated or down-regulated (**Figure 3**). Among those 271 proteins, 77 proteins were abundantly elevated in K279a CS treated cells, whereas 194 proteins were decreased (**Figure 2C**). A list of all identified and quantified proteins is presented in **Supplementary Table 1**.

Characterization of Classically Secreted Proteins

Proteins classically secreted via an ER/Golgi dependent pathway normally have an amino-terminal secretion signal peptide sequence (25). We screened for both non-classically secreted (ER/Golgi independent pathway) proteins using SecretomeP and classically secreted proteins utilizing SignalP software. Of the 271 proteins, 79 were categorized as non-classical whereas 101 were designated as classically secreted. The shared agreement among the algorithms was good, with 52 entries fulfilling the set criteria for secretion through the classical pathway (SignalP prediction). Only 3 proteins were predicted to have a transmembrane (TM) domain while 98 proteins were not using SignalP-TM and SignalP-noTM to predict those proteins that might include TM regions. In contrast, TMHMM (a transmembrane helix prediction tool) predicted that 42 proteins had a TM

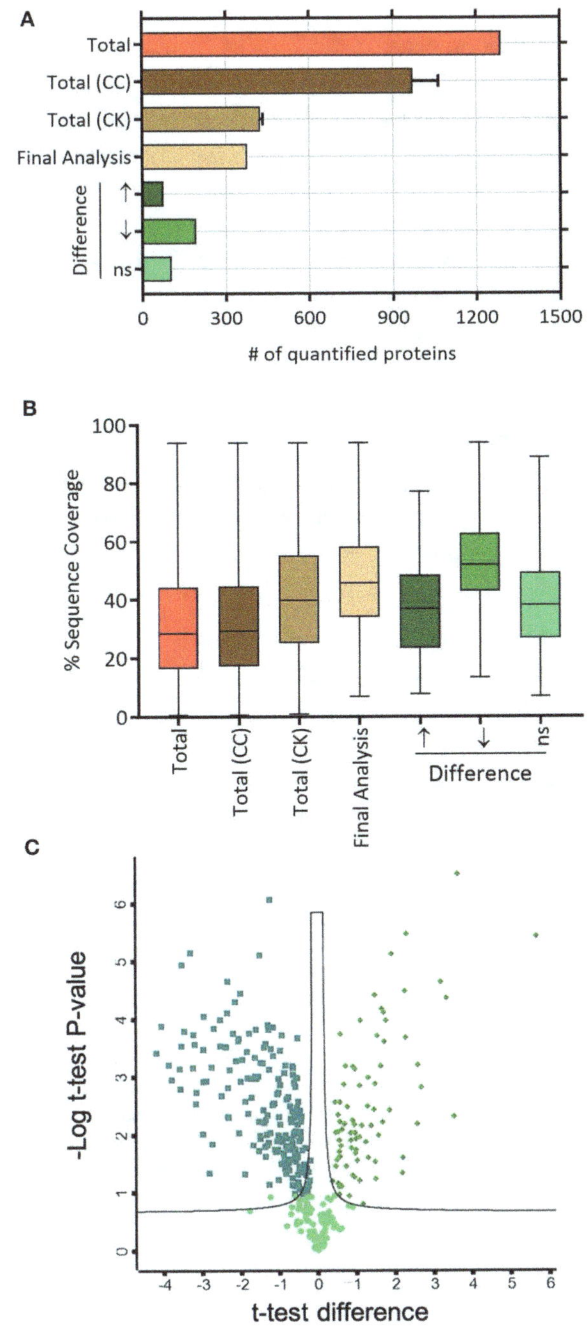

FIGURE 2 | Label-free mass spectrometry secretome analyses of CFBE41o- cells treated with K279a CS. **(A)** Number of quantified proteins in the indicated protein fractions and experimental conditions. The mean and standard deviation are shown where necessary. **(B)** Box and whisker plots depicting the distribution of protein sequence coverage (coverage of tryptic peptides per protein in %). **(C)** Of the 376 proteins identified, statistically significant differentially expressed proteins (Benjamini Hochberg false discovery ratio 0.05) are shown in the volcano plot. Volcano plot analysis reveals that 271 proteins are significantly differentially expressed. Among the 271 proteins, 77 proteins were significantly elevated in CFBE41o- cells treated with K279a CS (green diamonds), whereas 194 proteins were significantly decreased (green squares). Abbreviations: CC, CFBE41o- cell control; CK, CFBE41o- cells treated with K279a CS.

domain. Phobius, a combined transmembrane topology and signal peptide predictor, predicted that 32 proteins contained both a signal peptide and a TM domain. This correlated well with combined SignalP and TMHMM analysis with 34 overlapping proteins predicted to have both a signal peptide and a TM. WoLF Psort was used to determine the subcellular location of the identified proteins, 77 proteins were determined as extracellular and represented 28% of the total number of quantified proteins. The remaining proteins were located in the cytoplasm (32.84%), nucleus (11.44%), mitochondrion (9.59%), plasma membrane (5.54%), and endoplasmic reticulum (ER, 4.43%) (**Figure 4**).

Biological Significance of Identified Proteins

To understand the functional significance of the identified proteins, analyses of gene ontology for cellular component and biological function were classified using DAVID 6.8 (26). The analysis revealed major differences in the proteins that were differentially expressed in CFBE41o- cells treated with K279a CS compared to control. To enhance the power of disease-associated pathway detection, up-regulated and down-regulated proteins were analyzed separately [(27); **Supplementary Figure 3**]. Proteins residing in the extracellular region and extracellular matrix (ECM) were the most significantly altered in both groups but especially in the up-regulated proteins. Enrichment for cell junction was similar for both groups.

The terms biological adhesion, growth, and localization were enriched in the up-regulated proteins whereas cell killing, locomotion, and multi-organism process were enriched in down-regulated proteins. Notably, no significant differences in immune system processes were identified, indicating that the pathological response of CF bronchial epithelial cells in response to secreted *S. maltophilia* virulence factors may be structural rather than primarily immunostimulatory.

Identification of Candidate Disease Proteins From PPI Networks Based on Identified Differentially Regulated Proteins

Protein-protein interaction (PPI) networks are critical to comprehensively understand cellular mechanisms and function. They have emerged as an important resource for understanding data from proteomics experiments in order to identify proteins which could play important pathogenic roles in lung disease (28). The importance of PPIs in disease pathogenesis was recently demonstrated in CF. A detailed analysis of the CFTR interactome identified key novel interactors whose loss promoted enhanced CFTR channel function indicating that global remodeling of ΔF508 CFTR interactions is crucial for CFTR rescue (29).

Network analysis may reflect the biological processes more objectively than analyzing individual proteins. The first step is to identify proteins of interest and these inputs (or "seed proteins") are used to search for interactions from a curated PPI database. Constructing a PPI network (PPIN) using only the seed proteins may miss potentially important disease associated proteins and so completing the network with first order interactors by utilizing probabilistic PPINs improves the detection of

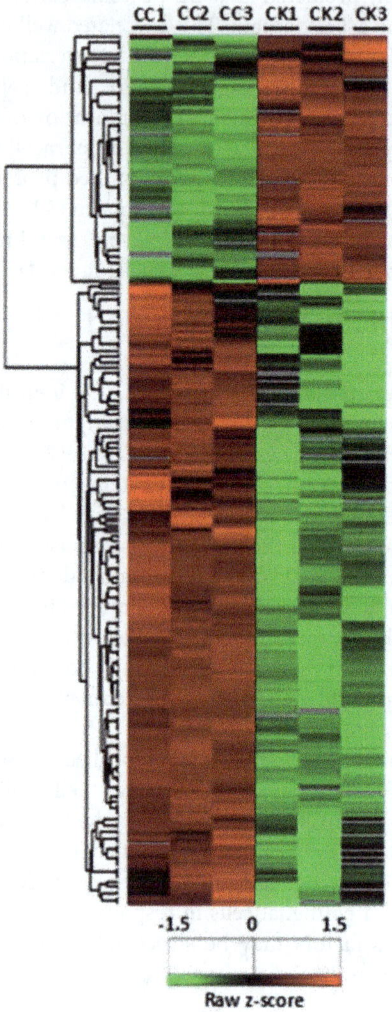

Increased

CD109	CD109	CTGF	FLNA	HNRNPC	LGALS3BP	PLXNB2	TFPI2
CD40	CD40	CYR61	FLNC	HNRNPH3	LTBP2	PPP1CA	TGFBI
CD44	CD44	DCBLD2	FN1	IGF2R	LYPD3	PRSS8	THBS1
CD59	CD59	EEF1G	FST	IGFL1	MAPRE1	PXDN	TMEM132A
CLDN6	CLDN6	EFNB2	GPR126	ILF2	NPM1	SEPT2	TNC
COCH	COCH	EGFR	H2AFY	LAMA3	NT5E	SFRP1	UGGT1
COPB2	COPB2	EPHA2	HIST1H2AJ	LAMB1	PAM	SOD1	XRCC6
CRIM1	CRIM1	FAM3C	HIST1H4A	LAMC2	PARP1	SSRP1	
CSNK2A1	CSNK2A1	FBLN2	HIST2H2BE	LCN2	PLAU	SUPT16H	
CSPG4	CSPG4	FKBP4	HIST2H3PS2	LGALS3	PLAUR	TAGLN2	

Decreased

ACTG1	CANT1	DDAH1	EZR	GLO1	HNRNPA2B1	ISYNA1	MYH9
AHCY	CFB	DDAH2	FBLN1	GLOD4	HNRNPK	KLK6	MYL6
AKR1B1	CFL1	DDT	FDPS	GNB2L1	HSP90AA1	L1CAM	NAP1L1
ALDOA	CLIC1	DKK3	FH	GOT1	HSP90B1	LAP3	NME1-NME2
ALDOC	CLIC4	DPP3	FKBP1A	GOT2	HSPA1B	LDHA	NPEPPS
APEX1	CLSTN1	DSG2	FLNB	GPC1	HSPA4	LDHB	NSFL1C
APOA1BP	CNBP	DSTN	FSCN1	GPI	HSPA5	LDLR	P4HB
ARHGDIA	COL4A2	DUT	FSTL3	GSN	HSPA8	LMNA	PAFAH1B1
ATRN	COL6A1	ECM1	FUCA2	GSS	HSPA9	LOXL2	PARK7
AXL	CS	EEF1A1P5	GANAB	GSTO1	HSPH1	LTA4H	PDIA3
B2M	CSRP1	EEF2	GAPDH	GSTP1	ICAM1	MAT2A	PDIA4
BCAM	CST3	EFEMP1	GDI1	HEXA	IGFBP7	MAT2B	PDIA6
BCAT2	CST6	EIF6	GDI2	HLA-A	ILF3	MDH1	PEBP1
CALM1	CTSD	ENO1	GGCT	HLA-B	INHBA	MDH2	PFN1
CALR	CTSZ	ERAP1	GGH	HNRNPA1	ISG15	MFI2	PGAM1

FIGURE 3 | Heat map of CFBE41o- cell secretome in response to K279a CS. Heatmap and dendrograms were produced by unsupervised hierarchical clustering (Euclidean distance with complete linkage) of the indicated 271 significantly differentially expressed proteins (two sample *t*-test <0.05). The row Z-score or scaled expression value of each feature is plotted in red–green color scale. The red color of the tile indicates high abundance and green indicates low abundance. Gray color in the heatmap indicates "not detected." The adjacent tables show the gene names of the proteins associated with the indicated clusters. CC, CFBE41o- cell control; CK, CFBE41o- cells treated with K279a CS.

candidate disease related proteins and disease pathways. This principle suggests that clues to the function of a protein can be obtained by seeing whether it interacts with another protein of known function (30). However, expanding a PPIN from a given set of "seed proteins" often leads to a complex PPIN lacking spatiotemporal consideration. To avoid this so-called "hairball" effect and to increase the robustness of our analysis we searched for shared candidate disease proteins among the top 100 interactors as ranked by three prioritization tools: NetworkAnalyst, GeneMANIA, and ToppGene.

In NetworkAnalyst, 161 up- and 348 down-regulated nodes were generated and the top 90 and 100 candidate proteins, respectively, were ranked. The interaction data from 100 related proteins generated using label propagation in GeneMANIA are summarized in **Supplementary Table 2.** Using ToppGene, 4,189 up- and 5,631 down-regulated first-order interactors of seed proteins were identified and ranked according to the network-based prioritization method (k-Step Markov, step size = 6) with a neighborhood distance of 1. The ranked list of the top 100 candidate proteins from the three prioritization tools are summarized in **Supplementary Tables 3–5.**

Overall comparison between the three networks identified 27 candidate proteins which were identified in two or more prioritization tools in both up-regulated and down-regulated networks. A list of these proteins and their basic information is described in **Supplementary Table 6.**

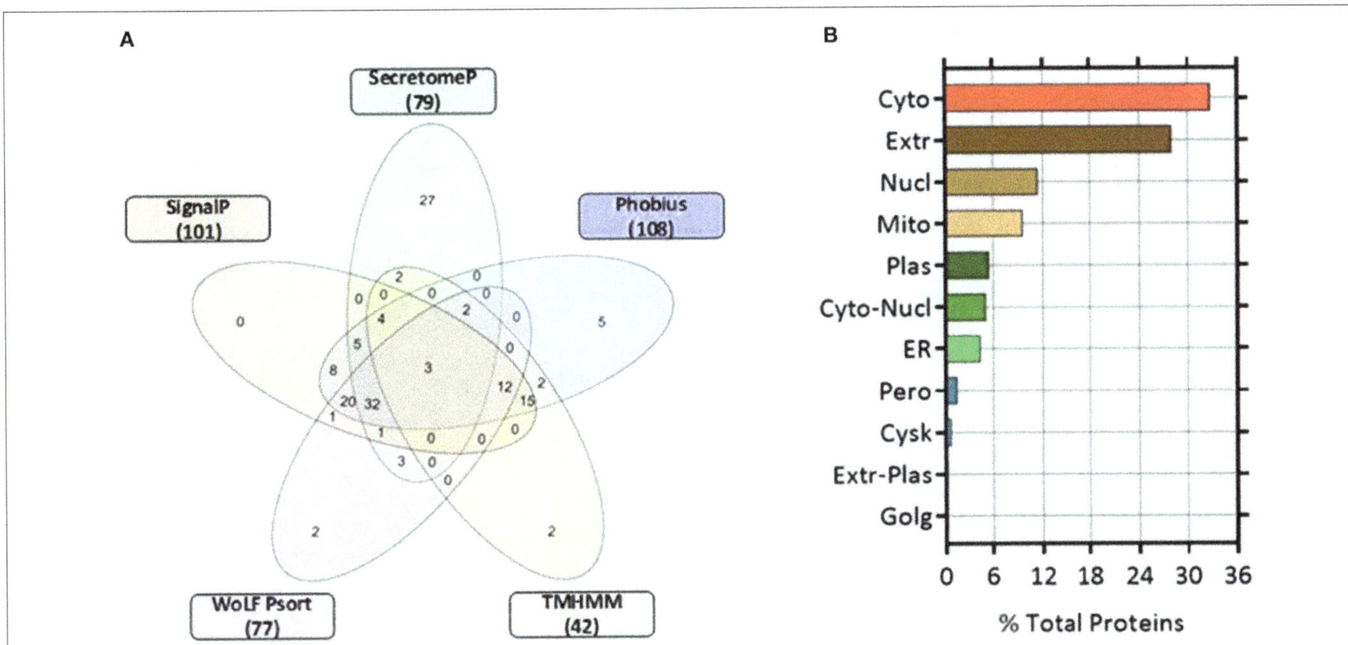

FIGURE 4 | Five-Venn diagram and cellular locations of the identified proteins as predicted by bioinformatic analyses. The significant differentially expressed proteins ($n = 271$) were submitted to SignalP, Secretome P, Phobius, TMHMM, and WoLF Psort servers as outlined in the Materials and Methods section. Results from each program were compiled and the numbers of proteins predicted by each program individually were tabulated (**Supplementary Table 1**). **(A)** The numbers of proteins predicted by each program and all possible combinations are indicated in the Venn diagram **(B)** Location analysis of the differentially secreted proteins was based on WoLF Psort. Results are represented as percentage of the total number of analyzed proteins. Cyto, cytoplasm; Extr, extracellular; Mito, mitochondrion; Plas, plasma membrane; ER, endoplasmic reticulum; Cysk, cytoskeleton; Golg, Golgi apparatus; Nucl, nucleus; Pero, peroxisome.

Functional Classification of Identified Proteins

To better understand the nature of the identified proteins, KEGG pathway annotations were obtained. Eighteen pathways were significantly over-represented in the KEGG database ($P < 0.01$), 12 in the up-regulated and 6 in the down-regulated network. In the up-regulated proteins focal adhesion, various cancers, ECM-receptor interaction, EGFR/GRB2/KRAS (annotated here as dorso-ventral axis formation), and Gap and adherens junctions featured, as did pathways related to bacterial and parasitic infection (**Supplementary Figure 4**). In contrast, in the down-regulated protein network, pathways related to metabolism, protein processing in the ER and Parkinson's disease featured (**Supplementary Figure 5**).

PPIN Module-Based Analysis Following Treatment of CFBE41o- Cells With K279a CS

Seed proteins and candidate proteins identified in both the up-regulated and down-regulated datasets were used for the construction of the final PPI network using STRING v10.0. Cluster analysis using the Reactome Functional Interaction (FI) app (Reactome FIViz) in Cytoscape v3.4.0 divided the up-regulated and down-regulated PPINs into five and seven modules, respectively (module 1 was excluded from further analysis secondary to an FDR > 0.01) (**Supplementary Figures 6, 7**). The most interesting terms are highlighted in bold; these relate to biological adhesion and bacterial infection. A summary of the over-represented KEGG pathways related to bacterial infection and their associated proteins can be found in **Table 1** and a summary of the over-represented KEGG pathways related to biological adhesion and their associated proteins can be found in **Table 2**.

Epithelial Barrier Integrity in CFBE41o- Cells Is Disrupted by Secreted K279a Serine Proteases

Using secretomics, we found that pathways related to biological adhesion and extracellular matrix components were significantly enriched following treatment with K279a CS. To extrapolate this further we sought to determine if serine proteases secreted by K279a had an effect on attachment of the CFBE41o- epithelial monolayer. Airway epithelial barrier function was determined by measuring TEER. In initial experiments, various concentrations of K279a CS with differing protease activity were added to the apical surface of CFBE41o- monolayers seeded in transwell permeable supports. Using repeated measures of analysis to evaluate the effect of K279a CS on TEER, apical treatment of CFBE41o- cell monolayers with K279a CS (protease activity of 5×10^3 RFU/min) significantly decreased monolayer resistance by 24 h ($p < 0.002$). The observed drop in TEER was protease

TABLE 1 | Proteins identified from KEGG pathways related to bacterial infection.

KEGG pathway	Network	Module	Proteins[a]	
			Seed	Candidate
Ep. cell signaling in *H. pylori* infection	↑	2	EGFR	SRC, TJP1
Legionellosis	↓	4	HSPA8, VCP	
Pathogenic *E. coli* infection	↓	5	ACTG1, EZR, TUBA1B	ACTB
		7	YWHAZ	YWHAQ
Shigellosis	↓	5	ACTG1, VCL, PFN1	ACTB
Salmonella infection	↓	5	ACTG1, MYH9, PFN1	ACTB
Bacterial invasion of epithelial cells	↓	5	ACTG1, VCL	ACTB

[a]*Proteins divided by (1) Seed proteins: identified from LFQ (label-free quantification) shotgun proteomics analysis and (2) Candidate proteins: Candidate disease proteins identified using prioritization tools.*
Ep, Epithelial; ↑, up-regulated network; ↓, down-regulated network.

TABLE 2 | Proteins identified from KEGG pathways related to biological adhesion.

KEGG Pathway	Network	Module(s)	Proteins[a]	
			Seed	Candidate
Focal adhesion	↑	2, 3, 5	COL4A2, EGFR, FLNA, FN1, LAMA3, LAMB1, LAMC2, PPP1CA, TNC, THBS1	COL1A1, CAV1, GRB2, LAMA5, SRC
Gap junction	↑	2	EGFR	GRB2, KRAS, SRC, TJP1
Tight junction	↑	2	CLDN6	KRAS, SRC, TJP1
	↓	5	ACTG1, MYH9, SPTAN1	ACTB
Adherens junction	↑	2	EGFR	SRC, TJP1
	↓	5	ACTG1, VCL	ACTB
ECM-receptor interaction	↑	5	AGRN, LAMA3, LAMB1, LAMC2	LAMA5
	↓	6	COL4A2, COL6A1, FN1	
ECM organization	↓	6	COL4A2, COL6A1, CTSD, EFEMP1, FBLN1, FN1, SERPINE1, SPARC, TIMP1	

[a]*Proteins divided by (1) Seed proteins: identified from LFQ (label-free quantification) shotgun proteomics analysis and (2) Candidate proteins: Candidate disease proteins identified using prioritization tools.*
↑, up-regulated network; ↓, down-regulated network.

mediated given the abrogation of the observed effects by PMSF ($p = 0.007$) (data not shown).

Further analysis of TEER kinetic curves demonstrated that addition of K279a CS to the apical surface of TEER monolayers resulted in a time-dependent decrease in monolayer resistance. TEER was significantly lower at 10 h in cells apically treated with K279a CS compared with controls cells ($p < 0.0001$) which indicated disruption of epithelial barrier integrity, the effect of which was prevented by PMSF ($p = 0.0004$). At 12 h, TEER was $60.1 \pm 11.75\%$ relative to the control ($p < 0.0001$; **Figure 5A**). In comparison, addition of K279a CS to the basolateral surface of CFBE41o- cell monolayers resulted in a significantly more rapid time-dependent decrease in monolayer resistance. After 4 h, cells treated with K279a CS had a lower TEER compared with controls ($p < 0.0001$). At 12 h, TEER was only $3.62 \pm 0.09\%$ relative to the control ($p < 0.0001$; **Figure 5B**). As observed in apically treated cells, this effect was abrogated in the presence of PMSF, which indicated that secreted serine protease(s) were responsible for this effect.

K279a CS Increase Paracellular Permeability to Macromolecular FITC-Dextran

We next assessed the permeability of K279a CS (protease activity $= 5 \times 10^3$ RFU/min) treated CFBE41o- monolayers with the macromolecular tracer, FITC-dextran (10 kDa), which can only transverse the monolayer via the paracellular route. At 12 h, when the development of TEER was significantly reduced in both apically and basolaterally treated cells, the permeability of FITC-dextran was measured. Apically treated monolayers displayed a 2.393 ± 0.2108-fold increase in permeability to FITC-dextran compared with control ($p = 0.009$) whereas a 15.54 ± 2.882-fold increase was observed in basolaterally treated monolayers ($p = 0.002$). In both instances, the permeability of FITC-dextran was prevented by PMSF, linking K279a protease activity to increased paracellular macromolecular transport (**Figure 6**).

Secreted K279a CS Degrade the Tight Junction Proteins ZO-1 and Occludin

Given that we observed a decline in TEER and increase in paracellular macromolecular permeability in CFBE41o- cell monolayers following treatment with K279a CS, we further investigated the integrity of tight junction proteins. Secretome analysis of CFBE41o- cells treated with K279a CS showed that the tight junction protein claudin-6 was up-regulated and that TJP1 or ZO-1 were identified as candidate disease associated proteins by PPIN analysis. We chose to examine the expression of ZO-1, occludin, JAM-A and claudin-1. Claudins 1, 3, 4, 5, 7, 8, and 18 are expressed in human bronchi and bronchioles whereas claudin-6 expression may be an effect of immortalization of the CFBE41o- epithelial cell line as it has been reported in non-small cell lung cancer (31) and in developing lung tissue (32). Therefore, we focussed on claudin-1 rather than claudin-6 as the expression of former is more constitutive in the adult lung epithelium.

CFBE41o- cells were either untreated (negative control) or treated with K279a CS (protease activity 5×10^3 RFU/min) in the presence or absence of PMSF (1 mM) for 4 h. Following normalization to negative controls and correction to β-actin (**Figure 7A**), ZO-1 ($p < 0.0001$) and occludin ($p = 0.003$) were

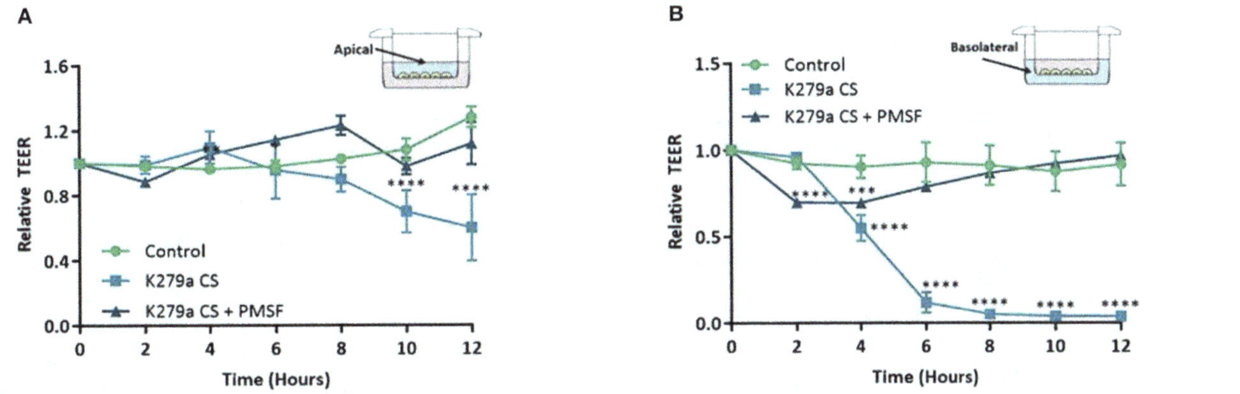

FIGURE 5 | TEER in CFBE41o- monolayers following treatment with K279a CS. CFBE41o- cells were seeded at a density of 5×10^5 cells/cm^2 onto clear permeable filter inserts (6.5 mm diameter, 0.4 μm pore size). Cells were grown for 7 days in MEM supplemented with 10% FCS and medium was changed on alternate days. Prior to treatment, cells were washed with DPBS to remove any residual FCS and the media replaced with serum free medium (SFM) and allowed to equilibrate for a further 48 h. The day before treatment cells were placed in fresh SFM overnight. CFBE41o- cell monolayers were left untreated (control) or treated with K279a CS (CS) (protease activity = 5×10^3 RFU/min) in the absence or presence of PMSF (1 mM). Transepithelial electrical resistance (TEER) was measured using an EVOM epithelial voltmeter in an Endohm-6 chamber. To construct TEER curves, measurements were taken every 2 h. **(A)** TEER curve of apically treated cells. **(B)** TEER curve of basolaterally treated cells. All results are representative of three independent experiments. Results are expressed as relative TEER to time zero (T0). Treatment vs. control: ****$p \leq 0.0001$, ***$p \leq 0.001$; Two-way-ANOVA followed by Tukey *post-hoc* test for multiple comparisons.

significantly degraded, effects that were prevented in the presence of PMSF (**Figures 7B,C**). No significant changes for JAM-A or claudin-1 were observed (**Figures 7D,E**). Therefore, we concluded that extracellular serine proteases from *S. maltophilia* degrade the tight junction proteins ZO-1 and occludin, but not JAM-A or claudin-1.

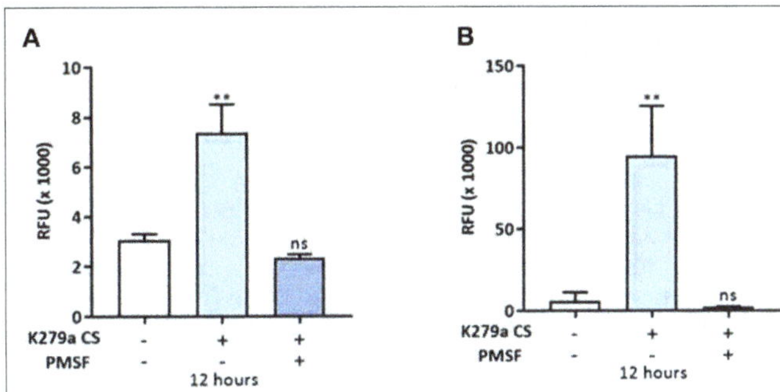

FIGURE 6 | *In vitro* permeability assay to FITC-dextran in CFBE41o- monolayers treated with K279a CS. FITC-dextran permeability (RFU × 1,000) in CFBE41o- cell monolayers was assessed in apically and basolaterally treated compartments after 12 h following treatment with K279a proteases (5×10^3 RFU/min) in the absence and presence of PMSF. Increased permeability to FITC dextran was observed in apically treated cells **(A)** but the effect was more pronounced when monolayers were treated basolaterally **(B)**. All measurements are means ± SEM from biological replicates. Treatment vs. control: **$p \leq 0.01$, one-way ANOVA followed by Tukey *post-hoc* test for multiple comparisons.

DISCUSSION

In this study, we analyzed the proteins secreted by CFBE41o- cells in response to treatment with *S. maltophilia* K279a CS. In total we identified 77 proteins which were significantly up-regulated and 194 proteins which were significantly down-regulated in response to treatment. Gene ontology and pathway analysis demonstrated that biological adhesion and assembly of extracellular matrix components were significantly enriched terms within the up-regulated proteins whereas cellular metabolism was over-represented in the down-regulated proteins. Using the seed proteins identified from this study we identified candidate disease proteins to determine the effect of *S. maltophilia* on CF bronchial epithelial cells using PPIN analysis from three prioritization tools: NetworkAnalyst, GeneMANIA, and ToppGene. Using modular analysis of the PPIN generated from the seed proteins and candidate disease proteins we identified six modules related to bacterial infection and five modules related to biological adhesion.

Stenotrophomonas maltophilia has been shown to preferentially adhere along intercellular junctions, raising the possibility that tight junction dysfunction may be an important pathogenic mechanism of this bacterium (14). In our analysis epithelial cell signaling related to *Helicobacter pylori* infection was significantly over-represented in the up-regulated PPIN. *H. pylori*, a spiral, gram negative rod plays an important role in the pathogenesis of peptic ulcer disease and like *S. maltophilia*, it preferentially attaches to cell-cell interfaces (33). *H. pylori* can alter the function of the apical junctional complex resulting in changes of structure, function and morphology of gastric epithelial cells. Translocation of the protein CagA into these cells induces recruitment of the tight junction proteins ZO-1 and JAM to the sites of bacterial attachment and may serve to target and retain *H. pylori* at epithelial cell-cell junctions (34). In addition to alterations in tight junction assembly, *H. pylori* can alter expression of tight junction proteins. ZO-1 expression is decreased whereas claudin-4 is increased in *H. pylori* infected

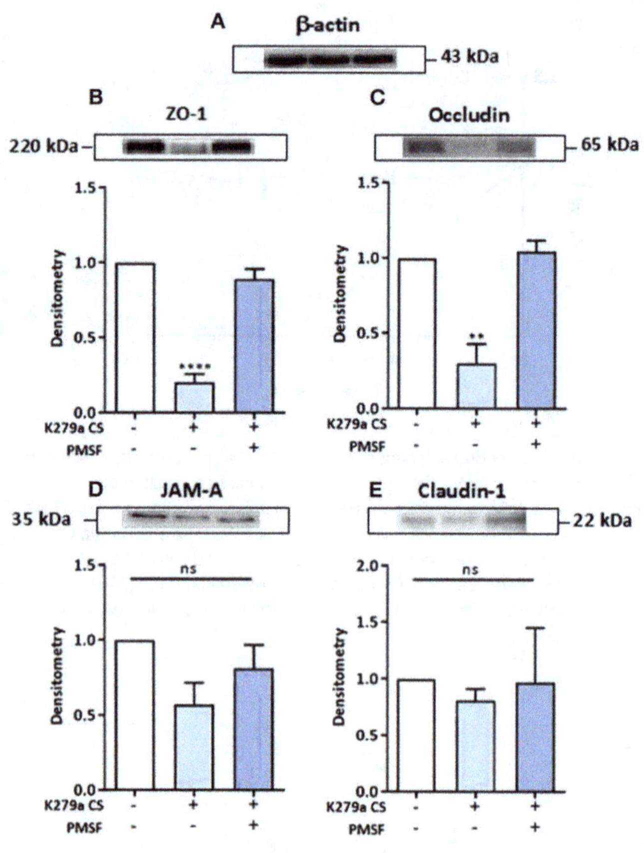

FIGURE 7 | Effect of K279a CS on the tight junction proteins: ZO-1, occludin, JAM-A and claudin-1. CFBE41o- cells were seeded at a density of 1×10^6 cells/ml onto 100 mm Triple Vented Tissue Culture Dishes. Cells were grown to 90% confluence in MEM supplemented with 10% FCS and medium was changed on alternate days. Prior to treatment, cells were washed with DPBS to remove any residual FCS and the media replaced with serum free medium (SFM) and allowed to equilibrate overnight. On the day of treatment, cells were placed in fresh SFM and treated for 4 h. Cells were left untreated (control) or treated with K279a proteases (5×10^3 RFU/min) in the absence or presence of PMSF (1 mM). Western blots were performed on whole-cell lysates (50 μg of protein) from CFBE41o- cells probed with antibodies to β-actin **(A)**, ZO-1 **(B)**, occludin **(C)**, JAM-A **(D)**, and claudin-1 **(E)**. Histograms represent the densitometric fold change in relative protein expression (relative to untreated controls) in response to treatment following correction with β-actin. All results (expressed as relative densitometry units) are representative of three independent experiments. All measurements are means ± SEM from biological replicates. ****$P < 0.001$, **$P \leq 0.01$; one-way-ANOVA with Tukey correction for multiple comparisons.

individuals indicating that damage to the gastric epithelial barrier function may be important in the pathogenesis of *H. pylori* peptic ulcer disease (35).

Stenotrophomonas maltophilia has been shown to induce morphological changes in fibroblast monolayers resulting in the cell layer partially condensing, formation of cell-free areas, and finally detachment from the culture plate (15). StmPR1 is a likely factor responsible for the clinical observation of lethal pulmonary hemorrhage in those who are immunocompromised (16). Although loss of structural components are important factors negatively affecting epithelial integrity, loss of function of key protease inhibitors and an increase in endogenous protease activity may also be relevant. TIMP1 and TIMP2, natural inhibitors of matrix metalloproteinases were down-regulated in response to K279a CS. We identified MMP2 (matrix metalloproteinase-2), a type IV collagenase as a candidate disease protein in the up-regulated protein network. *P. aeruginosa* has been shown to increase MMP-2 activity in CFBE41o- cells and a gain of functional MMP-2 and loss of function of TIMPs 1 and 2 are possible causes of epithelial damage in *S. maltophilia* lung disease (23). Other important anti-proteases which were down-regulated included alpha-1 antitrypsin and plasminogen activator inhibitor (PAI-1), an inhibitor of fibrinolysis, the absence of which predisposes the individual to a haemorrhagic diathesis. This is likely to have an important role in the pathogenesis of lung disease as *S. maltophilia* degrades the innate immune proteins: alpha-1 antitrypsin, secretory leukoprotease inhibitor and elafin (20).

In addition, the observed over enrichment of biological pathways involving biological adhesion indicated a possible causative role for secreted *S. maltophilia* proteases in disassembly of intercellular (tight, adherens, and gap) junctions. The cardinal work by Windhorst et al., examining the extracellular protease profile of *S. maltophilia* showed that the extracellular protease StmPR1 had significant pathological effects on fibroblasts and these effects were abrogated in the presence of the StmPR1 inhibitor chymostatin (15). Our observations using TEER measurements of CFBE41o- cell monolayers exposed to K279a CS are consistent with the suggested role of secreted extracellular proteases having a role in the pathogenesis of CF lung disease. Our conclusion is supported by several lines of evidence. Firstly, we demonstrated a significant disruption of the epithelial monolayer with morphological changes in cultured CFBE41o- cells which was abrogated in the presence of the protease inhibitor PMSF. Secondly, the TEER of CFBE41o- cells, which is higher than their non-CF counterparts, 16HBE14o- (36), was significantly reduced following treatment with K279a CS in comparison to the untreated control. Thirdly, the tight junction proteins ZO-1 and occludin but not JAM-A or claudin-1 were degraded in CFBE41o- cells following treatment with K279a CS, the effect of which was prevented by PMSF. The importance of this deleterious effect in the pathogenesis of CF has been demonstrated in other well-known CF pathogens, and disruption of epithelial barrier integrity may be one of the mechanisms inducing chronic inflammation in cystic fibrosis, similar to that observed in inflammatory bowel disease (37).

Like *S. maltophilia*, live *P. aeruginosa* is also capable of disrupting tight junctions in apically treated VA10 monolayers within 24 h of infection as measured by a gradual drop in TEER and a concomitant decrease in the expression of the tight junction protein, ZO-1 (22). *P. aeruginosa* have been shown to invade airway epithelial barriers by destroying tight junctions (38), while *Pseudomonas* elastase can disrupt the tight junction in human nasal epithelial cells by downregulating the transmembrane proteins claudin-1 and-4, occludin, and tricellulin (39). ER stress induced by *P. aeruginosa* has also been implicated as a cause of tight junction destruction in primary bronchial epithelial cells (40). More recently, a strong correlation between *in vitro* elastase activity of clinical isolates of *P. aeruginosa* and mucosal barrier dysfunction has been demonstrated. These changes were seen in conjunction with degradation of ZO-1, occludin and β-actin and implicate *P. aeruginosa* exoproteins in the pathophysiology of *P. aeruginosa* associated chronic rhinosinusitis by severely compromising mucosal barrier structure and function (41).

Others have shown similar effects using xps mutants of K279a, a key regulatory gene of the type II secretory system from *S. maltophilia*. DuMont et al. demonstrated rounding, detachment, and death of A549 cells, an adenocarcinoma human alveolar epithelial cell line, mediated via degradation of ECM components such as type I collagen and fibronectin by the major and minor extracellular proteases StmPr1 and StmPr2 (17, 42). More recently, we and others have identified an intermediate protease, StmPR3, as an additional potential virulence factor of *S. maltophilia* (18, 20). Interestingly, StmPr3 showed xps-mediated rounding and detachment of A549 cells, as well as xps-mediated degradation of fibronectin, fibrinogen, and interleukin-8 (IL-8), similar to StmPR1 and StmPR2 (18). Additionally, purified StmPR1 has been shown to degrade the tight junction protein occludin and the basolaterally expressed adherens junction protein E-cadherin. The observed ability of StmPR1 to degrade E-cadherin within 1 h of co-incubation may in part explain the relative increased speeds of TEER reduction seen here following treatment of the basolateral compartment with K279a CS compared to the apical one (18). From a clinical perspective, continued exposure of the immunocompetent host epithelium to *S. maltophilia* proteases may induce microbleeds in the lung such as in the context of CF. However, in the immunocompromised host the inability of the host to control the virulence of the pathogen could permit access to the basolateral compartment of the pulmonary epithelium leading to pulmonary hemorrhage.

The ability of extracellular serine proteases from *S. maltophilia* to denude the airway epithelium likely confers a growth advantage for the bacterium. K279a and other clinical isolates of *S. maltophilia* have siderophore-like activity when grown at 37 °C in low-iron media and a mutation in one of the predicted biosynthesis genes (entC) impairs the production of the siderophore and reduces bacterial growth in low-iron conditions (43). The ability of *S. maltophilia* to cause microbleeds within the CF lung likely has beneficial effects for growth of the organism *in vivo* but harmful effects for the host. Degradation of host iron-containing proteins by neutrophil elastase in the CF lung is a source of iron (44) that can promote growth of *S. maltophilia* via FecA mediated transport of exogenous siderophore ferric citrate from the environment into the bacterial periplasm (45). Moreover, release of haem can be harmful to the CF patient as haem can stimulate IL-8 from CFBE41o- cells (46).

This study has a number of limitations. Firstly, K279a, the reference clinical strain of *S. maltophilia* used in this work was isolated from the blood of a cancer patient and its virulence determinants may differ from CF strains of the bacterium (47). However, there is considerable overlap in the major extracellular protease gene (StmPR1) between CF *S. maltophilia* isolates and K279a with 70% of CF-derived strains carrying the 1,621-bp allelic variant of StmPr1 present in the K279a reference genome (48). Secondly, we did not specifically examine the ability of endogenous antiproteases [e.g., alpha-1 antitrypsin (AAT)] to abrogate the effect of extracellular proteases in K279a CS on epithelial barrier integrity. Thirdly, by maintaining CFBE41o- cell monolayers in a submerged culture rather than at an air-liquid interface there may have been a dilutional effect which may have reduced the inhibitory ability of endogenous antiproteases on K279a CS. Alpha-1 antitrypsin is an endogenous inhibitor of neutrophil elastase with an extracellular pulmonary epithelial concentration ~10% that of serum levels (49). While production of AAT and other antiproteases are normal in CF, the neutrophil elastase burden is so large that it overwhelms the normal anti–neutrophil elastase protection (50). We have recently shown that K279a CS is capable of degrading the endogenous proteases inhibitors AAT, SLPI, and elafin (20) and thus chronic colonization with *S. maltophilia* is an additional combatant to overwhelm the anti-protease armory within the CF lung. The use of aerosolised AAT is an attractive therapeutic option. Not only could it inhibit NE mediated IL-8, TNF-α, and LTB4 production (50), but it may also potentially inhibit extracellular bacterial proteases including those from *S. maltophilia*.

In conclusion, using secretomics we have provided a unique insight into the pathogenesis of *S. maltophilia* in CF lung disease. Using this data we have shown that one of the primary pathogenic mechanisms in *S. maltophilia* infection involves disruption of epithelial barrier integrity. We confirmed this by demonstrating a time dependent reduction in TEER and an increase in paracellular permeability, an effect mediated by degradation of the tight junction proteins ZO-1 and occludin. Future work to examine the relative contribution of purified StmPR1, StmPR2, and StmPR3 and mutant K279a strains lacking the aforementioned proteases will shed further light on the pathogenic potential of this emerging multi-drug resistant CF pathogen.

AUTHOR CONTRIBUTIONS

KM, CG, GC, ED, and NM contributed conception and design of the study. KM, GC, ED, and KW contributed to mass spectrometic analysis. KM performed the experiments, organized the data, performed the statistical analysis, and wrote the first draft of the manuscript. All authors contributed to manuscript revision, read, and approved the submitted version.

ACKNOWLEDGMENTS

We thank University College Cork for providing us with K279a, the reference clinical strain of *S. maltophilia* used in this work. We are especially grateful to GC, KW, and ED for their contribution in performing the secretomics/proteomics work at the School of Biomolecular and Biomedical Science, University College Dublin, Dublin, Ireland.

REFERENCES

1. Greene CM, Carroll TP, Smith SG, Taggart CC, Devaney J, Griffin S, et al. TLR-induced inflammation in cystic fibrosis and non-cystic fibrosis airway epithelial cells. *J Immunol.* (2005) 174:1638–46. doi: 10.4049/jimmunol.174.3.1638
2. Mcnally P, Coughlan C, Bergsson G, Doyle M, Taggart C, Adorini L, et al. Vitamin D receptor agonists inhibit pro-inflammatory cytokine production from the respiratory epithelium in cystic fibrosis. *J Cyst Fibros.* (2011) 10:428–34. doi: 10.1016/j.jcf.2011.06.013
3. Oglesby IK, Vencken SF, Agrawal R, Gaughan K, Molloy K, Higgins G, et al. miR-17 overexpression in cystic fibrosis airway epithelial cells decreases interleukin-8 production. *Eur Respir J.* (2015) 46:1350–60. doi: 10.1183/09031936.00163414
4. Schmidtchen A, Frick IM, Andersson E, Tapper H, Bjorck L. Proteinases of common pathogenic bacteria degrade and inactivate the antibacterial peptide LL-37. *Mol Microbiol.* (2002) 46:157–68. doi: 10.1046/j.1365-2958.2002.03146.x
5. Schmidtchen A, Holst E, Tapper H, Bjorck L. Elastase-producing *Pseudomonas aeruginosa* degrade plasma proteins and extracellular products of human skin and fibroblasts, and inhibit fibroblast growth. *Microb Pathog.* (2003) 34:47–55. doi: 10.1016/S0882-4010(02)00197-3
6. Guyot N, Bergsson G, Butler MW, Greene CM, Weldon S, Kessler E, et al. Functional study of elafin cleaved by *Pseudomonas aeruginosa* metalloproteinases. *Biol Chem.* (2010) 391:705–16. doi: 10.1515/bc.2010.066
7. Park PW, Pier GB, Preston MJ, Goldberger O, Fitzgerald ML, Bernfield M. Syndecan-1 shedding is enhanced by LasA, a secreted virulence factor of *Pseudomonas aeruginosa.* *J Biol Chem.* (2000) 275:3057–64. doi: 10.1074/jbc.275.5.3057
8. Nagano T, Hao JL, Nakamura M, Kumagai N, Abe M, Nakazawa T, et al. Stimulatory effect of pseudomonal elastase on collagen degradation by cultured keratocytes. *Invest Ophthalmol Vis Sci.* (2001) 42:1247–53.
9. Ranganathan S, Garg G. Secretome: clues into pathogen infection and clinical applications. *Genome Med.* (2009) 1:113. doi: 10.1186/gm113
10. Mukherjee P, Mani S. Methodologies to decipher the cell secretome. *Biochim Biophys Acta.* (2013) 1834:2226–32. doi: 10.1016/j.bbapap.2013.01.022
11. Lietzen N, Ohman T, Rintahaka J, Julkunen I, Aittokallio T, Matikainen S, et al. Quantitative subcellular proteome and secretome profiling of influenza a virus-infected human primary macrophages. *PLoS Pathog.* (2011) 7:e1001340. doi: 10.1371/journal.ppat.1001340
12. Li S, Li X, Wang Y, Yang J, Chen Z, Shan S. Global secretome characterization of A549 human alveolar epithelial carcinoma cells during *Mycoplasma pneumoniae* infection. *BMC Microbiol.* (2014) 14:27. doi: 10.1186/1471-2180-14-27
13. Fekkar A, Balloy V, Pionneau C, Marinach-Patrice C, Chignard M, Mazier D. Secretome of human bronchial epithelial cells in response to the fungal pathogen *Aspergillus fumigatus* analyzed by differential in-gel electrophoresis. *J Infect Dis.* (2012) 205:1163–72. doi: 10.1093/infdis/jis031
14. De Vidipo LA, De Marques EA, Puchelle E, Plotkowski MC. *Stenotrophomonas maltophilia* interaction with human epithelial respiratory cells *in vitro.* *Microbiol Immunol.* (2001) 45:563–9. doi: 10.1111/j.1348-0421.2001.tb01287.x
15. Windhorst S, Frank E, Georgieva DN, Genov N, Buck F, Borowski P, et al. The major extracellular protease of the nosocomial pathogen *Stenotrophomonas maltophilia*: characterization of the protein and molecular cloning of the gene. *J Biol Chem.* (2002) 277:11042–9. doi: 10.1074/jbc.M109525200
16. Mori M, Kitagawa T, Sasaki Y, Yamamoto K, Onaka T, Yonezawa A, et al. [Lethal pulmonary hemorrhage caused by *Stenotrophomonas maltophilia* pneumonia in a patient with acute myeloid leukemia]. *Kansenshogaku Zasshi.* (2012) 86:300–5. doi: 10.11150/kansenshogakuzasshi.86.300
17. Dumont AL, Karaba SM, Cianciotto NP. Type II secretion-dependent degradative and cytotoxic activities mediated by *Stenotrophomonas maltophilia* serine proteases StmPr1 and StmPr2. *Infect Immun.* (2015) 83:3825–37. doi: 10.1128/IAI.00672-15
18. Dumont AL, Cianciotto NP. *Stenotrophomonas maltophilia* serine protease StmPr1 induces matrilysis, anoikis, and protease-activated receptor 2 activation in human lung epithelial cells. *Infect Immun.* (2017) 85: e00544-17. doi: 10.1128/IAI.00544-17
19. Fouhy Y, Scanlon K, Schouest K, Spillane C, Crossman L, Avison MB, et al. Diffusible signal factor-dependent cell-cell signaling and virulence in the nosocomial pathogen Stenotrophomonas maltophilia. *J Bacteriol.* (2007) 189:4964–8. doi: 10.1128/JB.00310-07
20. Molloy K, Smith SG, Cagney G, Dillon ET, Greene CM, Mcelvaney NG. Characterisation of the major extracellular proteases of *Stenotrophomonas maltophilia* and their effects on pulmonary antiproteases. *Pathogens.* (2019) 8:E92. doi: 10.3390/pathogens8030092
21. Figueiredo PM, Furumura MT, Santos AM, Sousa AC, Kota DJ, Levy CE, et al. Cytotoxic activity of clinical *Stenotrophomonas maltophilia.* *Lett Appl Microbiol.* (2006) 43:443–9. doi: 10.1111/j.1472-765X.2006.01965.x
22. Halldorsson S, Gudjonsson T, Gottfredsson M, Singh PK, Gudmundsson GH, Baldursson O. Azithromycin maintains airway epithelial integrity during *Pseudomonas aeruginosa* infection. *Am J Respir Cell Mol Biol.* (2010) 42:62–8. doi: 10.1165/rcmb.2008-0357OC
23. Wright C, Pilkington R, Callaghan M, Mcclean S. Activation of MMP-9 by human lung epithelial cells in response to the cystic fibrosis-associated pathogen *Burkholderia cenocepacia* reduced wound healing *in vitro.* *Am J Physiol Lung Cell Mol Physiol.* (2011) 301:L575–586. doi: 10.1152/ajplung.00226.2010
24. Brown KJ, Seol H, Pillai DK, Sankoorikal BJ, Formolo CA, Mac J, et al. The human secretome atlas initiative: implications in health and disease conditions. *Biochim Biophys Acta.* (2013) 1834:2454–61. doi: 10.1016/j.bbapap.2013.04.007
25. Nickel W. The mystery of nonclassical protein secretion. *Eur J Biochem.* (2003) 270:2109–19. doi: 10.1046/j.1432-1033.2003.03577.x
26. Huang Da W, Sherman BT, Lempicki RA. Systematic and integrative analysis of large gene lists using DAVID bioinformatics resources. *Nat Protoc.* (2009) 4:44–57. doi: 10.1038/nprot.2008.211
27. Hong G, Zhang W, Li H, Shen X, Guo Z. Separate enrichment analysis of pathways for up- and downregulated genes. *J R Soc Interface.* (2014) 11:20130950. doi: 10.1098/rsif.2013.0950
28. Wu X, Chen L, Wang X. Network biomarkers, interaction networks and dynamical network biomarkers in respiratory diseases. *Clin Transl Med.* (2014) 3:16. doi: 10.1186/2001-1326-3-16
29. Pankow S, Bamberger C, Calzolari D, Martinez-Bartolome S, Lavallee-Adam M, Balch WE, et al. F508 CFTR interactome remodelling promotes rescue of cystic fibrosis. *Nature.* (2015) 528:510–6. doi: 10.1038/nature15729
30. Oliver S. Guilt-by-association goes global. *Nature.* (2000) 403:601–3. doi: 10.1038/35001165
31. Micke P, Mattsson JS, Edlund K, Lohr M, Jirstrom K, Berglund A, et al. Aberrantly activated claudin 6 and 18.2 as potential therapy targets in non-small-cell lung cancer. *Int J Cancer.* (2014) 135:2206–14. doi: 10.1002/ijc.28857
32. Jimenez FR, Lewis JB, Belgique ST, Wood TT, Reynolds PR. Developmental lung expression and transcriptional regulation of claudin-6 by TTF-1, Gata-6, and FoxA2. *Respir Res.* (2014) 15:70. doi: 10.1186/1465-9921-15-70
33. Heczko U, Smith VC, Mark Meloche R, Buchan AM, Finlay BB. Characteristics of *Helicobacter pylori* attachment to human primary antral epithelial cells. *Microbes Infect.* (2000) 2:1669–76. doi: 10.1016/S1286-4579(00)01322-8
34. Amieva MR, Vogelmann R, Covacci A, Tompkins LS, Nelson WJ, Falkow S. Disruption of the epithelial apical-junctional complex by *Helicobacter pylori* CagA. *Science.* (2003) 300:1430–4. doi: 10.1126/science.1081919
35. Li W, Shu X, Gu W, Peng K, Cai H, Jiang L, et al. [Tight junction protein expression of gastric mucosa and its significance in children with *Helicobacter pylori* infection]. *Zhonghua Er Ke Za Zhi.* (2015) 53:510–5.
36. Nilsson HE, Dragomir A, Lazorova L, Johannesson M, Roomans GM. CFTR and tight junctions in cultured bronchial epithelial cells. *Exp Mol Pathol.* (2010) 88:118–27. doi: 10.1016/j.yexmp.2009.09.018
37. Merga Y, Campbell BJ, Rhodes JM. Mucosal barrier, bacteria and inflammatory bowel disease: possibilities for therapy. *Dig Dis.* (2014) 32:475–83. doi: 10.1159/000358156

38. Rejman J, Di Gioia S, Bragonzi A, Conese M. *Pseudomonas aeruginosa* infection destroys the barrier function of lung epithelium and enhances polyplex-mediated transfection. *Hum Gene Ther.* (2007) 18:642–52. doi: 10.1089/hum.2006.192
39. Nomura K, Obata K, Keira T, Miyata R, Hirakawa S, Takano K, et al. *Pseudomonas aeruginosa* elastase causes transient disruption of tight junctions and downregulation of PAR-2 in human nasal epithelial cells. *Respir Res.* (2014) 15:21. doi: 10.1186/1465-9921-15-21
40. van't Wout EF, van Schadewijk A, Stolk J, Hiemstra PS. *Pseudomonas Aeruginosa* causes endoplasmic reticulum stress in primary bronchial epithelial cells which is associated with disruption of tight junctions. *Am J Respir Crit Care Med.* (2012) 185:A1068. doi: 10.1164/ajrccm-conference.2012.185.1_MeetingAbstracts.A1068
41. Li J, Ramezanpour M, Fong SA, Cooksley C, Murphy J, Suzuki M, et al. *Pseudomonas aeruginosa* exoprotein-induced barrier disruption correlates with elastase activity and marks chronic rhinosinusitis severity. *Front Cell Infect Microbiol.* (2019) 9:38. doi: 10.3389/fcimb.2019.00038
42. Karaba SM, White RC, Cianciotto NP. *Stenotrophomonas maltophilia* encodes a type II protein secretion system that promotes detrimental effects on lung epithelial cells. *Infect Immun.* (2013) 81:3210–9. doi: 10.1128/IAI.00546-13
43. Nas MY, Cianciotto NP. *Stenotrophomonas maltophilia* produces an EntC-dependent catecholate siderophore that is distinct from enterobactin. *Microbiology.* (2017) 163:1590–603. doi: 10.1099/mic.0.000545
44. Britigan BE, Hayek MB, Doebbeling BN, Fick RB Jr. Transferrin and lactoferrin undergo proteolytic cleavage in the *Pseudomonas aeruginosa*-infected lungs of patients with cystic fibrosis. *Infect Immun.* (1993) 61:5049–55. doi: 10.1128/IAI.61.12.5049-5055.1993
45. Huang TP, Wong AC. A cyclic AMP receptor protein-regulated cell-cell communication system mediates expression of a FecA homologue in *Stenotrophomonas maltophilia*. *Appl Environ Microbiol.* (2007) 73:5034–40. doi: 10.1128/AEM.00366-07
46. Cosgrove S, Chotirmall SH, Greene CM, Mcelvaney NG. Pulmonary proteases in the cystic fibrosis lung induce interleukin 8 expression from bronchial epithelial cells via a heme/meprin/epidermal growth factor receptor/Toll-like receptor pathway. *J Biol Chem.* (2011) 286:7692–704. doi: 10.1074/jbc.M110.183863
47. Crossman LC, Gould VC, Dow JM, Vernikos GS, Okazaki A, Sebaihia M, et al. The complete genome, comparative and functional analysis of *Stenotrophomonas maltophilia* reveals an organism heavily shielded by drug resistance determinants. *Genome Biol.* (2008) 9:R74. doi: 10.1186/gb-2008-9-4-r74
48. Nicoletti M, Iacobino A, Prosseda G, Fiscarelli E, Zarrilli R, De Carolis E, et al. *Stenotrophomonas maltophilia* strains from cystic fibrosis patients: genomic variability and molecular characterization of some virulence determinants. *Int J Med Microbiol.* (2011) 301:34–43. doi: 10.1016/j.ijmm.2010.07.003
49. Wewers MD, Casolaro MA, Sellers SE, Swayze SC, Mcphaul KM, Wittes JT, et al. Replacement therapy for alpha 1-antitrypsin deficiency associated with emphysema. *N Engl J Med.* (1987) 316:1055–62. doi: 10.1056/NEJM198704233161704
50. Mcelvaney NG. Alpha-1 antitrypsin therapy in cystic fibrosis and the lung disease associated with Alpha-1 antitrypsin deficiency. *Ann Am Thorac Soc.* (2016) 13(Suppl. 2):S191–6. doi: 10.1513/AnnalsATS.201504-245KV

9

Rhinovirus Infection Drives Complex Host Airway Molecular Responses in Children with Cystic Fibrosis

Kak-Ming Ling[1,2,3], *Luke W. Garratt*[2,3,4], *Erin E. Gill*[5], *Amy H. Y. Lee*[5], *Patricia Agudelo-Romero*[2,3], *Erika N. Sutanto*[2,3], *Thomas Iosifidis*[2,3], *Tim Rosenow*[2,3], *Stuart E. Turvey*[6], *Timo Lassmann*[3], *Robert E. W. Hancock*[5], *Anthony Kicic*[2,3,4,7,8,9*†] and *Stephen M. Stick*[2,3,4,8,9†] on behalf of the WAERP[3,8,10], AusREC[3,11,12], ARESTCF[3,8,13,14]

[1] Paediatrics, Medical School, Faculty of Healthy and Medical Science, The University of Western Australia, Nedlands, WA, Australia, [2] Telethon Kids Institute, Respiratory Research Centre, Nedlands, WA, Australia, [3] Telethon Kids Institute, Centre for Health Research, The University of Western Australia, Nedlands, WA, Australia, [4] School of Biomedical Sciences, The University of Western Australia, Nedlands, WA, Australia, [5] Centre for Microbial Diseases and Immunity Research, University of British Columbia, Vancouver, BC, Canada, [6] Department of Pediatrics, BC Children's Hospital, University of British Columbia, Vancouver, BC, Canada, [7] Occupation and Environment, School of Public Health, Curtin University, Perth, WA, Australia, [8] Department of Respiratory and Sleep Medicine, Perth Children's Hospital, Nedlands, WA, Australia, [9] Centre for Cell Therapy and Regenerative Medicine, School of Medicine and Pharmacology, The University of Western Australia, Nedlands, WA, Australia, [10] St. John of God Hospital, Subiaco, WA, Australia, [11] Priority Research Centre for Asthma and Respiratory Disease, Hunter Medical Research Institute, Newcastle, NSW, Australia, [12] Robinson Research Institute, University of Adelaide, North Adelaide, SA, Australia, [13] Murdoch Children's Research Institute, Melbourne, VIC, Australia, [14] Department of Paediatrics, University of Melbourne, Melbourne, VIC, Australia

***Correspondence:**
Anthony Kicic
anthony.kicic@telethonkids.org.au

† These authors share senior authorship

Early-life viral infections are responsible for pulmonary exacerbations that can contribute to disease progression in young children with cystic fibrosis (CF). The most common respiratory viruses detected in the CF airway are human rhinoviruses (RV), and augmented airway inflammation in CF has been attributed to dysregulated airway epithelial responses although evidence has been conflicting. Here, we exposed airway epithelial cells from children with and without CF to RV *in vitro*. Using RNA-Seq, we profiled the transcriptomic differences of CF and non-CF airway epithelial cells at baseline and in response to RV. There were only modest differences between CF and non-CF cells at baseline. In response to RV, there were 1,442 and 896 differentially expressed genes in CF and non-CF airway epithelial cells, respectively. The core antiviral responses in CF and non-CF airway epithelial cells were mediated through interferon signaling although type 1 and 3 interferon signaling, when measured, were reduced in CF airway epithelial cells following viral challenge consistent with previous reports. The transcriptional responses in CF airway epithelial cells were more complex than in non-CF airway epithelial cells with diverse over-represented biological pathways, such as cytokine signaling and metabolic and biosynthetic pathways. Network analysis highlighted that the differentially expressed genes of CF airway epithelial cells' transcriptional responses were highly interconnected and formed a more complex network than observed in non-CF airway epithelial cells. We corroborate observations in fully differentiated air–liquid interface (ALI) cultures, identifying genes involved in IL-1 signaling and mucin glycosylation that are only dysregulated in the

CF airway epithelial response to RV infection. These data provide novel insights into the CF airway epithelial cells' responses to RV infection and highlight potential pathways that could be targeted to improve antiviral and anti-inflammatory responses in CF.

Keywords: cystic fibrosis, RV, airway epithelial cells, transcriptomic, innate immune response

INTRODUCTION

Lung disease is the major cause of morbidity and mortality in cystic fibrosis (CF) (1). Progressive lung damage is associated with mucus obstruction, neutrophilic inflammation, and chronic airway infection and is already evident in the first years of life (2–6). Intermittent pulmonary exacerbations occur in individuals with CF who experience increased respiratory symptoms and reduction in pulmonary function that are responsive to therapy with antibiotics (7). Moreover, the frequency of exacerbations is a predictor of long-term morbidity and irreversible loss of lung function (8, 9). The triggers for these pulmonary exacerbations are not fully understood although it is recognized that lower respiratory infections caused by viruses are likely to play a significant role (10–14).

The most common virus detected in the airway of adults and children with CF is human rhinovirus (RV) (15–19). The clinical impact of RV includes reduction of lung function/FEV_1 (15, 20, 21), hospitalization (22), and increased requirement for intravenous antibiotic treatment (11, 14). Recent longitudinal data suggest that RV infection persists for a longer period in individuals with CF compared to non-CF controls (14), a finding consistent with *in vitro* observations that suggest a defective innate response of epithelial cells to RV (23, 24). The nature of any intrinsic deficiency still remains unclear although some explanations are now emerging (25).

In this study, we hypothesized that the antiviral responses of primary airway epithelial cells (AEC) from children with CF are dysregulated following RV infection. We utilized transcriptome sequencing (RNA-Seq) to assess the gene expression of CF (ΔPhe508del homozygous) and non-CF primary AEC pre- and post-RV infection. Differential expression analysis was carried out to compare the antiviral responses between CF and non-CF AEC. Functional analyses identified diverse biological pathways and complex networks in response to RV infection in CF AEC that were less apparent in non-CF AEC. We performed additional work to validate some of these unique biological pathways using primary differentiated AEC culture models, and data corroborates observations made from the RNA-Seq analysis. Overall, this study provides insights into the global transcriptomic response by non-CF and CF AEC to RV infection and has identified potential therapeutic targets that could reduce the harmful contribution of RV to progressive lung disease in individuals with CF.

MATERIALS AND METHODS

Patient Recruitment and Establishment of Primary Bronchial Epithelial Cells

The study was approved by the St. John of Gods Human Ethics Committee (SJOG#901) and Perth Children's Hospital Ethics Committee (#1762), and written informed consent was obtained from parents or guardians. Children without CF were recruited prior to undergoing elective surgery for non-respiratory-related conditions. Children with CF and homozygous for the Phe508del mutation were recruited during annual early surveillance visits (2, 3, 23). Subject demographic data for RNA-Seq analysis are provided in **Table 1**. Samples were obtained by brushing of the tracheal mucosa of children using a cytology brush as previously described (23, 26). Submerged monolayer primary airway epithelial (AEC) cultures from non-CF children and those with CF were then established, expanded in Bronchial Epithelial Basal Medium (BEBM®; LONZA™), supplemented with growth additives and 2% (v/v) Ultroser G (Pall Corporation) (23, 26–28), and used for experimentation. Subject demographic data for the validation experiments are provided in **Table 2**. Here, primary AECs were differentiated into ciliated pseudostratified AECs as described previously (29). Briefly, AECs were initially seeded on 0.4-µm polyester membrane culture inserts grown to confluence (Corning, NY, USA) and ALI cultures established. These were maintained for 28 days, and both beating cilia and mucus production were well-established. Prior to ALI validation experiments, inserts were confirmed to have a transepithelial electrical resistance (TEER) measurement $>800\ \Omega/cm^2$.

Human RV Infection and RNA Extraction

To emulate an acute RV infection episode *in vitro*, we exposed AEC with RV1b (courtesy of P. Wark, University of Newcastle) at MOI 12.5 (23, 30, 31). After 24 h, culture supernatant was collected for cytokine measurement and cell pellets for RNA extraction. RNA was extracted using a PureLink® RNA (Life Technologies) mini kit as per manufacturer instructions. Total RNA was eluted with 30 µL RNase free water with the addition

TABLE 1 | Patient demographic for subjects used for RNA sequencing analysis including five non-CF children and seven children with CF.

	Non-CF control[#]	Cystic fibrosis
Number of participants	5	7
Mean Age ± sd (yr)	3.5 ± 1.4	2.8 ± 2.3
Age range (yrs)	(1.7–5.4)	(0.2–5.6)
Male (%)	40	57
Genotype	Healthy non-CF	p. Phe508del/ p. Phe508del
NE Activity (%)	NA	43
IL-8 Detected in BALs (%)	NA	100
Microorganisms detected in BALf (%)	NA	14 (*Pseudomonas aeruginosa*)
PRAGMA Disease (%)	NA	3.44(2.24–4.16)

[#]Non-CF control were children who underwent elective surgery for non-respiratory-related conditions.

TABLE 2 | Patient demographics for subjects used for validation work including six non-CF children and six children with CF.

	Non-CF control[#]	Cystic fibrosis
Number of participants	6	6
Mean Age ± sd (yr)	3.3 ± 0.65	2.3 ± 2.3
Age range (yrs)	(2.4-4.0)	(0.2–5.9)
Male (%)	50	83
Genotype	Healthy non-CF	p. Phe508del/ p. Phe508del
NE Activity (%)	NA	50
IL-8 Detected in BALs (%)	NA	100
Microorganisms detected in BALf (%)	NA	50
PRAGMA Disease (%)	NA	3.53

[#] *Non-CF control were children who underwent elective surgery for non-respiratory related conditions.*

of 1 μL of RNase Inhibitor (Life Technologies). RNA purity and yield were determined using a NanoDrop, and integrity was assessed using an Agilent RNA 6000 Nanochip on an Agilent Bioanalyser.

RNA Sequencing (RNA-Seq) and Analysis

Samples identified with high purity (1.8–2.0 range A260/280) and quality (RIN > 8.0) were then processed for library preparation. Here, the KAPA Stranded mRNA-Seq kit (KAPABiosystems) was used for mRNA capture and fragmentation (~200–300 bp fragments). RNA fragments were then subsequently reverse transcribed into cDNA strands, followed by adapter ligation and library amplification. Sequencing of these libraries (100 bp, single-end) was performed on the Illumina HiSeq 2500 platform at an average depth of 5.08 ± 1.17 million reads (**Figure S1A**) per. The quality and quantity of the FASTQ sequence reads were assessed using FastQC (v0.11.3) (32), followed by mapping to the reference genome (Homo sapiens hg19/GRCh37 - Ensembl) using "hisat" (v0.1.6-beta) (33). Gene-level quantification (counts) of hisat alignments was performed using SummarizeOverlaps and, finally, post-alignment QC using Samstat (v1.5.2.) (34). Mapping rates to the human genome were within the expected rate for all samples at 88.2–91.2% (35), and post-alignment quality control using SAMStat 1.5.2 reported an average high quality (mapping quality score of thirty) mapping rate of 89.98% ± 0.67 (**Figure S1B**).

Bioinformatics and Statistical Analysis

Bioinformatics and statistical analyses were performed on five non-CF and seven CF samples. Statistical analysis was conducted in PRISM 8 (v8.1.2; GraphPad Software Inc., California, USA) and included the Mann–Whitney test to compare the statistical variance between genotype, and the Wilcoxon test was used to compare the statistical difference between paired samples. All subsequent bioinformatic analyses post-alignment were performed in R (v3.4.1) (36). To remove low-abundance genes, only those that had a minimum of 10 counts per sample in at least five or more samples were included, resulting in a total of 12,757 genes analyzed. The R package RUVseq (1.10.0) (37) was applied to normalize RNA-Seq read counts between samples to remove the unwanted variance. Differential gene expression was determined using DESeq2(v1.16.1) (38) after calculating variance-stabilizing transformation (VST) from the fitted dispersion mean relation to yield count data with constant variance along the range of mean values. We determined those genes with an adjusted p-value ≤ 0.05 and $\pm$ 1.5-fold change as statistically and biologically significant, respectively. To visualize the variance between samples, a principal component analysis plot was generated using the plotPCA function in DESeq2 and visualized using ggplot2 (v3.1.0) (39). Next, we identified non-infected baseline non-CF and CF enriched gene ontology (GO) terms from the biological process (BP) using Metascape (http://metascape.org) (40). Visualization of GO term analysis was performed using the GOPlot (v1.0.2) (41). The GoCircle function was used to highlight gene expression changes within each of the selected terms. The value of the z-score from GOPlot is calculated as zscore = (up - down) $\div \sqrt{count}$, where up and down were the number of up- and down-regulated genes respectively.

Pathway Analysis and Protein–Protein Interaction Network-Based Enrichment Analysis

Pathway analysis based upon Reactome repositories was performed using Signature Over-Representation Analysis (SIGORA) version 2.0.1. The pathway enrichment by SIGORA was identified according to statistically over-represented Pathway Gene-Pair Signatures (Pathway-GPS) (42). To expose the interactive associations among the DEGs at the protein level, genes obtained from both non-CF and CF responses were mapped using protein–protein interactions (PPI) via NetworkAnalyst (http://www.networkanalyst.ca/). Network Analyst (43, 44) and was based upon IMEX Interactome, a comprehensive, high-quality protein–protein interaction database curated from InnateDB (45) to characterize the relationships and interactions of input genes. The network was built by limiting the original seed proteins only and picking zero order interactions.

ELISA

Cytokine production of interleukin 8 (IL-8) (Becton Dickinson, Biosciences, San Diego, CA), interferon lambda 1, 2, 3 (IFNλ1, λ2, λ3), RANTES (CCL5), interleukin (IL)-1B, Interferon gamma-induced protein 10 (IP-10) (R&D, MN, Minneapolis) in culture supernatant was measured by ELISA. Production of interleukin 6 IL-6 was measured using a time-resolved fluorometry detection system (PerkinElmer, Waltham, MA). Expression of interferon beta (IFNβ) was measured using an AlphaLISA® bead-based assay (PerkinElmer).

Corroboration of RNA-Seq Observations in Fully Differentiated Cultures

Experiments were then performed to assess whether unique pathways identified from the initial RNA-Seq analysis were evident in fully differentiated 3-D cultures. Primary ALI cultures were established and, upon TEER confirmation, were rinsed three times with sterile room temperature 1× phosphate-buffered saline for 10 min at 37°C. Cultures were then subsequently infected with RV1b at MOI 0.1 in 200 μL for 24 h. An MOI of 0.1 was chosen based on the lowest infection dose from the literature with no reported cytopathic effects or major disruption to the epithelium (46–48) as this prevents assessment of mucin-related enzymes and other downstream analyses. After 24 h, inserts were harvested in RNA lysis buffer for RNA extraction using the PureLink® RNA (Life Technologies) mini kit as per manufacturer instructions. Total RNA was eluted with 30 μL RNase free water. Genes were chosen from at least two independent pathways identified to be uniquely expressed by AEC in children with CF in response to RV infection and included *IL1R2*, *STS8SIA4*, *ST6GALNAC2*, *MAN1A1*, and *B3GNT8*. Gene expression was determined via real-time qRT-PCR (refer to **Supplementary Materials** and Methods 1.1 and 1.2) using TaqMan® pre-designed primer/probes (ThermoFisher Scientific). Details on all primer probes are listed in **Table S8**.

RESULTS

Patient Demographics

The demographic information of children participating in this study is shown in **Table 1** (RNA sequencing) and **Table S1** (entire sample sets, including those additional samples used for ELISA). Non-CF controls were children who underwent elective surgery for non-respiratory-related conditions and did not possess existing lung disease. RNA samples of primary AECs obtained from these children ($n = 32$, 16 non-CF and 16 CF) were originally collected, both pre- and post-infection with RV *in vitro*. RNA sequencing was performed on all samples as summarized in the workflow diagram (**Figure 1A**). A sample elimination process was carried out to exclude unqualified samples (detailed in **Figure S3**). Samples that were run on a different sequencer did not pass rigorous quality control for RNA sequencing (mapping quality score >30, $n = 3$), and those with sequencing depth of less than one million reads ($n = 9$) were excluded from analysis. Finally, RNA sequencing samples from a total of seven CF and five non-CF children were included for the differential expression analysis by applying a fold change cutoff of ≥1.5-fold. Only one child with CF had detectable microorganisms in bronchioalveolar lavage fluid (BALf) during the time of AEC sampling. The PRAGMA CT score presented as percentage of disease was also conducted to demonstrate the quantitative measurement of disease progression during the time of sampling in children with CF.

Distinct Transcriptional Changes of AEC in Response to RV Infection

The normalized read counts matrix was used to build a non-supervised principal component analysis to visualize the major contributors to transcriptional variation within this data set (**Figure 1B**). The first principal component (PC1, 69% of the variance) completely separated RV-infected and non-infected AEC, and separation of uninfected or infected CF and non-CF AEC was observed on PC2 (8% of the variance), indicating that

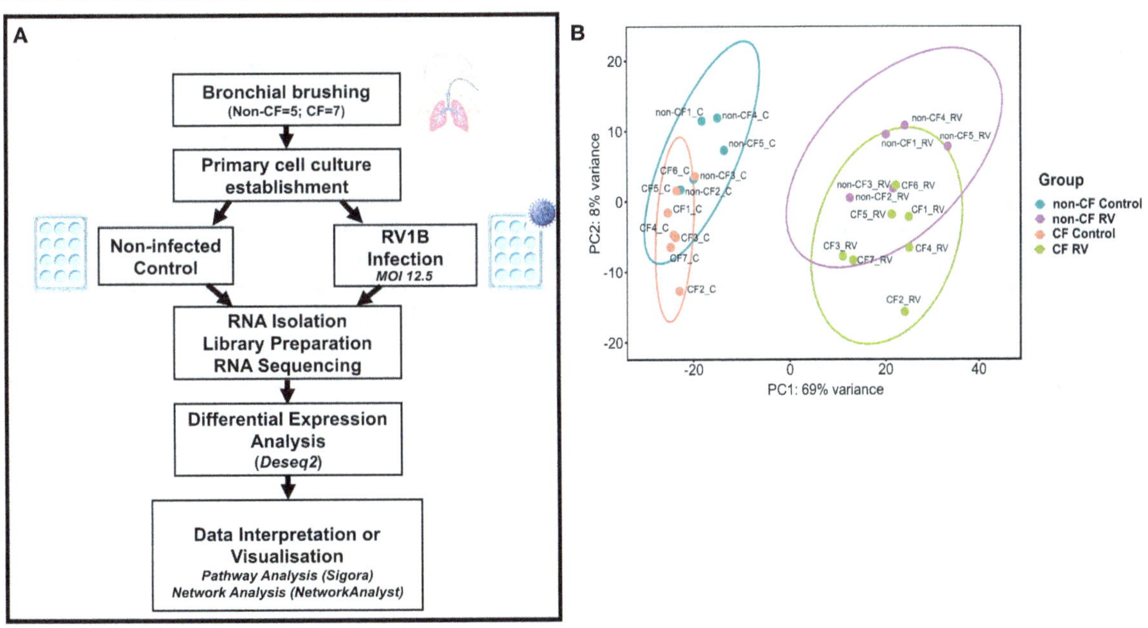

FIGURE 1 | Analytical methods. **(A)** Schematic workflow describing experimental procedure and transcriptomic analysis. Primary airway epithelial cells (AECs) from non-CF children ($n = 5$) and children with CF ($n = 7$) were obtained from bronchial brushings. AECs were established for infection with human rhinovirus 1B (RV1B) at MOI 12.5. At 24 h post-infection, RNA was isolated and processed for library preparation. Sample libraries were sequenced on the Illumina HiSeq 2500 platform as described in the methods section **(B)** Principal component analysis (PCA). Components 1 (PC1) and 2 (PC2) highlight distinct clustering of samples. PC1 shows the highest percentage of variance (69%) for all samples and completely separates the control and RV-infected samples. PC2 shows the second highest variance (8%) and separates non-CF and CF samples. Data points represent individual samples for non-CF controls (turquoise), non-CF infected (purple), CF control (coral), and CF infected (green).

patient genotype is the second largest source of variation within the data set.

Modest Transcriptional Differences Between Uninfected CF and Non-CF AEC

To determine whether the AECs transcriptional profiles from children with CF are intrinsically differed from non-CF controls, non-infected baseline CF and non-CF AECs were analyzed for differential gene expression. We observed a total of 162 DEGs with absolute fold change $\geq$1.5 between non-infected baseline CF and non-CF AECs. Among those, 92 genes were significantly downregulated, and 70 genes were significantly upregulated in CF AEC compared to non-CF AEC. To identify in which biological processes the 162 DEGs were involved, we performed gene ontology (GO) term enrichment analysis (41). The predominant enriched GO term in CF AEC is depicted by a circle plot (**Figure 2A**). The circle plot highlights the overall gene expression change by showing increased expression in red and decreased expression in blue. The *p*-value of the GO terms is represented by the height of the inner rectangle, which is also colored by *z*-score based on GOPlot formula (zscore = ([number of up-regulated genes] − [number of down-regulated genes]) ÷√[gene count]). Analysis identified the cytokine-mediated signaling pathway and type 1 interferon signaling pathway as the top enriched GO terms with decreased *z*-score and extracellular matrix as the GO term with an increased *z*-score. The full list of the top upregulated and downregulated genes is summarized in **Table S2**. The top DEG from differential expression analysis comparing non-infected baseline CF and non-CF AEC was *HLA-DQB1* (HLA Class II GWAS genes). We also identified the top 20 genes with the highest fold change between non-infected CF and non-CF AEC (**Figure 2B**). These genes were found to be involved in biological processes including type 1 interferon signaling pathway (*AIM2*, *BST2*, *IFI27*), keratin (*KRT14*), DNA methylation (*H19*), cell cycle (*BEX1*), extracellular matrix (*COL1A2*, *COL5A1*, *COL6A1*, *COL6A2*), cell–cell interaction (*LGALS7*), signal transduction (*FST*, *LRCH2*, *LRRN1*), calcium ion binding (*PCDH20*), potassium channel (*KCNJ5*), transferase activity (*NEURL3*), and phosphatase activity (*PTPRZ1*).

CF AEC Have More Transcriptional Changes in Response to RV Infection Than Non-CF AEC

We next analyzed the RNA-Seq data to assess the transcriptomic response of CF and non-CF AECs collected after infection with RV. Comparative analysis of response profiles indicates that AECs from both CF and non-CF differentially modulated the expression of several genes related to the innate antiviral immune response in response to RV infection. The Venn diagram (**Figure 3A**) was used to compare genes that were uniquely and commonly modulated between CF response (RV-infected CF AEC vs. uninfected CF AEC) and non-CF response (RV-infected non-CF AEC vs. uninfected non-CF AEC) to RV infection. A total of 896 (652 upregulated, 244 downregulated) DEGs were observed in the non-CF response to RV and 1442 DEGs (884 upregulated, 558 downregulated) in the CF response (**Figures 3A,B**). Candidate genes were ranked according to their extent of differential expression when compared to uninfected samples. Although there was considerable overlap between the groups (778 common DEGs, **Figure 3C**), there were significantly more unique DEGs (**Figures 3D,E**) specific to the CF response (664) compared with the non-CF response (118). A majority of overlapping DEGs were involved in the core immune response to RV infection, including interferon signaling, interferon regulation, cytokine signaling, cell death, and metabolism. The unique DEGs for both CF and non-CF AEC in response to RV infection are summarized (**Tables S3, S4**, respectively). The top unique DEG for the non-CF response was *CX3CL1*, which is an important chemoattractant to attract other immune cells, such as dendritic cells. Other top unique genes for the non-CF response were found to be associated with the cellular component *(FAXDC2, ARMCX4, RAB17, TMEM17*), DNA repair (*BRCA2*, *RMI2*), and cellular metabolism (*CBR3*, *B4GALNT3*, *HS3ST3B1*, *GIPR*). Nevertheless, 46% (664 out of 1442) of DEGs for the CF AEC response to RV infection were found to be unique with the *IL-1R2* gene, the IL-1 signaling decoy receptor, being the top unique DEG (4.8-fold change). Other unique genes for the CF AEC response were found to be associated with growth factor (*PTN*), immune response (*NOD2*, *CCRL2*, *HMOX1*, *SLC7A2*, *SERPINB4*), cellular metabolism *(MDGA1, ANGPT1*), cytoskeletal regulation (*LRCH2*), signal transduction (*MAPK8IP2*, *STK32A*), and transcription regulation (*SPDEF*, *ZNF488*).

RV Infection Drives Common Epithelium-Induced Innate Antiviral Response in CF and Non-CF AEC

Genes that were commonly modulated in CF and non-CF AECs (**Table S5**) were found to be key drivers of core epithelium-induced innate antiviral response to RV infection. Specifically, RV infection triggered a significant upregulation of type I and III interferons (*IFNB1*, *IFNL1*, *IFNL2*, *IFNL3*) in both CF and non-CF AECs (**Figure 3C**). However, it was evident that the fold changes (Log_2FC) of *IFNB1* (5.8-fold), *IFNL1* (5.8-fold), *IFNL2* (5.1-fold), and *IFNL3* (6.1-fold) in gene expression in response to RV infection were lower in the CF AEC response compared to the non-CF AEC response (*IFNB1*: 6.9-fold, *IFNL1*: 7.2-fold, *IFNL2*: 7-fold, *IFNL3*: 7.5-fold). Interferon signaling also triggered the induction of a variety of interferon-stimulated genes (ISGs), including *Mx1*; viperin (*RSDA2*); and the IFITM, IFIT, and OAS family in both CF and non-CF AECs (**Figure 3C**).

We extended our analysis to identify the biological pathways corresponding to all DEGs in CF and non-CF AECs in response to RV infection. The full list of enriched biological pathways for CF and non-CF AECs' antiviral responses are provided in **Tables S6, S7**, respectively. SIGORA pathway analysis was then performed using gene-pair signature pathway analysis, which only accounts for statistically significant gene pairs unique to the over-represented pathways. This analysis identified 52 and 31 biological pathways responsible for CF and non-CF AEC host responses to RV infection, respectively. Comparing the two, we identified 26 common significantly enriched biological

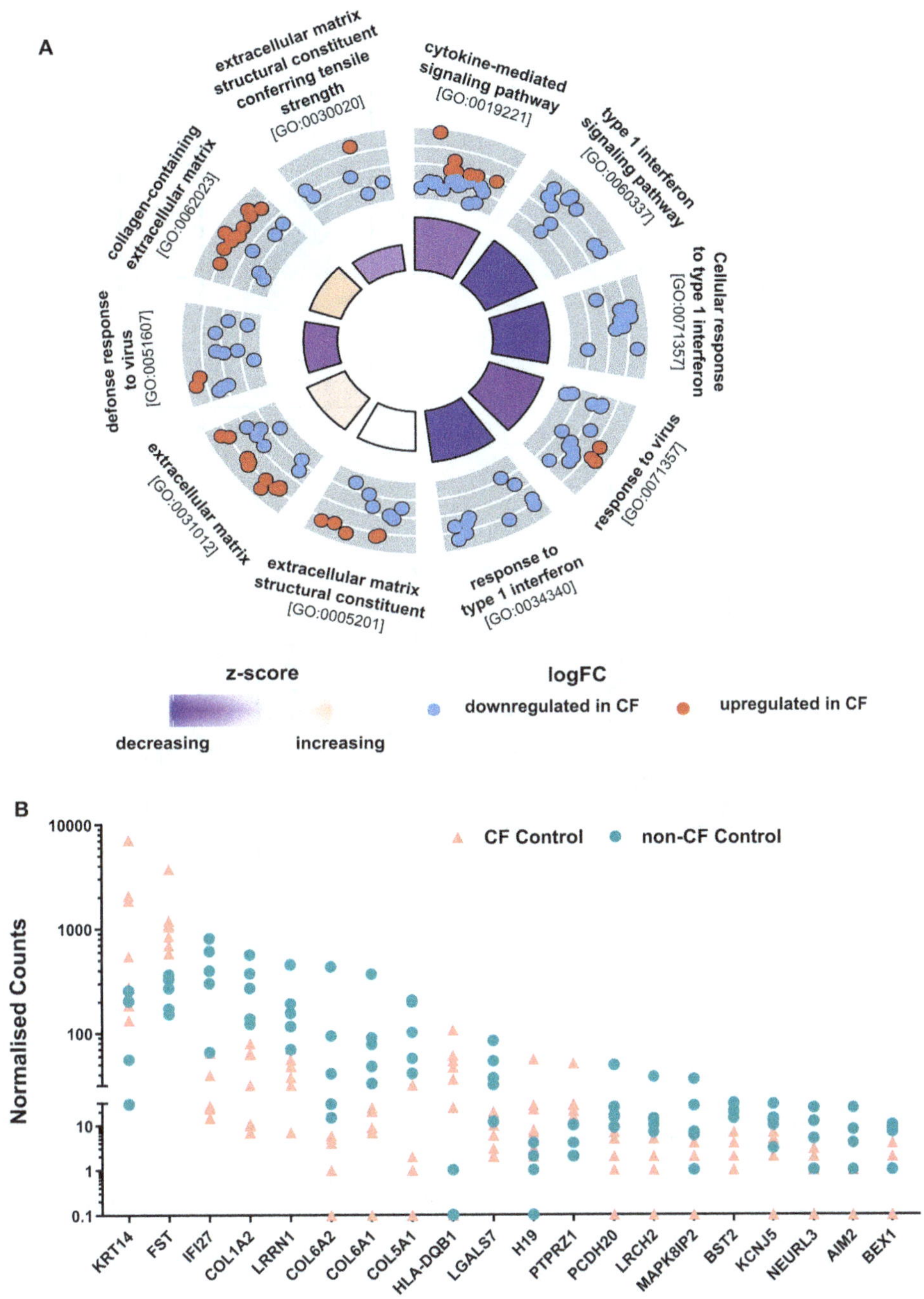

FIGURE 2 | Comparison of non-CF and CF non-infected baseline control. **(A)** Circular visualization of gene-annotation enrichment analysis of non-infected baseline samples. Statistically significant differentially expressed genes (DEGs) between non-infected CF and non-CF samples were annotated using gene ontology (GO). The circular plot combines gene expression and gene-annotation enrichment data. The outer circle shows a scatterplot for each enriched GO term of the Log2FC of the assigned genes. Red dots indicate upregulation, and blue dots indicate downregulation in CF non-infected control compared to non-CF. The inner ring is a bar plot where the height of the bar indicates the significance of GO terms (log10-adjusted *p*-value), and color corresponds to the *z*-score: blue, decreased; red, increased; and white, unchanged. **(B)** Normalized gene counts of the top 20 DEGs between CF and non-CF non-infected baseline samples with the highest fold change, data points represent individual samples for non-CF controls (turquoise; circle) and CF control (coral; triangle).

pathways (**Figure 4**), which are mainly categorized into five main functions, including (1) cytokine signaling in the immune system, (2) presentation to the adaptive immune system, (3) innate immune system, (4) metabolism or biosynthetic, and (5) signal transduction. Consistently, the core antiviral response was demonstrated by type I and III interferon and other antiviral factors as reported earlier with interferon-α/β signaling, interferon-γ signaling, and interferon signaling being the top

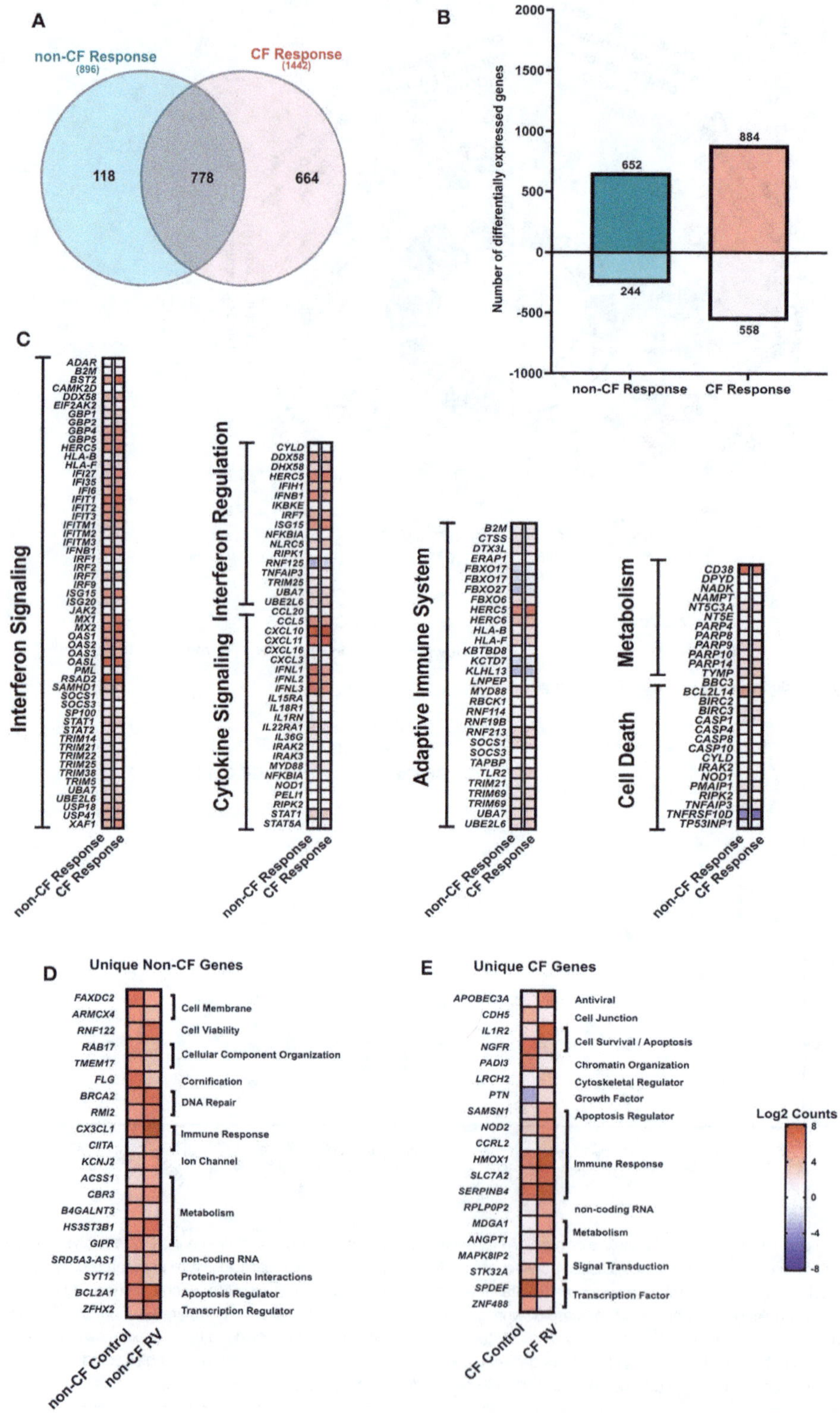

FIGURE 3 | Response to rhinovirus infection. **(A)** Venn diagram comparing the differentially expressed (DEGs) genes between non-CF (teal; *non-CF RV-infected* vs. *non-CF non-infected control*) and CF (pink; *CF RV-infected* vs. *CF non-infected control*) response to RV1B infection. A total of 778 DEGs were common between non-CF and CF response to RV1B infection. **(B)** The number (*y*-axis) and direction of change (upregulated = positive *y*-axis, downregulated = negative *y*-axis) of DEGs ($|Log_2FC|1.5$, adjusted *p*-value < 0.05) of non-CF and CF response to rhinovirus infection (*x*-axis). **(C)** The relative expression genes that are commonly differentially expressed ($|Log_2FC|>1.5$, adjusted *p*-value < 0.05) in airway epithelial cells (AECs) from non-CF and CF individuals when infected with rhinovirus. These

(Continued)

FIGURE 3 | genes are associated with immune response, including interferon signaling, cytokine signaling, adaptive immune system, cell death, and metabolism. **(D)** The normalized counts (Log_2Counts) of the top 20 genes that are uniquely differentially in AECs from non-CF children when infected with rhinovirus, including genes associated with cellular component, DNA repsir, immune response, ion channel and activity, cellular metabolism, protein–protein interactions and regulation of apoptotic process. **(E)** The normalized counts (Log_2Counts) of the top 20 genes that are uniquely differentially expressed in AECs from children with CF when infected with rhinovirus, these genes are involved in the apoptotic process, cell–cell junction, chromatin organization, cytoskeletal regulator, growth factor, immune response, cellular metabolism, signal transduction, and transcription regulation.

three most enriched pathways associated with cytokine signaling. Other common cytokine responses, such as interleukin 20 family signaling (**Figure 4A**, **Table S6**), was over-represented with upregulation of *IL22RA1*, STAT family (*STAT1, 2, 3*, and *5A*), JAK family (*JAK1, JAK2*), and the negative regulator of IFN signaling *SOCS3*. Infection with RV has also significantly increased gene expression of chemokines such as *CXCL10, CXCL11, CXCL3, CXCL16, CCL2, CCL5*, and *CCL20* in both CF and non-CF AECs. Additionally, we also detected transcriptional changes in pathogen recognition receptors, such as *TLR3, DDX58 (RIG-I)* and *IFIH (MDA5)*, and other key genes that regulate innate immune signaling, including *IKBKE, IRF7, ISG15, NFKBIA, UBE2L6, UBA7*, and *DDX58*. Genes involved in the over-represented pathway Class I MHC-mediated antigen processing and presentation, such as the gene set of F-box protein, TRIM, and the HERC family were the common DEGs in response to RV infection. The PARP protein family, including *PARP4, PARP8, PARP9, PARP10*, and *PARP14*, responsible for the regulation of nicotinamide metabolism and salvaging of cellular redox reactions, were also upregulated in response to RV infection. The changes of genes involved in nucleotide biosynthesis pathway pyrimidine catabolism were observed, including *NT5C3A, DPYD, TYMP*, and *NT5E*. Changes in gene expression of caspases (*CASP1, 4, 8, 10*), which provide pivotal links in cell regulatory networks controlling inflammation and cell death, were also observed in both CF and non-CF AEC post-RV infection.

CF AEC Transcriptome Reveals More Biological Pathways and a More Complex Network in Response to RV Infection Than for Non-CF AEC

In addition to the common over-represented pathways induced by RV infection, we observed an additional 26 enriched pathways specific to the CF response (**Figure 4A**). In addition to the five functions mentioned above, the unique over-represented pathways also fall under another two functions, including extracellular matrix organization and vesicle-mediated transport or transport of small molecules. Additional pathways categorized in cytokine signaling in the immune system, such as interleukin 1, 2, 7, 10, and 15 signaling pathways, were the unique enriched pathways specific to CF response. Genes associated with interleukin 1 family signaling–driven proinflammatory activity are *IL36G*; receptor antagonist *IL36RN*; *IL1R2*; *IL1RN*; receptor *IL18R1*; protein phosphatase *PTPN12*; pellino proteins *PELI1, PELI3*, and IRAK kinase *IRAK2, IRAK3*; and key immune and inflammatory response regulator *S100A12*. Other cytokines with essential immunomodulatory functions, including IL-7, IL-10, IL-15, and IL-2 family signaling, were the significantly over-represented pathways unique for CF response to RV infection. Furthermore, we observed a significant upregulation of the chemotactic factors for neutrophils *CXCL1* and *CXCL2* in the CF AEC response to RV infection. Downregulation of genes encoding E3 ubiquitin ligases, such as *TRIM45* (regulator of TNFα-induced NF-κB-mediated transcriptional activity) and *RNF128* (inhibitor of cytokine gene transcription), were also only observed in the CF response. The transcriptional change of the *HSPA5* gene was also observed in the CF response as part of major histocompatibility complex (MHC) class I molecules mediated adaptive immune regulation.

Several metabolism/biosynthetic pathways of notable interest to CF airway disease include nucleobase catabolism, inositol phosphate metabolism, synthesis of IP3 and IP4 in the cytosol and tryptophan catabolism, which were all altered in CF response to RV infection (**Figure 4A**). We observed transcriptional changes of ectonucleotidases in the nucleobase catabolism pathways, particularly ecto-nucleoside triphosphate diphosphohydrolases (ENTPDases) *ENTPD3* (downregulated) and *ENTPD6* (upregulated). The inositol phosphate metabolism pathway was also found to be altered in CF AECs, namely the downregulation of genes encoding phosphohydrolases *NUDT11*, phospholipase *PLCH2* and *PLCD4*, kinase *ITPKB*, and phosphatase *INPP4B*. We also observed a group of upregulated genes, including *KYNU, KMO, IDO1, AADAT*, and *CCBL1*, which are associated with the key biosynthetic process of tryptophan catabolism. Biological pathways regulating metabolism of proteins, notably mucin metabolism (O-linked Glycosylation of mucins and sialic acid metabolism), were also over-represented pathways for the CF response. Additionally, RV infection in CF AEC triggered transcriptional changes of transport of small molecules (including cellular hexose transport, metal ion SLC transporters, transport of amino acids, and SLC-mediated transmembrane transport). We noted transcriptional changes for genes involved in extracellular matrix organization, such as integrin α5 and β6 (*ITGA5, ITGA6*) and cell adhesion molecule *ICAM1*.

To better understand the potential functional interaction of DEGs, we also visualized expression and investigated the underlying molecular interactions between genes by generating zero-order PPI subnetworks (**Figures S2A,B**). The main CF and non-CF PPI subnetwork consisted of functionally enriched pathways that play imperative roles in the host antiviral response to RV infection. The non-CF AEC response subnetwork identified associations of 254 nodes and 565 edges (**Figure S2A**). We observed 172 genes with a degree more than one interactor, where 27 nodes were observed with $\geq$10 connections with other nodes. Key hub genes regulating the antiviral response

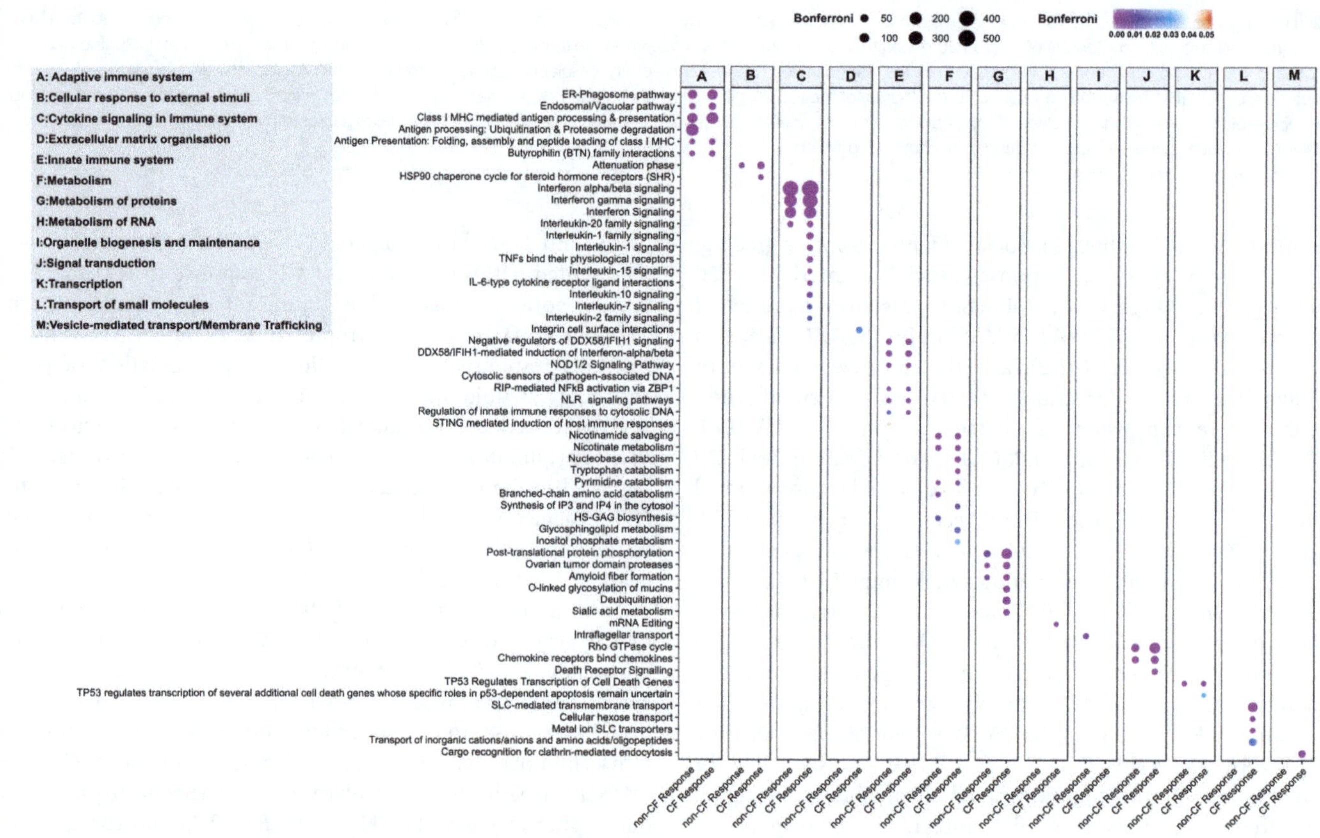

FIGURE 4 | Pathway and network analysis of non-CF and CF AECs response to rhinovirus infection. Pathway enrichment analysis results from 896 and 1,442 differentially expressed genes in non-CF and CF response to rhinovirus infection, respectively. Figure depicting the association of common and unique enriched pathways using Reactome database with the differentially expressed gene lists based on SIGORA successes metric (circle size) and the color bar depicting the significance of the association (Bonferroni < 0.05). The enriched biological pathways are categorized according to functions **(A)**, adaptive immuno system, **(B)** cellular response to external stimuli, **(C)** cytokine signaling in immune system, **(D)** extracellular matric organization, **(E)** innate immune system, **(F)** metabolism, **(G)** metabolism of proteins, **(H)** metabolism of RNA, **(I)** organelle biogenesis and maintenance, **(J)** signal transduction, **(K)** transcription, **(L)** transport of small molecules and **(M)** vesicle-mediated transport/membrane trafficking.

found included *STAT1*, *STAT2*, *IRF2*, *IRF1*, *ISG15*, *DDX58*, *IRF7*, *RIPK1*, *IKBKE*, and *CASP8*. Conversely, a more complex CF AEC response subnetwork projected the associations of 493 nodes and 1156 edges (**Figure S2B**). We observed 320 genes with a degree more than one, where 66 nodes were observed with ≥10 connections with other nodes. The key hub genes regulating the CF AEC response subnetwork included *IRF1*, *ISG15*, *STAT1*, *STAT3*, *HSAP1B*, *CASP8*, *TBK1*, *IKBKE*, *TRAF2*, and *CASP8*. The key hub genes of both CF and non-CF subnetworks are represented by key regulators related to the innate immune system and cytokine signaling.

Aberrant Cytokine Production of CF AECs to RV Infection

In order to validate the transcriptional changes of the enriched cytokine signaling pathways, we measured the levels of key innate and inflammatory cytokine production at 24 h post-RV infection (**Figure 5**). Although *IFNB1* was significantly induced upon RV infection in both cohorts, this is not reflected at the protein level with significantly lower levels (average 10.8-fold) of IFNβ1 (type 1 interferon) released by CF AEC (668.3 ± 576.2 pg/ml; $p < 0.05$) compared to non-CF AEC (7,265 ± 6,558 pg/ml). As shown in **Figure 3C**, all type 3 IFN genes (*IFNL1*, *IFNL2*, *IFNL2*) were upregulated post RV infection. Cytokine levels of the type III interferons IFNλ1, IFNλ2, and IFNλ3 were also significantly elevated in both CF and non-CF AEC infected with rhinovirus. However, levels of IFNλ1 (296.4 ± 293.3 pg/ml) and IFNλ2 (334.6 ± 642.8 pg/ml) produced by CF AEC in response to RV infection were significantly (3.5- to 5-fold) lower when compared to non-CF AEC (1,059 ± 1,170 pg/ml and 1,665 ± 1,932 pg/ml, respectively; $p < 0.05$). IFNλ3 produced by CF AEC (285.3 ± 287.3 pg/ml) following RV infection was somewhat but nonsignificantly lower compared to that produced by non-CF subject AEC (928.6 ± 997.9 pg/ml). Similar cytokine levels of antiviral chemokines CCL5 (RANTES) and IP10 and pro-inflammatory cytokines, including IL6 were detected in non-infected CF and non-CF AECs, and similar increases in these proteins occurred in response to RV infection. However, IL-8 and IL-1β cytokine production is significantly elevated in non-CF AECs in response to RV infection compared to CF AECs.

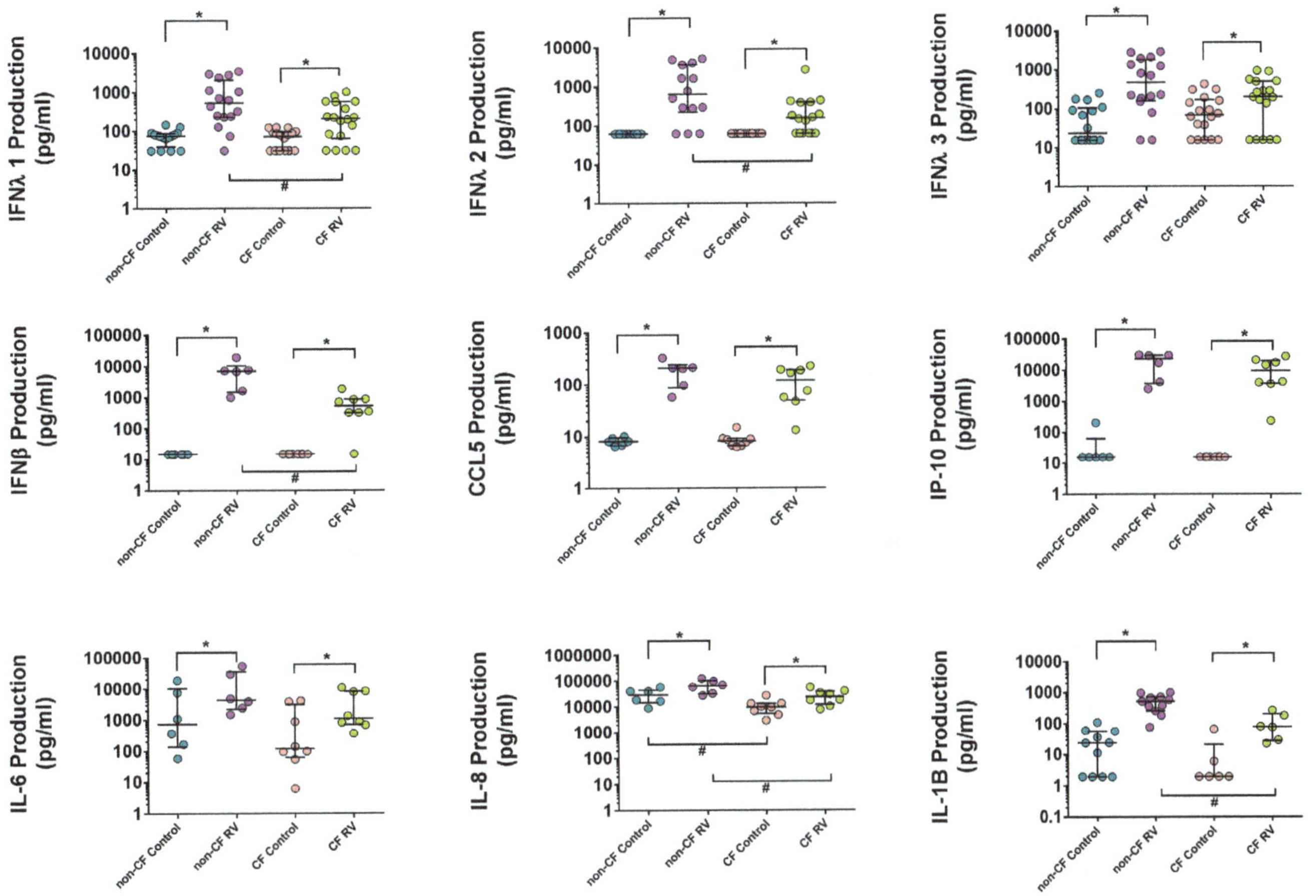

FIGURE 5 | Cytokine production in the supernatant AEC of non-CF individuals and children with CF following RV infection. Cytokine release was measured in cell culture supernatants using commercial ELISA kits and an in-house time-resolved fluorometry detection system. Type 1 and III interferons (IFN-β, IFN-λ1, and IFN-λ2) were significantly higher in non-CF AEC post-RV infection compared to CF AEC. Inflammatory cytokines IL-6, IL-8, and IL-1B were significantly increased in both CF and non-CF RV-infected samples with significantly higher IL-8 and IL-1B levels produced by non-CF RV-infected samples compared to CF RV-infected samples. RANTES (CCL5) and IP-10 were significantly elevated in CF and non-CF RV-infected samples but not significant between phenotype. Note: $n = 9$–11 for non-CF and 6–12 for CF. The data were represented as median ± IQR, symbols show statistical significance in RV-infected samples relative to paired non-infected control samples; *$p < 0.05$, determined using Wilcoxon test. Statistically significant for comparison between CF and non-CF non-infected samples determined using unpaired *t*-test or Mann–Whitney depending on Gaussian distribution, #$p < 0.05$.

Corroboration of Unique Gene Expression Patterns in Response to RV Infection in CF ALI Cultures

To validate results generated from the RNA-Seq in a model that better represents the airway, we assessed the expression of some unique DEGs identified in submerged CF cultures post- RV infection by challenging ALI cultures with the same RV and again assessing gene expression at 24 h (**Figure 6**). Expression of the top unique DEG for the CF response, *IL1R2*, was validated with a consistent increase in CF ALI post RV infection (9.4-fold over uninfected, $p < 0.05$; **Figure 6**). Upregulation of *IL1R2* appeared bimodal in non-CF ALI and was not significant ($p = 0.30$). Furthermore, expression of genes involved in glycosylation of mucins and sialic acid metabolisms, namely sialyltransferase *ST8SIA4*, *ST6GALNAC2*, mannosidase *MAN1A1*, and acetylglucosaminyltransferase *B3GNT8*, was also validated as unique to CF (**Figure 6**). A significantly higher level of sialyltransferase *ST8SIA4* expression (2.2-fold, $p < 0.05$) was observed in RV-infected CF ALI cultures while *ST6GALNAC2* was significantly downregulated (−1.4-fold, $p < 0.05$). The mannosidase *MAN1A1* were dramatically upregulated by 16.3-fold ($p < 0.05$) in CF ALI at 24 h post RV infection. *B3GNT8*, an acetylglucosaminyltransferase that adds N-acetylglucosamine (GlcNAc) to N-glycans was also increased by 1.9-fold ($p < 0.05$) in CF ALI in response to RV infection. Expressional changes of these genes were all consistent with the RNA-Seq data from submerged cultures. We observed that these genes did not change expression in non-CF ALI cultures upon infection with RV; *ST8SIA4* (3.6-fold, $p = 0.14$); *ST6GALNAC2* (−1.3-fold, $p = 0.09$); *MAN1A1* (5.4-fold; $p = 0.08$); *B3GNT8* (1-fold, $p = 0.28$).

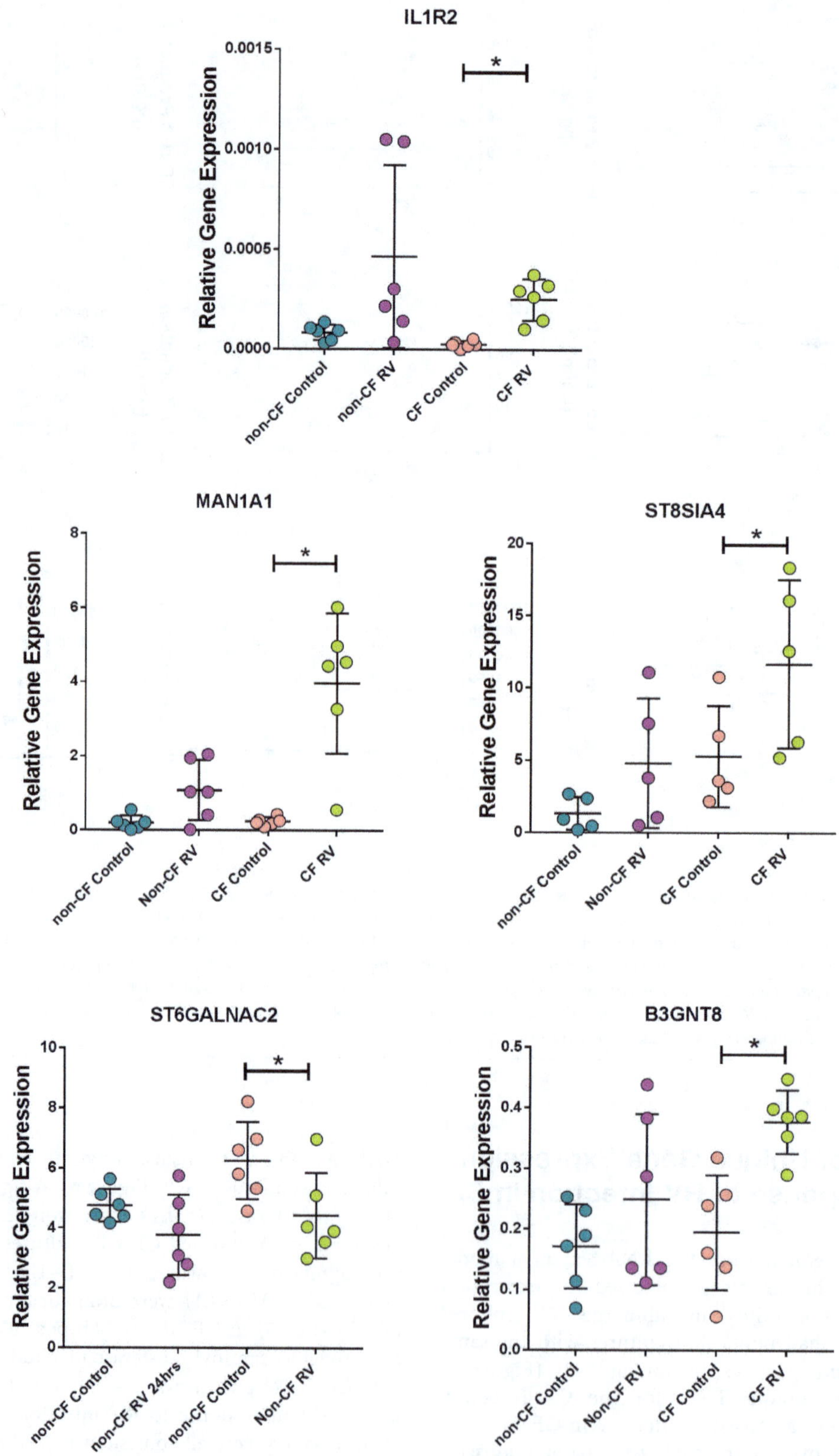

FIGURE 6 | Corroboration of uniquely expressed genes by CF AEC in fully differentiated cultures. Gene expression of the top unique gene *IL1R2* as well as mannosidase (*MAN1A1*), sialyltransferases (*ST8SIA4* and *ST6GALNAC2*), and acetylglucosaminyltransferase (*B3GNT8*), were uniquely altered in CF air–liquid interface cultures when infected with rhinovirus (RV) for 24 h. Data points represent individual samples for non-CF controls (turquoise), non-CF infected (purple), CF control (coral), and CF infected (green). Expression of all genes were normalized to the housekeeping gene PPIA (49). *Indicates $p < 0.05$ by one-way ANOVA following normal distribution test.

DISCUSSION

To improve knowledge of the underlying epithelial transcriptional responses during infection with rhinovirus, a major respiratory pathogen, we performed RNA sequencing on primary AEC from children with CF and non-CF controls *in vitro* at baseline and post-RV infection. There are five important findings from this study: (i) There were only modest baseline transcriptional differences between non-infected CF and non-CF AECs prior to exposure to RV, (ii) there was conservation in certain core antiviral responses (e.g., IFN signaling) of CF and non-CF AECs at the transcriptomic level but not the protein level, (iii) CF AECs elicited a larger and more complex transcriptional response compared to non-CF AECs with multiple unique biological pathways represented, (iv) key among these biological pathways are cytokine signaling and biosynthetic pathways (e.g., O-linked glycosylation of mucins) as they are highly relevant to CF lung pathology, (v) we corroborated observations made from the RNA-Seq analysis in fully differentiated cultures and identified genes involved in IL-1 signaling and mucin glycosylation that are only dysregulated in the CF airway epithelial response to RV infection. Collectively, these results identify potential biological pathways and processes that could be contributing to the adverse outcomes typically seen in people with CF during virus infection.

There were only modest baseline transcriptional differences between non-CF and CF AECs. This is most likely reflective of the very early and mild lung disease in the CF cohort. Minimal baseline differences also provide confidence that any difference in the antiviral transcriptional changes that we observed were due to infection. Nevertheless, the top differentially expressed baseline was HLA-DQB1, previously identified in a GWAS study with a high association signal to CF lung disease severity [reviewed in (50)]. Interestingly, the major enriched GO terms for the differentially expressed genes in non-infected baseline samples were denoted by the cytokine-mediated signaling pathway and type 1 interferon signaling pathway. Among these, *AIM2* inflammasome (associated with induction of pyroptosis, activation of pro-inflammatory cytokines, and viral suppression) (51, 52) *IFI27* (also known as *ISG12a*) contributes to IFN-dependent perturbation of normal mitochondrial function and enhanced cellular apoptosis (53), and the IFN-dependent antiviral factor *BST2* were all significantly downregulated in CF AECs. In response to RV infection, several common responses were found, including interferon signaling. However, the induction of type 1 and 3 interferon genes was lower in CF AEC. This was mirrored by reduced type 1 (IFNβ1) and type 3 interferon (IFNλ1 and IFNλ2) protein in supernatant. The reduction of type 1 and 3 interferon production of CF AECs in response to RV infection could be associated with the negative regulation of interferon signaling by the unique key gene, such as STAT3 (54, 55); however, this requires further characterization. Conversely, the IL-1 family signaling pathway was unique to the CF AECs response to RV infection, but in this case, IL-1β protein was significantly lower in CF supernatant compared to non-CF. This unusual observation could be, in part, mediated by negative regulators of IL-1 signaling expressed in CF AEC, including *IL1R2* and *IL1RN*, pellino protein genes *PELI1* and *PELI3*, together with interleukin 1 receptor-associated kinase *IRAK2* and *IRAK3*. We then assessed the expression of *IL1R2* pre- and post-RV infection in a differentiated culture model and made similar observations to those obtained using submerged cultures.

The IL-1 signaling pathway has been suggested as a link between hypoxic cell death and sterile neutrophilic inflammation in CF (56). Both IL-1α and IL-1β were detectable in bronchioalveolar lavage fluids (BALs) of young children with CF in the absence of bacterial infection, highlighting potential for inflammation of the CF airway under sterile inflammation (57). Since *S100A12* (key regulator of inflammatory process) is also part of the IL-1 family signaling pathway in CF response to RV infection, we postulate that the CF AECs could be directing from pro-inflammatory IL-1 signaling under sterile inflammation to a hyperinflammatory condition characterized by NF-κB signaling cascades during RV infection. Other evidence suggests the alteration of the inflammatory response with abundant cytokine signaling pathways (interleukin 1, 2, 7, 10, and 15 signaling) in CF AEC post-RV infection could be explained by downregulation of *RNF128* genes, which functions as an inhibitor of cytokine gene transcription and could interact with TBK1 (key hub of CF AEC response in our study here) kinase activity to enhance antiviral immunity. We also observed an elevated IL-8 production in both CF and non-CF AECs post-RV infection with higher amounts produced by non-CF AECs compared to CF AECs. Our IL-8 results agree with a previous study that also utilized primary AEC cultures in a similar infection setting (58) but contrasts with another that observed elevated inflammatory mediator release by the CF AECs (23). Overall, the over-represented cytokine signaling pathways suggest a unique and prominent role in regulating inflammation in CF AECs when infected with RV. However, with conflicting observations in this area, elucidating the complexity of the inflammatory response with associated cell death in CF AECs warrants further investigation.

We also identified over-represented metabolic pathways in CF AEC in response to RV infection specifically involved in the regulation of immunity, including inositol phosphate metabolism and synthesis of IP3 and IP4 in the cytosol, suggesting an altered CF airway microenvironment after RV infection. The induction of inositol phosphate has previously been related to endoplasmic reticulum expansion and Ca^{2+} storage, resulting in Ca^{2+}-dependent transcriptional activity of inflammatory mediators (59), which could contribute to hyperinflammatory responses seen in the CF AEC to viral infection (23). Upregulation of extracellular ectonucleotidase in the inositol phosphate metabolism pathway was found to cause depletion of ATP concentrations, reduction of air–surface liquid volume, ASL collapse, and failure in mucociliary clearance may trigger CF lung disease exacerbations as shown previously in a model of respiratory syncytial virus infection (60). Another metabolic pathway, trytophan catabolism, was also one of the over-represented pathways in the CF AECs following RV infection. Tryptophan metabolism has been previously found to be dysregulated in CF AEC (61) and has been implicated in *Pseudomonas aeruginosa* infection, oxidative stress, and Th17 hyperinflammation (62, 63). Alteration of tryptophan metabolism results in accumulation of kynurenine and anthranilate, which could subsequently disrupt the homeostatic balance of the host's innate immune system and reduce the antimicrobial activity of airway epithelium.

Other identified biosynthetic pathways associated with RV infection in CF include sialic acid metabolism and O-linked glycosylation of mucins. Sialic acids are a family of negatively charged monosaccharides that are commonly expressed as the terminal residues in glycans of the glycoconjugates on the epithelial cell surface lining the airways and are also major components of secreted mucins in the airway. Previous studies have identified increased fucoslyation and decreased sialylation in cultured AEC while a contrary observation was reported in CF sputum (64–67). As a key player that contributes to the rheological properties of mucus, aberrant sialic acid metabolism may worsen the pathological conditions of CF. O-linked glycosylation is a post-translational modification process and occurs within the endoplasmic reticulum (ER) and Golgi complex. The enzymes in ER and Golgi complex regulate glycosylation of N-glycans and O-glycans by successively adding to and then remodeling mucin oligosaccharides prior to transport to cell membranes for tethering or secretion. Here, alteration of genes encoding glycosyltransferases, such as N-acetylgalactosaminyltransferases, N-acetlyglucosaminyltransferase, and galactosyltransferases, were reported from our RNA-Seq analysis. We corroborated a number of these as unique to the AEC response to RV in children with CF. Changes in these glycosyltransferases could potentially alter the O-glycans on cell surfaces and, thus, affect interactions with airway pathogens and irritant exposures. Emerging evidence suggests alteration of mucin glycosylation is a response to infection and inflammation and might induce extended conformational changes to prevent damage from proteolytic enzymes (68). Although the impact that *CFTR* mutations has on mucin biomolecules is unknown, our results suggest that RV infection could be a potential mechanism that contributes to changes in mucin glycosylation that are exclusive to CF and that might influence mucosal barrier function. A previous investigation has demonstrated that a surplus of unfolded proteins that results from blocked glycosylation leads to prolonged ER stress and activation of the unfolded protein response (UPR) causing cell death (69). Previous *in vitro* work using an immortalized cell line discovered a pronounced reprogramming of host cell metabolism toward an anabolic state, including upregulation of glucose uptake, glycogenolysis, nucleotide synthesis, and lipogenesis (70). Considering most of the metabolic changes found in this study occur post-RV infection, future studies integrating the transcriptomic signature patterns with analyses of the metabolites produced by CF AEC in response to RV infection will provide significant insight into the exact metabolic changes that occur during infection.

Interestingly, RV infection in CF AECs results in the upregulation of a group of SLC transporter genes, including upregulation of *CP* (ferroxidase), *SLC41A2* (magnesium transporter), *SLC30A1* (zinc transporter), and *SLC39A8* (zinc transporter) and downregulation of *SLC39A10* (zinc transporter) and *SLC40A1* (iron-regulated transporter). Increasing total iron and zinc has previously been associated with airway inflammation in CF (71). These results suggest that RV infection in the CF airway is associated with the presence of redox active biometals. A previous study (72) has suggested that the dysregulation of iron homeostasis is accompanied by a respiratory virus infection, which, in turn, facilitates pseudomonas biofilm growth. Understanding the mechanistic link of virus infection to the alteration of the cellular microenvironment and instigation of secondary infection might aid in development of new treatment.

We acknowledge some limitations in the experimental design. First, we only analyzed transcriptomics at the 24-h time point, primarily due to the limited number and expansion of primary cells established from each patient. However, early optimization of our infection model did assess the transcriptional changes earlier (data not shown), and the greatest transcriptional change identified occurred at the 24-h time point. Although methodologies now exist to assist with primary AEC expansion *in vitro* (29), its effects at the transcriptomic level remain unknown and, thus, the use of unaltered primary airway cells remains a significant strength of this study. Future investigations could possibly include additional time points to better appreciate the transcriptional signature changes over the full course of RV infection as well as the long-term consequence of viral infection on CF AECs. Second, this study utilized a laboratory strain of rhinovirus (RV1b), which might exert differential effects on CF AEC compared to clinically derived isolates known to cause exacerbations in this cohort. With different RV serotypes causing infection in CF airways (10), future studies may identify whether innate immune responses may be serotype-specific. Similarly, comparison studies to other viruses (respiratory syncytial virus, influenza) would also assist in our understanding of the contribution of early-life viruses to CF disease progression. Finally, the simplified monolayer cell culture model of basal CF AECs may be regarded as a limitation, but basal cells are the primary target of RV (73). While monolayer cultures may oversimplify the multicellular interactions of epithelial (ciliated, goblet, basal, secretory cells) and immune cells (dendritic cells, neutrophils), it is an important, repeatable model with low methodological variation, and we were able to validate genes in differentiated AEC. Overall, we are highly confident that limitations are minor and that our results provide new insight into new therapeutic targets for treating acute viral infections in CF that can be validated in future transcriptomic studies assessing differentiated AEC models.

In conclusion, this study shows that, at the transcriptomic level, CF AECs induce a complex and unique set of responses when infected with RV *in vitro* that have implications for lung disease progression in CF. Despite type 1, II, and III interferon signaling being involved in the core CF antiviral response, IFNs protein levels were lower in CF AEC when compared to non-CF AEC. Metabolic and biosynthetic pathways were unexpectedly integrated with the core CF antiviral response, and multiple key regulatory molecules of antiviral response were dysregulated in CF AEC, revealing new potential to modulate CF AEC innate immunity to RV infection. Future work will explore whether these regulatory molecules are potential targets for therapy unique to RV and may be leveraged to reduce the impact viral infections have on lung disease progression CF.

AUTHOR CONTRIBUTIONS

Conceptualization: SS and AK. Funding acquisition: SS, AK, RH, and ST. Methodology: K-ML, EG, AL, TL, PA-R, TI, and TR. Supervision: SS, AK, TL, and LG. Validation: K-ML, ES, and LG. Manuscript writing: K-ML, LG, and AK. Manuscript review: SS, RH, TL, PA-R, ES, ST, TI, and EG. All authors contributed to the article and approved the submitted version.

ACKNOWLEDGMENTS

The authors thank the participants and their families in the Western Australian Epithelial Research Program (WAERP) and Australian Respiratory Early Surveillance Team for Cystic Fibrosis (AREST CF) for their contribution to this study. We also acknowledge Reza Falsafi for his technical support on performing the RNA-Seq. The members of WAERP are AK, SS, Darryl A. Knight, Elizabeth Kicic-Starcevich, LG, Marc Padros-Goosen, Ee-Lyn Tan, ES, Kevin Looi, Jessica Hillas, TI, Nicole C. Shaw, Samuel T. Montgomery, K-ML, Kelly M. Martinovich, Francis J. Lannigan, Ricardo Bergesio, Bernard Lee, Shyan Vijaya-Sekeran, Paul Swan, Mairead Heaney, Ian Forsyth, Tobias Schoep, Alexander Larcombe, Monica Hunter, Kate McGee, Nyssa Millington. The members of AREST CF are Georgia Banton, Luke Berry, Lisa Bennett, Luke Berry, Cindy Branch-Smith, Andrew Chong, Nick De Klerk, Rachel Foong, LG, Graham Hall, Alana HArper, Jessica Hillas, AK, Elizabeth Kicic-Starcevich, Ingrid Laing, K-ML, Kevin Looi, Kelly Martinovich, Samuel Montgomery, TR, Nicole Shaw, Peter Sly, ENS, Craig Schofield, Samantha McLean, Emma De Jong, PA-R, Joseph Bartlett, Samantha Grogan, Sally McCappin, Alexia Foti, Josh Beeson, Nat Eiffler, Eleanor Ferguson, Yuliya Karpievitch, Jaqueline Macpherson, Sally McCappin, Clara Mok, Rubi Nichin, Grace Pettigrew, Daniel Laucirica, Jasmine Grdrosic, Anoop Ramgolam, Kathryn Ramsey, Elizabeth Smith, Andrew Vaitekenas, Joshua Iszatt (Telethon Kids Institute, University of Western Australia, Perth, Australia); John Carlin, Rosemary Carzino, Nadeene Clarke, Jo Harrison, Katherine Holt, Louise King, Melanie Neeland, Roy Robins-Browne, Billy Skoric, Phil Sutton, Suzanna Vidmar, John Wong, Boris Vlottes, Shivanthan Shanthikumar and Hiep Pham (Murdoch Children's Research Institute, Melbourne, Australia) Barry Clements, Conor Murray, Stephen Oo, S. Stick (Department of Respiratory Medicine, Perth Children Hospital, Perth, Australia); and Jonathan Ajzner, J. Harrison, John Massie, Sarath Ranganathan, Phil Robinson, Colin Robertson (Department of Respiratory Medicine, Royal Children's Hospital, Melbourne, Australia). The Australian Respiratory Epithelium Consortium (AusREC) acknowledges the following members; AK, SS, Elizabeth Kicic-Starcevich, Luke W. Garratt, ES, Kevin Looi, Jessica Hillas, TI, Nicole C. Shaw, Samuel T Montgomery, K-ML, Kelly M. Martinovich, Matthew W.-P. Poh, Daniel R. Laucirica, Craig Schofield, Samantha McLean, Katherine Landwehr, Emma de Jong, Nigel Farrow, Eugene Roscioli, David Parsons, Darryl A. Knight, Christopher Grainge, Andrew T. Reid, Su-Kim Loo, and Punnam C. Veerati.

REFERENCES

1. Cutting GR. Cystic fibrosis genetics: from molecular understanding to clinical application. *Nat Rev Genet.* (2015) 16:45–56. doi: 10.1038/nrg3849
2. Sly PD, Brennan S, Gangell C, De Klerk N, Murray C, Mott L, et al. Lung disease at diagnosis in infants with cystic fibrosis detected by newborn screening. *Am J Respir Crit Care Med.* (2009) 180:146–52. doi: 10.1164/rccm.200901-0069OC
3. Stick SM, Brennan S, Murray C, Douglas T, von Ungern-Sternberg BS, Garratt LW, et al. Bronchiectasis in infants and preschool children diagnosed with cystic fibrosis after newborn screening. *J Pediatr.* (2009) 155:623–8.e1. doi: 10.1016/j.jpeds.2009.05.005
4. Sly PD, Gangell CL, Chen L, Ware RS, Ranganathan S, Mott LS, et al. Risk factors for bronchiectasis in children with cystic fibrosis. *N Engl J Med.* (2013) 368:1963–70. doi: 10.1056/NEJMoa1301725
5. Tang AC, Turvey SE, Alves MP, Regamey N, Tümmler B, Hartl D. Current concepts: host-pathogen interactions in cystic fibrosis airways disease. *Eur Respir Rev.* (2014) 23:320–32. doi: 10.1183/09059180.00006113
6. Esther CR, Muhlebach MS, Ehre C, Hill DB, Wolfgang MC, Kesimer M, et al. Mucus accumulation in the lungs precedes structural changes and infection in children with cystic fibrosis. *Sci Transl Med.* (2019) 11:eaav3488. doi: 10.1126/scitranslmed.aav3488
7. Fennell PB, Quante J, Wilson K, Boyle M, Strunk R, Ferkol T. Use of high-dose ibuprofen in a pediatric cystic fibrosis center. *J Cyst Fibros.* (2007) 6:153–8. doi: 10.1016/j.jcf.2006.06.003
8. Sanders DB, Bittner RCL, Rosenfeld M, Hoffman LR, Redding GJ, Goss CH. Failure to recover to baseline pulmonary function after cystic fibrosis pulmonary exacerbation. *Am J Respir Crit Care Med.* (2010) 182:627–32. doi: 10.1164/rccm.200909-1421OC
9. Asner S, Waters V, Solomon M, Yau Y, Richardson SE, Grasemann H, et al. Role of respiratory viruses in pulmonary exacerbations in children with cystic fibrosis. *J Cyst Fibros.* (2012) 11:433–9. doi: 10.1016/j.jcf.2012.04.006
10. de Almeida MB, Zerbinati RM, Tateno AF, Oliveira CM, Romão RM, Rodrigues JC, et al. Rhinovirus C and respiratory exacerbations in children with cystic fibrosis. *Emerg Infect Dis.* (2010) 16:996–9. doi: 10.3201/eid1606.100063
11. Kieninger E, Singer F, Tapparel C, Alves MP, Latzin P, Tan HL, et al. High rhinovirus burden in lower airways of children with cystic fibrosis. *Chest.* (2013) 143:782–90. doi: 10.1378/chest.12-0954
12. Goffard A, Lambert V, Salleron J, Herwegh S, Engelmann I, Pinel C, et al. Virus and cystic fibrosis: rhinoviruses are associated with exacerbations in adult patients. *J Clin Virol.* (2014) 60:147–53. doi: 10.1016/j.jcv.2014.02.005
13. Stelzer-Braid S, Johal H, Skilbeck K, Steller A, Alsubie H, Tovey E, et al. Detection of viral and bacterial respiratory pathogens in patients with cystic fibrosis. *J Virol Methods.* (2012) 186:109–12. doi: 10.1016/j.jviromet.2012.08.008
14. Dijkema JS, Ewijk BE van, Wilbrink B, Wolfs TFW, Kimpen JLL, Ent CK van der. Frequency and duration of rhinovirus infections in children with cystic fibrosis and healthy controls: a longitudinal cohort study. *Pediatr Infect Dis J.* (2016) 35:379–83. doi: 10.1097/INF.0000000000001014
15. Flight WG, Bright-Thomas RJ, Tilston P, Mutton KJ, Guiver M, Morris J, et al. Incidence and clinical impact of respiratory viruses in adults

with cystic fibrosis. *Thorax.* (2014) 69:247–53. doi: 10.1136/thoraxjnl-2013-204000
16. Shah A, Connelly M, Whitaker P, McIntyre C, Etherington C, Denton M, et al. Pathogenicity of individual rhinovirus species during exacerbations of cystic fibrosis. *Eur Respir J.* (2015) 45:1748–51. doi: 10.1183/09031936.00229114
17. Esposito S, Daleno C, Scala A, Castellazzi L, Terranova L, Sferrazza Papa S, et al. Impact of rhinovirus nasopharyngeal viral load and viremia on severity of respiratory infections in children. *Eur J Clin Microbiol Infect Dis.* (2014) 33:41–48. doi: 10.1007/s10096-013-1926-5
18. Gangell CL, Shackleton C, Poreddy S, Kappers J, Gaydon JE, Sloots TP, et al. Feasibility of parental collected nasal swabs for virus detection in young children with cystic fibrosis. *J Cyst Fibros.* (2014) 13:661–6. doi: 10.1016/j.jcf.2014.02.009
19. Deschamp AR, Hatch JE, Slaven JE, Gebregziabher N, Storch G, Hall GL, et al. Early respiratory viral infections in infants with cystic fibrosis. *J Cyst Fibros.* (2019) 18:844–50. doi: 10.1016/j.jcf.2019.02.004
20. Etherington C, Naseer R, Conway SP, Whitaker P, Denton M, Peckham DG. The role of respiratory viruses in adult patients with cystic fibrosis receiving intravenous antibiotics for a pulmonary exacerbation. *J Cyst Fibros.* (2014) 13:49–55. doi: 10.1016/j.jcf.2013.06.004
21. Cousin M, Molinari N, Foulongne V, Caimmi D, Vachier I, Abely M, et al. Rhinovirus-associated pulmonary exacerbations show a lack of FEV 1 improvement in children with cystic fibrosis. *Influenza Other Respi Viruses.* (2016) 10:109–12. doi: 10.1111/irv.12353
22. Armstrong D, Grimwood K, Carlin JB, Carzino R, Hull J, Olinsky A, et al. Severe viral respiratory infections in infants with cystic fibrosis. *Pediatr Pulmonol.* (1998) 26:371–9. doi: 10.1002/(sici)1099-0496(199812)26:6<371::aid-ppul1>3.0.co;2-n
23. Sutanto EN, Kicic A, Foo CJ, Stevens PT, Mullane D, Knight DA, et al. Innate inflammatory responses of pediatric cystic fibrosis airway epithelial cells: effects of nonviral and viral stimulation. *Am J Respir Cell Mol Biol.* (2011) 44:761–7. doi: 10.1165/rcmb.2010-0368OC
24. Schögler A, Stokes AB, Casaulta C, Regamey N, Edwards MR, Johnston SL, et al. Interferon response of the cystic fibrosis bronchial epithelium to major and minor group rhinovirus infection. *J Cyst Fibros.* (2016) 15:332–9. doi: 10.1016/j.jcf.2015.10.013
25. Schögler A, Caliaro O, Brügger M, Oliveira Esteves BI, Nita I, Gazdhar A, et al. Modulation of the unfolded protein response pathway as an antiviral approach in airway epithelial cells. *Antiviral Res.* (2019) 162:44–50. doi: 10.1016/j.antiviral.2018.12.007
26. Kicic A, Sutanto EN, Stevens PT, Knight DA, Stick SM. Intrinsic biochemical and functional differences in bronchial epithelial cells of children with asthma. *Am J Respir Crit Care Med.* (2006) 174:1110–18. doi: 10.1164/rccm.200603-392OC
27. Lane C, Burgess S, Kicic A, Knight DA, Stick S. The use of non-bronchoscopic brushings to study the paediatric airway. *Respir Res.* (2005) 6:53. doi: 10.1186/1465-9921-6-53
28. McNamara PS, Kicic A, Sutanto EN, Stevens PT, Stick SM. Comparison of techniques for obtaining lower airway epithelial cells from children. *Eur Respir J.* (2008) 32:763–8. doi: 10.1183/09031936.00162507
29. Martinovich KM, Iosifidis T, Buckley AG, Looi K, Ling KM, Sutanto EN, et al. Conditionally reprogrammed primary airway epithelial cells maintain morphology, lineage and disease specific functional characteristics. *Sci Rep.* (2017) 7:17971. doi: 10.1038/s41598-017-17952-4
30. Garratt LW, Sutanto EN, Foo CJ, Ling KM, Looi K, Kicic-Starcevich E, et al. Determinants of culture success in an airway epithelium sampling program of young children with cystic fibrosis. *Exp Lung Res.* (2014) 40:447–59. doi: 10.3109/01902148.2014.946631
31. Kicic A, Stevens PT, Sutanto EN, Kicic-Starcevich E, Ling K-M, Looi K, et al. Impaired airway epithelial cell responses from children with asthma to rhinoviral infection. *Clin Exp Allergy.* (2016) 46:1441–55. doi: 10.1111/cea.12767
32. Andrews S. *FastQC A Quality Control tool for High Throughput Sequence Data.* (2017) Available online at: https://www.bioinformatics.babraham.ac.uk/projects/fastqc/ (accessed June 01, 2017).
33. Kim D, Langmead B, Salzberg S. HISAT: hierarchical indexing for spliced alignment of transcripts. *Nat Methods.* (2014) 12:357–60. doi: 10.1101/012591
34. Lassmann T, Hayashizaki Y, Daub CO. SAMStat: monitoring biases in next generation sequencing data. *Bioinformatics.* (2011) 27:130–31. doi: 10.1093/bioinformatics/btq614
35. Conesa A, Madrigal P, Tarazona S, Gomez-Cabrero D, Cervera A, McPherson A, et al. A survey of best practices for RNA-seq data analysis. *Genome Biol.* (2016) 17:13. doi: 10.1186/s13059-016-0881-8
36. Dalgaard P. *R Development Core Team: R: A Language and Environment for Statistical Computing* (2010).
37. Risso D, Ngai J, Speed TP, Dudoit S. Normalization of RNA-seq data using factor analysis of control genes or samples. *Nat Biotechnol.* (2014) 32:896–902. doi: 10.1038/nbt.2931
38. Love MI, Huber W, Anders S. Moderated estimation of fold change and dispersion for RNA-seq data with DESeq2. *Genome Biol.* (2014) 15:550. doi: 10.1186/s13059-014-0550-8
39. Wickham H. *Ggplot2 : Elegant Graphics for Data Analysis.* New York, NY: Springer-Verlag (2016). Available online at: https://ggplot2.tidyverse.org (accessed June 15, 2017).
40. Zhou Y, Zhou B, Pache L, Chang M, Khodabakhshi AH, Tanaseichuk O, et al. Metascape provides a biologist-oriented resource for the analysis of systems-level datasets. *Nat Commun.* (2019) 10:1523. doi: 10.1038/s41467-019-09234-6
41. Walter W, Sánchez-Cabo F, Ricote M. GOplot: An R package for visually combining expression data with functional analysis. *Bioinformatics.* (2015) 31:2912–14. doi: 10.1093/bioinformatics/btv300
42. Foroushani ABK, Brinkman FSL, Lynn DJ. Pathway-GPS and SIGORA: identifying relevant pathways based on the over-representation of their gene-pair signatures. *PeerJ.* (2013) 1:e229. doi: 10.7717/peerj.229
43. Xia J, Benner MJ, Hancock REW. NetworkAnalyst - integrative approaches for protein–protein interaction network analysis and visual exploration. *Nucleic Acids Res.* (2014) 42:W167–74. doi: 10.1093/nar/gku443
44. Xia J, Gill EE, Hancock REW. NetworkAnalyst for statistical, visual and network-based meta-analysis of gene expression data. *Nat Protoc.* (2015) 10:823–44. doi: 10.1038/nprot.2015.052
45. Breuer K, Foroushani AK, Laird MR, Chen C, Sribnaia A, Lo R, et al. InnateDB: systems biology of innate immunity and beyond—recent updates and continuing curation. *Nucleic Acids Res.* (2013) 41:D1228–33. doi: 10.1093/nar/gks1147
46. Oliver BGG, Lim S, Wark P, Laza-Stanca V, King N, Black JL, et al. Rhinovirus exposure impairs immune responses to bacterial products in human alveolar macrophages. *Thorax.* (2008) 63:519–25. doi: 10.1136/thx.2007.081752
47. Stokes CA, Kaur R, Edwards MR, Mondhe M, Robinson D, Prestwich EC, et al. Human rhinovirus-induced inflammatory responses are inhibited by phosphatidylserine containing liposomes. *Mucosal Immunol.* (2016) 9:1303–16. doi: 10.1038/mi.2015.137
48. Singanayagam A, Loo S-L, Calderazzo M, Finney LJ, Trujillo Torralbo M-B, Bakhsoliani E, et al. Antiviral immunity is impaired in COPD patients with frequent exacerbations. *Am J Physiol Lung Cell Mol Physiol.* (2019) 317:893–903. doi: 10.1152/ajplung.00253.2019
49. He JQ, Sandford AJ, Wang IM, Stepaniants S, Knight DA, Kicic A, et al. Selection of housekeeping genes for real-time PCR in atopic human bronchial epithelial cells. *Eur Respir J.* (2008) 32:755–62. doi: 10.1183/09031936.00129107
50. O'neal WK, Knowles MR. Cystic fibrosis disease modifiers: complex genetics defines the phenotypic diversity in a monogenic disease. *Annu Rev Genom Hum Genet.* (2018) 19:201–22. doi: 10.1146/annurev-genom-083117-021329
51. Cesur MF, Durmuş S. Systems biology modeling to study pathogen–host interactions. *Methods Mol Biol.* (2018) 1734:97–112. doi: 10.1007/978-1-4939-7604-1_10
52. Yogarajah T, Ong KC, Perera D, Wong KT. AIM2 inflammasome-mediated pyroptosis in enterovirus A71-infected neuronal cells restricts viral replication. *Sci Rep.* (2017) 7:5845. doi: 10.1038/s41598-017-05589-2
53. Rosebeck S, Leaman DW. Mitochondrial localization and pro-apoptotic effects of the interferon-inducible protein ISG12a. *Apoptosis.* (2008) 13:562–72. doi: 10.1007/s10495-008-0190-0
54. Ho HH, Ivashkiv LB. Role of STAT3 in type i interferon responses. *J Biol Chem.* (2006) 281:14111–18. doi: 10.1074/jbc.M511797200
55. Wang W-B, Levy DE, Lee C-K. STAT3 negatively regulates type I IFN-mediated antiviral response. *J Immunol.* (2011) 187:2578–85. doi: 10.4049/jimmunol.1004128

56. Montgomery ST, Mall MA, Kicic A, Stick SM. Hypoxia and sterile inflammation in cystic fibrosis airways: mechanisms and potential therapies. *Eur Respir J.* (2017) 49:1600903. doi: 10.1183/13993003.00903-2016
57. Montgomery ST, Dittrich AS, Garratt LW, Turkovic L, Frey DL, Stick SM, et al. Interleukin-1 is associated with inflammation and structural lung disease in young children with cystic fibrosis. *J Cyst Fibros.* (2018) 17:715–22. doi: 10.1016/j.jcf.2018.05.006
58. Kieninger E, Vareille M, Kopf BS, Blank F, Alves MP, Gisler FM, et al. Lack of an exaggerated inflammatory response on virus infection in cystic fibrosis. *Eur Respir J.* (2012) 39:297–304. doi: 10.1183/09031936.00054511
59. Ribeiro CMP, Paradiso AM, Carew MA, Shears SB, Boucher RC. Cystic fibrosis airway epithelial Ca2+ I signaling: the mechanism for the larger agonist-mediated Ca2+ I signals in human cystic fibrosis airway epithelia. *J Biol Chem.* (2005) 280:10202–9. doi: 10.1074/jbc.M410617200
60. Tarran R, Button B, Picher M, Paradiso AM, Ribeiro CM, Lazarowski ER, et al. Normal and cystic fibrosis airway surface liquid homeostasis. *J Biol Chem.* (2005) 280:35751–9. doi: 10.1074/jbc.M505832200
61. Wetmore DR, Joseloff E, Pilewski J, Lee DP, Lawton KA, Mitchell MW, et al. Metabolomic profiling reveals biochemical pathways and biomarkers associated with pathogenesis in cystic fibrosis cells. *J Biol Chem.* (2010) 285:30516–22. doi: 10.1074/jbc.M110.140806
62. Tiringer K, Treis A, Fucik P, Gona M, Gruber S, Renner S, et al. A Th17- and Th2-skewed cytokine profile in cystic fibrosis lungs represents a potential risk factor for *Pseudomonas aeruginosa* infection. *Am J Respir Crit Care Med.* (2013) 187:621–9. doi: 10.1164/rccm.201206-1150OC
63. Bortolotti P, Hennart B, Thieffry C, Jausions G, Faure E, Grandjean T, et al. Tryptophan catabolism in *Pseudomonas aeruginosa* and potential for inter-kingdom relationship. *BMC Microbiol.* (2016) 16:137. doi: 10.1186/s12866-016-0756-x
64. Rhim AD, Kothari VA, Park PJ, Mulberg AE, Glick MC, Scanlin TF. Terminal glycosylation of cystic fibrosis airway epithelial cells. *Glycoconj J.* 17:385–91. doi: 10.1023/A:1007156014384
65. Glick MC, Kothari VA, Liu A, Stoykova LI, Scanlin TF. Activity of fucosyltransferases and altered glycosylation in cystic fibrosis airway epithelial cells. *Biochimie.* (2001) 83:743–7. doi: 10.1016/S0300-9084(01)01323-2
66. Stoykova LI, Liu A, Scanlin TF, Glick MC. α1,3Fucosyltransferases in cystic fibrosis airway epithelial cells. *Biochimie.* (2003) 85:363–7. doi: 10.1016/S0300-9084(03)00061-0
67. Virella-Lowell I, Herlihy J-D, Liu B, Lopez C, Cruz P, Muller C, et al. Effects of CFTR, interleukin-10, and *Pseudomonas aeruginosa* on gene expression profiles in a CF bronchial epithelial cell Line. *Mol Ther.* (2004) 10:562–73. doi: 10.1016/j.ymthe.2004.06.215
68. Linden SK, Sutton P, Karlsson NG, Korolik V, McGuckin MA. Mucins in the mucosal barrier to infection. *Mucosal Immunol.* (2008) 1:183–97. doi: 10.1038/mi.2008.5
69. Hsu J-L, Chiang P-C, Guh J-H. Tunicamycin induces resistance to camptothecin and etoposide in human hepatocellular carcinoma cells: role of cell-cycle arrest and GRP78. *Naunyn Schmiedebergs Arch Pharmacol.* (2009) 380:373–82. doi: 10.1007/s00210-009-0453-5
70. Gualdoni GA, Mayer KA, Kapsch A-M, Kreuzberg K, Puck A, Kienzl P, et al. Rhinovirus induces an anabolic reprogramming in host cell metabolism essential for viral replication. *Proc Natl Acad Sci USA.* (2018) 115:E7158–65. doi: 10.1073/pnas.1800525115
71. Gray RD, Duncan A, Noble D, Imrie M, O'Reilly DSJ, Innes JA, et al. Sputum trace metals are biomarkers of inflammatory and suppurative lung disease. *Chest.* (2010) 137:635–41. doi: 10.1378/chest.09-1047
72. Hendricks MR, Lashua LP, Fischer DK, Flitter BA, Eichinger KM, Durbin JE, et al. Respiratory syncytial virus infection enhances *Pseudomonas aeruginosa* biofilm growth through dysregulation of nutritional immunity. *Proc Natl Acad Sci USA.* (2016) 113:1642–7. doi: 10.1073/pnas.1516979113
73. Jakiela B, Brockman-Schneider R, Amineva S, Lee W-M, Gern JE. Basal cells of differentiated bronchial epithelium are more susceptible to rhinovirus infection. *Am J Respir Cell Mol Biol.* (2008) 38:517–23. doi: 10.1165/rcmb.2007-0050OC

10

More than Just a Barrier: The Immune Functions of the Airway Epithelium in Asthma Pathogenesis

Andreas Frey[1,2], Lars P. Lunding[2,3], Johanna C. Ehlers[2,4], Markus Weckmann[2,5], Ulrich M. Zissler[6,7] and Michael Wegmann[2,3]*

[1] Division of Mucosal Immunology and Diagnostics, Research Center Borstel, Borstel, Germany, [2] Airway Research Center North, German Center for Lung Research (DZL), Borstel, Germany, [3] Division of Asthma Exacerbation & Regulation, Research Center Borstel, Borstel, Germany, [4] Division of Experimental Pneumology, Research Center Borstel, Borstel, Germany, [5] Department of Pediatric Pulmonology and Allergology, University Children's Hospital, Lübeck, Germany, [6] Center of Allergy & Environment (ZAUM), Technical University of Munich and Helmholtz Center Munich, German Research Center for Environmental Health, Munich, Germany, [7] Member of the German Center for Lung Research (DZL), CPC-M, Munich, Germany

***Correspondence:**
Michael Wegmann
mwegmann@fz-borstel.de

Allergic bronchial asthma is a chronic disease of the airways that is characterized by symptoms like respiratory distress, chest tightness, wheezing, productive cough, and acute episodes of broncho-obstruction. This symptom-complex arises on the basis of chronic allergic inflammation of the airway wall. Consequently, the airway epithelium is central to the pathogenesis of this disease, because its multiple abilities directly have an impact on the inflammatory response and thus the formation of the disease. In turn, its structure and functions are markedly impaired by the inflammation. Hence, the airway epithelium represents a sealed, self-cleaning barrier, that prohibits penetration of inhaled allergens, pathogens, and other noxious agents into the body. This barrier is covered with mucus that further contains antimicrobial peptides and antibodies that are either produced or specifically transported by the airway epithelium in order to trap these particles and to remove them from the body by a process called mucociliary clearance. Once this first line of defense of the lung is overcome, airway epithelial cells are the first cells to get in contact with pathogens, to be damaged or infected. Therefore, these cells release a plethora of chemokines and cytokines that not only induce an acute inflammatory reaction but also have an impact on the alignment of the following immune reaction. In case of asthma, all these functions are impaired by the already existing allergic immune response that *per se* weakens the barrier integrity and self-cleaning abilities of the airway epithelium making it more vulnerable to penetration of allergens as well as of infection by bacteria and viruses. Recent studies indicate that the history of allergy- and pathogen-derived insults can leave some kind of memory in these cells that can be described as imprinting or trained immunity. Thus, the airway epithelium is in the center of processes that lead to formation, progression and acute exacerbation of asthma.

Keywords: asthma, inflammation, barrier, mucus, polarization, imprinting, trained immunity

INTRODUCTION

With more than 300 million people affected bronchial asthma is one of the most common chronic inflammatory diseases worldwide (1). Actually, 1 out of 250 deaths is associated with asthma and it causes annual direct medical (drugs, care, hospitalization) and indirect economic (productivity loss, early retirement) costs of about €34 Billion for the EU (2) and over 80 Billion for the United States (3, 4), making it a major burden for public healthcare systems (5).

Asthma is characterized by acute broncho-obstruction, in combination with additional symptoms such as cough, chest tightness, shortness of breath, and wheezing, which vary in extent and over time. These symptoms arise on the basis of chronic airway inflammation in response to a trigger, most commonly inhaled allergen(s), that causes airway hyperresponsiveness (AHR), airway remodeling and mucus hypersecretion (6). Due to the complexity and variation of the symptoms along with its pathogenesis, asthma is nowadays described as a heterogeneous syndrome with distinct sub- or endotypes. However, the majority of asthma patients displays allergic inflammation of the airways, which can be classified by profiles of several characteristic mediators in "TH2 high" or "TH2 low" subtypes (7). Thus, in sensitized individuals T helper 2 (TH2) cells orchestrate allergic inflammation by releasing a typical array of cytokines including interleukins (IL)-4, -5, -9, and -13 and granulocyte-macrophage colony stimulating factor (GM-CSF). These mediators induce the production of allergen-specific immunoglobulin (Ig) E, TH2 cell development, goblet cell differentiation, submucosal gland activity, as well as recruitment, maturation, and activation of eosinophils and its precursors (8). Activation of mast cells and eosinophils via IgE-bound allergens results in their degranulation and, thus, in the release of a plethora of effector molecules and growth factors that on the one hand destroy airway tissue and on the other hand conduct its repair. Chronic activation of these processes ultimately lead to signs of airway remodeling such as increased smooth muscle mass, subepithelial fibrosis, and epithelial desquamation, which in turn give rise to the pathological changes and clinical symptoms characteristic for asthma (9).

Allergic sensitization against aeroallergens represents the strongest factor predisposing for the development of asthma, indicating a hyperreaction of the immune system to be the central event within the pathogenesis of this disease. Nevertheless, structural cells and particularly airway epithelial cells also appear to be of critical importance. This is not surprising since these cells represent the barrier that first encounters environmental stress factors like air pollutants, bacterial and viral pathogens, as well as allergens, and markedly contributes to their neutralization by a mechanism called mucociliary clearance (MCC). Besides these barrier and cleaning functions airway epithelial cells also exert a number of immunological tasks interweaving the role of the epithelium with that of the above-mentioned cells of the immune system. Here we aim to review these immune functions of the airway epithelium against the background of asthma pathogenesis.

THE BARRIER FUNCTION OF THE AIRWAY EPITHELIAL CELL LAYER ITSELF

The main purpose of mucosae is to separate the body from its environment and therefore they are essential for the maintenance of the inner homeostasis. Though this task is not commonly regarded as an "active" or "typical" immune function, it is absolutely central for the defense against allergens, pathogens and other harmful environmental factors. In order to fulfill this function the airway epithelium forms a continuous, self-cleaning barrier with a considerable resistance against biological, chemical or physical stressors (10). Together with the physical barriers of the MCC and glycocalyx, this is achieved by three types of intercellular epithelial junctions that form the structural adhesion forces of the airway mucosa by linking the intracellular structures of the cytoskeleton of one epithelial cell to that of its neighbors. These junctions involve adherens junctions (AJs), hemidesmosomes, and tight junctions (TJs).

AJs can appear as spots (adhesion plaques) or as bands encircling the cell (zonula adherens). In the junctional zone AJs interconnect the actin filaments of the adherent cells via homotypic transmembrane E-cadherin adhesions and anchor proteins like actinin, vinculin, and α-, β-, and p120 catenins, while adhesion plaques attach the cells to the extracellular matrix (11).

Similarly, hemidesmosomes are focal structures that form adhesive bonds between the cytoskeleton of epithelial cells and the lamina lucida, which is a part of the lamina propria. Hemidesmosomes utilize integrin α6β4, plectin 1a and the tetraspanin CD151 connecting laminin and fibronectin of the extracellular matrix to the intermediate filaments of the cytoskeleton (12).

In contrast, TJs form a multiprotein junctional complex called zonula occludens (ZO) that in turn appears as the main regulator of the paracellular permeability. These complexes are formed by several transmembrane and cytoplasmic proteins that are attached to actin filaments of the cytoskeleton. The main components of TJs are claudins and occludins, proteins with four transmembrane domains, as well as so-called junctional adhesion molecules (JAMs) belonging to the immunoglobulin superfamily with only one transmembrane domain. These proteins are connected to actin filaments by cingulin and ZO proteins 1, -2, and -3 (13).

In the airways of healthy individuals, the TJs of the zonula occludens and AJs of the zonula adherens constitute dense protein networks that interconnect the basolateral sides of epithelial cells in such a way that they prevent the paracellular passage of basically all molecules, including water, ions and proteins, as well as of pathogens or other inhaled particulate matter. Several findings strongly indicate that in asthma patients the barrier function is impaired by epithelial disruption. For example, endobronchial biopsies revealed a fragile or even injured airway mucosa with partially or completely uncovered areas and detachment of columnar, ciliated cells (14). Epithelial desquamation is further indicated by the presence of epithelial cells in bronchoalveolar lavage (BAL) and of creola bodies (epithelial cell aggregates) in sputum of asthmatics (15). Furthermore, bronchial biopsies of asthmatic subjects displayed patchy disruption of TJs (16) and the expression of a number of proteins that are essential for the formation of TJs and AJs has been shown to be markedly reduced. Among these proteins are α-catenin (17), β-catenin (18), occluding (16), ZO-1 (16, 17), and E-cadherin (17, 19). The levels of the latter one in sputum also correlate with asthma severity (20). These data are further supported by *in vitro* studies where primary bronchial epithelial cells are kept in air liquid interface (ALI) culture, a method that allows the cells to differentiate and form a pseudo-stratified epithelial monolayer largely resembling the physiological structure of the airway mucosa. Once this structure has been established, *in vitro* barrier integrity can be assessed by measuring the transepithelial electrical resistance (TEER), a characteristic that is indicative of the tightness of a cell layer (21). Several studies showed that ALI cultured airway epithelia from asthma patients display a decreased TEER in comparison to epithelia derived from healthy controls (16, 22, 23).

IMPAIRMENT OF CELLULAR BARRIER FUNCTIONS IN ASTHMA PATHOGENESIS

To date, three different factors are discussed to have a harmful impact on the barrier integrity of the airway epithelium in asthma pathogenesis: allergens themselves, viral infection, and (allergic) inflammation. According to the "protease hypothesis" allergens with an inherent protease activity are capable of cleaving the protein components of the aforementioned intercellular epithelial junctions so that the barrier function is disrupted and allergens can penetrate the airway mucosa on the paracellular route, which eventually could result in sensitization against them. Accordingly, a considerable number of allergens has been tested *in vitro* for proteolytic potential and for an effect on epithelial barrier integrity. Several studies provided evidence for a direct cleavage of e.g., occludin and ZO-1 proteins by the major allergen from house dust mites (*Dermatophagoides*), Der p 1 (24, 25). House dust mite extracts as well as Der p 1 have been shown to increase the permeability and to decrease TEER of epithelial layers *in vitro* (23, 25, 26). Comparable effects have been shown for extracts of the allergenic fungus *Alternaria alternata* that reduced TEER of human bronchial epithelial cells *in vitro* (27) or the *Aspergillus fumigatus*-derived alkaline protease 1 (Alp-1) (28). Similarly, a variety of different pollen extracts has been investigated for their effect on the barrier integrity of epithelial cells *in vitro*. Diffusates of Italian cypress (*Cupressus sempervirens*), Orchard grass (*Dactylis glomerata*), Olive (*Olivia europaea*), and *Scots pine* (*Pinus sylvestris*) have been shown to affect claudin-1, E-cadherin, and occludin expression and thus to disrupt epithelial junctions in ALI cultures of Calu-3 cells, an effect which could be suppressed by protease inhibitors (29). Japanese hop (*Humulus japonicus*) extract also reduced expression of occludin in a comparable setting (30). Another study provided evidence for proteolytic activity of Giant ragweed (*Ambrosia trifida*), Kentucky bluegrass (*Poa pratensis*), and White birch (*Betula pendula*) as shown by reduced expression of claudin-1, occludin, and ZO-1 in Calu-3 as well as in MDCK cells (31).

However, an inherent protease activity appears not to be the only way, by which allergens can impair the barrier integrity of the airway epithelium. Cockroach, HDM, fungus, and mold extracts have also been shown to activate the protease-activated receptor (PAR-) 1 and/or 2, which in turn leads to degradation of AJ components (25, 32–34).

The effect of viral infections on airway barrier function is even more pronounced than that of allergens. Respiratory viruses cause junction dysfunction by different mechanisms: human rhinoviruses (HRV), respiratory syncytial virus (RSV), human metapneumovirus (HMPV), influenza and parainfluenza viruses bind to their entry receptor, which are typically protein or sugar structures expressed on the cellular surface for other purposes, leading to endocytosis of the virus. Once the virus has been internalized, it uncoats and initiates the viral replication process, which has certain consequences for infected cells. On the one hand, the cell starts with the production of type I interferons (IFN) in order to slow down the internal virus replication and to activate the cellular immune response against the virus. In consequence, infected airway epithelial cells are killed by virus-specific, cytotoxic CD8 + T cells. On the other hand, the virus itself also kills epithelial cells, since it induces morphological alteration of the cells summarized as cytopathic effect (CPE). For HRV and influenza viruses, the CPE manifests in rounding and detachment of airway epithelial cells that are ultimately lysed by the virus in order to release freshly produced viruses. Paramyxoviruses such as RSV and HMPV induce cell fusion so that four or more cells form typical syncytia (35, 36). Additionally, at least HRV and RSV affect the barrier integrity of the airway epithelium by reducing the expression of epithelial junction proteins (37–40). It could be shown that HRV increases epithelial permeability by a reduction of occludin and ZO-1 expression (41, 42). RSV also disrupts junctional complex structures by fostering the activity of protein kinase D (PKD) (43).

The antiviral immune response also includes the release of cytokines that directly affect epithelial barrier function as well. This is especially true for IL-1β, IFN-γ and tumor necrosis factor (TNF). These cytokines have been shown to support epithelial permeability and to decrease expression of claudins, JAM, occludin, and ZO-1 in several *in vitro* studies (44–46). In case of asthma, these effects are even more pronounced because of the allergic inflammatory response that already exists before the viral infection of the airway epithelium. Hence, TH2 type cytokines like IL-4 and IL-13 also increase barrier permeability by inhibiting the surface expression of β-catenin, E-cadherin, occludin, and ZO-1 (45, 47). In addition to cytokines, mast cell derived mediators also appear to have an effect on the barrier function of the airway mucosa. Histamine for example has been shown to contribute to transient disruption of apical junctional complex integrity and thus to increase epithelial permeability *in vitro* (48).

Allergens, viruses, and the inflammatory response to their exposure represent extrinsic factors that impair the barrier integrity of the airway epithelium. However, some studies suggest that epithelial cells of asthma patients inherently predispose for an increased permeability. As already mentioned above, airway epithelial cells that have been isolated from asthmatics and propagated *in vitro* to form an epithelial monolayer under ALI culture conditions, display a decreased TEER as compared to cells from healthy donors (23, 45). This observation indicates that the cellular properties leading to an increased barrier permeability are somehow imprinted within the cells. Whether this is a matter of genetic predisposition encoded in epithelial stem cells or whether epithelial cells from asthma patients "remember" previous insults by epigenetic modifications that predispose for asthma development in later life remains elusive.

PASSIVE LUMINAL BARRIER STRUCTURE ON THE AIRWAY EPITHELIUM

Besides the barrier function of the epithelium provided by the mere presence of the sealed cell layer itself, two additional barrier structures are "exported" onto the luminal surface by the airway epithelium, a static one dubbed glycocalyx or periciliary layer (PCL) and a mobile one termed mucus.

STRUCTURE AND FUNCTION OF THE PERICILIARY LAYER

The glycocalyx or PCL is a sponge/fleece-like, cell membrane-anchored layer of glycolipids and glycoproteins - mainly mucins (see below) - that vertically stick out of the apical epithelial cell membrane. Although mainly attributed to the gut epithelium where it can extend up to 1500 nm (49) and to the vascular endothelium (50, 51) a glycocalyx/PCL is also present throughout the airway epithelium even down to the alveoli (52), again with heights up to 1500 nm in certain areas (53) (**Figure 1**). This static glycoprotein and glycolipid coat stores water to control mucus hydration but also serves as a protective zone against the compression of the mucus lying above in order to allow persistent cilia beating for ongoing functionality of the mucociliary clearance (MCC; see below) (53, 54). Beyond that, the glycocalyx/PCL regulates receptor specificity by architectural means and prevents the progression of viruses through the occasionally patchy mucus layer. It has been shown that the height and density of the epithelial glycocalyx can determine whether a ligand-equipped nanoparticle may attach to its membrane receptor or not (49, 55). In line with this, the inefficiency of adenovirus-mediated gene transfer into the airway epithelium was found to be caused by the membrane-tethered glycocalyx/PCL proteins that put a halt to the advance of the viral vectors (56, 57). Consequently, the susceptibility of the airway epithelium toward infection is at least to some extent controlled by the glycocalyx/PCL. Very small viruses such as bocavirus (HBoV1) and HRV, which are 20–30 nm in size (58, 59) should readily advance through the PCL to the epithelial plasma membrane as has been observed with nanoparticles of the respective size (53). Consequently, those viruses should be able to luminally infect airway epithelial cells as long as their receptor is present on the apical side. Little is known about receptor distribution *in vivo* but at least on cultured airway epithelial cells apical receptor expression and/or infectivity has been demonstrated for both viruses (60–63). Larger particles of about 100 nm and above, on the other hand, are efficiently blocked by the PCL (53). Hence, viruses such as RSV, HMPV, influenza and parainfluenza viruses, adenovirus or coronavirus, which are in this size range (64–67), should be hindered efficiently by the PCL to infect the host. Yet, those viruses often are associated with respiratory infections and asthma exacerbations (68, 69). One possibility for them to infect the airway epithelium may be the presence of the viral receptor on structures that extend from the PCL such as the tips of the cilia. An example for this is chemokine receptor CX3CR1 via which RSV can infect its host. In differentiated human airway epithelial cells this molecule is highly abundant on cilia (70, 71). Another possibility is the preceding action of a door-opener such as HBoV1 which may pave the way for further viral infections. HBoV1 was shown to persist for several months in the human airway epithelium (72) and causes pyroptotic cell death, epithelial cell hypertrophy, loss of cilia and disruption of the tight junction barrier (60, 61). Such a predamaged epithelial barrier may then readily fall victim to an influenza, parainfluenza or HPMV infection. With up to 13% of asthma exacerbations in small children found to be associated with HBoV1 infection (73) it may be worthwhile to further investigate possible coinfections with HBoV1 in asthma exacerbation cases. In this context, it may also be of interest that the treatment of chronic inflammatory diseases of the airways such as asthma with corticosteroids (CS) seems to reduce the glycocalyx/PCL height on the alveolar epithelium (74) thereby rendering the lung more susceptible to e.g., *Pneumocystis carinii* infection. Consequently, alleviating chronic inflammation in asthma with CS may make the patient more susceptible to certain infections, which in turn may enhance inflammation again, clearly a two-edged outcome of CS therapy in asthma.

Although the glycocalyx appears to be static on the architectural level, it may not be invariant in terms of its molecular composition. It was shown that lipopolysaccharide exposure could lead to heparan sulfate shedding from the airway epithelium thereby causing increased lung permeability (52). Allergen exposure of experimental animals resulted in different glycosylation patterns of the glycocalyx (75), which may result in a deviant presentation of viral and bacterial receptors on the cell surface. In light of the above, the airway epithelial glycocalyx seems to play a so far underestimated but possibly important role in airway epithelial defense. Whether or not the molecular composition

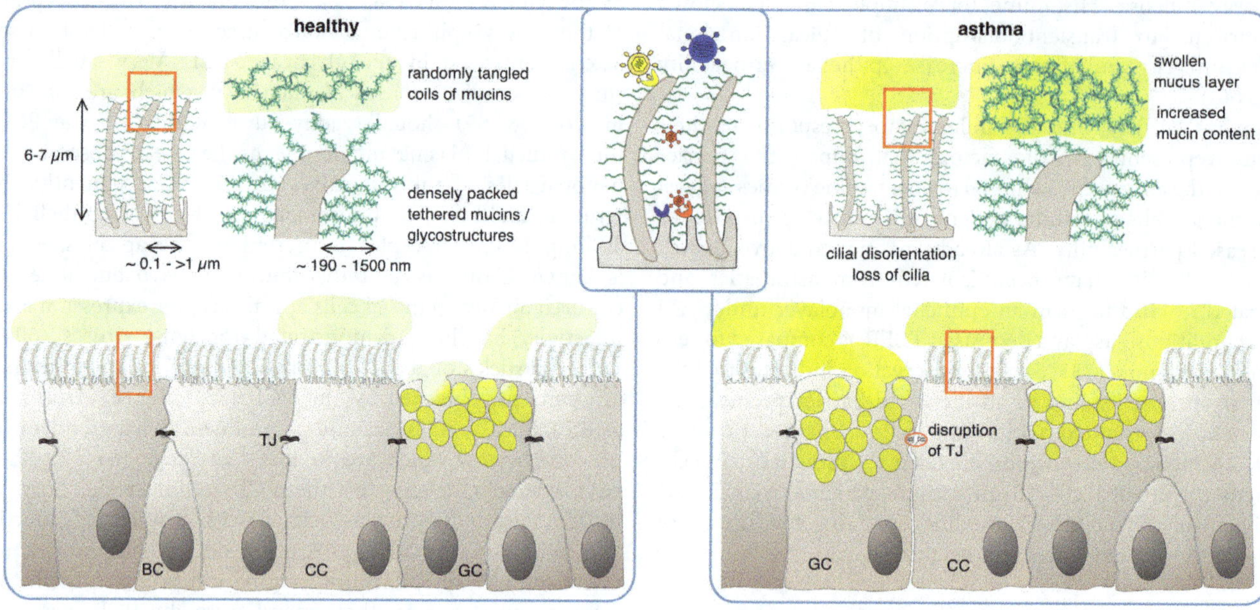

FIGURE 1 | Protection of epithelial surfaces by physical barriers. In the healthy state, ciliated cells (CC) form a tight epithelial layer where paracellular passage is prevented by sealing of lateral intercellular spaces with tight junctions (TJ). The apical epithelial cell surface, including the cilia, is covered by a layer of membrane-anchored glycoproteins and glycolipids, the glycocalyx. The dense meshwork of glycostructures restricts access of luminal matter to the apical cell surface; depending on their size, larger pathogens can be cut off from their receptor if it is not present on cilia (inset). Goblet cells (GC) secrete mucus, consisting of highly glycosylated mucins which absorb large quantities of water to form a viscous gel. The mucus – and any matter trapped within – is transported upward in the airway lumen by the coordinated beating of the cilia. BC, basal cells. In the asthmatic state, barrier functions can be compromised by partial disruption of tight junctions and gaps in the PCL/glycocalyx meshwork due to loss of cilia. Mucus clearance is impeded by increased mucus viscosity and swelling of the gel matrix, and by disturbance of ciliar beating due to disorganization and dykinesia of cilia.

of this static cell coat is different in asthma, remains to be investigated.

COMPOSITION AND FUNCTION OF MUCUS

While the role of the glycocalyx/PCL is still subject of debate, the importance of mucus in airway luminal defense is unchallenged. Mucus is an unstirred discontinuous sheet of secreted mucous hydrogel which floats on top of the epithelium and is transported toward the oral cavity like the cargo on a conveyor due to the constant and coordinated beating of underlying ciliated cells (76). The mucus carried upward by this mucociliary clearance (MCC) mechanism can be swallowed or expectorated. As the mucus layer separates the airway lumen from the epithelium only objects that diffuse faster "vertically" toward the epithelial surface than the mucus is transported "horizontally" toward the oral cavity can reach the epithelial cell membranes. Thus, only nanoscalar objects and smaller, like gases, water, salts and nutrients are able to reach the epithelial cells (77, 78). This way the mucus carpet provides a protective line of defense against pathogens, dust and other harmful objects that might be inhaled by an individual. In addition to that, the sticky texture of the mucus slows down airborne objects and further prevents their advance to the epithelial cell layer. In order to exert these functions properly, mucus requires a specific composition. Mucus consists mainly of water, further components are salts, lipids and proteins. Among those, antimicrobial proteins like lysozyme, immunoglobulins and antimicrobial peptides are major molecular scavengers distributed within the mucus layer (79–81). The characteristic viscous, elastic and sticky properties of the mucus are provided by a group of macromolecules named mucins (82, 83).

To date, 21 genes coding for mucins have been described (84). Their protein products are secreted either to form mucus or remain immobile on the apical membranes of the airway epithelial cells where they become part of the glycocalyx/PCL. MUC5AC and MUC5B are the major secreted mucins in the airways. In addition, MUC2 and MUC19 are also part of airway mucus, albeit to a considerably smaller proportion, and thus belong to the family of secreted mucins (83). In contrast, MUC1, MUC4 and MUC16 are tethered to the cells of the airway epithelium (**Figure 1**) thereby contributing to the static luminal epithelial barrier, which resides underneath the mobile mucus layer (85, 86).

The viscous and elastic properties of the mucous gel are primarily given by the secreted polymeric mucins MUC5AC and MUC5B (83). These mucins are highly O-glycosylated proteins enriched with amino acids like proline, serine or threonine (87). Although both have a similar structure, MUC5B and MUC5AC differ in charge due to differential glycosylations (88). Their production depends on cell type and site of production. In the upper airways, MUC5AC is produced by epithelial goblet cells while MUC5B is secreted from mucous cells in submucosal glands from secretory cells in the tracheal and bronchial epithelium. In the distal airways, MUC5B is also produced by secretory cells of the epithelium and seems to be the major mucin of this airway region (83, 89, 90). Before secretion, polymeric proteins are stored in secretory granules in a compacted, dehydrated state. Upon release, they switch to a hydrated form, which is necessary for the mucous gel-like properties (91, 92). Whether the two different mucins have different functions restricted to their site of production or whether the two mucins mingle to create a novel type of barrier structure is not clear yet. At least some studies analyzing airways of piglets have shown that MUC5B strands are becoming coated with MUC5AC to some extent after release at the epithelial surface (93, 94). A possible role of MUC2 and MUC19 has not been identified yet.

Howsoever, under healthy conditions, the viscous mucus traps noxious substances, which are then removed from the airway via cilial beating by the MCC (95). In asthma, the MCC is impaired leading to mucus plug formation which in turn results in the characteristic obstruction observed in asthmatics. This is already a feature of mild stable asthma and the dysfunction worsens during aggravation of asthma and in asthma exacerbations (96–98). One reason is an increased mucin content of the mucus thereby disturbing its regular composition. Normally, the airways' mucus consists of ~98% water and only ~2% solid factors mainly mucins. In obstructive diseases, the amounts of mucins rise up to 8–15% (54, 86). Due to its hygroscopic nature, this leads to acquisition of water from the underlying PCL/glycocalyx and shrinking of this static layer. The now protruding cilia either project into the mucus or get bend (54). Both effects impede passing on of the mucus to the next cell. Loss and/or disorientation of cilia as it is typical for asthmatics will further disturb the "bucket chain"-like transport process (99). On the cargo side enhanced intermolecular crosslinking of mucus constituents by oxidative processes may further complicate forwarding. It will also increase mucus viscosity eventually leading to plug formation. Oxidative intramolecular crosslinking of biomolecules is predominantly caused by cysteines whose thiol side chains can form disulfide bridges. All mucins are rich in cysteines, especially in their less glycosylated carboxy- and amino terminal regions. In the "normal" mucous gel of healthy individuals these cysteines are believed to be only moderately crosslinked, forming a lightly entangled network. In asthma, however, the degree of crosslinking and the density of the mucin network increases considerably (100, 101) (**Figure 1**). Increased oxidative stress appears to play an important role in this respect with eosinophils being the main suspects for oxidant production. The abnormally high levels of eosinophil peroxidase detected in the sputum of asthma patients may form an oxidative milieu. This would also bring the widely observed correlation between airway eosinophilia and airway obstruction into a causative relationship (102). Lastly, the MUC5AC of asthmatics tends to tether to the epithelium, which also complicates mucus forwarding (103).

In asthmatics not only the amount but also the composition of the mucus changes, especially the ratio of MUC5AC to MUC5B as well as the posttranslational modification of MUC5B. Mucus from healthy individuals contains predominantly MUC5B, which is essential for the MCC and protection against pathogens (104–106). In asthma, the proportion of MUC5B relative to MUC5AC often decreased (104, 105) along with the expression of a low-charge form of MUC5B. Consequently, there was a changed ratio between the two differently glycosylated forms of MUC5B (104, 107). The importance of MUC5B is indicated by *Muc5b*-deficient mice, which showed an accumulation of undesired substances e.g., bacteria, resulting in severe inflammation and airway obstruction (106).

The ratio between MUC5B and MUC5AC changes dramatically in asthma because MUC5AC expression and protein production are substantially upregulated in asthmatic patients (104, 105, 107). Especially patients with an eosinophilic type 2 asthmatic phenotype showed a shifted ratio toward higher MUC5AC concentrations (105, 108). This is in line with the assumption that MUC5AC seems to be important for the defense against enteric nematodal and influenza infections (109, 110). The increased expression of MUC5AC seems to depend on substantially increased levels of IL-13. The IL-13 signaling pathway activates the signal transducer and activator of transcription 6 (STAT6), which induces the expression of MUC5AC via various regulators (111) and appears to be involved in AHR development (112, 113). Several studies using *in vitro* systems with human epithelial cells or murine models validated this mechanism (114–117). Furthermore, EGFR, which is also overexpressed in asthma, also induces the expression of MUC5AC (118–121). This excessive production of mucins in the asthmatic airway epithelium leads to an increased volume of intracellular stored mucins, a mucus metaplasia (122). Thus, a higher number of goblet cells compared to the healthy situation appears in case of asthma (122). It is not exactly understood, whether this switch from a muco-ciliary phenotype to a mucous metaplastic phenotype develops from goblet cell hyperplasia, metaplasia or both as reviewed before (123). In animal models, goblet cell metaplasia/hyperplasia arises from an increased expression of primarily IL-13, but also of IL-4 and IL-9 (124–127). These cytokines are highly upregulated in asthmatic individuals (128–131). One important factor for the development of the goblet cell metaplasia is Notch2 regulated by IL-13 (132). Studies analyzing the function of SAM-pointed domain containing ETS transcription factor (SPDEF) highlighted its essential role in the development of goblet cell differentiation, hyperplasia and mucous metaplasia (133–135). Therefore, SPDEF seems to inhibit the expression of Forkhead box protein A2 (FOXA2) which is an important negative regulator of genes associated with mucous metaplasia and goblet cell hyperplasia (111, 121, 133, 136, 137).

Thus, the physical barriers provided by the airway epithelial layer seem to be deeply disturbed in asthmatic individuals. Although mucin is one of the most important barrier molecules in the airways its unbalanced overproduction is clearly detrimental to the desired outcome. Mucus plugging impedes egress of the active luminal defense molecules necessary to eliminate invaders.

ACTIVE LUMINAL DEFENSE MECHANISMS ON THE AIRWAY EPITHELIUM

Although strong walls (tight junctionally sealed epithelial cell layer) surrounded by a glacis (pericilial layer/glycocalyx) and a moat filled with flowing liquid (MCC) are crucial to prevent invaders from entering a castle, active defenses are necessary to end the siege. This is of particular importance when the besieger can replicate and thus may increase continuously by number, as is the case when pathogenic bacteria colonize the luminal side of the airway epithelium.

DEFENSIVE MOLECULES PRODUCED BY THE EPITHELIUM

In order to get rid of a potential invader the airway epithelium possesses a battery of defense molecules, with which a potential microbial enemy can be attacked, destroyed or removed out of the airway lumen. Prominent innate molecular scavengers are lysozyme, transferrin and antimicrobial peptides. Lysozyme is produced in large amounts (20 mg/day) by serous cells of the upper human airway epithelium (138) and is able to destroy the polysaccharide capsules of many bacterial species. It has been shown that the production of lysozyme by serous cells residing in the serous glands of the upper airways is crucial for defending against bacterial airway invaders (139). Once the polysaccharide capsule is destroyed or damaged, so called defensins or antimicrobial peptides may exert the lethal hit to the invader. Defensins can form holes or pores into a bacterial cell membrane thereby killing a pathogen that aims to enter the body (79, 140, 141). In addition, lactoferrin is produced and secreted by serous cells (142), and transferrin is expressed by alveolar type I cells (143). These ferrins are iron-binding proteins, which deplete their environment from iron ions that are essential for the growth of a self-replicating organism (143, 144). Consequently, the pathogen is starved out.

THE ROLE OF SECRETORY IgA IN EPITHELIAL DEFENSE

Besides this innate "rapid response team," the polarized epithelium of the human airways is also able to transport and apically release immunoglobulins that carry a J-chain (joining chain) by using its poly Ig receptor (pIgR) (145–147) that is expressed by all non-stratified epithelial cells (**Figure 2**). Only IgM and multimeric IgA are equipped with J-chains (148, 149). These two immunoglobulin classes not only circulate in the bloodstream but are also produced directly underneath the airway epithelium by B cells, given those lymphocytes express the J-chain (150, 151). Functionally, IgM can substitute for multimeric IgA. For that reason IgA-deficient individuals do not show a strong phenotype concerning susceptibility to infection. Nevertheless, secreted IgA (sIgA) outperforms IgM in terms of mucosal protection as it usually displays a higher affinity toward its antigen and, more importantly, is able to crosslink with mucins upon target binding (152, 153). This way an incoming viral or bacterial pathogen becomes trapped in mucus and is removed from the airway surface via the MCC. The protective function of secreted IgA has been demonstrated with various model systems, both for the gastrointestinal mucosa as well as for the airways, using passively administered monoclonal IgA (154–157), injected hybridoma cells whose target specific, dimeric IgAs are then transported across the mucosae ("backpack tumor model") (158–160) and by neutralization of preexisting mucosal IgA immunity with mucosally administered anti-IgA immunoglobulins (80). Although adaptive multivalent target binding via its hypervariable regions is probably the main mode of protection in those models, sIgA is also able to bind in an innate manner to luminal pathogens via its carbohydrate components by presenting decoy structures that mimic target cell surface receptors (161). If both modes of repelling fail and a pathogen has nonetheless invaded an epithelial cell, dimeric IgA may still be able to protect the infected cell, this time from inside. This is possible whenever the respective pathogen does not directly infect the cytosol of its target cell or inject its nucleic acids directly into the cytosol but rather uses an initial endocytosis step for infection. Depending on the infected organelle, vesicles, which concurrently translocate IgA toward the apical site, may fuse with the infected organelle, bind to the invader and carry it away into the lumen. In addition to this removal activity, mucus crosslinking and the tricking of pathogens by offering decoy receptors, sIgA also scavenges IL-8 and thereby inhibits IL-8-driven neutrophil chemotaxis (162).

In addition to these molecular interactions with a pathogenic target, IgA also binds to numerous cell types that patrol at the airway epithelium. The most important cellular partner seems to be the eosinophil as this cell possesses a total of five different receptors for IgA: FcαRI (CD89), transferrin receptor (TfR) (CD71), pIgR, asialoglycoprotein receptor (ASGPR) and a receptor for secretory component (SCR) with the integrin Mac-1 (CD11b/CD18) serving as a coreceptor for FcαRI (163, 164). Depending on the receptor addressed and the form of IgA offered, i.e., soluble versus target-bound and cross-linked, eosinophils are either calmed down or activated (165–167). Yet, eosinophils are not only manipulated by IgA, they also influence IgA production themselves (168, 169). Thus, immunoglobulin A and eosinophils share a really intimate relationship.

Equipped with less receptors but still responsive to IgA are neutrophils, dendritic cells, macrophages, basophils and even epithelial lining cells that express the transferrin receptor such as alveolar-type 2 cells (170). An additional, so far unidentified receptor is present on M cells (microfold cells) (171, 172). M cells are a specialized epithelial lining cell type that is responsible for antigen sampling at mucosal surfaces and predominantly occurs in the epithelium above organized mucosa-associated lymphoid tissue (173, 174). This receptor senses the distance between two heavy chain domains in IgA. Thus, it is not able to bind IgA1, an IgA subclass present only in primates. IgA1 is different from IgA2 in that it contains a mucin-like, highly glycosylated

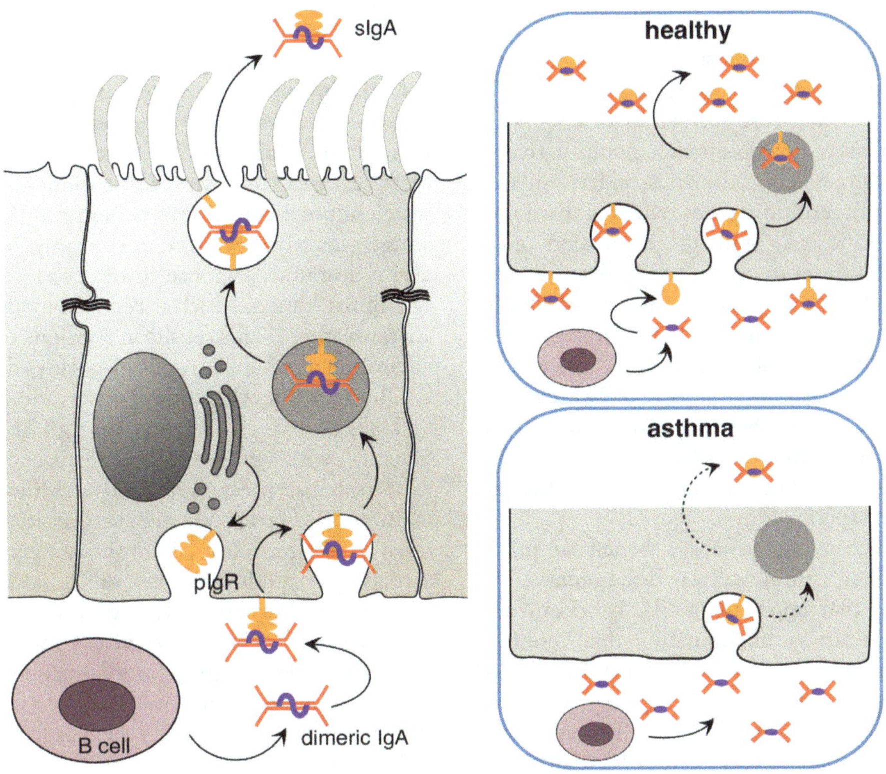

FIGURE 2 | Release of immunoglobulin A at epithelial surfaces. Dimeric IgA is released submucosally by B cells and binds to the poly Ig receptor (pIgR) which is found in high amounts in the basolateral membrane of the epithelium in the healthy state. The complex of pIgR and dimeric IgA is transported in secretory vesicles to the apical side, where it is released into the lumen as secreted IgA (sIgA) to bind target antigens/allergens/pathogens and entrap them in mucus. In the asthmatic state, the amount of pIgR in the epithelium appears to be reduced, resulting in diminished secretion of sIgA and futile accumulation of IgA in the subepithelial compartment.

extension of its hinge region. It is believed that this hinge region also serves as a ligand for yet other IgA receptors (163). If this holds true, subclass switching may be another adjusting wheel for IgA function. The class switch from IgA1 to IgA2 depends on the presence of the cytokines APRIL and BAFF which were shown to be produced by the epithelial layer itself, at least in case of the gut, upon bacterial stimulation (175). This way the microbiome as sparring partner of the epithelium comes into play as the true master of this adjusting wheel. In contrast to the gut where IgA2 prevails, IgA1 is the predominant IgA subclass in the airways (176). This, however, does not imply that IgA2 is of less importance for airway defense. IgA1 simply may be the first class formed after pathogen challenge. Those initial secretory IgA (sIgA) responses are believed to be not very mature. Upon pathogen challenge the human body apparently rapidly switches its current IgM repertoire to IgA even if most of such "first line of defense" IgA are of low affinity (177). This can be regarded as just a "better than nothing" attempt; yet it creates a window of opportunity for the body to develop more powerful sIgA via affinity maturation. Such optimized immunological scavengers are then able to block and eventually clear a microbial infection. Thus, the IgA system in which the transporting epithelium plays a key role is a complex defense machinery that combines innate with adaptive immune responses. It is therefore not surprising that the role of secretory IgA attracted attention in asthma research in recent years.

sIgA IN CHRONIC INFLAMMATION OF THE LUNG

The role of sIgA in chronic inflammatory lung diseases is still ambiguous. Some studies show that sIgA is necessary to maintain immune homeostasis, other reports claim that sIgA may play a detrimental role in asthma. A harmful effect of IgA in asthma may be explained by its ability to activate eosinophils and neutrophils because both cell types play a central role in the pathogenesis and persistence of asthma (178). When IgA is able to activate those cell types, this would readily lead to the hypothesis that in case of allergic asthma, allergen-specific IgA is responsible for this activation upon allergen exposure. This assumption is supported by the finding that increased levels of both, allergen-specific IgE and IgA were observed in the airway mucosa of patients with atopic asthma and/or rhinitis (179–183), and it was shown that allergen-specific IgA levels were positively correlated to eosinophil activation marker release after segmental lung challenge of asthmatic patients (166). Yet, coincidence and correlation do not necessarily imply a causative relationship.

In the abovementioned study, where a positive correlation of allergen-specific IgA and eosinophil activation was observed, the non-allergic control patients also displayed allergen-specific IgA in their airways; but in contrast, they did not have any allergen-specific IgE as was the case for asthmatics. Either so the allergen-specific IgE was responsible for eosinophil activation in asthmatics or the eosinophils of asthmatics underwent some kind of imprinting or immune training that rendered them more sensitive to allergen-specific IgA. With the expression of five different IgA receptors on the eosinophil described so far (163), locked-in differences in IgA receptor expression in eosinophils of asthmatics versus healthy individuals are not impossible. On the other hand, a coincidence of allergen-specific IgA and IgE does not necessarily imply a pathological role of IgA either. It may still be the case that IgA are beneficial to chronic airway inflammation, and the concomitant production of allergen-specific IgA can also be interpreted as a rescue attempt of the body to counteract the allergen-specific IgE.

In fact, more evidence points toward a beneficial role of IgA in asthma and other chronic airway inflammations. It was shown for instance that upon aging IgA knockout mice tend to develop chronic airway inflammation that resembles chronic obstructive pulmonary disease (COPD) in humans (184). A COPD-like phenotype also develops in pIgR knockout mice upon exogenous bacterial challenge (185), and it has been shown in the past that COPD patients have an impaired pIgR expression (186) and reduced sIgA levels on the airway epithelium (187). Recently a similar phenomenon was reported for asthma (188) and rhinosinusitis (189). In the study of Ladjemi et al., asthmatics show a reduced immunostaining of pIgR in airway epithelia, with IL-4 and IL-13 being the suppressors of pIgR formation in the airway epithelium. Notably, there were no significant differences in the pIgR gene expression rate among asthmatics and healthy individuals (188). Thus, a posttranslational event such as proteolytic degradation of pIgR in the epithelium may be responsible for the observed differences.

A beneficial effect of allergen-specific IgA in the airway lumen was highlighted by Schwarze et al. (190). They showed that local application of a human monoclonal IgA antibody directed against the ragweed allergen Amb a attenuated the proinflammatory response to allergen inhalation in mice sensitized to Amb a I, whereas a control IgA against ovalbumin did not. Notably, the instilled anti-ragweed IgA induced the formation of Amb a I-specific IgG2a in the animals upon allergen challenge which indicates a shift toward Th1. Thus, IgA residing in the airways may have an anti-allergic/anti-asthmatic immunomodulatory activity. This effect may be explained by the IgA feedback loop, via which a secretory IgA response is adjusted to current needs. In order to provide an optimal defense against luminal noxa luminal IgA are continuously sampled at the epithelium and transported to the basolateral side, where it is inspected by immune cells whether it is loaded with antigen or not. If this is the case, an immune response is mounted or boosted (191). Although this type of transcytotic event has been attributed primarily to M cells, the set-up of the ragweed-study rather precludes that route in this specific case in as much as a human IgA1 against Amb a I was used and this type of IgA does not bind to murine M cells (172). However, with a plethora of IgA receptors known, other epithelial cell types may have taken over the task. The IgA-binding transferrin receptor, for instance, is expressed by type II pneumocytes and was shown to transport transferrin conjugates to the basolateral site (192). In addition, similar to the gut, airway dendritic cells, which also carry IgA receptors, send protrusions to the epithelial layer via which luminal antigen can be sampled (193, 194). Yet, sampling antigen-loaded IgA from the airway lumen and driving the airway immune response toward Th1 requires the presence of IgA in the lumen, which is reduced by the Th2 micro-milieu in allergic asthma. This results in a vicious circle of a locked-in Th2 environment where a lack of IgA causes a further lack of IgA.

This is in line with clinical observations on asthmatic patients that suggests a critical role for IgA in asthma pathogenesis. Patients with selective IgA deficiency tend to bronchial hyperresponsiveness (195) and children that show a delay in maturation of IgA production display atopic manifestations more often (196). Moreover, immunotherapy against the respective aeroallergen result in higher specific mucosal IgA levels along with lower skin prick test sensitivity (197) or lower airway hyperreactivity (198). Nevertheless, most of the above suggests a prominent role of sIgA or, more precisely, the lack thereof in the pathogenesis and chronicity of atopic asthma. Whether a lack of sIgA also plays a prominent role in asthma exacerbations remains to be elucidated.

THE AIRWAY EPITHELIUM AS MEDIATOR OF AN ACUTE INFLAMMATORY REACTION

In addition to all the homeostatic defense functions like the maintenance of barrier integrity, transcytosis, and the mucosal clearance the airway epithelium also plays a major role against inhaled materials by producing several defense proteins such as mucins, defensins, antimicrobial peptides, cytokines, and chemokines (199). Thus, it contributes to local acute inflammatory reactions by regulating early inflammatory events via transcription and secretion of antimicrobial and pro-inflammatory proteins and by activating of mucin production (200, 201). Consequently, it is also a critical player during sensitization processes, asthma pathogenesis and acute exacerbations of the established disease (**Figure 3**).

DANGER AND PATHOGEN ASSOCIATED MOLECULAR PATTERN (DAMP AND PAMP) RECOGNITION BY PATTERN RECOGNITION RECEPTORS (PRR) OF THE AIRWAY EPITHELIUM

Inhaled pathogens that are not cleared by MCC are recognized by airway epithelial cells (202). Equipped with a large number of PRRs such as cytoplasmic NOD like receptors (NLR) and transmembrane toll like receptors (TLR) that can respond to

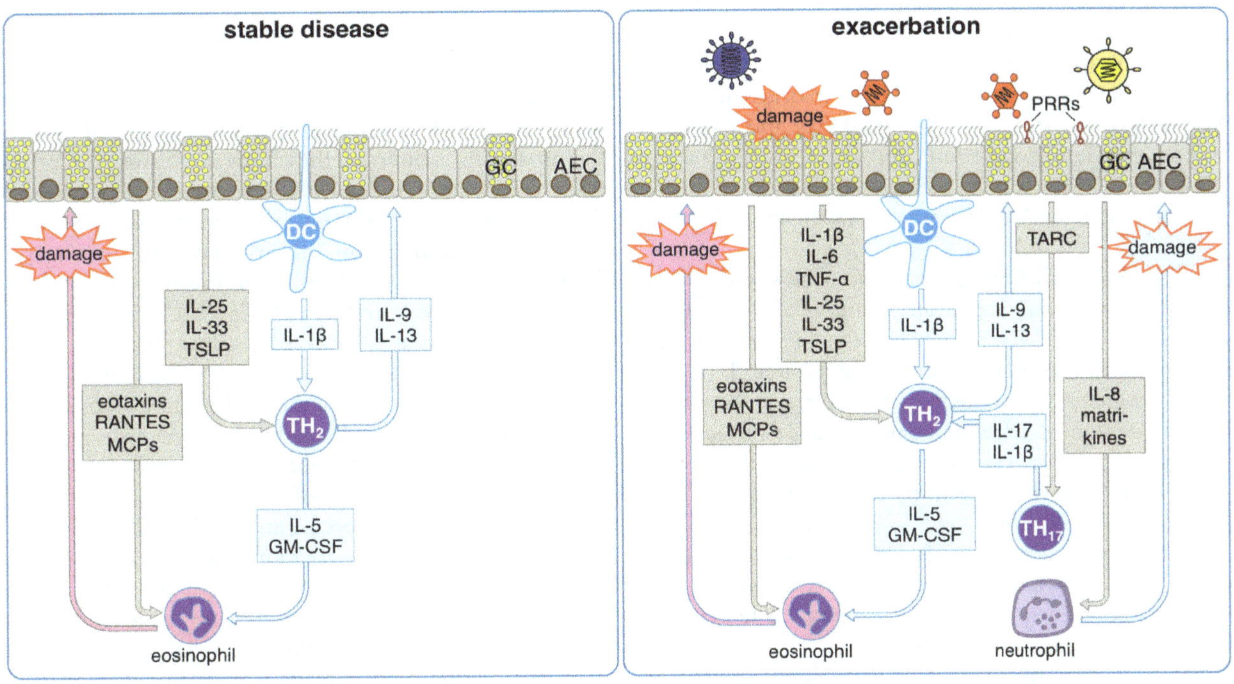

FIGURE 3 | Inflammatory response of the airway epithelium during stable allergic asthma and exacerbation. During stable allergic asthma airway epithelial cells (AECs) release IL-25, IL-33 and TSLP supporting differentiation of T helper (TH) 2 cells that are activated by dendritic cells (DCs). Th2 cells in turn secrete IL-5 and GM-CSF that together with AEC-derived eotaxins, RANTES and MCPs regulate the production, maturation, recruitment and activation of eosinophils. Local degranulation of eosinophils in the lung eventually leads to damage of the airway epithelium. In parallel, the TH2-type cytokines IL-9 and IL-13 induce goblet cell (GC) metaplasia in airway epithelium. During viral induced asthma exacerbations, several other additional factors lead to an aggravation of this inflammatory response. Viral infection can be detected by the airway epithelium via pattern recognition receptors (PRR). Subsequently, AECs secrete on the one hand TARC, the main chemokine for the recruitment of Th17 cells that amplifies the proinflammatory effects of Th2 cells via release of IL-17, and on the other hand IL-8, which leads to the recruitment of neutrophils. Local degranulation of neutrophils in the lung eventually leads to additional damage of the airway epithelium. Viral infection of AECs also directly leads to damage of the airway epithelium. In summary, these conditions result in a markedly increased damage of the airway epithelium compared to the stable disease, which further impairs barrier integrity and leads to release of matrikines further amplifying the ongoing inflammation.

DAMPs and PAMPs AECs represent the first line of cells, which can respond to pathogens and other danger signals like cell stress and cell death in the lung (203).

DAMPs are molecules that are release from injured cells. Their presence is a clear sign for the loss of homeostatic integrity of specific cell compartments or even whole cells. Hence, they originate from the cytoplasm (S100 proteins, heat shock proteins, defensins, galectins, uric acid), the nucleus (High-Mobility-Group-Protein (HMGB1)), the endoplasmic reticulum (calreticulin), mitochondria (ATP, mitochondrial DNA, N-formylated peptides) or from the extracellular matrix (fibronectin, hyaluronan, versican) (204). Airway epithelial cells are both, responder to and producer of DAMPs (205, 206). The DNA binding protein HMGB1 for example, set free during necrosis of one cell can be detected from nearby cells by binding to their receptor AGE (RAGE), which leads to activation of nuclear factor kappa b (NFκB) and thereby to the production of pro-inflammatory mediators and consequently the recruitment of immune cells.

In turn, PAMPs are preserved molecules and structures from pathogens and toxins. They can originate from such different sources as bacteria, mycobacteria, viruses, fungi and parasites (207).

PAMPs and DAMPs activate signaling pathways resulting in the transcription and production of cytokines and chemokines. In brief, signal transduction through MyD88 and MyD88-independent mechanisms leads to the activation of NFκB, mitogen-activated protein (MAP) kinases, and interferon regulatory factor (IRF) 3 (203). Based on the nature of the triggering PAMPs and DAMPs and a possible preexisting inflammatory environment in the lung its signals can result in protective effects or pathological effects for the host organism (208). Repeated cell stress and exposure to pathogens trigger chronic activation of PRR pathways in airway epithelial cells that are highly active and play an important role in chronic airways diseases (204).

PRR-TRIGGERED CYTOKINE AND CHEMOKINE REACTION OF THE AIRWAY EPITHELIUM

Activation of PRRs by DAMPs leads to a massive secretion of proinflammatory mediators like IL-6, CXCL8, TNF that consequently entail infiltration of activated immune cells. Some of these cells like dendritic cells (DC), lymphocytes and mast cells are also involved in the pathogenesis of asthma (204, 209, 210). After contact for example with HDM extracts, representing a major source of asthma associated allergens, TLR4 dependent activation of NFκB and protease induced injuries in airway epithelial cells lead to secretion of chemokines and cytokines like thymic stromal lymphopoietin (TSLP), GM-CSF, IL-25, and IL-33 (211–215). This results in the activation and infiltration of DCs, innate lymphoid cells type 2 (ILC2) and Th2 cells (216–218).

During infection with bacterial pathogens airway epithelial cells can sense bacterial cell wall components via TLR2 (recognizing e.g., LTA), TLR4 (recognizing e.g., LPS), nucleotide-binding oligomerization domain-containing protein 1 (Nod1) and Nod2 (recognizing peptidoglycans) leading to activation of NFκB and subsequent immune responses and consequently to regulation of bacterial clearance (219, 220). Nucleic acid patterns arising during viral infection can be sensed via TLR3, TLR7/8, retinoic acid inducible gene I (RIG-1), and melanoma differentiation-associated protein 5 (MDA-5) (221–225). In response to TLR activation airway epithelial cells can also produce antimicrobial peptides such as human β-Defensin 2 (HBD-2) after TLR2 activation (201, 226).

The signals of different PRRs like TLRs, NLRs, and RAGE cooperate to regulate cellular immune responses to cell stress, infection and inflammation, which can amplify or dampen their effects (227).

Airway epithelial cells are very potent producers of cytokines and chemokines. The presence of aggressors like toxins and pathogens leads to production and fast and early secretion of IL-1β, IL-6, TNF, CXCL8, CCL11, and CCL20 (202, 228–230). Thereby, airway epithelial cells regulate and orchestrate local immunity by interacting with the recruitment of DCs, T-cells, and B-cells (CCL20), eosinophils (CCL11), and neutrophils (CXCL8). During viral infections they constitutively produce IFNβ to reduce viral replication and to support epithelial apoptosis (231). Thereby, airway epithelial cells represent the frontline of antiviral defense mechanisms. As mentioned earlier, increased concentrations of proinflammatory cytokines like IL-1β, IL-4, IL-13, and TNF can directly lead to damage of the barrier function of the airway epithelium (44–47, 232, 233).

In allergic asthma airway epithelial cells are one of the main producers of proinflammatory cytokines and chemokines like IL-13, IL-33, TSLP, CCL5 (Rantes), CCL7 (MCP-3), CCL17 (TARC), CCL22, and several eotaxins. All of these cytokines strongly direct or support the development of a Th2 polarized inflammation (234). The chemokines CCL17 and CCL22 play a prominent role in the recruitment of Th2 cells by binding to the CCR4 receptor, since activation of it is a key event for Th2 cell specific chemoattraction (235, 236). As a highly potent producer of TSLP the airway epithelium can create a local micro-milieu that supports and maintains a Th2 polarized inflammation (234, 237). In response to different epithelial injuries, airway epithelial cells secrete so-called alarmins like TSLP, IL-25, and IL-33 that direct T helper cell differentiation toward an Th2 phenotype (238). Additionally, secreted GM-CSF from airway epithelial cells leads to maturation and survival of eosinophils (239–241). Both effects are supporting allergic inflammation in asthma.

Taken together the airway epithelium plays a major role for the recognition of PAMPs and DAMPs in the lung. Binding of these molecules to their respective receptors enables the airway epithelium to regulate pathways important for barrier function, MCC and local immune responses. Functional disorders of the airway epithelium in the ability to answer the presence of PAMPs and DAMPs favor the development of chronic airways diseases. Viral infections and exposure to bacteria in early life modulate the acquisition of Th1 and Th2 immunity during further development and influence the responses to following exposures. These effects could play an even greater role in patients with asthma since they show disrupted MCC that could amplify the disease morbidity (242, 243). A cytokine induced Th2 polarization of the epithelium in combination with a barrier dysfunction induced by the same cytokines augments barrier impairment, further infiltration of proinflammatory cells, and enhanced penetration of inhaled allergens, which can be described as a self-reinforcing mechanism that predisposes for the development and perpetuation of allergic asthma (244–246).

Consequently, it has been suggested that an abnormal programming of the airway epithelium in general paired with an impaired capability to produce anti-inflammatory mediators such as IL-37 or α melanocyte stimulating hormone (α-MSH) may be the origin of chronic inflammatory airway diseases (247, 248).

THE AIRWAY EPITHELIUM IN VIRAL EXACERBATIONS OF ASTHMA

Viral infections of the airways is of critical importance for the pathogenesis of allergic bronchial asthma: On the one hand recurrent respiratory viral infections during early childhood represent one of the strongest factors increasing the risk for the development of asthma in later life (249–253). On the other hand such infections are by far the most common cause for acute exacerbation of already established asthma leading to acute aggravation of disease symptoms and necessitating increased medication, GP visits, and can lead to hospitalization and critical care measures under certain conditions (254). Indeed, the airway epithelium is in the center of action during such an exacerbation, since it is not only the barrier that first comes into contact with viral pathogens, but its cells are also the target for their infection and the site of their replication. Thus, viral infection of the airway epithelium does not only impair the barrier integrity as already mentioned before, but also triggers the release of chemokines, cytokines, alarmins, and matrikines of the epithelial layer that affect the pre-existing inflammatory response in the asthmatic airway, which largely contributes to the formation of an acute exacerbation.

The viruses that have been implicated in asthma pathogenesis and especially the formation of acute exacerbation are HRV, RSV, influenza and parainfluenza viruses, human metapneumovirus, corona and adenoviruses, however, HRV infections appear to be the most common cause (255, 256). HRV is a non-enveloped, icosahedral virus, which belongs to the family of picornaviridae (genus enterovirus) and is subdivided into three clades (A, B, and C). The single-stranded positive RNA genome of HRV is constituted of ca. 7200 nucleotides (257, 258).

Clades A and B, which comprise the 100 most common serotypes, are further subdivided into a major and minor group. The major group utilizes the intracellular adhesion molecule-1 (ICAM-1) to bind to and transfect the host cell (259–261). The minor group HRV bind to the low density lipoprotein (LDL) receptor (262–265) and are considered to be more infectious. Clade C consists of 50 serotypes (266), which all bind to the cadherin-related family member 3 (CDHR3). All species of HRV have been shown to infect and replicate in airway epithelial cells (267).

Viral engagement with the specific receptor leads to transfection of the host cell (e.g., bronchial epithelial cells) and subsequently to a multitude of cellular responses. It is this cellular response that is believed to facilitate acute asthma exacerbation.

The cellular response to the virus is initiated by the detection of single-stranded RNA via TLRs -3, -7, and -8, MAD5, and RIG-I (221, 268). Activation of these receptors ultimately leads to the secretion of cytokines such as IL-1, IL-6, IL-8, IL-11, chemokines like CXCL10, CCL11 (eotaxin), CCL5 and anti-viral interferons of type I and III (268–274). The interferons have not only innate but also adaptive immune-system functionality to keep the viral infection locally at bay by mobilizing the adaptive immune response for effective viral clearance (275). Furthermore, proinflammatory cytokines like IL-1β and IL-6 are not specific for special types of immune response and thus, not only support the immune response against the invading virus but also promote the allergic immune response already established in the airways. Consequently, augmentation of the allergic immune response results in acute amplification of tissue damage, mucus production, and mediator release, and therefore in acute symptom aggravation.

Especially, the interferon response is thought to be an early post-infection event. In asthmatics epithelial interferon responses are believed to be hampered and as a consequence antiviral responses lack sufficient clearance (275). Not only interferons seem to be differently expressed in epithelial cells from asthmatics but also TSLP, which promotes Th2 responses (276). Another critical cytokine elevated in humans after HRV infections is IL-33, which also augments Th2 cell development (277).

AIRWAY REMODELING IS A FEATURE OF HUMAN RHINOVIRUS INFECTION

It is of note that viral infections not only initiate an immune response but also drive remodeling of the epithelial barrier and the subepithelial extracellular matrix (ECM). Hence, HRV16 induces perlecan, collagen V, tenascin c and matrix-associated (ma-) VEGF expression in an either TLR-3 or TLR-3/-7 associated manner *in vitro* (278, 279). Elevated expression of ma-VEGF and tenascin c was replicated in a mouse model of HRV infection, in which also Collagen I and fibronectin was found to be increased (278, 279). In addition, our group found human nasal epithelial cells infected with RV-16 *in vitro* to significantly downregulated genes associated with ECM receptor interaction and focal adhesion (280).

After infection and viral replication, the release of a vast array of mediators is among the earliest responses. In tissue culture a pneumocyte cell line expresses large amounts of IL-8 and CCL20 readily after 6 h post-infection (281). Also, the interferon response is thought to be an early post-infection event. In asthmatics epithelial interferon responses have been suggested to be hampered and as a consequence antiviral responses lack sufficient clearance (275). But not only interferons seem to be differently expressed in epithelial cells from asthmatics but also TSLP, which promotes Th2 responses (276). Another critical cytokine elevated in humans after HRV infections is IL-33. In line with that, Jackson et al. impressively showed, that the release of IL-33 by bronchial epithelial cells induces IL-4, IL-5, IL-13, and GATA3 expression in Th0 cells. An effect, which could be entirely blocked by an antibody against the IL-33 receptor (277).

Recently, active fragments from epithelial deposited ECM molecules have gained some recognition in asthma and asthma exacerbation. Matrikines are a class of molecules derived from ECM proteins (e.g., via proteolysis) with different properties from the parent molecule (282–284).

In 2010, Burgess et al. reported diminished levels of the collagen IV isoform alpha 3 (COL4A3) in airways from asthmatic subjects. The non-collagenous domain of COL4A3 is referred to as tumstatin and a biologically active matrikine. Treatment of mice with experimental allergic asthma with human recombinant tumstatin let to a significant reduction of hallmark disease features (e.g., airway hyperresponsiveness, ma-VEGF, eosinophil influx, IL13) (285). In another study, Van der Velden et al. identified an anti-angiogenic effect of tumstatin in a sheep model of asthma (286). Further investigations revealed a novel active region in Tumstatin (CP17), which significantly reduced neutrophil influx, mucus production in a mouse model of viral asthma exacerbation and reduced migrational speed and production of reactive oxygen species of neutrophils *in vitro* (287, 288). While the matrikine tumstatin conveys protection from experimental features of asthma and asthma exacerbation, a collagen I derived matrikine (PGP, Acetylated-(Ac) PGP) has been shown to be a more potent inducer of neutrophil chemotaxis then IL-8 and is found to be increased in severe asthmatics, a group of patients prone to develop exacerbations (283, 289).

Albeit ECM derived matrikines follow a different kinetical pathway (deposited first, released during inflammation) as compared to cytokines and chemokines (*de novo* production after viral infection), they can serve as protective or aggravating factors in asthma exacerbations.

In addition, the notion of epigenetic modification due to HRV infection in epithelial cells in asthma has gained attraction. McErlean et al. infected nasal epithelial cells from asthmatics and found evidence of reproducible changes to the methylome (290). We confirmed these results, which may unriddle how asthmatic airway epithelial cells may be able to respond differently to the same stimuli as compared to healthy epithelial cells (280). First studies to investigate this effect *in vivo* are underway (291, 292).

E2-POLARIZED AIRWAY EPITHELIUM

Infection associated stimuli appear not to be the only factors that imprint mucosal immune reactions of the airway epithelium. In addition, the interaction between epithelial cells and leukocytes can lead to sustained alteration of respiratory epithelial cell biology. Even though these cells are definitely not able to constitute an immunological memory, it becomes more and more obvious that especially epithelial cells somehow memorize their exposure to certain environmental factors and the following insults and thereby develop some kind of trained immunity. We are just at the beginning to understand these processes and questions of which parts of the epithelium are trained and of how long the training effects sustain in the mucosa remain to be answered.

Thus, respiratory epithelial cells are constantly exposed to many types of challenges, including pathogens, allergens and environmental pollutants. Consequently, they are able to respond quickly and effectively to cellular damage such as the local cytokine production, lateral transport by ion exchanges, wide arrays of mucus compositions, secretion of antimicrobial peptides, and epithelial shedding. To date, it appears possible that different inflammatory environments as originated by for example typical Th1- or Th2-directed immune responses have a different impact on the biology of the respiratory epithelium and lead to some kind of E1- or E2- polarization of the respective epithelial cells (293) (**Figure 4**).

There is *in vivo* evidence for the inhibitory role of IFN-γ on asthma pathogenesis at the epithelial level indicating that type-1 responses counteract allergy (294, 295). The direct implication of airway epithelial cells was demonstrated by selective transgenic expression of the IFN-γ receptor on the airway epithelium and showed that IFN-γ inhibits mucus secretion, release of chitinases and eosinophilia independent of the activation of Th2 cells (296). In turn, GATA-3 inhibition causes an increase of T-BET und IFN-γ expression levels, leading to a dampened allergic phenotype (297). In addition, an increase in DNA-methylation of IFN-γ was observed during allergic sensitization (298), while perinatal prevention of allergy mediated by *Acinetobacter* does not show the anticipated drop in H4 acetylation in the IFN-γ promoter (299). The immunological consequence of epithelial differentiation becomes increasingly interesting, as sensitization, but also recovery processes and airway remodeling could open new options for intervention and prevention of lung damage. Increasing evidence of mechanisms involving epithelial cytokine production such as CCL-26, and the epithelium-derived alarmins TSLP and IL-33 are substantiating the current focus on the cross talk between airway epithelium and immune cells in allergy research.

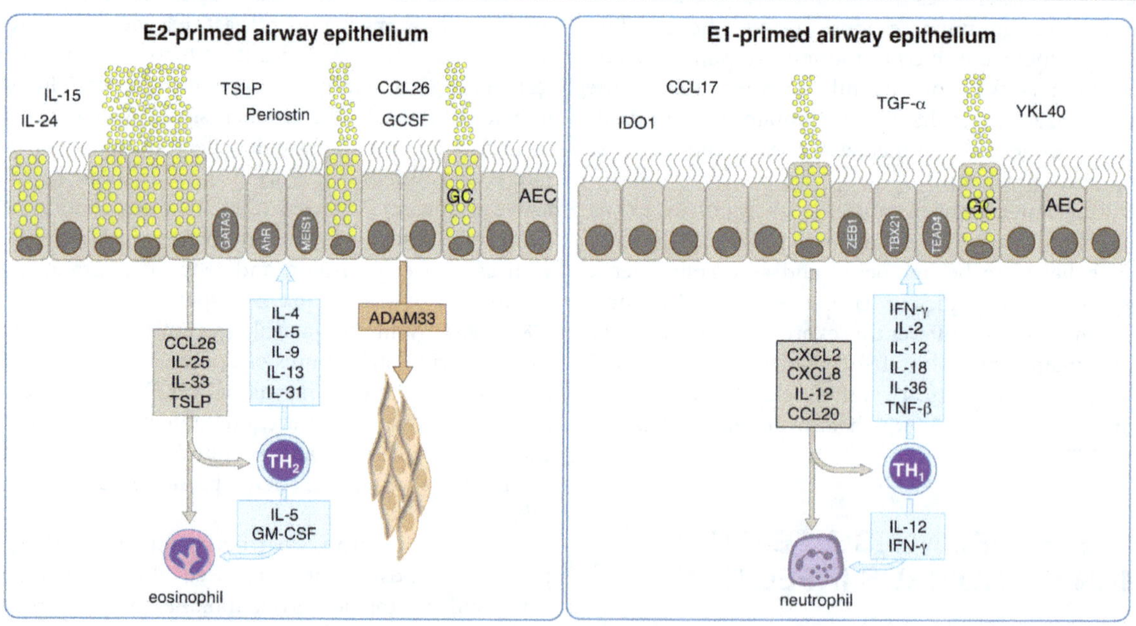

FIGURE 4 | Mechanisms of allergic inflammation in epithelial cells. The role of tissue cells in the early phase of disease is largely unknown, but could provide important information about the pathologic development and could help to identify the causal relationships. However, bronchial epithelial cells are pre-committed to a type-2 (E2) or type-1 (E1) like phenotype. E2 epithelial cell activation by allergens takes place and their pro-inflammatory cytokines and chemokines induce inflammation and contribute to an epithelial type-2 response, so called "E2 response" with epithelial alarmins TSLP, IL-31, CCL-26, IL-25, and IL-33. Local type-2 responses involve multiple cytokines such as IL-4, IL-5, IL-9, IL-13, IL-25, IL-33, and increase of eosinophils. A series of chemokines are produced and migration of inflammatory cells to the allergic tissues takes place. The activation of e.g., smooth muscle cells by ADAM33 lead to remodeling. Bronchial hyperreactivity takes place leading to an enhanced susceptibility to bronchoconstriction. E1 epithelial cells respond to an infection releasing CXCL2, CXCL8, IL12 and CCL20, thus stimulating the local synthesis of IFN-γ, IL-2, IL-12, IL-18, IL-36, and TNF-α that present a wide range of antiviral activities, inducing up-regulation of MHC-I molecules and antiviral resistance in uninfected cells. Neutrophils respond to the infection signals IL-12 and IFN-γ by releasing pro-inflammatory cytokines, leading to the containment of the infection, rise of body temperature and to the recruitment of further phagocytic cells.

However, it is unknown whether epithelial cells are influenced by IL-4 prior or with entry into terminal differentiation. This early influence could imprint the offspring cells that populate the epithelial surface and therefore have major consequences for the physiology of the airways. IL-4 was shown to have a major effect on the epithelium, as mice overexpressing this cytokine under the Club cell-secretory protein 10 (CC10) promoter show increased cellular infiltration, epithelial hypertrophy, mucus cell hyperplasia, secretion of gastric mucins and surfactant proteins (SP) A and B (300). While this model effectively demonstrated all hallmarks of experimental allergic asthma, it did not demonstrate whether IL-4 itself is inducing differentiation of basal cells or whether secondary effects trigger epithelial differentiation. However, the differentiation effects could also be observed in human primary epithelial cells of the nose, where IL-13 modulates the differentiation toward less ciliated and more secretory cells (114). To date, it is controversially discussed, whether IL-4 and IL-13 can also affect fully differentiated epithelial cells in air liquid-interphase cultures or whether this is only possible in immature submerged cultures (301, 302). However, during the epithelial differentiation process induced by air-liquid exposure, the addition of IL-4 enhances expression of certain antimicrobial peptides (303) and eicosanoids (304). Furthermore, it was demonstrated that IL-4 and IL-13, through inhibition of TLR3 expression and signaling (IRF3), impair immune responses to HRV infection (305). This is in line with the finding that chronic house dust mite exposure in the airways not only causes a strong Th2-directed inflammation but also diminishes anti-rhinovirus responses and local IFN expression, particularly of epithelial IFN-λ (306). In line with this, transgenic IL-4 expression in the lungs reduces cytotoxic T cell responses against Influenza viruses (307). On the level of secreted factors, it was shown that cytokines such as Wnt5a (Wingless-Type MMTV Integration Site Family, Member 5a) or IL-24 are expressed as response to IL-4 stimulation only, while proteins with known pathological roles such as the IL-4 induced protein CCL-26 or periostin were shown to be upregulated by IL-4 and down-regulated in IFN-γ environment. These results were consistent when comparing upper and lower airway secretions, thus confirming nasal lining fluids as a proxy for the lower respiratory tract, particularly for epithelial type-2 biomarker like CCL-26 and IL24 (308, 309). The E2-related transcription factor network contained the E2 hub-transcription factors *GATA3, NFE2, MEIS1, HEY2,* and *AHR*: *GATA3* is well known as the master transcription factor of type-2 response in immune cells, however it was also shown to be expressed in airway epithelial cells. *NFE2* was demonstrated to have a cytoprotective activity against epithelial cell injury by cigarette smoke, which could hint on a protective role in an IL-4 dominated micro-milieu (310). For *MEIS1,* it has been demonstrated that its inactivation produces an increase in airway smooth muscle mass and a corresponding decrease in cartilage and suggesting an important role in allergic airway diseases. A loss of Hox gene function, however, does not preclude airway repair, but regenerated epithelium displays goblet cell metaplasia and less SCGB1A1-positive cells, demonstrating the essential role of Hoxa5 for correct differentiation. This goblet cell metaplasia is further associated with increased Notch signaling activity. Consistent with these findings, expression levels of activated NOTCH1 and the effector gene HEY2 are in turn enhanced in patients with allergic disease (293, 311, 312). Taken together, E2-polarization has a marked impact on the barrier and especially immune functions of the airway epithelium and at least supports impairment of the MCC and antiviral responses, both factors that are critical in asthma pathogenesis.

CONCLUSION

In summary, the airway epithelium exerts a broad variety of immune functions that range from passive barrier over MCC, active production and transport of pathogen-neutralizing molecules to pathogen recognition and targeting as well as cytokine and chemokine release. The airway epithelium is usually the first tissue that is exposed to inhaled allergens, pathogens or pollutants. Since it is able to react on this contact by inducing local inflammatory reactions, it is clearly a central part of the local immune response and bridges innate and adaptive immune functions against all types of harmful intruders entering the respiratory system. Therefore, the airway epithelium is a key factor in asthma pathogenesis and plays a critical role in the development as well as in the progression and exacerbation of the disease: Hence, a disturbed cellular barrier enables allergens to enter the body and to induce a sensitization reaction, which is widely regarded as the starting point of an asthma career. Down the line, the protective mucus and PCL layers provided by the epithelium as physical barriers are compromised and the release of pathogen deterring molecules such as secretory Iimmunoglobulins becomes impaired. As a consequence, this frontline toward invading pathogens can be breached and airway epithelial cells are infected and even destroyed by respiratory pathogens. A vicious cycle is started where barrier disturbance and infection promote each other. The latter, in particular with certain viruses, is also one of the strongest factors predisposing toward asthma development in early childhood.

Once asthma has been established, the airway epithelium responds to further viral infection with the release of manifold factors promoting not only the antiviral response but also augmenting the already present allergic inflammation and thus promoting acute asthma exacerbations. Finally yet importantly, it is also impaired and polarized by products released from cells of the chronified allergic immune response in the airways, which leads to impairment of mucus production, MCC, and the anti-inflammatory IFN-response in E2-polarized airway epithelial cells. Recent studies indicate that, in addition to this E2-polarization, also the history of allergy- and pathogen-derived insults does not only have a transient effect on the airway epithelium, but leaves some kind of memory in these cells that can be described as "imprinting" or "trained immunity." Understanding the mechanisms underlying these processes would not only help to further understand the key role of airway epithelial cells in asthma pathogenesis but also could identify new targets for the treatment or even prevention of allergic asthma.

AUTHOR CONTRIBUTIONS

All authors listed have made a substantial, direct and intellectual contribution to the work, and approved it for publication.

REFERENCES

1. Network GA. *The Global Asthma Report 2018*. Auckland: Global Asthma Network (2018).
2. Gibson GJ, Loddenkemper R, Lundbäck B, Sibille Y. Respiratory health and disease in Europe: the new European Lung white book. *Eur Respir J.* (2013) 42:559–63.
3. Nunes C, Pereira AM, Morais-Almeida M. Asthma costs and social impact. *Asthma Res Pract.* (2017) 3:1.
4. Nurmagambetov T, Kuwahara R, Garbe P. The economic burden of asthma in the United States, 2008-2013. *Ann Am Thorac Soc.* (2018) 15:348–56.
5. Eder W, Ege MJ, von Mutius E. The asthma epidemic. *N Engl J Med.* (2006) 355:2226–35.
6. Taylor DR, Bateman, Boulet L-P, Boushey HA, Busse WW, Casale TB, et al. A new perspective on concepts of asthma severity and control. *Eur Respir J.* (2008) 32:545–54.
7. Peters MC, Mekonnen ZK, Yuan S, Bhakta NR, Woodruff PG, Fahy JV. Measures of gene expression in sputum cells can identify TH2-high and TH2-low subtypes of asthma. *J Allergy Clin Immunol.* (2014) 133:388–94.
8. Papi A, Brightling C, Pedersen SE, Reddel HK. Asthma. *Lancet.* (2018) 391:783–800.
9. Fehrenbach H, Wagner C, Wegmann M. Airway remodeling in asthma: what really matters. *Cell Tissue Res.* (2017) 367:551–69.
10. Gon Y, Hashimoto S. Role of airway epithelial barrier dysfunction in pathogenesis of asthma. *Allergol Int.* (2018) 67:12–7.
11. Garcia MA, Nelson WJ, Chavez N. Cell-cell junctions organize structural and signaling networks. *Cold Spring Harb Perspect Biol.* (2018) 10:029181. doi: 10.1101/cshperspect.a029181
12. Walko G, Castañón MJ, Wiche G. Molecular architecture and function of the hemidesmosome. *Cell Tissue Res.* (2015) 360:363–78.
13. Buckley A, Turner JR. Cell biology of tight junction barrier regulation and mucosal disease. *Cold Spring Harb Perspect Biol.* (2018) 10:29314. doi: 10. 1101/cshperspect.a029314
14. Chanez P, Bourdin A. Pathophysiology of Asthma. *Clinical Asthma.* (2008) 7:23–34. doi: 10.1016/b978-032304289-5 10003-7
15. Yoshihara S, Yamada Y, Abe T, Lindén A, Arisaka O. Association of epithelial damage and signs of neutrophil mobilization in the airways during acute exacerbations of paediatric asthma. *Clin Exp Immunol.* (2006) 144:212–6.
16. Xiao C, Puddicombe SM, Field S, Haywood J, Broughton-Head V, Puxeddu I, et al. Defective epithelial barrier function in asthma. *J Allergy Clin Immunol.* (2011) 128:549–56.
17. de Boer WI, Sharma HS, Baelemans SMI, Hoogsteden HC, Lambrecht BN, Braunstahl GJ. Altered expression of epithelial junctional proteins in atopic asthma: possible role in inflammation. *Can J Physiol Pharmacol.* (2008) 86:105–12.
18. Hackett T-L, de Bruin HG, Shaheen F, van den Berge M, van Oosterhout AJ, Postma DS, et al. Caveolin-1 controls airway epithelial barrier function. Implications for asthma. *Am J Respir Cell Mol Biol.* (2013) 49:662–71.
19. Hackett T-L, Singhera GK, Shaheen F, Hayden P, Jackson GR, Hegele RG, et al. Intrinsic phenotypic differences of asthmatic epithelium and its inflammatory responses to respiratory syncytial virus and air pollution. *Am J Respir Cell Mol Biol.* (2011) 45:1090–100.
20. Masuyama K, Morishima Y, Ishii Y, Nomura A, Sakamoto T, Kimura T, et al. Sputum E-cadherin and asthma severity. *J Allergy Clin Immunol.* (2003) 112:208–9.
21. Rezaee F, Georas SN. Breaking barriers. New insights into airway epithelial barrier function in health and disease. *Am J Respir Cell Mol Biol.* (2014) 50:857–69.
22. Blume C, Swindle EJ, Dennison P, Jayasekera NP, Dudley S, Monk P, et al. Barrier responses of human bronchial epithelial cells to grass pollen exposure. *Eur Respir J.* (2013) 42:87–97. doi: 10.1183/09031936.00075612
23. Post S, Nawijn MC, Jonker MR, Kliphuis N, van den Berge M, van Oosterhout AJM, et al. House dust mite-induced calcium signaling instigates epithelial barrier dysfunction and CCL20 production. *Allergy.* (2013) 68:1117–25.
24. Wan H, Winton HL, Soeller C, Gruenert DC, Thompson PJ, Cannell MB, et al. Quantitative structural and biochemical analyses of tight junction dynamics following exposure of epithelial cells to house dust mite allergen Der p 1. *Clin Exp Allergy.* (2000) 30:685–98.
25. Wan H, Winton HL, Soeller C, Tovey ER, Gruenert DC, Thompson PJ, et al. Der p 1 facilitates transepithelial allergen delivery by disruption of tight junctions. *J Clin Invest.* (1999) 104:123–33.
26. Heijink IH, Brandenburg SM, Noordhoek JA, Postma DS, Slebos D-J, van Oosterhout AJM. Characterisation of cell adhesion in airway epithelial cell types using electric cell-substrate impedance sensing. *Eur Respir J.* (2010) 35:894–903. doi: 10.1183/09031936.00065809
27. Leino MS, Loxham M, Blume C, Swindle EJ, Jayasekera NP, Dennison PW, et al. Barrier disrupting effects of alternaria alternata extract on bronchial epithelium from asthmatic donors. *PLoS One.* (2013) 8:e71278. doi: 10.1371/ journal.pone.0071278
28. Balenga NA, Klichinsky M, Xie Z, Chan EC, Zhao M, Jude J, et al. A fungal protease allergen provokes airway hyper-responsiveness in asthma. *Nat Commun.* (2015) 6:6763.
29. Vinhas R, Cortes L, Cardoso I, Mendes VM, Manadas B, Todo-Bom A, et al. Pollen proteases compromise the airway epithelial barrier through degradation of transmembrane adhesion proteins and lung bioactive peptides. *Allergy.* (2011) 66:1088–98.
30. Lee SI, Pham LD, Shin YS, Suh DH, Park H-S. Environmental changes could enhance the biological effect of Hop J pollens on human airway epithelial cells. *J Allergy Clin Immunol.* (2014) 134:470–2.
31. Runswick S, Mitchell T, Davies P, Robinson C, Garrod DR. Pollen proteolytic enzymes degrade tight junctions. *Respirology.* (2007) 12:834–42.
32. Winter MC, Shasby SS, Ries DR, Shasby DM. PAR2 activation interrupts E-cadherin adhesion and compromises the airway epithelial barrier: protective effect of beta-agonists. *Am J Physiol Lung Cell Mol Physiol.* (2006) 291:L628–35.
33. Jacquet A. Interactions of airway epithelium with protease allergens in the allergic response. *Clin Exp Allergy.* (2011) 41:305–11.
34. Li B, Zou Z, Meng F, Raz E, Huang Y, Tao A, et al. Dust mite-derived Der f 3 activates a pro-inflammatory program in airway epithelial cells via PAR-1 and PAR-2. *Mol Immunol.* (2019) 109:1–11. doi: 10.1016/j.molimm.2019.02.018
35. Nam HH, Ison MG. Respiratory syncytial virus infection in adults. *BMJ.* (2019) 366:l5021. doi: 10.1136/bmj.l5021
36. Soto JA, Gálvez NMS, Benavente FM, Pizarro-Ortega MS, Lay MK, Riedel C, et al. Human Metapneumovirus: mechanisms and molecular targets used by the virus to avoid the immune system. *Front Immunol.* (2018) 9:2466.
37. Singh D, McCann KL, Imani F. MAPK and heat shock protein 27 activation are associated with respiratory syncytial virus induction of human bronchial epithelial monolayer disruption. *Am J Physiol Lung Cell Mol Physiol.* (2007) 293:L436–45.
38. Comstock AT, Ganesan S, Chattoraj A, Faris AN, Margolis BL, Hershenson MB, et al. Rhinovirus-induced barrier dysfunction in polarized airway epithelial cells is mediated by NADPH oxidase 1. *J Virol.* (2011) 85:6795–808.
39. Faris AN, Ganesan S, Chattoraj A, Chattoraj SS, Comstock AT, Unger BL, et al. Rhinovirus delays cell repolarization in a model of injured/regenerating human airway epithelium. *Am J Respir Cell Mol Biol.* (2016) 55:487–99.
40. Looi K, Troy NM, Garratt LW, Iosifidis T, Bosco A, Buckley AG, et al. Effect of human rhinovirus infection on airway epithelium tight junction protein disassembly and transepithelial permeability. *Exp Lung Res.* (2016) 42:380–95.
41. Rezaee F, DeSando SA, Ivanov AI, Chapman TJ, Knowlden SA, Beck LA, et al. Sustained protein kinase D activation mediates respiratory syncytial virus-induced airway barrier disruption. *J Virol.* (2013) 87:11088–95.

42. Sajjan U, Wang Q, Zhao Y, Gruenert DC, Hershenson MB. Rhinovirus disrupts the barrier function of polarized airway epithelial cells. *Am J Respir Crit Care Med.* (2008) 178:1271–81.
43. Rezaee F, Meednu N, Emo JA, Saatian B, Chapman TJ, Naydenov NG, et al. Polyinosinic:polycytidylic acid induces protein kinase D-dependent disassembly of apical junctions and barrier dysfunction in airway epithelial cells. *J Allergy Clin Immunol.* (2011) 128:1216–24.e11.
44. Coyne CB, Vanhook MK, Gambling TM, Carson JL, Boucher RC, Johnson LG. Regulation of airway tight junctions by proinflammatory cytokines. *Mol Biol Cell.* (2002) 13:3218–34.
45. Soyka MB, Wawrzyniak P, Eiwegger T, Holzmann D, Treis A, Wanke K, et al. Defective epithelial barrier in chronic rhinosinusitis: the regulation of tight junctions by IFN-γ and IL-4. *J Allergy Clin Immunol.* (2012) 130:1087–96.e10.
46. Hardyman MA, Wilkinson E, Martin E, Jayasekera NP, Blume C, Swindle EJ, et al. TNF-α-mediated bronchial barrier disruption and regulation by src-family kinase activation. *J Allergy Clin Immunol.* (2013) 132:665–75.e8.
47. Saatian B, Rezaee F, Desando S, Emo J, Chapman T, Knowlden S, et al. Interleukin-4 and interleukin-13 cause barrier dysfunction in human airway epithelial cells. *Tissue Barriers.* (2013) 1:e24333. doi: 10.4161/tisb.24333
48. Zabner J, Winter M, Excoffon KJDA, Stoltz D, Ries D, Shasby S, et al. Histamine alters E-cadherin cell adhesion to increase human airway epithelial permeability. *J Appl Physiol.* (2003) 95:394–401. doi: 10.1152/japplphysiol.01134.2002
49. Ramaker K, Bade S, Röckendorf N, Meckelein B, Vollmer E, Schultz H, et al. Absence of the epithelial glycocalyx as potential tumor marker for the early detection of colorectal cancer. *PLoS One.* (2016) 11:e0168801. doi: 10.1371/journal.pone.0168801
50. Mehta D, Ravindran K, Kuebler WM. Novel regulators of endothelial barrier function. *Am J Physiol Lung Cell Mol Physiol.* (2014) 307:L924–35.
51. Van Teeffelen JW, Brands J, Stroes ES, Vink H. Endothelial glycocalyx: sweet shield of blood vessels. *Trends Cardiovasc Med.* (2007) 17:101–5.
52. Haeger SM, Liu X, Han X, McNeil JB, Oshima K, McMurtry SA, et al. Epithelial heparan sulfate contributes to alveolar barrier function and is shed during lung injury. *Am J Respir Cell Mol Biol.* (2018) 59:363–74.
53. Kesimer M, Ehre C, Burns KA, Davis CW, Sheehan JK, Pickles RJ. Molecular organization of the mucins and glycocalyx underlying mucus transport over mucosal surfaces of the airways. *Mucosal Immunol.* (2013) 6:379–92.
54. Button B, Cai L-H, Ehre C, Kesimer M, Hill DB, Sheehan JK, et al. A periciliary brush promotes the lung health by separating the mucus layer from airway epithelia. *Science.* (2012) 337:937–41.
55. Frey A, Giannasca KT, Weltzin R, Giannasca PJ, Reggio H, Lencer WI, et al. Role of the glycocalyx in regulating access of microparticles to apical plasma membranes of intestinal epithelial cells: implications for microbial attachment and oral vaccine targeting. *J Exp Med.* (1996) 184:1045–59.
56. Pickles RJ, Fahrner JA, Petrella JM, Boucher RC, Bergelson JM. Retargeting the coxsackievirus and adenovirus receptor to the apical surface of polarized epithelial cells reveals the glycocalyx as a barrier to adenovirus-mediated gene transfer. *J Virol.* (2000) 74:6050–7.
57. Stonebraker JR, Wagner D, Lefensty RW, Burns K, Gendler SJ, Bergelson JM, et al. Glycocalyx restricts adenoviral vector access to apical receptors expressed on respiratory epithelium in vitro and in vivo: role for tethered mucins as barriers to lumenal infection. *J Virol.* (2004) 78:13755–68.
58. Qiu J, Söderlund-Venermo M, Young NS. Human Parvoviruses. *Clin Microbiol Rev.* (2017) 30:43–113.
59. Oliveira MA, Zhao R, Lee WM, Kremer MJ, Minor I, Rueckert RR, et al. The structure of human rhinovirus 16. *Structure.* (1993) 1:51–68.
60. Deng X, Yan Z, Luo Y, Xu J, Cheng F, Li Y, et al. In vitro modeling of human bocavirus 1 infection of polarized primary human airway epithelia. *J Virol.* (2013) 87:4097–102.
61. Deng X, Zou W, Xiong M, Wang Z, Engelhardt JF, Ye SQ, et al. Human parvovirus infection of human airway epithelia induces pyroptotic cell death by inhibiting apoptosis. *J Virol.* (2017) 91:e1533–1517. doi: 10.1128/JVI.01533-17
62. Jakiela B, Gielicz A, Plutecka H, Hubalewska-Mazgaj M, Mastalerz L, Bochenek G, et al. Th2-type cytokine-induced mucus metaplasia decreases susceptibility of human bronchial epithelium to rhinovirus infection. *Am J Respir Cell Mol Biol.* (2014) 51:229–41.
63. Griggs TF, Bochkov YA, Basnet S, Pasic TR, Brockman-Schneider RA, Palmenberg AC, et al. Rhinovirus C targets ciliated airway epithelial cells. *Respir Res.* (2017) 18:84.
64. Lamb RA, Choppin PW. The gene structure and replication of influenza virus. *Annu Rev Biochem.* (1983) 52:467–506. doi: 10.1146/annurev.bi.52.070183.002343
65. van den Hoogen BG, de Jong JC, Groen J, Kuiken T, de Groot R, Fouchier RA, et al. newly discovered human pneumovirus isolated from young children with respiratory tract disease. *Nat Med.* (2001) 7:719–24.
66. Bracken MK, Hayes BC, Kandel SR, Scott-Shemon D, Ackerson L, Hoffman MA. Viral protein requirements for assembly and release of human parainfluenza virus type 3 virus-like particles. *J Gen Virol.* (2016) 97:1305–10.
67. Ke Z, Dillard RS, Chirkova T, Leon F, Stobart CC, Hampton CM, et al. The morphology and assembly of respiratory syncytial virus revealed by cryo-electron tomography. *Viruses.* (2018) 10:446. doi: 10.3390/v10080446
68. McErlean P, Greiman A, Favoreto S Jr., Avila PC. Viral diversity in asthma. *Immunol Allergy Clin North Am.* (2010) 30:481–95.
69. Zheng X-Y, Xu Y-J, Guan W-J, Lin L-F. Regional, age and respiratory-secretion-specific prevalence of respiratory viruses associated with asthma exacerbation: a literature review. *Arch Virol.* (2018) 163:845–53.
70. Johnson SM, McNally BA, Ioannidis I, Flano E, Teng MN, Oomens AG, et al. Respiratory Syncytial Virus Uses CX3CR1 as a Receptor on Primary Human Airway Epithelial Cultures. *PLoS Pathog.* (2015) 11:e1005318. doi: 10.1371/journal.ppat.1005318
71. Anderson CS, Chu C-Y, Wang Q, Mereness JA, Ren Y, Donlon K, et al. CX3CR1 as a respiratory syncytial virus receptor in pediatric human lung. *Pediatr Res.* (2019) 87:862–7. doi: 10.1038/s41390-019-0677-0
72. Broccolo F, Falcone V, Esposito S, Toniolo A. Human bocaviruses: Possible etiologic role in respiratory infection. *J Clin Virol.* (2015) 72:75–81. doi: 10.1016/j.jcv.2015.09.008
73. Vallet C, Pons-Catalano C, Mandelcwajg A, Wang A, Raymond J, Lebon P, et al. Human bocavirus: a cause of severe asthma exacerbation in children. *J Pediatr.* (2009) 155:286–8.
74. Yoneda K, Walzer PD. The effect of corticosteroid treatment on the cell surface glycocalyx of the rat pulmonary alveolus: relevance to the host-parasite relationship in pneumocystis carinii infection. *Br J Exp Pathol.* (1984) 65:347–54.
75. Mariassy AT, Abraham WM, Wanner A. Effect of antigen on the glycoconjugate profile of tracheal secretions and the epithelial glycocalyx in allergic sheep. *J Allergy Clin Immunol.* (1994) 93:585–93.
76. Houtmeyers E, Gosselink R, Gayan-Ramirez G, Decramer M. Regulation of mucociliary clearance in health and disease. *Eur Respir J.* (1999) 13:1177–88.
77. Ernst M, John T, Guenther M, Wagner C, Schaefer UF, Lehr C-MA. Model for the transient subdiffusive behavior of particles in mucus. *Biophys J.* (2017) 112:172–9.
78. Lieleg O, Ribbeck K. Biological hydrogels as selective diffusion barriers. *Trends Cell Biol.* (2011) 21:543–51.
79. Hiemstra PS, Amatngalim GD, van der Does AM, Taube C. Antimicrobial peptides and innate lung defenses: role in infectious and noninfectious lung diseases and therapeutic applications. *Chest.* (2016) 149:545–51.
80. Renegar KB, Small PA Jr., Boykins LG, Wright PF. Role of IgA versus IgG in the control of influenza viral infection in the murine respiratory tract. *J Immunol.* (2004) 173:1978–86.
81. Jacquot J, Hayem A, Galabert C. Functions of proteins and lipids in airway secretions. *Eur Respir J.* (1992) 5:343–58.
82. Ridley C, Thornton DJ. Mucins: the frontline defence of the lung. *Biochem Soc Trans.* (2018) 46:1099–106.
83. Thornton DJ, Rousseau K, McGuckin MA. Structure and function of the polymeric mucins in airways mucus. *Annu Rev Physiol.* (2008) 70:459–86.
84. Gene group. *HUGO Gene Nomenclature Committee.* (2020) Available online at: https://www.genenames.org/data/genegroup/#!/group/648 (accessed January 15, 2020).
85. Hattrup CL, Gendler SJ. Structure and function of the cell surface (tethered) mucins. *Annu Rev Physiol.* (2008) 70:431–57.
86. Fahy JV, Dickey BF. Airway mucus function and dysfunction. *N Engl J Med.* (2010) 363:2233–47.

87. Dekker J, Rossen JWA, Büller HA, Einerhand AWC. The MUC family: an obituary. *Trends Biochem Sci.* (2002) 27:126–31.
88. Raclawska DS, Ttofali F, Fletcher AA, Harper DN, Bochner BS, Janssen WJ, et al. Mucins and Their Sugars. Critical Mediators of Hyperreactivity and Inflammation. *Ann Am Thorac Soc.* (2016) 13(Suppl. 1):S98–9.
89. Hovenberg HW, Davies JR, Carlstedt I. Different mucins are produced by the surface epithelium and the submucosa in human trachea: identification of MUC5AC as a major mucin from the goblet cells. *Biochem J.* (1996) 318(Pt 1):319–24.
90. Wickström C, Davies JR, Eriksen GV, Veerman EC, Carlstedt I. MUC5B is a major gel-forming, oligomeric mucin from human salivary gland, respiratory tract and endocervix: identification of glycoforms and C-terminal cleavage. *Biochem J.* (1998) 334(Pt 3):685–93.
91. Verdugo P. Mucin exocytosis. *Am Rev Respir Dis.* (1991) 144:S33–7.
92. Forstner G. Signal transduction, packaging and secretion of mucins. *Annu Rev Physiol.* (1995) 57:585–605. doi: 10.1146/annurev.ph.57.030195.003101
93. Ermund A, Meiss LN, Rodriguez-Pineiro AM, Bähr A, Nilsson HE, Trillo-Muyo S, et al. The normal trachea is cleaned by MUC5B mucin bundles from the submucosal glands coated with the MUC5AC mucin. *Biochem Biophys Res Commun.* (2017) 492:331–7.
94. Ostedgaard LS, Moninger TO, McMenimen JD, Sawin NM, Parker CP, Thornell IM, et al. Gel-forming mucins form distinct morphologic structures in airways. *Proc Natl Acad Sci USA.* (2017) 114:6842–7.
95. Bustamante-Marin XM, Ostrowski LE. Cilia and mucociliary clearance. *Cold Spring Harb Perspect Biol.* (2017) 9:a028241. doi: 10.1101/cshperspect.a028241
96. Bateman JR, Pavia D, Sheahan NF, Agnew JE, Clarke SW. Impaired tracheobronchial clearance in patients with mild stable asthma. *Thorax.* (1983) 38:463–7.
97. O'Riordan TG, Zwang J, Smaldone GC. Mucociliary clearance in adult asthma. *Am Rev Respir Dis.* (1992) 146:598–603. doi: 10.1164/ajrccm/146.3.598
98. Messina MS, O'Riordan TG, Smaldone GC. Changes in mucociliary clearance during acute exacerbations of asthma. *Am Rev Respir Dis.* (1991) 143:993–7.
99. Thomas B, Rutman A, Hirst RA, Haldar P, Wardlaw AJ, Bankart J, et al. Ciliary dysfunction and ultrastructural abnormalities are features of severe asthma. *J Allergy Clin Immunol.* (2010) 126:722–9.e2.
100. Innes AL, Carrington SD, Thornton DJ, Kirkham S, Rousseau K, Dougherty RH, et al. Ex vivo sputum analysis reveals impairment of protease-dependent mucus degradation by plasma proteins in acute asthma. *Am J Respir Crit Care Med.* (2009) 180:203–10.
101. Yuan S, Hollinger M, Lachowicz-Scroggins ME, Kerr SC, Dunican EM, Daniel BM, et al. Oxidation increases mucin polymer cross-links to stiffen airway mucus gels. *Sci Transl Med.* (2015) 7:276ra27. doi: 10.1126/scitranslmed.3010525
102. Dunican EM, Elicker BM, Gierada DS, Nagle SK, Schiebler ML, Newell JD, et al. Mucus plugs in patients with asthma linked to eosinophilia and airflow obstruction. *J Clin Invest.* (2018) 128:997–1009. doi: 10.1172/jci95693
103. Bonser LR, Zlock L, Finkbeiner W, Erle DJ. Epithelial tethering of MUC5AC-rich mucus impairs mucociliary transport in asthma. *J Clin Invest.* (2016) 126:2367–71.
104. Welsh KG, Rousseau K, Fisher G, Bonser LR, Bradding P, Brightling CE, et al. MUC5AC and a Glycosylated Variant of MUC5B Alter Mucin Composition in Children With Acute Asthma. *Chest.* (2017) 152:771–9.
105. Lachowicz-Scroggins ME, Yuan S, Kerr SC, Dunican EM, Yu M, Carrington SD, et al. Abnormalities in MUC5AC and MUC5B Protein in Airway Mucus in Asthma. *Am J Respir Crit Care Med.* (2016) 194:1296–9.
106. Roy MG, Livraghi-Butrico A, Fletcher AA, McElwee MM, Evans SE, Boerner RM, et al. Muc5b is required for airway defence. *Nature.* (2014) 505:412–6.
107. Kirkham S, Sheehan JK, Knight D, Richardson PS, Thornton DJ. Heterogeneity of airways mucus: variations in the amounts and glycoforms of the major oligomeric mucins MUC5AC and MUC5B. *Biochem J.* (2002) 361:537–46.
108. Woodruff PG, Modrek B, Choy DF, Jia G, Abbas AR, Ellwanger A, et al. helper type 2-driven inflammation defines major subphenotypes of asthma. *Am J Respir Crit Care Med.* (2009) 180:388–95.
109. Hasnain SZ, Evans CM, Roy M, Gallagher AL, Kindrachuk KN, Barron L, et al. Muc5ac: a critical component mediating the rejection of enteric nematodes. *J Exp Med.* (2011) 208:893–900. doi: 10.1084/jem.20102057
110. Ehre C, Worthington EN, Liesman RM, Grubb BR, Barbier D, O'Neal WK, et al. Overexpressing mouse model demonstrates the protective role of Muc5ac in the lungs. *Proc Natl Acad Sci USA.* (2012) 109:16528–33.
111. Erle DJ, Sheppard D. The cell biology of asthma. *J Cell Biol.* (2014) 205:621–31.
112. Tomkinson A, Kanehiro A, Rabinovitch N, Joetham A, Cieslewicz G, Gelfand EW. The failure of STAT6-deficient mice to develop airway eosinophilia and airway hyperresponsiveness is overcome by interleukin-5. *Am J Respir Crit Care Med.* (1999) 160:1283–91.
113. Hoshino A, Tsuji T, Matsuzaki J, Jinushi T, Ashino S, Teramura T, et al. STAT6-mediated signaling in Th2-dependent allergic asthma: critical role for the development of eosinophilia, airway hyper-responsiveness and mucus hypersecretion, distinct from its role in Th2 differentiation. *Int Immunol.* (2004) 16:1497–505.
114. Laoukili J, Perret E, Willems T, Minty A, Parthoens E, Houcine O, et al. IL-13 alters mucociliary differentiation and ciliary beating of human respiratory epithelial cells. *J Clin Invest.* (2001) 108:1817–24.
115. Kuperman DA, Huang X, Koth LL, Chang GH, Dolganov GM, Zhu Z, et al. Direct effects of interleukin-13 on epithelial cells cause airway hyperreactivity and mucus overproduction in asthma. *Nat Med.* (2002) 8:885–9.
116. Whittaker L, Niu N, Temann U-A, Stoddard A, Flavell RA, Ray A, et al. Interleukin-13 mediates a fundamental pathway for airway epithelial mucus induced by CD4 T cells and interleukin-9. *Am J Respir Cell Mol Biol.* (2002) 27:593–602. doi: 10.1165/rcmb.4838
117. Kuperman DA, Lewis CC, Woodruff PG, Rodriguez MW, Yang YH, Dolganov GM, et al. Dissecting asthma using focused transgenic modeling and functional genomics. *J Allergy Clin Immunol.* (2005) 116:305–11.
118. Amishima M, Munakata M, Nasuhara Y, Sato A, Takahashi T, Homma Y, et al. Expression of epidermal growth factor and epidermal growth factor receptor immunoreactivity in the asthmatic human airway. *Am J Respir Crit Care Med.* (1998) 157:1907–12.
119. Takeyama K, Dabbagh K, Lee HM, Agustí C, Lausier JA, Ueki IF, et al. Epidermal growth factor system regulates mucin production in airways. *Proc Natl Acad Sci USA.* (1999) 96:3081–6.
120. Perrais M, Pigny P, Copin M-C, Aubert J-P, Van Seuningen I. Induction of MUC2 and MUC5AC mucins by factors of the epidermal growth factor (EGF) family is mediated by EGF receptor/Ras/Raf/extracellular signal-regulated kinase cascade and Sp1. *J Biol Chem.* (2002) 277:32258–67.
121. Zhen G, Park SW, Nguyenvu LT, Rodriguez MW, Barbeau R, Paquet AC, et al. 13 and epidermal growth factor receptor have critical but distinct roles in epithelial cell mucin production. *Am J Respir Cell Mol Biol.* (2007) 36:244–53.
122. Ordoñez CL, Khashayar R, Wong HH, Ferrando R, Wu R, Hyde DM, et al. Mild and moderate asthma is associated with airway goblet cell hyperplasia and abnormalities in mucin gene expression. *Am J Respir Crit Care Med.* (2001) 163:517–23.
123. Boucherat O, Boczkowski J, Jeannotte L, Delacourt C. Cellular and molecular mechanisms of goblet cell metaplasia in the respiratory airways. *Exp Lung Res.* (2013) 39:207–16.
124. Temann UA, Prasad B, Gallup MW, Basbaum C, Ho SB, Flavell RA, et al. novel role for murine IL-4 in vivo: induction of MUC5AC gene expression and mucin hypersecretion. *Am J Respir Cell Mol Biol.* (1997) 16:471–8.
125. Grünig G, Warnock M, Wakil AE, Venkayya R, Brombacher F, Rennick DM, et al. Requirement for IL-13 independently of IL-4 in experimental asthma. *Science.* (1998) 282:2261–3.
126. Temann UA, Geba GP, Rankin JA, Flavell RA. Expression of interleukin 9 in the lungs of transgenic mice causes airway inflammation, mast cell hyperplasia, and bronchial hyperresponsiveness. *J Exp Med.* (1998) 188:1307–20.
127. Dabbagh K, Takeyama K, Lee HM, Ueki IF, Lausier JA, Nadel JAIL-. 4 induces mucin gene expression and goblet cell metaplasia in vitro and in vivo. *J Immunol.* (1999) 162:6233–7.
128. Saha SK, Berry MA, Parker D, Siddiqui S, Morgan A, May R, et al. Increased sputum and bronchial biopsy IL-13 expression in severe asthma. *J Allergy Clin Immunol.* (2008) 121:685–91.

129. Humbert M, Durham SR, Kimmitt P, Powell N, Assoufi B, Pfister R, et al. Elevated expression of messenger ribonucleic acid encoding IL-13 in the bronchial mucosa of atopic and nonatopic subjects with asthma. *J Allergy Clin Immunol.* (1997) 99:657–65.
130. Leonard C, Tormey V, Burke C, Poulter LW. Allergen-induced cytokine production in atopic disease and its relationship to disease severity. *Am J Respir Cell Mol Biol.* (1997) 17:368–75.
131. Shimbara A, Christodoulopoulos P, Soussi-Gounni A, Olivenstein R, Nakamura Y, Levitt RC, et al. IL-9 and its receptor in allergic and nonallergic lung disease: increased expression in asthma. *J Allergy Clin Immunol.* (2000) 105:108–15.
132. Danahay H, Pessotti AD, Coote J, Montgomery BE, Xia D, Wilson A, et al. Notch2 is required for inflammatory cytokine-driven goblet cell metaplasia in the lung. *Cell Rep.* (2015) 10:239–52.
133. Chen G, Korfhagen TR, Xu Y, Kitzmiller J, Wert SE, Maeda Y, et al. SPDEF is required for mouse pulmonary goblet cell differentiation and regulates a network of genes associated with mucus production. *J Clin Invest.* (2009) 119:2914–24.
134. Park K-S, Korfhagen TR, Bruno MD, Kitzmiller JA, Wan H, Wert SE, et al. SPDEF regulates goblet cell hyperplasia in the airway epithelium. *J Clin Invest.* (2007) 117:978–88.
135. Rajavelu P, Chen G, Xu Y, Kitzmiller JA, Korfhagen TR, Whitsett JA. Airway epithelial SPDEF integrates goblet cell differentiation and pulmonary Th2 inflammation. *J Clin Invest.* (2015) 125:2021–31.
136. Wan H, Kaestner KH, Ang S-L, Ikegami M, Finkelman FD, Stahlman MT, et al. Foxa2 regulates alveolarization and goblet cell hyperplasia. *Development.* (2004) 131:953–64.
137. Vock C, Yildirim AÖ, Wagner C, Schlick S, Lunding LP, Lee CG, et al. Distal airways are protected from goblet cell metaplasia by diminished expression of IL-13 signalling components. *Clin Exp Allergy.* (2015) 45:1447–58.
138. Duszyk M. CFTR and lysozyme secretion in human airway epithelial cells. *Pflugers Arch.* (2001) 443(Suppl. 1):S45–9.
139. Dajani R, Zhang Y, Taft PJ, Travis SM, Starner TD, Olsen A, et al. Lysozyme secretion by submucosal glands protects the airway from bacterial infection. *Am J Respir Cell Mol Biol.* (2005) 32:548–52.
140. Beisswenger C, Bals R. Antimicrobial peptides in lung inflammation. *Chem Immunol Allergy.* (2005) 86:55–71. doi: 10.1159/000086651
141. Schutte BC, McCray PB Jr. [beta]-defensins in lung host defense. *Annu Rev Physiol.* (2002) 64:709–48.
142. Basbaum CB, Jany B, Finkbeiner WE. The serous cell. *Annu Rev Physiol.* (1990) 52:97–113.
143. Chen J, Chen Z, Chintagari NR, Bhaskaran M, Jin N, Narasaraju T, et al. Alveolar type I cells protect rat lung epithelium from oxidative injury. *J Physiol.* (2006) 572:625–38.
144. Kim K-J, Malik AB. Protein transport across the lung epithelial barrier. *Am J Physiol Lung Cell Mol Physiol.* (2003) 284:L247–59.
145. Mostov KE. Transepithelial transport of immunoglobulins. *Annu Rev Immunol.* (1994) 12:63–84. doi: 10.1146/annurev.iy.12.040194.000431
146. Johansen FE, Braathen R, Brandtzaeg P. The J chain is essential for polymeric Ig receptor-mediated epithelial transport of IgA. *J Immunol.* (2001) 167:5185–92.
147. Turula H, Wobus CE. The Role of the Polymeric Immunoglobulin Receptor and Secretory Immunoglobulins during Mucosal Infection and Immunity. *Viruses.* (2018) 10:237. doi: 10.3390/v10050237
148. Mestecky J, Zikan J, Butler WT. Immunoglobulin M and secretory immunoglobulin A: presence of a common polypeptide chain different from light chains. *Science.* (1971) 171:1163–5.
149. Johansen FE, Braathen R, Brandtzaeg P. Role of J chain in secretory immunoglobulin formation. *Scand J Immunol.* (2000) 52:240–8.
150. Brandtzaeg P, Johansen F-E. Mucosal B cells: phenotypic characteristics, transcriptional regulation, and homing properties. *Immunol Rev.* (2005) 206:32–63. doi: 10.1111/j.0105-2896.2005.00283.x
151. Castro CD, Flajnik MF. Putting J chain back on the map: how might its expression define plasma cell development? *J Immunol.* (2014) 193:3248–55.
152. Gibbins HL, Proctor GB, Yakubov GE, Wilson S, Carpenter GH. SIgA binding to mucosal surfaces is mediated by mucin-mucin interactions. *PLoS One.* (2015) 10:e0119677. doi: 10.1371/journal.pone.0119677
153. Phalipon A, Cardona A, Kraehenbuhl JP, Edelman L, Sansonetti PJ, Corthésy B. Secretory component: a new role in secretory IgA-mediated immune exclusion in vivo. *Immunity.* (2002) 17:107–15.
154. Weltzin R, Traina-Dorge V, Soike K, Zhang JY, Mack P, Soman G, et al. Intranasal monoclonal IgA antibody to respiratory syncytial virus protects rhesus monkeys against upper and lower respiratory tract infection. *J Infect Dis.* (1996) 174:256–61.
155. Blanchard TG, Czinn SJ, Maurer R, Thomas WD, Soman G, Nedrud JG. Urease-specific monoclonal antibodies prevent *Helicobacter* felis infection in mice. *Infect Immun.* (1995) 63:1394–9.
156. Weltzin R, Hsu SA, Mittler ES, Georgakopoulos K, Monath TP. Intranasal monoclonal immunoglobulin A against respiratory syncytial virus protects against upper and lower respiratory tract infections in mice. *Antimicrob Agents Chemother.* (1994) 38:2785–91.
157. Mazanec MB, Nedrud JG, Lamm ME. Immunoglobulin A monoclonal antibodies protect against Sendai virus. *J Virol.* (1987) 61:2624–6.
158. Winner L III, Mack J, Weltzin R, Mekalanos JJ, Kraehenbuhl JP, Neutra MR. New model for analysis of mucosal immunity: intestinal secretion of specific monoclonal immunoglobulin A from hybridoma tumors protects against *Vibrio cholerae* infection. *Infect Immun.* (1991) 59:977–82.
159. Michetti P, Mahan MJ, Slauch JM, Mekalanos JJ, Neutra MR. Monoclonal secretory immunoglobulin A protects mice against oral challenge with the invasive pathogen *Salmonella* typhimurium. *Infect Immun.* (1992) 60:1786–92.
160. Apter FM, Michetti P, Winner LS III, Mack JA, Mekalanos JJ, Neutra MR. Analysis of the roles of antilipopolysaccharide and anti-cholera toxin immunoglobulin A (IgA) antibodies in protection against *Vibrio cholerae* and cholera toxin by use of monoclonal IgA antibodies in vivo. *Infect Immun.* (1993) 61:5279–85.
161. Royle L, Roos A, Harvey DJ, Wormald MR, van Gijlswijk-Janssen D, Redwan E-RM, et al. Secretory IgA N- and O-glycans provide a link between the innate and adaptive immune systems. *J Biol Chem.* (2003) 278:20140–53.
162. Marshall LJ, Perks B, Ferkol T, Shute JK. IL-. 8 released constitutively by primary bronchial epithelial cells in culture forms an inactive complex with secretory component. *J Immunol.* (2001) 167:2816–23.
163. Wines BD, Hogarth PM. IgA receptors in health and disease. *Tissue Antigens.* (2006) 68:103–14.
164. Van Spriel AB, Leusen JHW, Vilé H, Van De Winkel JGJ. Mac-1 (CD11b/CD18) as accessory molecule for Fc alpha R (CD89) binding of IgA. *J Immunol.* (2002) 169:3831–6.
165. Bartemes KR, Cooper KM, Drain KL, Kita H. Secretory IgA induces antigen-independent eosinophil survival and cytokine production without inducing effector functions. *J Allergy Clin Immunol.* (2005) 116:827–35.
166. Peebles RS Jr., Liu MC, Adkinson NF Jr., Lichtenstein LM, Hamilton RG. Ragweed-specific antibodies in bronchoalveolar lavage fluids and serum before and after segmental lung challenge: IgE and IgA associated with eosinophil degranulation. *J Allergy Clin Immunol.* (1998) 101: 265–73.
167. Abu-Ghazaleh RI, Fujisawa T, Mestecky J, Kyle RA, Gleich GJ. IgA-induced eosinophil degranulation. *J Immunol.* (1989) 142:2393–400.
168. Chu VT, Beller A, Rausch S, Strandmark J, Zänker M, Arbach O, et al. Eosinophils promote generation and maintenance of immunoglobulin-A-expressing plasma cells and contribute to gut immune homeostasis. *Immunity.* (2014) 40:582–93.
169. Jung Y, Wen T, Mingler MK, Caldwell JM, Wang YH, Chaplin DD, et al. IL-1β in eosinophil-mediated small intestinal homeostasis and IgA production. *Mucosal Immunol.* (2015) 8:930–42.
170. Kobayashi K, Suzukawa M, Watanabe K, Arakawa S, Igarashi S, Asari I, et al. Secretory IgA accumulated in the airspaces of idiopathic pulmonary fibrosis and promoted VEGF, TGF-β and IL-8 production by A549 cells. *Clin Exp Immunol.* (2019) 199:326–36. doi: 10.1111/cei.13390
171. Weltzin R, Lucia-Jandris P, Michetti P, Fields BN, Kraehenbuhl JP, Neutra MR. Binding and transepithelial transport of immunoglobulins by intestinal M cells: demonstration using monoclonal IgA antibodies against enteric viral proteins. *J Cell Biol.* (1989) 108:1673–85.
172. Mantis NJ, Cheung MC, Chintalacharuvu KR, Rey J, Corthésy B, Neutra MR. Selective adherence of IgA to murine Peyer's patch M cells: evidence for a novel IgA receptor. *J Immunol.* (2002) 169:1844–51.

173. Neutra MR, Pringault E, Kraehenbuhl JP. Antigen sampling across epithelial barriers and induction of mucosal immune responses. *Annu Rev Immunol.* (1996) 14:275–300. doi: 10.1146/annurev.immunol.14.1.275
174. Kimura S. Molecular insights into the mechanisms of M-cell differentiation and transcytosis in the mucosa-associated lymphoid tissues. *Anat Sci Int.* (2018) 93:23–34. doi: 10.1007/s12565-017-0418-6
175. He B, Xu W, Santini PA, Polydorides AD, Chiu A, Estrella J, et al. Intestinal bacteria trigger T cell-independent immunoglobulin A(2) class switching by inducing epithelial-cell secretion of the cytokine APRIL. *Immunity.* (2007) 26:812–26.
176. Burnett D, Crocker J, Stockley RA. Cells containing IgA subclasses in bronchi of subjects with and without chronic obstructive lung disease. *J Clin Pathol.* (1987) 40:1217–20.
177. Stoel M, Evenhuis WNH, Kroese FGM, Bos NA. Rat salivary gland reveals a more restricted IgA repertoire than ileum. *Mol Immunol.* (2008) 45:719–27.
178. Fahy JV. Eosinophilic and neutrophilic inflammation in asthma: insights from clinical studies. *Proc Am Thorac Soc.* (2009) 6:256–9.
179. Peebles RS Jr., Hamilton RG, Lichtenstein LM, Schlosberg M, Liu MC, Proud D, et al. Antigen-specific IgE and IgA antibodies in bronchoalveolar lavage fluid are associated with stronger antigen-induced late phase reactions. *Clin Exp Allergy.* (2001) 31:239–48.
180. Aghayan-Ugurluoglu R, Ball T, Vrtala S, Schweiger C, Kraft D, Valenta R. Dissociation of allergen-specific IgE and IgA responses in sera and tears of pollen-allergic patients: a study performed with purified recombinant pollen allergens. *J Allergy Clin Immunol.* (2000) 105:803–13.
181. Nahm DH, Kim HY, Park HS. Elevation of specific immunoglobulin A antibodies to both allergen and bacterial antigen in induced sputum from asthmatics. *Eur Respir J.* (1998) 12:540–5.
182. Xiao SF, Okuda M, Ohnishi M, Okubo K. Specific IgA and IgG antibodies to house dust mite Dermatophagoides farinae in nasal secretions. *Arerugi.* (1994) 43:634–44.
183. Reed CE, Bubak M, Dunnette S, Blomgren J, Pfenning M, Wentz-Murtha P, et al. Ragweed-specific IgA in nasal lavage fluid of ragweed-sensitive allergic rhinitis patients: increase during the pollen season. *Int Arch Allergy Appl Immunol.* (1991) 94:275–7.
184. Richmond BW, Brucker RM, Han W, Du R-H, Zhang Y, Cheng D-S, et al. Airway bacteria drive a progressive COPD-like phenotype in mice with polymeric immunoglobulin receptor deficiency. *Nat Commun.* (2016) 7:11240.
185. Richmond BW, Du R-H, Han W, Benjamin JT, van der Meer R, Gleaves L, et al. Bacterial-derived Neutrophilic Inflammation Drives Lung Remodeling in a Mouse Model of Chronic Obstructive Pulmonary Disease. *Am J Respir Cell Mol Biol.* (2018) 58:736–44.
186. Polosukhin VV, Cates JM, Lawson WE, Zaynagetdinov R, Milstone AP, Massion PP, et al. Bronchial secretory immunoglobulin a deficiency correlates with airway inflammation and progression of chronic obstructive pulmonary disease. *Am J Respir Crit Care Med.* (2011) 184:317–27.
187. Polosukhin VV, Richmond BW, Du R-H, Cates JM, Wu P, Nian H, et al. Secretory IgA Deficiency in Individual Small Airways Is Associated with Persistent Inflammation and Remodeling. *Am J Respir Crit Care Med.* (2017) 195:1010–21.
188. Ladjemi MZ, Gras D, Dupasquier S, Detry B, Lecocq M, Garulli C, et al. Bronchial Epithelial IgA Secretion Is Impaired in Asthma. Role of IL-4/IL-13. *Am J Respir Crit Care Med.* (2018) 197:1396–409.
189. Hupin C, Rombaux P, Bowen H, Gould H, Lecocq M, Pilette C. Downregulation of polymeric immunoglobulin receptor and secretory IgA antibodies in eosinophilic upper airway diseases. *Allergy.* (2013) 68:1589–97.
190. Schwarze J, Cieslewicz G, Joetham A, Sun LK, Sun WN, Chang TW, et al. Antigen-specific immunoglobulin-A prevents increased airway responsiveness and lung eosinophilia after airway challenge in sensitized mice. *Am J Respir Crit Care Med.* (1998) 158:519–25.
191. Rochereau N, Pavot V, Verrier B, Jospin F, Ensinas A, Genin C, et al. Delivery of antigen to nasal-associated lymphoid tissue microfold cells through secretory IgA targeting local dendritic cells confers protective immunity. *J Allergy Clin Immunol.* (2016) 2016:214–22.e2.
192. Widera A, Kim K-JJ, Crandall, Shen W-C. Transcytosis of GCSF-transferrin across rat alveolar epithelial cell monolayers. *Pharm Res.* (2003) 20:1231–8.
193. Rescigno M, Urbano M, Valzasina B, Francolini M, Rotta G, Bonasio R, et al. Dendritic cells express tight junction proteins and penetrate gut epithelial monolayers to sample bacteria. *Nat Immunol.* (2001) 2:361–7.
194. Jahnsen FL, Strickland DH, Thomas JA, Tobagus IT, Napoli S, Zosky GR, et al. Accelerated antigen sampling and transport by airway mucosal dendritic cells following inhalation of a bacterial stimulus. *J Immunol.* (2006) 177:5861–7.
195. Papadopoulou A, Mermiri D, Taousani S, Triga M, Nicolaidou P, Priftis KN. Bronchial hyper-responsiveness in selective IgA deficiency. *Pediatr Allergy Immunol.* (2005) 16:495–500. doi: 10.1111/j.1399-3038.2005.00316.x
196. Lúdvíksson BR, Eiríksson TH, Ardal B, Sigfússon A, Valdimarsson H. Correlation between serum immunoglobulin A concentrations and allergic manifestations in infants. *J Pediatr.* (1992) 121:23–7.
197. Huoman J, Papapavlou G, Pap A, Alm J, Nilsson LJ, Jenmalm MC. Sublingual immunotherapy alters salivary IgA and systemic immune mediators in timothy allergic children. *Pediatr Allergy Immunol.* (2019) 30:522–30.
198. Liu Y-H, Tsai J-J. Production of salivary immunoglobulin A and suppression of Dermatophagoides pteronyssinus-induced airway inflammation by local nasal immunotherapy. *Int Arch Allergy Immunol.* (2005) 138:161–8.
199. Gohy ST, Hupin C, Pilette C, Ladjemi MZ. Chronic inflammatory airway diseases: the central role of the epithelium revisited. *Clin Exp Allergy.* (2016) 46:529–42.
200. Bals R, Hiemstra PS. Innate immunity in the lung: how epithelial cells fight against respiratory pathogens. *Eur Respir J.* (2004) 23:327–33.
201. Parker D, Prince A. Innate immunity in the respiratory epithelium. *Am J Respir Cell Mol Biol.* (2011) 45:189–201. doi: 10.1165/rcmb.2011-0011rt
202. Hallstrand TS, Hackett TL, Altemeier WA, Matute-Bello G, Hansbro PM, Knight DA. Airway epithelial regulation of pulmonary immune homeostasis and inflammation. *Clin Immunol.* (2014) 151:1–15. doi: 10.1016/j.clim.2013.12.003
203. Lambrecht BN, Hammad H. The airway epithelium in asthma. *Nat Med.* (2012) 18:684–92.
204. Pouwels SD, Heijink IH, Hacken NHT, Vandenabeele P, Krysko DV, Nawijn MC, et al. DAMPs activating innate and adaptive immune responses in COPD. *Mucosal Immunol.* (2014) 7:215–26.
205. Kang JH, Hwang SM, Chung IY. S100A8, S100A9 and S100A12 activate airway epithelial cells to produce MUC5AC via extracellular signal-regulated kinase and nuclear factor-κB pathways. *Immunology.* (2015) 144:79–90. doi: 10.1111/imm.12352
206. Ellson CD, Dunmore R, Hogaboam CM, Sleeman MA, Murray LA. Danger-associated molecular patterns and danger signals in idiopathic pulmonary fibrosis. *Am J Respir Cell Mol Biol.* (2014) 51:163–8.
207. Kawai T, Akira S. Toll-like receptors and their crosstalk with other innate receptors in infection and immunity. *Immunity.* (2011) 34:637–50.
208. Parker D, Prince A. Type I interferon response to extracellular bacteria in the airway epithelium. *Trends Immunol.* (2011) 32:582–8.
209. Willart MAM, Lambrecht BN. The danger within: endogenous danger signals, atopy and asthma. *Clin Exp Allergy.* (2009) 39:12–9.
210. Holgate ST. Innate and adaptive immune responses in asthma. *Nat Med.* (2012) 18:673–83.
211. Hammad H, Chieppa M, Perros F, Willart MA, Germain RN, Lambrecht BN. House dust mite allergen induces asthma via Toll-like receptor 4 triggering of airway structural cells. *Nat Med.* (2009) 15:410–6.
212. Kouzaki H, Tojima I, Kita H, Shimizu T. Transcription of interleukin-25 and extracellular release of the protein is regulated by allergen proteases in airway epithelial cells. *Am J Respir Cell Mol Biol.* (2013) 49:741–50.
213. Tan AM, Chen H-C, Pochard P, Eisenbarth SC, Herrick CA, Bottomly HK. TLR4 signaling in stromal cells is critical for the initiation of allergic Th2 responses to inhaled antigen. *J Immunol.* (2010) 184:3535–44.
214. Willart MAM, Deswarte K, Pouliot P, Braun H, Beyaert R, Lambrecht BN, et al. Interleukin-1α controls allergic sensitization to inhaled house dust mite via the epithelial release of GM-CSF and IL-33. *J Exp Med.* (2012) 209:1505–17.
215. Kouzaki H, O'Grady SM, Lawrence CB, Kita H. Proteases induce production of thymic stromal lymphopoietin by airway epithelial cells through protease-activated receptor-2. *J Immunol.* (2009) 183:1427–34.
216. Lambrecht BN, Hammad H. Allergens and the airway epithelium response: gateway to allergic sensitization. *J Allergy Clin Immunol.* (2014) 134:499–507. doi: 10.1016/j.jaci.2014.06.036

217. Hill DA, Siracusa MC, Abt MC, Kim BS, Kobuley D, Kubo M, et al. Commensal bacteria-derived signals regulate basophil hematopoiesis and allergic inflammation. *Nat Med.* (2012) 18:538–46.
218. Monticelli LA, Sonnenberg GF, Artis D. Innate lymphoid cells: critical regulators of allergic inflammation and tissue repair in the lung. *Curr Opin Immunol.* (2012) 24:284–9.
219. Regueiro V, Moranta D, Campos MA, Margareto J, Garmendia J, Bengoechea JA. *Klebsiella pneumoniae* increases the levels of Toll-like receptors 2 and 4 in human airway epithelial cells. *Infect Immun.* (2009) 77:714–24.
220. Uehara A, Fujimoto Y, Fukase K, Takada H. Various human epithelial cells express functional Toll-like receptors, NOD1 and NOD2 to produce antimicrobial peptides, but not proinflammatory cytokines. *Mol Immunol.* (2007) 44:3100–11.
221. Wang Q, Nagarkar DR, Bowman ER, Schneider D, Gosangi B, Lei J, et al. Role of double-stranded RNA pattern recognition receptors in rhinovirus-induced airway epithelial cell responses. *J Immunol.* (2009) 183:6989–97.
222. Bertolusso R, Tian B, Zhao Y, Vergara L, Sabree A, Iwanaszko M, et al. Dynamic cross talk model of the epithelial innate immune response to double-stranded RNA stimulation: coordinated dynamics emerging from cell-level noise. *PLoS One.* (2014) 9:e93396. doi: 10.1371/journal.pone.0093396
223. Groskreutz DJ, Monick MM, Powers LS, Yarovinsky TO, Look DC, Hunninghake GW. Respiratory syncytial virus induces TLR3 protein and protein kinase R, leading to increased double-stranded RNA responsiveness in airway epithelial cells. *J Immunol.* (2006) 176:1733–40.
224. Le Goffic R, Pothlichet J, Vitour D, Fujita T, Meurs E, Chignard M, et al. Cutting Edge: Influenza A virus activates TLR3-dependent inflammatory and RIG-I-dependent antiviral responses in human lung epithelial cells. *J Immunol.* (2007) 178:3368–72.
225. Shornick LP, Wells AG, Zhang Y, Patel AC, Huang G, Takami K, et al. Airway epithelial versus immune cell Stat1 function for innate defense against respiratory viral infection. *J Immunol.* (2008) 180:3319–28.
226. Hertz CJ, Wu Q, Porter EM, Zhang YJ, Weismüller K-H, Godowski PJ, et al. Activation of Toll-like receptor 2 on human tracheobronchial epithelial cells induces the antimicrobial peptide human beta defensin-2. *J Immunol.* (2003) 171:6820–6.
227. Ibrahim ZA, Armour CL, Phipps S, Sukkar MB. RAGE and TLRs: relatives, friends or neighbours? *Mol Immunol.* (2013) 56:739–44.
228. Gao W, Li L, Wang Y, Zhang S, Adcock IM, Barnes PJ, et al. Bronchial epithelial cells: The key effector cells in the pathogenesis of chronic obstructive pulmonary disease? *Respirology.* (2015) 20:722–9.
229. Hirota K, Yoshitomi H, Hashimoto M, Maeda S, Teradaira S, Sugimoto N, et al. Preferential recruitment of CCR6-expressing Th17 cells to inflamed joints via CCL20 in rheumatoid arthritis and its animal model. *J Exp Med.* (2007) 204:2803–12.
230. Hirota JA, Gold MJ, Hiebert PR, Parkinson LG, Wee T, Smith D, et al. The nucleotide-binding domain, leucine-rich repeat protein 3 inflammasome/IL-1 receptor I axis mediates innate, but not adaptive, immune responses after exposure to particulate matter under 10 μm. *Am J Respir Cell Mol Biol.* (2015) 52:96–105. doi: 10.1165/rcmb.2014-0158oc
231. Hsu AC-Y, Parsons K, Barr I, Lowther S, Middleton D, Hansbro PM, et al. Critical role of constitutive type I interferon response in bronchial epithelial cell to influenza infection. *PLoS One.* (2012) 7:e32947. doi: 10.1371/journal.pone.0032947
232. Parker JC, Thavagnanam S, Skibinski G, Lyons J, Bell J, Heaney LG, et al. Chronic IL9 and IL-13 exposure leads to an altered differentiation of ciliated cells in a well-differentiated paediatric bronchial epithelial cell model. *PLoS One.* (2013) 8:e61023. doi: 10.1371/journal.pone.0061023
233. Petecchia L, Sabatini F, Usai C, Caci E, Varesio L, Rossi GA. Cytokines induce tight junction disassembly in airway cells via an EGFR-dependent MAPK/ERK1/2-pathway. *Lab Invest.* (2012) 92:1140–8.
234. Ziegler SF, Artis D. Sensing the outside world: TSLP regulates barrier immunity. *Nat Immunol.* (2010) 11:289–93.
235. Perros F, Hoogsteden HC, Coyle AJ, Lambrecht BN, Hammad H. Blockade of CCR4 in a humanized model of asthma reveals a critical role for DC-derived CCL17 and CCL22 in attracting Th2 cells and inducing airway inflammation. *Allergy.* (2009) 64:995–1002. doi: 10.1111/j.1398-9995.2009.02095.x
236. Vijayanand P, Durkin K, Hartmann G, Morjaria J, Seumois G, Staples KJ, et al. Chemokine receptor 4 plays a key role in T cell recruitment into the airways of asthmatic patients. *J Immunol.* (2010) 184:4568–74.
237. Kato A, Favoreto S Jr., Avila PC, Schleimer RP. TLR3- and Th2 cytokine-dependent production of thymic stromal lymphopoietin in human airway epithelial cells. *J Immunol.* (2007) 179:1080–7.
238. Gras D, Chanez P, Vachier I, Petit A, Bourdin A. Bronchial epithelium as a target for innovative treatments in asthma. *Pharmacol Ther.* (2013) 140:290–305. doi: 10.1016/j.pharmthera.2013.07.008
239. Sedgwick JB, Quan SF, Calhoun WJ, Busse WW. Effect of interleukin-5 and granulocyte-macrophage colony stimulating factor on in vitro eosinophil function: comparison with airway eosinophils. *J Allergy Clin Immunol.* (1995) 96:375–85.
240. Gold MJ, Antignano F, Halim TYF, Hirota JA, Blanchet M-R, Zaph C, et al. Group 2 innate lymphoid cells facilitate sensitization to local, but not systemic. TH2-inducing allergen exposures. *J Allergy Clin Immunol.* (2014) 133:1142–8.
241. Halim TYF, Krauss RH, Sun AC, Takei F. Lung natural helper cells are a critical source of Th2 cell-type cytokines in protease allergen-induced airway inflammation. *Immunity.* (2012) 36:451–63.
242. Sze MA, Dimitriu PA, Hayashi S, Elliott WM, McDonough JE, Gosselink JV, et al. The lung tissue microbiome in chronic obstructive pulmonary disease. *Am J Respir Crit Care Med.* (2012) 185:1073–80.
243. Hansel TT, Johnston SL, Openshaw PJ. Microbes and mucosal immune responses in asthma. *Lancet.* (2013) 381:861–73.
244. Georas SN, Rezaee F. Epithelial barrier function: at the front line of asthma immunology and allergic airway inflammation. *J Allergy Clin Immunol.* (2014) 134:509–20.
245. Busse WW, Lemanske RF Jr., Gern JE. Role of viral respiratory infections in asthma and asthma exacerbations. *Lancet.* (2010) 376:826–34.
246. Ege MJ, Mayer M, Normand A-C, Genuneit J, Cookson WOCM, Braun-Fahrländer C, et al. GABRIELA Transregio 22 Study Group. Exposure to environmental microorganisms and childhood asthma. *N Engl J Med.* (2011) 364:701–9.
247. Lunding L, Webering S, Vock C, Schröder A, Raedler D, Schaub B, et al. 37 requires IL-18Rα and SIGIRR/IL-1R8 to diminish allergic airway inflammation in mice. *Allergy.* (2015) 70:366–73.
248. Webering S, Lunding LP, Vock C, Schröder A, Gaede KI, Herzmann C, et al. The alpha-melanocyte-stimulating hormone acts as a local immune homeostasis factor in experimental allergic asthma. *Clin Exp Allergy.* (2019) 49:1026–39.
249. Stein RT, Sherrill D, Morgan WJ, Holberg CJ, Halonen M, Taussig LM, et al. Respiratory syncytial virus in early life and risk of wheeze and allergy by age 13 years. *Lancet.* (1999) 354:541–5.
250. Sigurs N, Bjarnason R, Sigurbergsson F, Kjellman B. Respiratory syncytial virus bronchiolitis in infancy is an important risk factor for asthma and allergy at age 7. *Am J Respir Crit Care Med.* (2000) 161:1501–7.
251. Lemanske RF Jr., Jackson DJ, Gangnon RE, Evans MD, Li Z, Shult PA, et al. Rhinovirus illnesses during infancy predict subsequent childhood wheezing. *J Allergy Clin Immunol.* (2005) 116:571–7.
252. Kusel MMH, de Klerk NH, Kebadze T, Vohma V, Holt PG, Johnston SL, et al. Early-life respiratory viral infections, atopic sensitization, and risk of subsequent development of persistent asthma. *J Allergy Clin Immunol.* (2007) 119:1105–10.
253. Jackson DJ, Gangnon RE, Evans MD, Roberg KA, Anderson EL, Pappas TE, et al. Wheezing rhinovirus illnesses in early life predict asthma development in high-risk children. *Am J Respir Crit Care Med.* (2008) 178: 667–72.
254. Barnett SBL, Nurmagambetov TA. Costs of asthma in the United States: 2002-2007. *J Allergy Clin Immunol.* (2011) 127:145–52.
255. Jackson DJ, Sykes A, Mallia P, Johnston SL. Asthma exacerbations: origin, effect, and prevention. *J Allergy Clin Immunol.* (2011) 128:1165–74.
256. Friedlander SL, Busse WW. The role of rhinovirus in asthma exacerbations. *J Allergy Clin Immunol.* (2005) 116:267–73.
257. Turner RB, Lee W-M. Rhinovirus. 3rd ed. *Clinical Virology.* 3rd eds Richman DD, Whitley RJ, and Hayden FG, Washington, DC: American Society of Microbiology (2019) p. 1063–82.

258. Palmenberg AC, Spiro D, Kuzmickas R, Wang S, Djikeng A, Rathe JA, et al. Sequencing and analyses of all known human rhinovirus genomes reveal structure and evolution. *Science.* (2009) 324:55–9.
259. Tomassini JE, Graham D, DeWitt CM, Lineberger DW, Rodkey JA, Colonno RJ. cDNA cloning reveals that the major group rhinovirus receptor on HeLa cells is intercellular adhesion molecule 1. *Proc Natl Acad Sci USA.* (1989) 86:4907–11.
260. Greve JM, Davis G, Meyer AM, Forte CP, Yost SC, Marlor CW, et al. The major human rhinovirus receptor is ICAM-1. *Cell.* (1989) 56:839–47.
261. Colonno RJ, Condra JH, Mizutani S, Callahan PL, Davies ME, Murcko MA. Evidence for the direct involvement of the rhinovirus canyon in receptor binding. *Proc Natl Acad Sci USA.* (1988) 85:5449–53.
262. Suzuki T, Yamaya M, Kamanaka M, Jia YX, Nakayama K, Hosoda M, et al. Type 2 rhinovirus infection of cultured human tracheal epithelial cells: role of LDL receptor. *Am J Physiol Lung Cell Mol Physiol.* (2001) 280:L409–20.
263. Mosser AG, Brockman-Schneider R, Amineva S, Burchell L, Sedgwick JB, Busse WW, et al. Similar frequency of rhinovirus-infectible cells in upper and lower airway epithelium. *J Infect Dis.* (2002) 185:734–43.
264. Olson NH, Kolatkar PR, Oliveira MA, Cheng RH, Greve JM, McClelland A, et al. Structure of a human rhinovirus complexed with its receptor molecule. *Proc Natl Acad Sci USA.* (1993) 90:507–11.
265. Vlasak M, Roivainen M, Reithmayer M, Goesler I, Laine P, Snyers L, et al. The minor receptor group of human rhinovirus (HRV) includes HRV23 and HRV25, but the presence of a lysine in the VP1 HI loop is not sufficient for receptor binding. *J Virol.* (2005) 79:7389–95.
266. Bochkov YA, Watters K, Ashraf S, Griggs TF, Devries MK, Jackson DJ, et al. Cadherin-related family member 3, a childhood asthma susceptibility gene product, mediates rhinovirus C binding and replication. *Proc Natl Acad Sci USA.* (2015) 112:5485–90.
267. Papadopoulos NG, Bates PJ, Bardin PG, Papi A, Leir SH, Fraenkel DJ, et al. Rhinoviruses infect the lower airways. *J Infect Dis.* (2000) 181: 1875–84.
268. Slater L, Bartlett NW, Haas JJ, Zhu J, Message SD, Walton RP, et al. Co-ordinated role of TLR3, RIG-I and MDA5 in the innate response to rhinovirus in bronchial epithelium. *PLoS Pathog.* (2010) 6:e1001178. doi: 10.1371/journal.ppat.1001178
269. Schroth MK, Grimm E, Frindt P, Galagan DM, Konno SI, Love R, et al. Rhinovirus replication causes RANTES production in primary bronchial epithelial cells. *Am J Respir Cell Mol Biol.* (1999) 20:1220–8.
270. Einarsson O, Geba GP, Zhu Z, Landry M, Elias JA. Interleukin-11: stimulation in vivo and in vitro by respiratory viruses and induction of airways hyperresponsiveness. *J Clin Invest.* (1996) 97:915–24.
271. Terajima M, Yamaya M, Sekizawa K, Okinaga S, Suzuki T, Yamada N, et al. Rhinovirus infection of primary cultures of human tracheal epithelium: role of ICAM-1 and IL-1beta. *Am J Physiol.* (1997) 273:L749–59.
272. Griego SD, Weston CB, Adams JL, Tal-Singer R, Dillon SB. Role of p38 mitogen-activated protein kinase in rhinovirus-induced cytokine production by bronchial epithelial cells. *J Immunol.* (2000) 165:5211–20.
273. Triantafilou K, Vakakis E, Richer EAJ, Evans GL, Villiers JP, Triantafilou M. Human rhinovirus recognition in non-immune cells is mediated by Toll-like receptors and MDA-5, which trigger a synergetic pro-inflammatory immune response. *Virulence.* (2011) 2:22–9.
274. Lunding LP, Webering S, Vock C, Behrends J, Wagner C, Hölscher C, et al. Poly(inosinic-cytidylic) acid-triggered exacerbation of experimental asthma depends on IL-17A produced by NK cells. *J Immunol.* (2015) 194:5615–25.
275. Ritchie AI, Jackson DJ, Edwards MR, Johnston SL. Airway epithelial orchestration of innate immune function in response to virus infection. A focus on asthma. *Ann Am Thorac Soc.* (2016) 13(Suppl. 1):S55–63.
276. Uller L, Leino M, Bedke N, Sammut D, Green B, Lau L, et al. Double-stranded RNA induces disproportionate expression of thymic stromal lymphopoietin versus interferon-beta in bronchial epithelial cells from donors with asthma. *Thorax.* (2010) 65:626–32.
277. Jackson DJ, Makrinioti H, Rana BMJ, Shamji BWH, Trujillo-Torralbo M-B, Footitt J, et al. IL-33-dependent type 2 inflammation during rhinovirus-induced asthma exacerbations in vivo. *Am J Respir Crit Care Med.* (2014) 190:1373–82.
278. Kuo C, Lim S, King NJC, Johnston SL, Burgess JK, Black JL, et al. Rhinovirus infection induces extracellular matrix protein deposition in asthmatic and nonasthmatic airway smooth muscle cells. *Am J Physiol Lung Cell Mol Physiol.* (2011) 300:L951–7.
279. Mills JT, Schwenzer A, Marsh EK, Edwards MR, Sabroe I, Midwood KS, et al. Airway Epithelial Cells Generate Pro-inflammatory Tenascin-C and Small Extracellular Vesicles in Response to TLR3 Stimuli and Rhinovirus Infection. *Front Immunol.* (2019) 10:1987.
280. Pech M, Weckmann M, König IR, Franke A, Heinsen F-A, Oliver B, et al. Rhinovirus infections change DNA methylation and mRNA expression in children with asthma. *PLoS One.* (2018) 13:e0205275. doi: 10.1371/journal.pone.0205275
281. Reza Etemadi M, Ling K-H, Zainal Abidin S, Chee H-Y, Sekawi Z. Gene expression patterns induced at different stages of rhinovirus infection in human alveolar epithelial cells. *PLoS One.* (2017) 12:e0176947. doi: 10.1371/journal.pone.0176947
282. Burgess JK, Weckmann M. Matrikines and the lungs. *Pharmacol Ther.* (2012) 134:317–37.
283. Patel DF, Peiró T, Shoemark A, Akthar S, Walker SA, Grabiec AM, et al. An extracellular matrix fragment drives epithelial remodeling and airway hyperresponsiveness. *Sci Transl Med.* (2018) 10:eaaq0693. doi: 10.1126/scitranslmed.aaq0693
284. Gaggar A, Weathington N. Bioactive extracellular matrix fragments in lung health and disease. *J Clin Invest.* (2016) 126:3176–84.
285. Burgess JK, Boustany S, Moir LM, Weckmann M, Lau JY, Grafton K, et al. Reduction of tumstatin in asthmatic airways contributes to angiogenesis, inflammation, and hyperresponsiveness. *Am J Respir Crit Care Med.* (2010) 181:106–15.
286. Van der Velden J, Harkness LM, Barker DM, Barcham GJ, Ugalde CL, Koumoundouros E, et al. The effects of tumstatin on vascularity, airway inflammation and lung function in an experimental sheep model of chronic asthma. *Sci Rep.* (2016) 6:26309.
287. Weckmann M, Moir LM, Heckman CA, Black JL, Oliver BG, Burgess JK. Lamstatin–a novel inhibitor of lymphangiogenesis derived from collagen IV. *J Cell Mol Med.* (2012) 16:3062–73.
288. Nissen G, Hollaender H, Tang FSM, Wegmann M, Lunding L, Vock C, et al. Tumstatin fragment selectively inhibits neutrophil infiltration in experimental asthma exacerbation. *Clin Exp Allergy.* (2018) 48:1483–93. doi: 10.1111/cea.13236
289. Gaggar A, Jackson PL, Noerager BD, O'Reilly PJ, McQuaid DB, Rowe SM, et al. novel proteolytic cascade generates an extracellular matrix-derived chemoattractant in chronic neutrophilic inflammation. *J Immunol.* (2008) 180:5662–9.
290. McErlean P, Favoreto S, Costa FF, Shen J, Quraishi J, Biyasheva A, et al. Human rhinovirus infection causes different DNA methylation changes in nasal epithelial cells from healthy and asthmatic subjects. *BMC Med Genomics.* (2014) 7:37.
291. Lund RJ, Osmala M, Malonzo M, Lukkarinen M, Leino A, Salmi J, et al. Atopic asthma after rhinovirus-induced wheezing is associated with DNA methylation change in the SMAD3 gene promoter. *Allergy.* (2018) 73:1735–40.
292. Forno E, Wang T, Qi C, Yan Q, Xu C-J, Boutaoui N, et al. DNA methylation in nasal epithelium, atopy, and atopic asthma in children: a genome-wide study. *Lancet Respir Med.* (2019) 7:336–46.
293. Zissler UM, Chaker AM, Effner R, Ulrich M, Guerth F, Piontek G, et al. Interleukin-4 and interferon-γ orchestrate an epithelial polarization in the airways. *Mucosal Immunol.* (2016) 9:917–26.
294. Cohn L, Homer RJ, Niu N, Bottomly KT. helper 1 cells and interferon gamma regulate allergic airway inflammation and mucus production. *J Exp Med.* (1999) 190:1309–18.
295. Huang TJ, MacAry PA, Eynott P, Moussavi A, Daniel KC, Askenase PW, et al. Allergen-specific Th1 cells counteract efferent Th2 cell-dependent bronchial hyperresponsiveness and eosinophilic inflammation partly via IFN-gamma. *J Immunol.* (2001) 166:207–17.
296. Mitchell C, Provost K, Niu N, Homer R, Cohn L. IFN. -γ acts on the airway epithelium to inhibit local and systemic pathology in allergic airway disease. *J Immunol.* (2011) 187:3815–20.
297. Sel S, Wegmann M, Dicke T, Sel S, Henke W, Yildirim AO, et al. Effective prevention and therapy of experimental allergic asthma using a GATA-3-specific DNAzyme. *J Allergy Clin Immunol.* (2008) 121:910–6.e5.

298. Brand S, Kesper DA, Teich R, Kilic-Niebergall E, Pinkenburg O, Bothur E, et al. DNA methylation of TH1/TH2 cytokine genes affects sensitization and progress of experimental asthma. *J Allergy Clin Immunol.* (2012) 129:1602–10.e6.
299. Brand S, Teich R, Dicke T, Harb H, Yildirim AÖ, Tost J, et al. Epigenetic regulation in murine offspring as a novel mechanism for transmaternal asthma protection induced by microbes. *J Allergy Clin Immunol.* (2011) 128:618–25.
300. Jain-Vora S, Wert SE, Temann UA, Rankin JA, Whitsett JA. Interleukin-4 alters epithelial cell differentiation and surfactant homeostasis in the postnatal mouse lung. *Am J Respir Cell Mol Biol.* (1997) 17: 541–51.
301. van Wetering S, Zuyderduyn S, Ninaber DK, van Sterkenburg MAJA, Rabe KF, Hiemstra PS. Epithelial differentiation is a determinant in the production of eotaxin-2 and -3 by bronchial epithelial cells in response to IL-4 and IL-13. *Mol Immunol.* (2007) 44:803–11.
302. Kikuchi T, Shively JD, Foley JS, Drazen JM, Tschumperlin DJ. Differentiation-dependent responsiveness of bronchial epithelial cells to IL-4/13 stimulation. *Am J Physiol Lung Cell Mol Physiol.* (2004) 287:L119–26.
303. Zuyderduyn S, Ninaber DK, Schrumpf JA, van Sterkenburg MA, Verhoosel RM, Prins FA, et al. IL-4 and IL-13 exposure during mucociliary differentiation of bronchial epithelial cells increases antimicrobial activity and expression of antimicrobial peptides. *Respir Res.* (2011) 12:59.
304. Jakiela B, Gielicz A, Plutecka H, Hubalewska M, Mastalerz L, Bochenek G, et al. Eicosanoid biosynthesis during mucociliary and mucous metaplastic differentiation of bronchial epithelial cells. *Prostaglandins Other Lipid Mediat.* (2013) 106:116–23.
305. Contoli M, Ito K, Padovani A, Poletti D, Marku B, Edwards MR, et al. Th2 cytokines impair innate immune responses to rhinovirus in respiratory epithelial cells. *Allergy.* (2015) 70:910–20.
306. Rochlitzer S, Hoymann H-G, Müller M, Braun A. U-BIOPRED consortium. No exacerbation but impaired anti-viral mechanisms in a rhinovirus-chronic allergic asthma mouse model. *Clin Sci.* (2014) 126:55–65. doi: 10.1042/cs20130174
307. Bot A, Holz A, Christen U, Wolfe T, Temann A, Flavell R, et al. Local IL-4 expression in the lung reduces pulmonary influenza-virus-specific secondary cytotoxic T cell responses. *Virology.* (2000) 269:66–77. doi: 10.1006/viro.2000.0187
308. Zissler UM, Ulrich M, Jakwerth CA, Rothkirch S, Guerth F, Weckmann M, et al. Biomatrix for upper and lower airway biomarkers in patients with allergic asthma. *J Allergy Clin Immunol.* (2018) 142:1980–3.
309. Zissler UM, Jakwerth CA, Guerth FM, Pechtold L, Aguilar-Pimentel JA, Dietz K, et al. Early IL-10 producing B-cells and coinciding Th/Tr17 shifts during three year grass-pollen AIT. *EBioMedicine.* (2018) 36:475–88.
310. Tan LH, Bahmed K, Lin C-R, Marchetti N, Bolla S, Criner GJ, et al. The cytoprotective role of DJ-1 and p45 NFE2 against human primary alveolar type II cell injury and emphysema. *Sci Rep.* (2018) 8:3555.
311. Boucherat O, Chakir J, Jeannotte L. The loss of Hoxa5 function promotes Notch-dependent goblet cell metaplasia in lung airways. *Biol Open.* (2012) 1:677–91.
312. Zissler UM, Esser-von Bieren J, Jakwerth CA, Chaker AM, Schmidt-Weber CB. Current and future biomarkers in allergic asthma. *Allergy.* (2016) 71:475–94.

11

Gestational Exposure to Cigarette Smoke Suppresses the Gasotransmitter H_2S Biogenesis and the Effects are Transmitted Transgenerationally

*Shashi P. Singh[1], Dinesh Devadoss[2], Marko Manevski[2], Aryaz Sheybani[1], Teodora Ivanciuc[3], Vernat Exil[4], Hemant Agarwal[4], Veena Raizada[4], Roberto P. Garofalo[3], Hitendra S. Chand[2] and Mohan L. Sopori[1]**

[1] Respiratory Immunology Division, Lovelace Respiratory Research Institute, Albuquerque, NM, United States, [2] Department of Immunology and Nanomedicine, Herbert Wertheim College of Medicine, Florida International University, Miami, FL, United States, [3] Department of Microbiology and Immunology, Galveston, TX, United States, [4] Department of Pediatrics, University of New Mexico Health Sciences Center, Albuquerque, NM, United States

***Correspondence:**
Mohan L. Sopori
msopori@lrri.org

Rationale: Gestational cigarette smoke (CS) impairs lung angiogenesis and alveolarization, promoting transgenerational development of asthma and bronchopulmonary dysplasia (BPD). Hydrogen sulfide (H_2S), a proangiogenic, pro-alveolarization, and anti-asthmatic gasotransmitter is synthesized by cystathionine-γ-lyase (CSE), cystathionine-β-synthase (CBS), and 3-mercaptopyruvate sulfur transferase (3MST).

Objective: Determine if gestational CS exposure affected the expression of H_2S synthesizing enzymes in the mouse lung and human placenta.

Methods: Mice were exposed throughout gestational period to secondhand CS (SS) at approximating the dose of CS received by a pregnant woman sitting in a smoking bar for 3 h/days during pregnancy. Lungs from 7-days old control and SS-exposed pups and human placenta from mothers who were either non-smokers or smokers during pregnancy were analyzed for expression of the enzymes.

Measurements: Mouse lungs and human placentas were examined for the expression of CSE, CBS, and 3MST by immunohistochemical staining, qRT-PCR and/or Western blot (WB) analyses.

Results: Compared to controls, mouse lung exposed gestationally to SS had significantly lower levels of CSE, CBS, and 3MST. Moreover, the SS-induced suppression of CSE and CBS in F1 lungs was transmitted to the F2 generation without significant change in the magnitude of the suppression. These changes were associated with impaired epithelial-mesenchymal transition (EMT)—a process required for normal lung angiogenesis and alveolarization. Additionally, the placentas from mothers who smoked during pregnancy, expressed significantly lower levels of CSE, CBS, and 3MST, and the effects were partially moderated by quitting smoking during the first trimester.

Conclusions: Lung H_2S synthesizing enzymes are downregulated by gestational CS and the effects are transmitted to F2 progeny. Smoking during pregnancy decreases H_2S synthesizing enzymes is human placentas, which may correlate with the increased risk of asthma/BPD in children.

Keywords: gestational cigarette smoke, H_2S biogenesis, human placenta, lungs, transgenerational effect

INTRODUCTION

Maternal smoking during pregnancy remains relatively common (1, 2) and about 1/4th of mothers, who smoke during pregnancy, misreport as quitters (3). Epidemiological data and animal studies suggest that exposure to CS, including secondhand CS (SS) during pregnancy increases the risk of allergic asthma (AA) and BPD in the progeny (4–7); the latter encompasses alveolar simplification (8). Gestational exposure of mice to CS/SS impairs angiogenesis, exacerbates AA, and induces BPD-like alveolar simplification through downregulation of HIF-1α; this phenotype is transmitted to the F2 progeny (9–11). The mechanisms by which gestation CS promotes AA and BPD are unclear. H_2S is the newest member of gasotransmitter that affects many physiological systems (12). H_2S is an anti-inflammatory that promotes angiogenesis/vascularization and wound healing (7, 13). In the lung, H_2S attenuates lipopolysaccharide-induced acute lung injury (14), confers protection against ventilation-induced pulmonary inflammation and injury (15), promotes alveolarization and airway development (16), and protects against asthma and allergic inflammation (17, 18).

In mammals, H_2S is mainly produced from L-cysteine by three enzymes: cystathionine γ-lyase (CSE), cystathionine β-synthase (CBS), and 3-mercaptopyruvate sulfur transferase (3MST) (19, 20). The distribution of these enzymes in various tissue is somewhat uncertain. It is generally believed that CSE and CBS are the two most prominent H_2S synthesizing enzymes, where CBS is primarily localized to the brain and CSE in non-neuronal tissues (21, 22). However, this is not an inflexible rule. For example, adult rat lung expresses CSE and 3MST, but insignificant levels of CBS (23), but CBS has been reported in airway vasculature and lung epithelial cells, and CSE is present in the lung parenchyma (16). All three H_2S synthesizing enzymes (CSE, CBS, and 3MST) are present in the lungs of cows and sea lions (24) and lung biopsies from non-small cell lung cancer patients (25) and the lung epithelial cell line A549 (26) also express all the three enzymes. In a recent report, 3MST was shown to be upregulated in the lung adenocarcinoma (27). Similarly, while the portal vein and thoracic aorta contain CSE, ileum expresses both CSE and CBS (28). Thus, the expression of H_2S enzymes depends on the tissue type and the state of cell differentiation.

Epithelial mesenchymal transition (EMT) is an important process for cell differentiation during development, organogenesis, and carcinogenesis (29, 30). While dysregulated EMT in the adult lung promotes multiple respiratory diseases, it is indispensable for the development of lung epithelium (31), where the TGF-β/Smad pathway plays a key role (31, 32). Although, H_2S has been shown to inhibit EMT in lung cancers through Wnt/Catenin signaling and the activation of HIF-1α (25, 33), HIF-1α is dramatically downregulated by gestational CS in the 7-days old mouse lung (11, 34) and, in some lung injuries, H_2S promotes EMT and lung repair (35, 36). Moreover, HIF-1α mediates cellular differentiation through TGF-β (37, 38)—a key participant in EMT (39, 40). Thus, EMT is important in lung development and organogenesis, and requires H2S-induced HIF-1α/TGF-β.

In this communication we demonstrate that gestational SS suppresses TGF-β, EMT, and anti-asthmatic factors, and the 7-days old mouse lung and human placentas contains all the three H_2S synthesizing enzymes. Gestational exposure to CS suppresses the expression of these enzymes in the mouse lung and human placentas from mothers' who smoke during pregnancy. The latter prompts the possibility that the placental levels of H_2S synthesizing enzymes may correlate with the risk of AA and BPD in children.

MATERIALS AND METHODS

Animals

Pathogen-free BALB/c mice were purchased from the FCR Facility (Frederick, MD). The animals were housed at the Animal Facility of Lovelace Respiratory Research Institute, Albuquerque, NM in accordance with the Guidelines from the Association for the Assessment and Accreditation for Laboratory Animal Care International. Animals were kept in exposure chambers maintained at 26 ± 2°C with 12-h light/dark cycle. Food and water were provided *ad libitum*.

Study Approval

All animal protocols were approved by the Institutional Animal Care and Use Committee in accordance with the Guide for Laboratory Animal Practice under the Association for the Assessment and Accreditation for Laboratory Animal Care International.

Abbreviations: AA, allergic asthma; BPD, bronchopulmonary dysplasia; CBS, cystathionine-β-synthase; CCSP, Clara-cell secretory protein; COPD, chronic obstructive pulmonary disease; CS, cigarette smoke; CSE, cystathionine-γ-lyase; CS, cigarette smoke; EMT, epithelial mesenchymal transition; FA, filtered air; GesCS, gestational cigarette smoke; GesCS1/3, mothers who quit smoking during the 1st trimester; HIF-1α, hypoxia Inducible factor-1α; H_2S, Hydrogen sulfide; 3MST, 3-mercaptopyruvate sulfur transferase; MFI, mean fluorescence intensity; NaHS, sodium hydrosulfide; SS, secondhand CS; SP-C, surfactant protein-C; TGF-β, transforming growth factor beta; ZO-1, zonula occludens-1.

Gestational Exposure to Sidestream Cigarette Smoke (SS)

Adult (3–4 months old) male and female mice (BALB/c) were separately acclimatized to SS or filtered air (FA) for 2 weeks before being paired for mating under the same exposure conditions. Briefly, mice were exposed to whole-body SS or FA for 6 h/days, 7 days/weeks (total particulate matter 1.52 ± 0.41 mg/m^3) using Type 1,300 smoking machine (AMESA Electronics, Geneva, Switzerland) that generated two 70 cm^3 puffs/min from 2R1 cigarettes as described previously (9, 10). The dose of SS was approximately equivalent to the amount of SS a pregnant woman would receive by sitting in a smoking bar for 3 h/days throughout the gestational period (10). After pregnancy was established, male mice were removed and the pregnant mice continued to receive SS or FA until the pups were born. Immediately after the birth of pups the exposures were stopped. On the postnatal day 7, some animals were sacrificed by an intraperitoneal injection of 0.2 ml Euthasol. Some adult F1 mice from FA and SS groups were mated to obtain the F2 progeny as described previously (10). Representative results are presented using animal from two different sets of SS-exposure. At least 15 animals per group were used; each analysis used 5 mice/group and the analysis was repeated twice. Specific details are given under figure legends.

Human Placenta Samples

Placentas were collected at the University of New Mexico Hospital (UNMH), Albuquerque, NM according to protocol #17-064 approved by the University of New Mexico Medical Center Institutional Review Board and Human Research Protection Office in accordance with the NIH guidelines. All donors had agreed to donate the tissues. We were able to collect 10 placentas in a span of 7 months (by Dr. A. Sheybani and Dr. V. Exil, both from UNMH) representing three controls (mothers who did not smoke during the pregnancy), 4 CS-exposed (mothers who smoked throughout the pregnancy), two first-trimester quitters (mothers who stopped smoking during the first trimester of pregnancy), one false-control (mother who claimed to have quitted smoking during pregnancy, but the placenta had high level of cotinine). A 3 cm^3 section of each placenta was dissected and frozen immediately for RNA and protein assays. Rest of the placentas were kept at $-80°$Cuntil use. Tissue slides (5 μm) were prepared by the institutional Pathology Core.

Determination of Cotinine Levels in Placentas

The smoking status of the mothers was confirmed by determining the cotinine levels in the placental tissues using the cotinine ELISA kit (Calbiotech Inc., CA) with a sensitivity of 5 ng/ml. Immunoblots were developed using placental homogenates.

Assays for H_2S Synthesizing Enzymes

The expression of CSE, CBS, and 3MST was determined by WB analysis, IF-IHC, and/or qPCR. Assay details are given under relevant figure legends.

Immunostaining and Immunofluorescent Imaging

For immunohistochemical (IHC) staining, deparaffinized and hydrated lung and placental tissue sections were washed in 0.05% v Brij-35 in PBS (pH 7.4) and immunostained for antigen expression as described previously (41). Briefly, the antigens were unmasked by steaming the sections in 10 mM Citrate buffer (pH 6.0) followed by incubation in a blocking solution containing 3% BSA, 1% Gelatin and 1% normal donkey serum with 0.1% Triton X-100 and 0.1% Saponin. Serial sections were stained with antibodies to Vimentin, E-cadherin, and ZO-1 (Invitrogen Inc., Carlsbad, CA), or isotype control antibodies. The immunolabelled tissues were detected using respective secondary antibodies conjugated with fluorescent dyes (Jackson ImmunoResearch Lab Inc., West Grove, PA). Where indicated, the sections were stained with 4′,6-diamidino-2-phenylindole (DAPI) containing Fluormount-G (SouthernBiotech, Birmingham, AL) to visualize nuclei. Immunofluorescent images were captured with BZX700 Microscopy system (Keyence, Tokyo, Japan). Specific details are given under appropriate figure legends.

Western Blot Analysis

Western blot (WB) analysis of mouse lung and human placenta homogenates was carried out as described previously (10). Briefly, lung or placental tissues were homogenized in RIPA buffer and the protein content of the extracts was determined by the BCA Protein Assay Kit (Pierce, Rockford, IL). The homogenates were run on SDS-PAGE on 10% precast polyacrylamide gels (BioRad Lab, Hercules CA). The gels were transferred electrophoretically to nitrocellulose membranes (BioRad Lab). The blots were incubated with the respective antibodies. The mouse anti-β actin antibody (Santa Cruz Biotech) was used as the house-keeping protein. After incubating with an appropriate secondary antibody, the blots were developed with Amersham ECL Western Blotting Detection Reagent (GE Healthcare Bio-Science Corp. Piscataway, NJ) and the images were captured by Fujiform LAS-4000 luminescent image analyzer (FUJIFILM Corporation, Tokyo). Densitometry was used to quantitate the expression of specific proteins and expressed as the protein/β-actin band ratio.

Quantitative Real-Time PCR (qPCR)

Total RNA was extracted by using a ToTALLY RNA kit (catalog number AM1910; Ambion, Austin, TX, USA). RNA samples were quantified by using a NanoDrop spectrophotometer and quality was analyzed on an RNA Nano-drop by using the Agilent 2100 bioanalyzer (Agilent Technologies). Synthesis of cDNA used 1 μg of total RNA in a 20 μl reaction mixture and TaqMan Reverse Transcription Reagents kit from ABI (catalog number N8080234; Applied Biosystems). qPCR amplification (performed in triplicate) used 1 μl of cDNA in a total volume of 25 μl of Faststart Universal SYBR green master mix (Roche Applied Science #04913850001). The mRNA sequences for CSE, and CBS for mouse and human reported under GenBank accession numbers NM145953 (CSE mouse), NM144855.3 (CBS mouse), NM_001902 (CSE human), and NM000071 (CBS (human) and were used to design primers for qRT-PCR assay (42–44). Expression of 3MST mRNA was performed using total RNA from lung and placental tissues by qPCR analysis and One-Step Real-Time PCR MasterMix containing TaqMan probes and a specific-labeled primer/probe set (Applied Biosystems). 18S RNA was used as housekeeping gene for normalization. PCR assays were run in the ABI Prism 7500 Sequence Detection System. Triplicate cycle threshold (C_T) values were analyzed using the comparative C_T ($\Delta\Delta C_T$) method as per manufacturer's instructions (Applied Biosystems). The amount of target ($2^{-\Delta\Delta CT}$) was obtained by normalization to the endogenous reference (18S) sample. RNA isolation, primer design, and qRT-PCR assays were performed using the Molecular Genomic Core, UTMB, Galveston, TX.

Statistical Analysis

Grouped results were expressed as mean ± SD and $p \leq 0.05$ were considered significant. The data were normalized via natural log transformations and when the data was normally distributed, statistical significance among the groups was determined by one-way ANOVA with Bonferroni correction with multiple pairwise comparisons. When the data was not normally distributed, we used Kruskal-Wallis assessment on ranks followed by Dunn's multiple comparison tests. Student's *t*-test was employed for comparison between two groups at 95% confidence interval using Prizm software (GraphPad Software Inc., San Diego, CA). $p \leq 0.05$ was considered statistically significant.

RESULTS AND DISCUSSION

Gestational SS Inhibits EMT in the F1-Progeny Lung

Gestational exposure to SS impairs alveolarization and promotes BPD in the progeny, and these effects are transmitted to the F2 progeny and associated with suppressed levels of HIF-1α (11, 34). EMT is a biological process that allows epithelial cells to assume mesenchymal phenotype, which is critical for normal alveolarization (45) and regulated by HIF-1α, TGF-β, and VEGF (38, 39, 46, 47). VEGF promotes angiogenesis that stimulates EMT and alveolarization (48, 49) and intratracheal transplantation of mesenchymal stem cells attenuate lung injury in newborn mice (50). During embryogenesis and organ development, epithelial markers such as E-cadherin and ZO-1 are decreased and mesenchymal markers such as vimentin are increased (48, 51). The transcription factor HIF-1α promotes synthesis of TGF-β–the most potent inducer of EMT (52, 53) and HIF-1α is potently reduced in gestationally SS-exposed lungs (11). To determine whether gestational SS affected EMT, we determined the lung levels of epithelial (E-cadherin and ZO-1) and mesenchymal (vimentin) cell markers by IHC and Western blot analysis in 7-days old lungs from control and gestationally SS-exposed mice. Compared to control lungs, levels of E-cadherin (**Figure 1A**) and ZO-1 (**Figure 1B**) were significantly higher than those of vimentin (**Figures 1A,C**) in gestationally SS-exposed lungs. Moreover, the concentrations of TGF-β by Western blot analysis (**Figure 1D**) and of the anti-asthmatic factor SOX2 by IHC (**Figure 1E**), were significantly lower in gestationally SS-exposed lungs. SOX2 is a pluripotent transcription factor in bronchoalveolar progenitors, which promotes the Club cells to express Clara-cell secretory protein (CCSP) and surfactant protein-C (SP-C) (54). CCSP and SP-C are suppressed by gestational SS (10) and reduced SOX2 and CCSP levels are associated with higher risk of asthma (55); humans and mice deficient in CCSP, exhibit airway hyperresponsiveness (56). Together, these results suggest that gestational exposure to CS inhibits EMT and is associated with decreased numbers of SOX2-positive Clara cell progenitors.

Gestational SS Suppresses CSE and CBS in the F1 and F2 Progeny Lungs

H_2S is required for normal angiogenesis and alveolarization (16, 25) and produced in the periphery mainly by CSE and CBS (12). H_2S attenuates lung injury (15, 57) and CSE deficiency exacerbates airway hyperreactivity (44) and impairs alveolarization. Impaired angiogenesis and alveolarization in CSE- and CBS-deficient mice are partially restored by H_2S donor compounds (16). Moreover, H_2S levels are lower in the exhaled air from asthma and COPD patients and correlates with lower FEV_1 (58). Expression level of H_2S enzymes is reported to be tissue specific. Thus, the brain and the vascular endothelium have a strong expression of CBS and CSE, respectively; however, both tissues also express 3MST (22). The situation in the lung is somewhat confusing. Lungs were reported to primarily express CSE (21); however, human lung cell lines such as A549 (26) and the lungs from cow and sea lions express all the three H_2S synthesizing enzymes (24).

To ascertain whether gestational SS affected H_2S production in the lung, we determined the mRNA levels of CSE (**Figure 2A**) and CBS (**Figure 2B**) and 3MST (**Figure 2C**) by qPCR in 7-day-old lungs from control and SS-exposed mice. Gestational CS inhibited mRNA levels of CSE, CBS, and 3MST, which would decrease the level of H2S in the lung and increase the risk of inflammatory lung diseases in these animals.

Gestational CS/SS/nicotine increases the risk of asthma and/or BPD transgenerationally in humans and animals (10, 59–61). To determine whether the transgenerational pro-asthmatic/pro-BDP effects of gestational SS were related to changes in H_2S, 7-days old lungs from control and gestationally SS-exposed F1 and F2 mice were analyzed for CSE (**Figure 2D**) and CBS (**Figure 2E**) levels by IHC staining. Results showed that control lungs contained about equal numbers (~25%of total cells) of CSE- and CBS-positive cells, and gestational exposure to SS significantly reduced the number CSE/CBS-positive cells in both F1 and F2 animals. Thus, as reported for HIF-1α, angiogenesis, and alveolar volumes (11), gestational SS suppresses the levels of CSE and CBS in F1 progeny and the effects are transmitted to F2. Given the relationship between HIF-1α, TGF-β, EMT, angiogenesis, alveolarization, BPD, AA, and H_2S, it is likely that the CS-induced proinflammatory lung responses in F1 and F2 progenies are related to

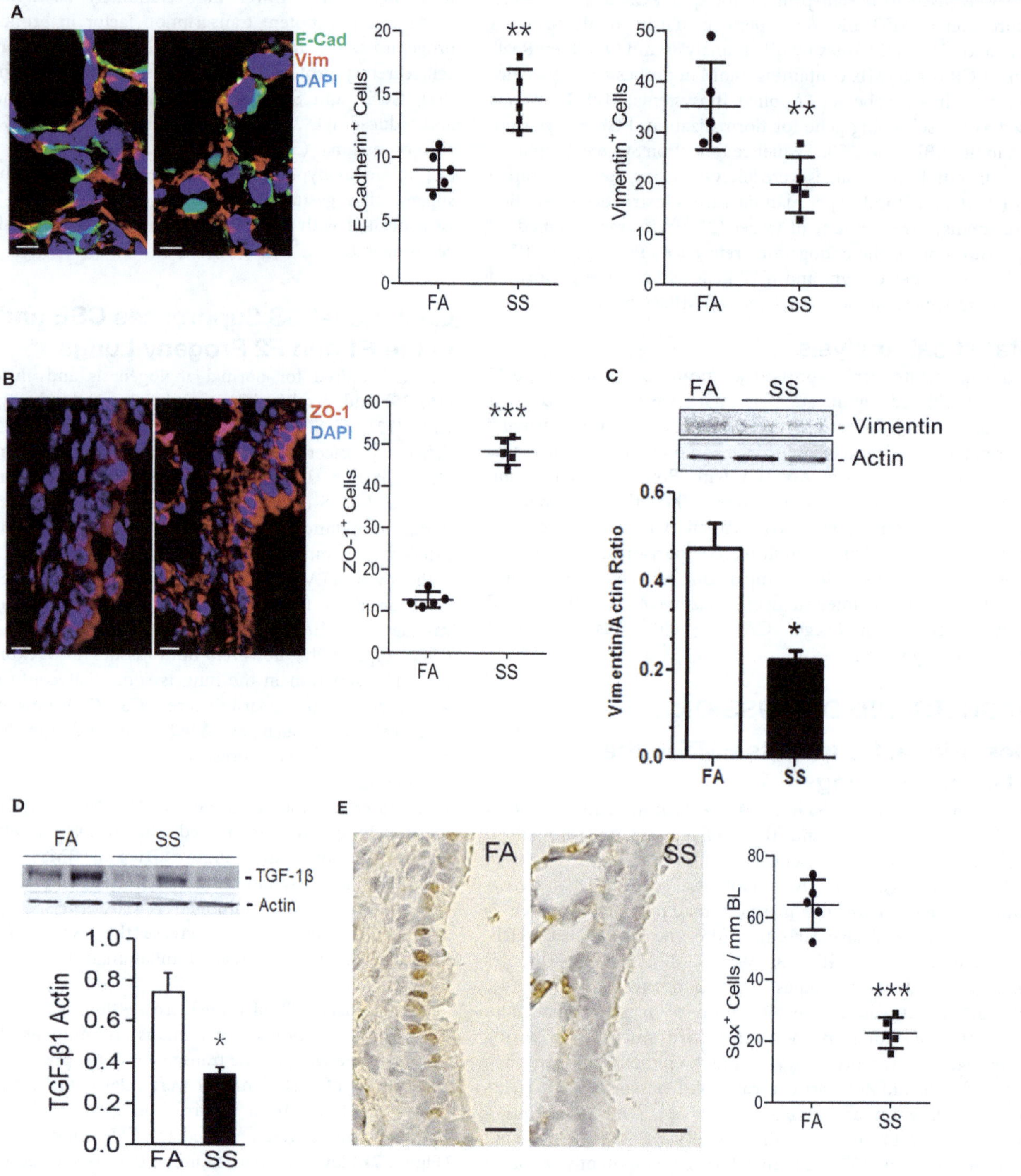

FIGURE 1 | Gestational exposure to SS inhibits EMT in the mouse F1 lung. **(A)** Representative micrographs of lung sections from mice exposed gestationally to filtered-air (FA) or side-stream cigarette smoke (SS) and co-stained with vimentin (red) and cadherin (green); DAPI-stained nuclei (blue). E-Cadherin$^+$ and Vimentin$^+$ cells per unit area (18,000 μm^2) were counted blind using NDP View on a Nanozoomer (Hamamatsu Photonics Inc.). **(B)** Representative micrographs of lung sections from gestationally FA or SS-exposed mice and stained with ZO-1 (red). ZO-1$^+$ cells (12,400 μm^2; NDP scanner). **(C)** Representative Western blot of lung tissue homogenates (70 μg) from FA or SS-exposed mice and probed with anti-vimentin antibody. Lower panel is the densitometry of the blot and expressed as Vimentin/Actin ratio. **(D)** Western blot analysis of lung tissue homogenates (70 μg) from FA or SS-exposed lungs probed with anti-TGF-β1 antibody (Cat# ab92486, Abcam). Lower panel is densitometry of the blot presented as TGF-β1/Actin ratio. **(E)** Representative image of the lung sections (5 μm) stained with anti-Sox2 antibody and detected by immunohistochemical staining. Right panel shows Sox$^+$ cells (17,000 μm^2; NDP scanner) counted blind. Data shown as mean±SD ($n = 5$/gp; $^*p < 0.05$; $^{**}p < 0.01$; $^{***}p < 0.001$).

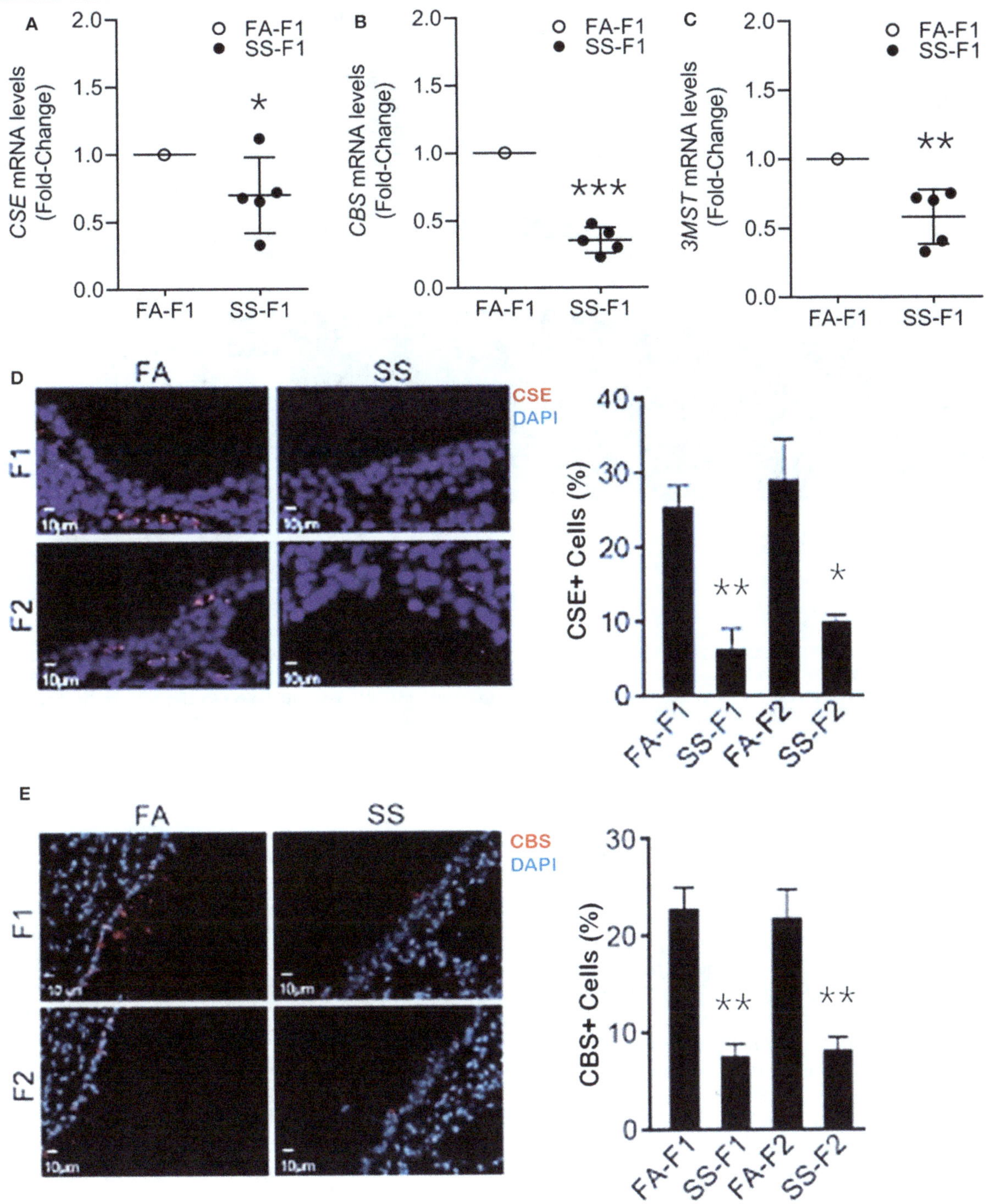

FIGURE 2 | Gestational SS suppresses H2S biogenesis enzymes, CSE, CBS and 3MST in 7d old F1 mouse lung. Relative mRNA levels of *CSE* **(A)**, *CBS* **(B)**, and *3MST* **(C)** in F1 lungs exposed gestationally to FA or SS. **(D)** Representative micrographs of lung sections from F1 and F2 progenies exposed gestationally to SS or FA. Sections were stained for CSE (red) and DAPI (blue). Right pane is quantitation of CSE$^+$ cells (%) in each group. **(E)** Micrographs of lung sections from F1 and F2 stained for CBS (red) and DAPI (blue). Right panel shows quantitation of CBS$^+$ cells (%) in each group. Data shown as mean ± SD (n = 5/gp; $^*p < 0.05$; $^{**}p < 0.01$; $^{***}p < 0.001$).

changes in H_2S levels regulated by H_2S synthesizing enzymes. These data suggest that mouse lungs contain all three H_2S synthesizing enzymes and gestational exposure to CS suppresses their expression. Reduced levels of these enzymes has the potential to promote lung diseases such as asthma and BPD.

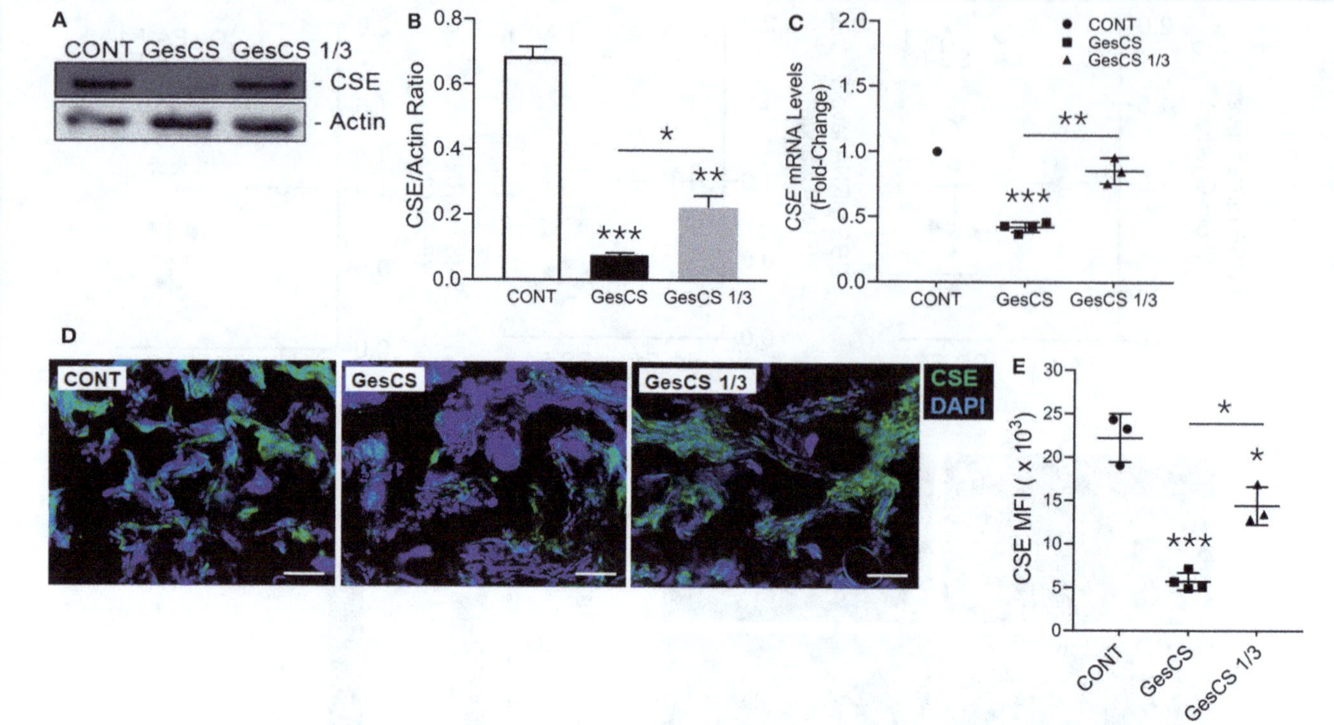

FIGURE 3 | Gestational exposure to CS suppresses H2S biosynthetic enzyme CSE in human placenta. Placentas were analyzed for CSE expression using WB, qPCR and IF-IHC staining. **(A)** Western blot analysis of the placental tissue homogenate (150 µg protein) with anti-CSE antibody (Abcam, MA, USA). **(B)** Densitometry of CBS normalized to β-actin levels. **(C)** *CSE* mRNA detection by qPCR and expressed relative to CONT group. **(D)** Representative micrographs showing placental CSE (green) along with DAPI-stained nuclei (blue), scale–10 µ. **(E)** Quantification of CSE expression by MFIs (mean fluorescence intensity). CONT, control non-smoker; GesCS, cigarette smoking during whole pregnancy; GesCS1/3, CS exposure during first trimester; Data shown as mean ± SD (n = 3–4/gp; *$p < 0.05$; **$p < 0.01$; ***$p < 0.001$).

Placentas From Women Who Smoked During Pregnancy Express Low Levels of H_2S Synthesizing Enzymes

Children from women who smoke during pregnancy have increased risk of AA and BPD (4–7) and herein our results suggest that the increased susceptibility may correlate with decreased levels of H_2S synthesizing enzymes. Thus, the lung levels of H_2S enzymes at birth may predict the risk of AA and BPD in children; however, it is unrealistic to obtain lung samples from newborn babies. Because, H_2S synthesizing enzymes are present in most tissues (12, 62), we ascertained whether the enzymes were present in human placentas and, if so, whether smoking during pregnancy affected their expression. We were able to obtain 10 human placentas representing 3 controls (mothers who did not smoke during the pregnancy), four CS-exposed (mothers who smoked throughout the pregnancy), two first-trimester quitters (mothers who stopped smoking during the first trimester of pregnancy), one false-control (mother who claimed to have quitted smoking during pregnancy, but the placental showed high cotinine). Cotinine was determined on all placentas by ELISA to ensure that the tissues were from smoking/non-smoking mothers. CSE expression was determined by WB analysis, qPCR, and IF-IHC; CBS by WB and IF-IHC, and 3MST by qPCR analysis.

Immunoblot analysis of the placental homogenates from mothers who smoked throughout the pregnancy (GesCS) showed very low expression of CSE as compared to control non-smokers (CONT) or the mothers who quit during the 1st trimester (GesCS1/3) (**Figures 3A,B**). Similarly, as determined by qPCR analysis, CSE-specific mRNA content of GesCS placentas was significantly lower than CONT and GesCS1/3 (**Figure 3C**). Although the protein content of CSE in GesCS1/3 was higher than GesCS, it was still significantly lower than CONT (**Figure 3B**), suggesting that quitting smoking during the first trimester may be beneficial; however, the effects are not totally reversible and may persists after the birth. CSE expression was further confirmed by immunostaining of placental sections showing a 4-fold lower expression of CSE in GesCS than CONT; CSE expression in GesCS1/3 placentas was intermediate between CONT and GesCS (**Figures 3D,E**).

WB analysis also indicated that the expression of CBS was lower in GesCS than CONT or GesCS1/3 (**Figures 4A,B**). Furthermore, IHC analysis of CBS in placentas showed the expression was 3-fold lower in GesCS than CONT; however, the difference between CONT and GesCS 1/3 groups was not statistically significant (**Figures 4C,D**). We also examined the status of 3MST mRNA expression in human placentas by qPCR. Like CSE and CBS, exposure to cigarette smoke significantly

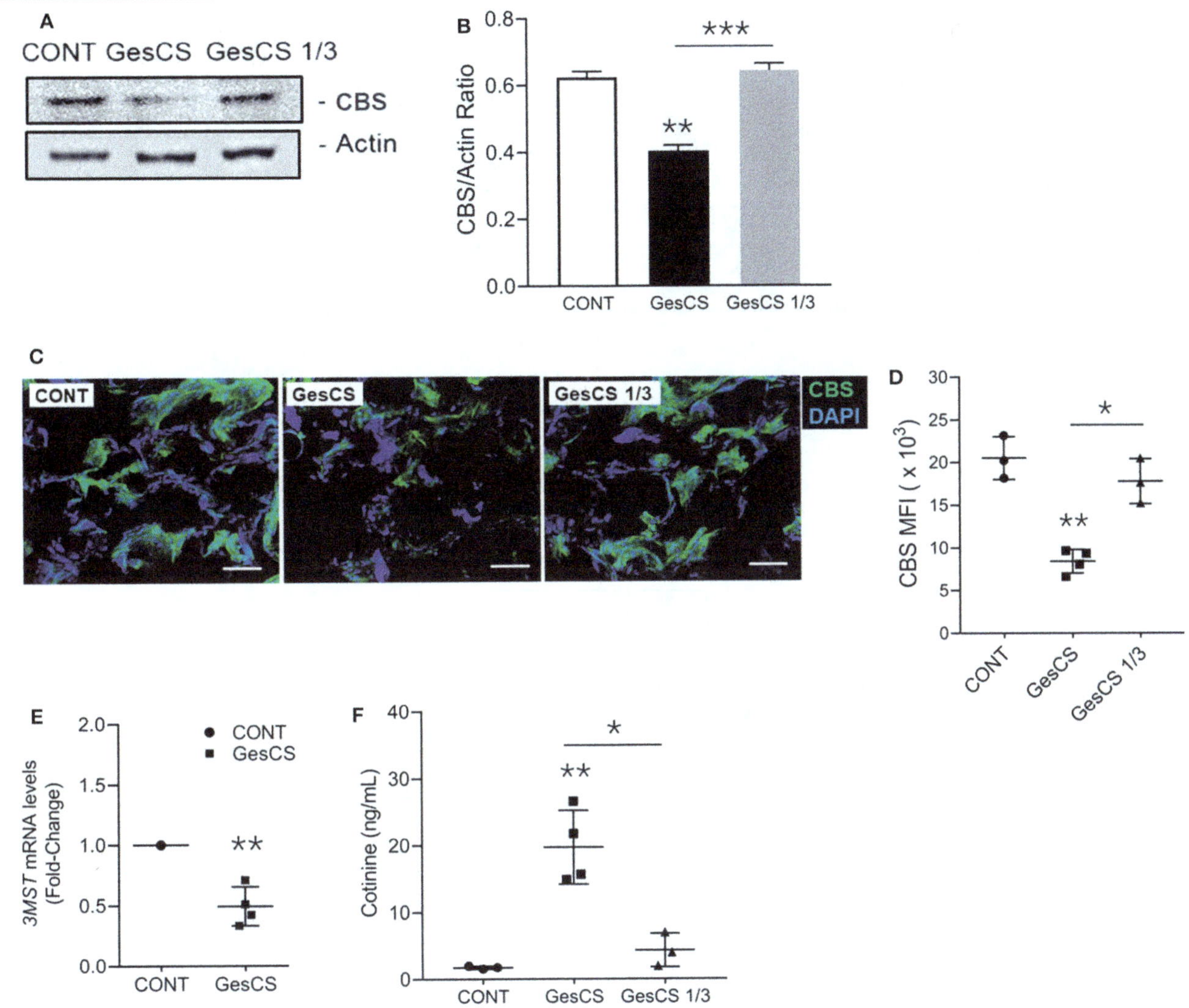

FIGURE 4 | Gestational exposure to CS suppresses CBS and 3MST in human placenta. **(A)** Western blot analysis of placental tissue homogenates (150 μg protein) probed with anti-CBS antibody (Abcam, MA). **(B)** Densitometry of CBS normalized to β-actin. **(C)** Representative micrographs showing placental CBS (green) and DAPI-stained nuclei (blue), scale–10 μ. **(D)** Quantification of CBS expression by MFI (mean fluorescence intensity) of CBS-immunoreactive fluorescence. **(E)** Quantitative RT-PCR of *3MST* mRNA expression ($n = 5$). **(F)** The smoking status of mother's was ascertained by the cotinine levels in the placental homogenate using cotinine ELISA kit (Calbiotech Inc., CA) with sensitivity of 5 ng/ml. CONT, non-smoker control; GesCS, cigarette smoker during pregnancy; GesCS1/3, CS exposure during first trimester; Data shown as mean ± SD ($n = 3$–4/gp; $^*p < 0.05$; $^{**}p < 0.01$; $^{***}p < 0.001$).

inhibited the expression of 3MST (**Figure 4E**) indicating that, like CSE and CBS, gestational CS also downregulates 3MST expression in human placentas.

The smoking status of the mothers who donated the placentas was verified by measuring the cotinine levels (**Figure 4F**) and, in general, corroborated their assertion. However, we observed one outlier, where the WB and qPCR analyses of the placenta indicated very low levels of CSE (data not shown), yet the donor claimed to have quitted smoking during the pregnancy. The placenta contained high cotinine levels and was not included in the analyses. Sadly, it is not uncommon for the mothers to falsely assert quitting smoking during the pregnancy (3, 63).

The current study does not clearly define the stage(s) of pregnancy, where the fetus is completely resistant to the effects of CS on placental H_2S enzymes. While the epidemiological evidence strongly suggests that CS exposure during pregnancy promotes wheeze and asthma in children (64), but the identity of the susceptible stage(s) of the pregnancy is not unequivocal and may vary from first trimester (6) to third trimester (5). Our data with placental levels of H_2S enzymes suggest that the effects of smoking during first trimester are moderate, but not negligible; however, we have not correlated these levels to the actual incidence of asthma in the progeny. Interestingly, perinatal exposure to nicotine induces asthma in rats (61), suggesting that late stages of embryonic development might be more sensitive

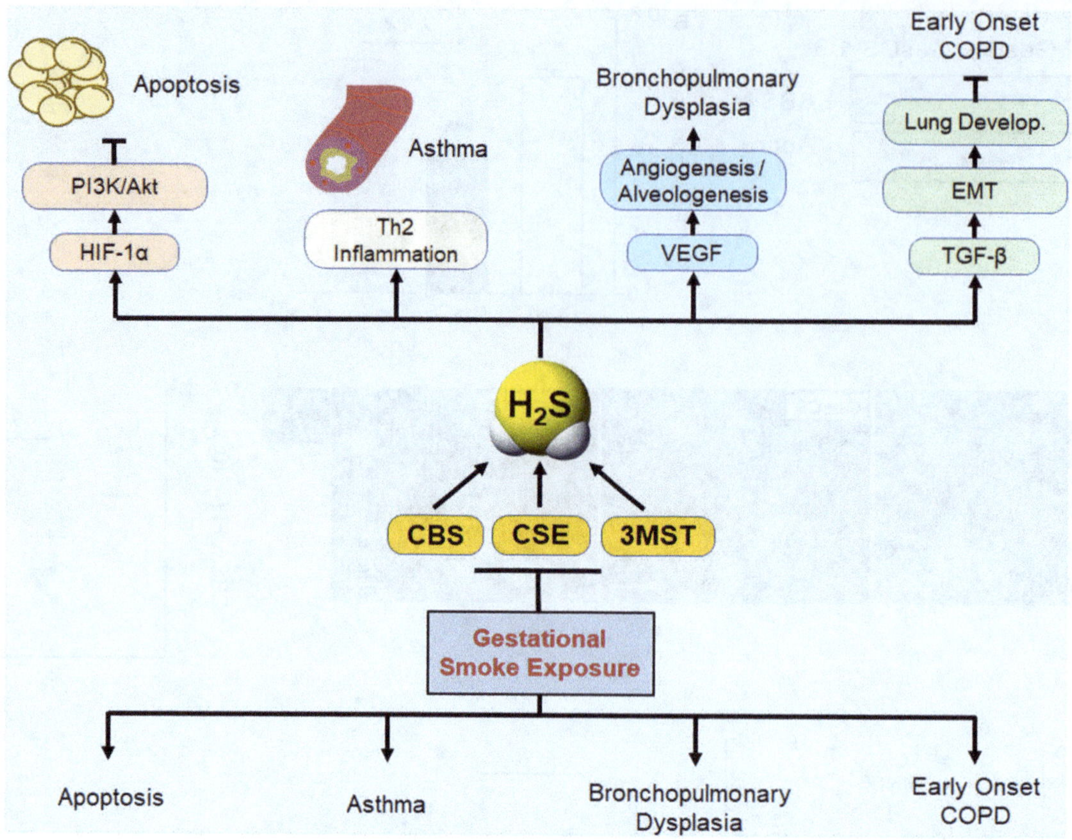

FIGURE 5 | Schematic representation of potential protective role of biosynthesized H_2S in basic lung pathophysiologies that are disrupted by gestational exposure to CS. Gestational exposure to CS is primarily linked to four major pulmonary predicaments: cell apoptosis, asthma, BPD, and susceptibility to early development of COPD. Lung cell apoptosis is associated with allergic inflammation (18) and decreased levels of HIF-1α and PI3K/Akt (34). PI3K/Akt inhibits apoptosis and promotes cell proliferation (67), and activation of Akt protects the neonatal lung against injuries (68). H2S donors inhibit apoptosis, attenuate lung damage, and promote normal lung development (21, 69). Asthma development as a consequence of gestational CS exposure or the deficiency of H_2S enzymes is associated with increased Th2 inflammation (9, 17, 70), and exogenous H_2S was shown to reverse the exacerbated asthma response in CSE-deficient mice (17). Gestation SS suppresses VEGF and angiogenesis, leading to impaired alveolarization and BPD (11, 34), and H_2S stimulates VEGF expression and angiogenesis, (71), and alveolarization (72, 73). Maternal smoking affects lung development and has been linked to early onset of COPD in the progeny (74, 75). TGF-β is critical for EMT and normal lung development (31, 53) and herein we have shown that gestational CS downregulates TGF-β and inhibits EMT. Thus, gestational exposure to CS downregulates H_2S synthesizing enzymes that in turn may increase the susceptibility of children to respiratory diseases associated with gestational exposure to CS.

to gestational CS. Nonetheless, it is highly likely that there is a correlation between placental levels of H_2S enzymes and the risk of asthma/BPD in children and H_2S or H_2S-donor compounds may have therapeutic value to reduce this risk. The manner by which H_2S inhibits allergic asthma is related to its ability to suppress Th2 immune responses (65) and CSE deficient mice have elevated GATA3 nuclear content, higher levels of Th2 cytokines, and exaggerated asthma response; H_2S donors attenuate asthma (17, 66). Thus, gestational exposure to CS downregulates H_2S synthesizing enzymes that in turn may increase the susceptibility of children to respiratory diseases associated with gestational exposure to CS. Taken together, the data presented herein provide a basic outline of the potential interaction between gestational CS exposure, *de novo* synthesis of H_2S, and development of lung developmental diseases as described schematically in **Figure 5**.

RESEARCH IMPACT

Exposure to cigarette smoke (CS) during pregnancy impairs epithelial-mesenchymal transition (EMT) and angiogenesis in the lung, increasing the risk of allergic asthma and bronchopulmonary dysplasia (BPD), transgenerationally. Hydrogen sulfide (H2S), a recently recognized gasotransmitter, promotes angiogenesis and inhibits asthma and alveolar simplification. H_2S is synthesized by cystathionine-β-synthase (CBS), cystathionine-γ-lyase (CSE), and 3-mercaptopyruvate sulfur transferase (3MST). Results presented herein show that exposure of mice to CS during pregnancy suppressed the lung expression of CSE, CBS, 3-MST, and the CS-induced suppression of CSE and CBS was transmitted to F2. Similarly, smoking during pregnancy downregulated the expression of CSE, CBS, and 3MST in human placentas; the downregulated expression of the enzymes might be a biomarker for asthma susceptibility in children.

AUTHOR CONTRIBUTIONS

SS performed the experiments, analyzed the data, and wrote the manuscript, DD, MM, AS, and TI analyzed the data, VE, HA, and VR performed the sample analysis and analyzed the data. RG analyzed the data and wrote the manuscript. HC performed the sample analysis, analyzed the data, and wrote the manuscript. MS designed the studies, analyzed the data, and wrote the manuscript. All authors reviewed the manuscript.

ACKNOWLEDGMENTS

We thank the staff and veterinarians of the Inhalation Core and Histology Core facility of Lovelace Respiratory Research Institute.

REFERENCES

1. Hylkema MN, Blacquiere MJ. Intrauterine effects of maternal smoking on sensitization, asthma, and chronic obstructive pulmonary disease. *Proc Am Thorac Soc.* (2009) 6:660–2. doi: 10.1513/pats.200907-065DP
2. Mazurek JM, England LJ. Cigarette smoking among working women of reproductive age-United States, 2009-2013. *Nicotine Tob Res.* (2016) 18:894–9. doi: 10.1093/ntr/ntv292
3. England LJ, Grauman A, Qian C, Wilkins DG, Schisterman EF, Yu KF, et al. Misclassification of maternal smoking status and its effects on an epidemiologic study of pregnancy outcomes. *Nicotine Tob Res.* (2007) 9:1005–13. doi: 10.1080/14622200701491255
4. Hu FB, Persky V, Flay BR, Zelli A, Cooksey J, Richardson J. Prevalence of asthma and wheezing in public schoolchildren: association with maternal smoking during pregnancy. *Ann Allergy Asthma Immunol.* (1997) 79:80–4. doi: 10.1016/S1081-1206(10)63090-6
5. Xepapadaki P, Manios Y, Liarigkovinos T, Grammatikaki E, Douladiris N, Kortsalioudaki C, et al. Association of passive exposure of pregnant women to environmental tobacco smoke with asthma symptoms in children. *Pediatr Allergy Immunol.* (2009) 20:423–9. doi: 10.1111/j.1399-3038.2008.00820.x
6. Neuman A, Hohmann C, Orsini N, Pershagen G, Eller E, Kjaer HF, et al. Maternal smoking in pregnancy and asthma in preschool children: a pooled analysis of eight birth cohorts. *Am J Respir Crit Care Med.* (2012) 186:1037–43. doi: 10.1164/rccm.201203-0501OC
7. Wang G, Li W, Chen Q, Jiang Y, Lu X, Zhao X. Hydrogen sulfide accelerates wound healing in diabetic rats. *Int J Clin Exp Pathol.* (2015) 8:5097–104.
8. Martinez S, Garcia-Meric P, Millet V, Aymeric-Ponsonnet M, Alagha K, Dubus JC. Tobacco smoke in infants with bronchopulmonary dysplasia. *Eur J Pediatr.* (2015) 174:943–8. doi: 10.1007/s00431-015-2491-y
9. Singh SP, Gundavarapu S, Pena-Philippides JC, Rir-Sima-ah J, Mishra NC, Wilder JA, et al. Prenatal secondhand cigarette smoke promotes Th2 polarization and impairs goblet cell differentiation and airway mucus formation. *J Immunol.* (2011) 187:4542–52. doi: 10.4049/jimmunol.1101567
10. Singh SP, Gundavarapu S, Smith KR, Chand HS, Saeed AI, Mishra NC, et al. Gestational exposure of mice to secondhand cigarette smoke causes bronchopulmonary dysplasia blocked by the nicotinic receptor antagonist mecamylamine. *Environ Health Perspect.* (2013) 121:957–64. doi: 10.1289/ehp.1306611
11. Singh SP, Chand HS, Langley RJ, Mishra N, Barrett T, Rudolph K, et al. Gestational exposure to Sidestream (Secondhand) cigarette smoke promotes transgenerational epigenetic transmission of exacerbated allergic Asthma and Bronchopulmonary Dysplasia. *J Immunol.* (2017) 198:3815–22. doi: 10.4049/jimmunol.1700014
12. Polhemus DJ, Lefer DJ. Emergence of hydrogen sulfide as an endogenous gaseous signaling molecule in cardiovascular disease. *Circ Res.* (2014) 114:730–7. doi: 10.1161/CIRCRESAHA.114.300505
13. Katsouda A, Bibli SI, Pyriochou A, Szabo C, Papapetropoulos A. Regulation and role of endogenously produced hydrogen sulfide in angiogenesis. *Pharmacol Res.* (2016) 113(Pt A):175–85. doi: 10.1016/j.phrs.2016.08.026
14. Ali FF, Abdel-Hamid HA, Toni ND. H2S attenuates acute lung inflammation induced by administration of lipopolysaccharide in adult male rats. *Gen Physiol Biophys.* (2018) 37:421–31. doi: 10.4149/gpb_2018002
15. Spassov SG, Faller S, Hummel M, Helo K, Ihle A, Ryter SW, et al. Hydrogen sulfide confers lung protection during mechanical ventilation via cyclooxygenase 2, 15-deoxy Delta12,14-Prostaglandin J2, and peroxisome proliferator-activated receptor gamma. *Crit Care Med.* (2017) 45:e849–57. doi: 10.1097/CCM.0000000000002440
16. Madurga A, Golec A, Pozarska A, Ishii I, Mizikova I, Nardiello C, et al. The H2S-generating enzymes cystathionine beta-synthase and cystathionine gamma-lyase play a role in vascular development during normal lung alveolarization. *Am J Physiol Lung Cell Mol Physiol.* (2015) 309:L710–24. doi: 10.1152/ajplung.00134.2015
17. Zhang G, Wang P, Yang G, Cao Q, Wang R. The inhibitory role of hydrogen sulfide in airway hyperresponsiveness and inflammation in a mouse model of asthma. *Am J Pathol.* (2013) 182:1188–95. doi: 10.1016/j.ajpath.2012.12.008
18. Mendes JA, Ribeiro MC, Reis Filho G, Rocha T, Muscara MN, Costa SKP, et al. Hydrogen sulfide inhibits apoptosis and protects the bronchial epithelium in an allergic inflammation mice model. *Int Immunopharmacol.* (2019) 73:435–41. doi: 10.1016/j.intimp.2019.05.041
19. Szabo C. Hydrogen sulphide and its therapeutic potential. *Nat Rev Drug Discov.* (2007) 6:917–35. doi: 10.1038/nrd2425
20. Kimura H. Hydrogen sulfide: its production, release and functions. *Amino Acids.* (2011) 41:113–21. doi: 10.1007/s00726-010-0510-x
21. Bazhanov N, Ansar M, Ivanciuc T, Garofalo RP, Casola A. Hydrogen sulfide: a novel player in airway development, pathophysiology of respiratory diseases, and antiviral defenses. *Am J Respir Cell Mol Biol.* (2017) 57:403–10. doi: 10.1165/rcmb.2017-0114TR
22. Kimura H. Production and physiological effects of hydrogen sulfide. *Antioxid Redox Signal.* (2014) 20:783–93. doi: 10.1089/ars.2013.5309
23. Madden JA, Ahlf SB, Dantuma MW, Olson KR, Roerig DL. Precursors and inhibitors of hydrogen sulfide synthesis affect acute hypoxic pulmonary vasoconstriction in the intact lung. *J Appl Physiol.* (1985) (2012) 112:411–8. doi: 10.1152/japplphysiol.01049.2011
24. Olson KR, Whitfield NL, Bearden SE, St Leger J, Nilson E, Gao Y, et al. Hypoxic pulmonary vasodilation: a paradigm shift with a hydrogen sulfide mechanism. *Am J Physiol Regul Integr Comp Physiol.* (2010) 298:R51–60. doi: 10.1152/ajpregu.00576.2009
25. Wang M, Yan J, Cao X, Hua P, Li Z. Hydrogen sulfide modulates epithelial-mesenchymal transition and angiogenesis in non-small cell lung cancer via HIF-1α activation. *Biochem Pharmacol.* (2020) 172:113775. doi: 10.1016/j.bcp.2019.113775
26. Wang M, Cao X, Luan C, Li Z. Hydrogen sulfide attenuates hydrogen peroxide-induced injury in human lung Epithelial A549 cells. *Int J Mol Sci.* (2019) 20:3975. doi: 10.3390/ijms20163975
27. Augsburger F, Szabo C. Potential role of the 3-mercaptopyruvate sulfurtransferase (3-MST)-hydrogen sulfide (H2S) pathway in cancer cells. *Pharmacol Res.* (2020) 154:104083. doi: 10.1016/j.phrs.2018.11.034

28. Hosoki R, Matsuki N, Kimura H. The possible role of hydrogen sulfide as an endogenous smooth muscle relaxant in synergy with nitric oxide. *Biochem Biophys Res Commun.* (1997) 237:527–31. doi: 10.1006/bbrc.1997.6878
29. Chen T, You Y, Jiang H, Wang ZZ. Epithelial-mesenchymal transition (EMT): a biological process in the development, stem cell differentiation, and tumorigenesis. *J Cell Physiol.* (2017) 232:3261–72. doi: 10.1002/jcp.25797
30. Pei D, Shu X, Gassama-Diagne A, Thiery JP. Mesenchymal-epithelial transition in development and reprogramming. *Nat Cell Biol.* (2019) 21:44–53. doi: 10.1038/s41556-018-0195-z
31. Jolly MK, Ward C, Eapen MS, Myers S, Hallgren O, Levine H, et al. Epithelial-mesenchymal transition, a spectrum of states: role in lung development, homeostasis, and disease. *Dev Dyn.* (2018) 247:346–58. doi: 10.1002/dvdy.24541
32. Guan S, Xu W, Han F, Gu W, Song L, Ye W, et al. Ginsenoside Rg1 attenuates cigarette smoke-induced pulmonary epithelial-mesenchymal transition via inhibition of the TGF- β1/Smad pathway. *Biomed Res Int.* (2017) 2017:7171404. doi: 10.1155/2017/7171404
33. Guo L, Peng W, Tao J, Lan Z, Hei H, Tian L, et al. Hydrogen sulfide inhibits transforming growth factor-β1-induced EMT via Wnt/catenin pathway. *PLoS One.* (2016) 11:e0147018. doi: 10.1371/journal.pone.0147018
34. Singh SP, Chand HS, Gundavarapu S, Saeed AI, Langley RJ, Tesfaigzi Y, et al. HIF-1α plays a critical role in the gestational sidestream smoke-induced Bronchopulmonary Dysplasia in mice. *PLoS One.* (2015) 10:e0137757. doi: 10.1371/journal.pone.0137757
35. Pan Y, Zhou C, Yuan D, Zhang J, Shao C. Radiation exposure promotes Hepatocarcinoma cell invasion through epithelial mesenchymal transition mediated by H2S/CSE pathway. *Radiat Res.* (2016) 185:96–105. doi: 10.1667/RR14177.1
36. Zhang H, Song Y, Zhou C, Bai Y, Yuan D, Pan Y, et al. Blocking endogenous H2S signaling attenuated radiation-induced long-term metastasis of residual HepG2 cells through inhibition of EMT. *Radiat Res.* (2018) 190:374–84. doi: 10.1667/RR15074.1
37. Caniggia I, Mostachfi H, Winter J, Gassmann M, Lye SJ, Kuliszewski M, et al. Hypoxia-inducible factor-1 mediates the biological effects of oxygen on human trophoblast differentiation through TGFβ(3). *J Clin Invest.* (2000) 105:577–87. doi: 10.1172/JCI8316
38. Yoshimoto S, Tanaka F, Morita H, Hiraki A, Hashimoto S. Hypoxia-induced HIF-1α and ZEB1 are critical for the malignant transformation of ameloblastoma via TGF-β-dependent EMT. *Cancer Med.* (2019) 8:7822–32. doi: 10.1002/cam4.2667
39. Xu J, Lamouille S, Derynck R. TGF-β-induced epithelial to mesenchymal transition. *Cell Res.* (2009) 19:156–72. doi: 10.1038/cr.2009.5
40. Lamouille S, Xu J, Derynck R. Molecular mechanisms of epithelial-mesenchymal transition. *Nat Rev Mol Cell Biol.* (2014) 15:178–96. doi: 10.1038/nrm3758
41. Chand HS, Harris JF, Tesfaigzi Y. IL-13 in LPS-induced inflammation causes Bcl-2 expression to sustain hyperplastic mucous cells. *Sci Rep.* (2018) 8:436. doi: 10.1038/s41598-017-18884-9
42. Li H, Ma Y, Escaffre O, Ivanciuc T, Komaravelli N, Kelley JP, et al. Role of hydrogen sulfide in paramyxovirus infections. *J Virol.* (2015) 89:5557–68. doi: 10.1128/JVI.00264-15
43. Ivanciuc T, Sbrana E, Casola A, Garofalo RP. Protective role of nuclear factor erythroid 2-related factor 2 against respiratory syncytial virus and human Metapneumovirus infections. *Front Immunol.* (2018) 9:854. doi: 10.3389/fimmu.2018.00854
44. Ivanciuc T, Sbrana E, Casola A, Garofalo RP. Cystathionine gamma-lyase deficiency enhances airway reactivity and viral-induced disease in mice exposed to side-stream tobacco smoke. *Pediatr Res.* (2019) 86:39–46. doi: 10.1038/s41390-019-0396-6
45. Morrisey EE, Hogan BL. Preparing for the first breath: genetic and cellular mechanisms in lung development. *Dev Cell.* (2010) 18:8–23. doi: 10.1016/j.devcel.2009.12.010
46. Hines EA, Sun X. Tissue crosstalk in lung development. *J Cell Biochem.* (2014) 115:1469–77. doi: 10.1002/jcb.24811
47. Duan L, Ye L, Zhuang L, Zou X, Liu S, Zhang Y, et al. VEGFC/VEGFR3 axis mediates TGFbeta1-induced epithelial-to-mesenchymal transition in non-small cell lung cancer cells. *PLoS One.* (2018) 13:e0200452. doi: 10.1371/journal.pone.0200452
48. Fantozzi A, Gruber DC, Pisarsky L, Heck C, Kunita A, Yilmaz M, et al. VEGF-mediated angiogenesis links EMT-induced cancer stemness to tumor initiation. *Cancer Res.* (2014) 74:1566–75. doi: 10.1158/0008-5472.CAN-13-1641
49. Jakkula M, Le Cras TD, Gebb S, Hirth KP, Tuder RM, Voelkel NF, et al. Inhibition of angiogenesis decreases alveolarization in the developing rat lung. *Am J Physiol Lung Cell Mol Physiol.* (2000) 279:L600–7. doi: 10.1152/ajplung.2000.279.3.L600
50. Kim YE, Park WS, Ahn SY, Sung DK, Chang YS. Intratracheal transplantation of mesenchymal stem cells attenuates hyperoxia-induced lung injury by down-regulating, but not direct inhibiting formyl peptide receptor 1 in the newborn mice. *PLoS One.* (2018) 13:e0206311. doi: 10.1371/journal.pone.0206311
51. Kalluri R, Weinberg RA. The basics of epithelial-mesenchymal transition. *J Clin Invest.* (2009) 119:1420–8. doi: 10.1172/JCI39104
52. Nahomi RB, Nagaraj RH. The role of HIF-1α in the TGF-β2-mediated epithelial-to-mesenchymal transition of human lens epithelial cells. *J Cell Biochem.* (2018) 119:6814–27. doi: 10.1002/jcb.26877
53. Saito A, Horie M, Nagase T. TGF-β signaling in lung health and disease. *Int J Mol Sci.* (2018) 19:2460. doi: 10.3390/ijms19082460
54. Archer F, Abi-Rizk A, Desloire S, Dolmazon C, Gineys B, Guiguen F, et al. Lung progenitors from lambs can differentiate into specialized alveolar or bronchiolar epithelial cells. *BMC Vet Res.* (2013) 9:224. doi: 10.1186/1746-6148-9-224
55. Laing IA, Hermans C, Bernard A, Burton PR, Goldblatt J, Le Souef PN. Association between plasma CC16 levels, the A38G polymorphism, and asthma. *Am J Respir Crit Care Med.* (2000) 161:124–7. doi: 10.1164/ajrccm.161.1.9904073
56. Zhai J, Insel M, Addison KJ, Stern DA, Pederson W, Dy A, et al. Club cell secretory protein deficiency leads to altered lung function. *Am J Respir Crit Care Med.* (2019) 199:302–12. doi: 10.1164/rccm.201807-1345OC
57. Esechie A, Kiss L, Olah G, Horvath EM, Hawkins H, Szabo C, et al. Protective effect of hydrogen sulfide in a murine model of acute lung injury induced by combined burn and smoke inhalation. *Clin Sci (Lond).* (2008) 115:91–7. doi: 10.1042/CS20080021
58. Zhang J, Wang X, Chen Y, Yao W. Exhaled hydrogen sulfide predicts airway inflammation phenotype in COPD. *Respir Care.* (2015) 60:251–8. doi: 10.4187/respcare.03519
59. Li YF, Langholz B, Salam MT, Gilliland FD. Maternal and grandmaternal smoking patterns are associated with early childhood asthma. *Chest.* (2005) 127:1232–41. doi: 10.1016/S0012-3692(15)34472-X
60. Accordini S, Calciano L, Johannessen A, Portas L, Benediktsdottir B, Bertelsen RJ, et al. A three-generation study on the association of tobacco smoking with asthma. *Int J Epidemiol.* (2018) 47:1106–17. doi: 10.1093/ije/dyy031
61. Rehan VK, Liu J, Sakurai R, Torday JS. Perinatal nicotine-induced transgenerational asthma. *Am J Physiol Lung Cell Mol Physiol.* (2013) 305:L501–7. doi: 10.1152/ajplung.00078.2013
62. Levitt MD, Abdel-Rehim MS, Furne J. Free and acid-labile hydrogen sulfide concentrations in mouse tissues: anomalously high free hydrogen sulfide in aortic tissue. *Antioxid Redox Signal.* (2011) 15:373–8. doi: 10.1089/ars.2010.3525
63. Burstyn I, Kapur N, Shalapay C, Bamforth F, Wild TC, Liu J, et al. Evaluation of the accuracy of self-reported smoking in pregnancy when the biomarker level in an active smoker is uncertain. *Nicotine Tob Res.* (2009) 11:670–8. doi: 10.1093/ntr/ntp048
64. Silvestri M, Franchi S, Pistorio A, Petecchia L, Rusconi F. Smoke exposure, wheezing, and asthma development: a systematic review and meta-analysis in unselected birth cohorts. *Pediatr Pulmonol.* (2015) 50:353–62. doi: 10.1002/ppul.23037
65. Xu S, Liu Z, Liu P. Targeting hydrogen sulfide as a promising therapeutic strategy for atherosclerosis. *Int J Cardiol.* (2014) 172:313–7. doi: 10.1016/j.ijcard.2014.01.068
66. Wang P, Wu L, Ju Y, Fu M, Shuang T, Qian Z, et al. Age-dependent allergic asthma development and cystathionine gamma-lyase deficiency. *Antioxid Redox Signal.* (2017) 27:931–44. doi: 10.1089/ars.2016.6875
67. Krasilnikov MA. Phosphatidylinositol-3 kinase dependent pathways: the role in control of cell growth, survival, and malignant transformation. *Biochemistry (Mosc).* (2000) 65:68–78.

68. Alphonse RS, Vadivel A, Coltan L, Eaton F, Barr AJ, Dyck JR, et al. Activation of Akt protects alveoli from neonatal oxygen-induced lung injury. *Am J Respir Cell Mol Biol.* (2011) 44:146–54. doi: 10.1165/rcmb.2009-0182OC
69. Liu WL, Liu ZW, Li TS, Wang C, Zhao B. Hydrogen sulfide donor regulates alveolar epithelial cell apoptosis in rats with acute lung injury. *Chin Med J (Engl).* (2013) 126:494–9. doi: 10.3760/cma.j.issn.0366-6999.20120809
70. Ivanciuc T, Sbrana E, Ansar M, Bazhanov N, Szabo C, Casola A, et al. Hydrogen sulfide is an antiviral and antiinflammatory endogenous gasotransmitter in the airways. Role in respiratory syncytial virus infection. *Am J Respir Cell Mol Biol.* (2016) 55:684–96. doi: 10.1165/rcmb.2015-0385OC
71. Longchamp A, Mirabella T, Arduini A, MacArthur MR, Das A, Trevino-Villarreal JH, et al. Amino acid restriction triggers angiogenesis via GCN2/ATF4 regulation of VEGF and H2S production. *Cell.* (2018) 173:117–29.e14. doi: 10.1016/j.cell.2018.03.001
72. Madurga A, Mizikova I, Ruiz-Camp J, Vadasz I, Herold S, Mayer K, et al. Systemic hydrogen sulfide administration partially restores normal alveolarization in an experimental animal model of bronchopulmonary dysplasia. *Am J Physiol Lung Cell Mol Physiol.* (2014) 306:L684–97. doi: 10.1152/ajplung.00361.2013
73. Vadivel A, Alphonse RS, Ionescu L, Machado DS, O'Reilly M, Eaton F, et al. Exogenous hydrogen sulfide (H2S) protects alveolar growth in experimental O2-induced neonatal lung injury. *PLoS One.* (2014) 9:e90965. doi: 10.1371/journal.pone.0090965
74. Bush A. Lung development and aging. *Ann Am Thorac Soc.* (2016) 13(Suppl. 5):S438–46. doi: 10.1513/AnnalsATS.201602-112AW
75. Savran O, Ulrik CS. Early life insults as determinants of chronic obstructive pulmonary disease in adult life. *Int J Chron Obstruct Pulmon Dis.* (2018) 13:683–93. doi: 10.2147/COPD.S153555

12

Expression and Roles of Antimicrobial Peptides in Innate Defense of Airway Mucosa: Potential Implication in Cystic Fibrosis

Regina Geitani[1*†], *Carole Ayoub Moubareck*[1,2†], *Zhengzhong Xu*[3,4,5], *Dolla Karam Sarkis*[1] *and Lhousseine Touqui*[4,5*]

[1] Microbiology Laboratory, School of Pharmacy, Saint Joseph University, Beirut, Lebanon, [2] College of Natural and Health Sciences, Zayed University, Dubai, United Arab Emirates, [3] Jiangsu Key Laboratory of Zoonosis, Yangzhou University, Yangzhou, China, [4] Sorbonne Université, INSERM UMR_S 938, Centre de Recherche Saint Antoine (CRSA), Paris, France, [5] "Mucoviscidose and Bronchopathies Chroniques", Pasteur Institute, Paris, France

***Correspondence:**
Regina Geitani
regina.geitani@net.usj.edu.lb
Lhousseine Touqui
lhousseine.touqui@pasteur.fr

† These authors have contributed equally to this work and share first authorship

The treatment of respiratory infections is associated with the dissemination of antibiotic resistance in the community and clinical settings. Development of new antibiotics is notoriously costly and slow; therefore, alternative strategies are needed. Antimicrobial peptides (AMPs), the central effector molecules of the immune system, are being considered as alternatives to conventional antibiotics. Most AMPs are epithelium-derived and play a key role in host defense at mucosal surfaces. They are classified on the basis of their structure and amino acid motifs. These peptides display a range of activities, including not only direct antimicrobial activity, but also immunomodulation and wound repair. In the lung, airway epithelial cells and neutrophils, in particular, contribute to AMP synthesis. The relevance of AMPs for host defense against infection has been demonstrated in animal models and is supported by observations in patient studies, showing altered expression and/or unfavorable circumstances for their action in a variety of lung diseases. Of note, AMPs are active against bacterial strains that are resistant to conventional antibiotics, including multidrug-resistant bacteria. Several strategies have been proposed to use these peptides in the treatment of infections, including direct administration of AMPs. In this review, we focus on studies related to direct bactericidal effects of AMPs and their potential clinical applications with a particular focus on cystic fibrosis.

Keywords: respiratory infections, antibiotic resistance, antimicrobial peptides, antimicrobial effect, immune modulation, cystic fibrosis

HISTORICAL OVERVIEW AND DEFINITION

In the early 1920s, Fleming independently discovered both AMPs and penicillin. In 1922, he identified, in his nasal discharge, an antimicrobial substance, later named lysozyme, which was able to kill certain bacteria in few minutes. Seven years later, penicillin was carried forward for clinical application (1). After that, several AMPs were isolated and identified as having activity against both Gram-positive and Gram-negative bacteria. In 1939, gramicidin was the first natural peptide-based drug to be introduced in the market. It was isolated from *Bacillus brevis* and was active against a wide range of Gram-positive and some Gram-negative bacteria but was not devoid of toxicity (2). The real explosion of therapeutic potential of AMPs began in the early 1980s when Hans Boman isolated and characterized AMPs, known as cecropins, from the hemolymph of silk moth (*Hyalophora cecropia*) (3). Later in 1987, the significance of AMPs was increased when Zasloff discovered magainins in frog skin (*Xenopus laevis*) (4) and showed for the first time that AMPs are present not only in lower invertebrates but also in higher vertebrates (5). Antimicrobial activities in fluids such as blood, saliva, plasma, sweat, leucocytes secretions, and granule extracts were discovered at that period, suggesting the natural production of AMPs in humans (6). Since then, more than 3,000 naturally occurring AMPs have been isolated from different kingdoms (bacteria, archea, protists, fungi, plants, animals, and humans) and were registered in the AMP database (http://aps.unmc.edu/AP/main.php). Thus, AMPs were discovered at the same time as antibiotics (ATBs) but were eclipsed by the success of those drugs. Now that the emergence of ATB resistance is a major threat to human health, global voices are calling for solutions. Among the existing research lines for alternatives to conventional ATBs, AMPs, both natural and synthetic, seem to be promising candidates (7).

AMPs, also referred to as host defense peptides, are biologically active molecules with a rapid and broad spectrum of activity against bacteria, yeast, viruses, and fungi in addition to immunomodulatory activities, wound healing, and cytotoxic effects on cancer cells (8, 9). To date, the large majority of identified AMPs are antibacterial peptides representing 83% of all AMPs (10). AMPs, evolutionarily conserved in the genome, are produced by most living organisms as an essential component of their innate immune system, representing an ancient host defense mechanism to eliminate invading pathogens and boost immune response. In mammals, the primary site at which a host encounters a pathogen is classically the skin or the mucosal surface, such as the respiratory tract, the gastrointestinal tract, and the urogenital tract (11). Infections at these sites are prevented by the innate host defense responses intended to maintain host integrity (12). AMPs, being an important component of the innate immune system, constitute one of the early, rapid, nonspecific mechanisms by which the host immune system provides protection against infections (13). Studies using knockout mice and transgenic (Tg) expression systems have confirmed that AMPs play a major role in limiting microbial proliferation to skin and mucosal surfaces, therefore preventing spread to the deep tissues where serious infection may occur (14). AMPs are produced by epithelial cells of vertebrates as a first line of defense against microbial pathogens.

Abbreviations: AMPs, Antimicrobial peptides; ARDS, Acute respiratory distress syndrome; ASL, Airways surface liquid; ATBs, Antibiotics; cDNA, complimentary DNA; CF, Cystic fibrosis; CFTR, cystic fibrosis transmembrane conductance regulator; EGR1, Early growth response gene-1; GBS, Group B Streptococcus; HBD, Human β-defensin; HIV, Human immunodeficiency virus; HNP, Human neutrophil defensin; HSV, Herpes simplex virus; IL, Interleukin; KLF, Krüppel-like transcription factor; LPS, Lipopolysaccharides; MCP, Monocyte chemoattractant protein; MIC, Minimum Inhibitory Concentration; MOA, Mechanism of action; MRSA, methicillin-resistant *Staphylococcus aureus*; PAMP, Pathogen-associated molecular pattern; sPLA2, secreted phospholipase A2; sPLA2-IIA, Type-IIA secreted phospholipase A_2; TNF-α, Tumor necrosis factor alfa; Tg, Transgenic; VRE, vancomycin-resistant *Enterococci;* WT, Wild-type.

AMPs: STRUCTURE AND CLASSIFICATION

Despite their extreme diversity in terms of composition and length, AMPs share several common structural characteristics (15). The most studied AMPs are short polypeptides of fewer than 50 amino acids, cationic with an average net charge of +3, and having a hydrophobic content of 42% on average. Both the net positive charge and the hydrophobicity of these AMPs generate the observed amphipathic structure. This structure determines their conformational flexibility, enables electrostatic attraction between these cationic peptides and the anionic bacterial membranes, and allows penetration into bacterial cells inducing membrane lysis. Cationic AMPs, however, do not affect the neutrally charged mammalian cells; this chemical property favors their use as future drugs (7, 15). The differences in composition between bacterial cell membranes rich in phosphatidylglycerols and human cell membranes dominated by zwitterionic phospholipids is believed to be the major reason of the selectivity of AMPs (**Figure 1**) (7).

Based on structural features, AMPs can be classified into three subgroups: α-helical, β-sheet, and extended AMPs (16–18). These structures are highly correlated with the functional specificity of each peptide. Some of these peptides demonstrate no secondary structure in aqueous solution but become structured when exposed to a lipid, such as the bacterial cell membrane (19). In addition to that, some peptides might have mixed α-helical and β-sheet structures; classification is then based on the predominant one (20).

The first subgroup contains AMPs that form α-helical structures and are predominately found in the extracellular matrix of frogs and insects in addition to the extensively studied human AMP LL-37, which is a member of the cathelicidins. Cathelicidins, originally isolated from granule extracts of bovine neutrophils (21), are among the most diverse AMPs of vertebrates; they can adopt a variety of structures and play, in addition to their antimicrobial activity, an important immunomodulatory role (22). Magainins, which are active against a broad spectrum of microbial agents, present another example of AMPs with an α-helical structure. They have been extensively studied and are among the first ones to have been tested clinically (23). Cecropin is a prototype of this group and is active against Gram-negative bacteria. Other cecropins, which can act synergistically against both Gram-negative and Gram-positive bacteria, have been recently identified (24). Another final example of the α-helical AMPs is the aureins that are secreted from the granular dorsal glands of the Australian Green and Golden Bell Frog *Litoria aurea* and the southern Bell Frog *L. raniformis*. The aurein family is mostly active against Gram-positive bacteria, such as *Staphylococcus aureus* and *S. epidermidis*, and have anti-cancer activities (20).

The second subgroup includes cyclic AMPs that adopt a β-sheet structure, such as protegrins, defensins, and tachyplesins. Although they have antifungal properties in some cases, they are often considered to be antibacterial peptides (19). Defensins, the largest group of AMPs produced by mammals, were first discovered in human neutrophils as small cationic molecules. They have been found later in mammals, insects, plants,

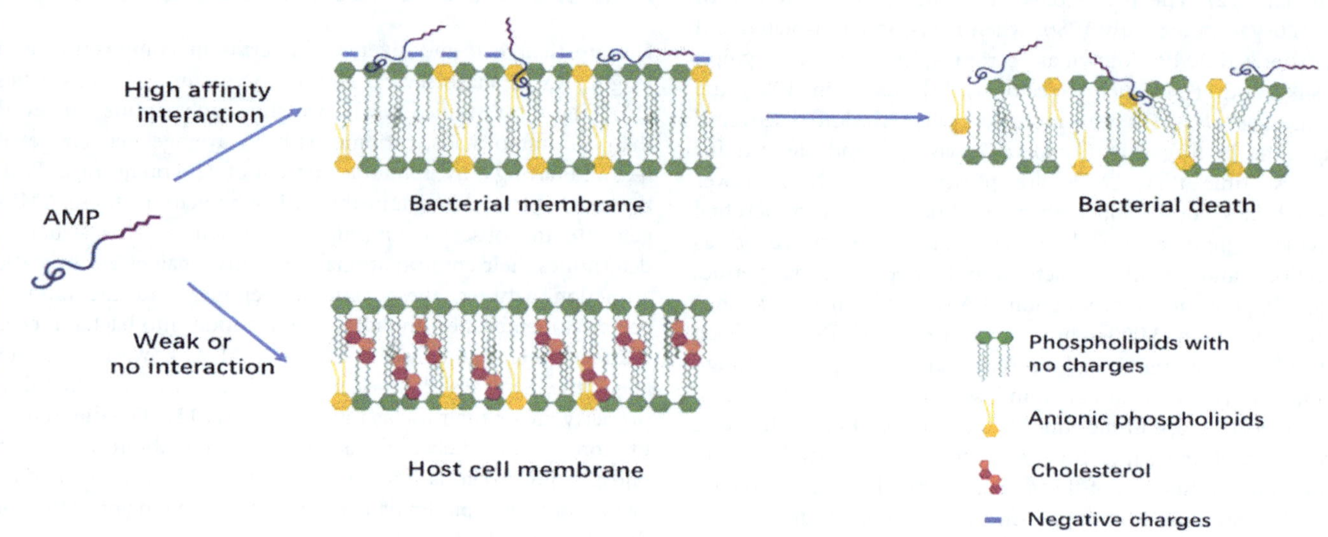

FIGURE 1 | Early interactions of cationic antimicrobial peptides with bacterial or host cell membrane. The anionic molecules in the membranes of Gram-negative and Gram-positive bacteria attract cationic AMPs via electrostatic and hydrophobic interactions. In contrast to bacteria, the cytoplasmic membrane of host cells with a neutral net charge connects with cationic AMPs via hydrophobic interactions, which are relatively weak.

parasites, and fungi. Defensins are also involved in immune and inflammation responses (25). Although most defensins lose much of their antimicrobial activity at the physiological concentrations of Na^+, Mg^{2+}, or Ca^{2+}, they have been shown to exhibit broad-spectrum antimicrobial activity against bacteria, fungi, and enveloped viruses *in vitro*. Of note, electrolytes may have a more complex effect on peptide-induced antimicrobial effects (25). Another example of β-sheet AMPs are tachyplesins, isolated from hemocytes of horseshoe crabs (20).

The third and last subgroup comprises peptides with a unique extended/random coil structure. In this category, most of the AMPs are from the cathelicidin family, which are known to have linear structure rather than secondary structure due to the presence of proline residues. One of the best studied peptides in this subgroup is indolicidin, which is produced by bovine leucocytes and consists of only 13 amino acids (17, 20).

Sources of some AMPs, their classes, and chemical structures are shown in **Table 1**.

TABLE 1 | Classification of some antimicrobial peptides along with their chemical structure and origin.

Classification	AMP	Origin	Chemical structure
α-helix	LL-37	Human	GIGAVLKVLTTGLPALISWIKRKRQQ
	Melittin	Honey bee	GIGKFLHSAGKFGKAFVGEIMKS
	Dermaseptin-		LLGDFFRKSKEIGEFKRIVQRIKDFLR
	S1	Frog	NLVPRTES
β-helix		Pig	RGGRLC[1]YC[2]RRRFC[2]VC[1]VGR
	Protegrin-1	Human	AC[1]YC[2]RIPAC[3]IAGGRRYGTC[2]I
	HNP-1	Human	YGGRKWAFC[3]C[1]
	HBD-1		DHYNC[1]VSSGGQC[2]LYASC[3]PIF
			TKIQGTC[2]YRGKAKC[1]C[3]K
Extended structure	PR-39	Pig	RRRPRPPYLPRRPRPPFFPPLRLPPR
	Indolicidin	Cow	IPPGFPPRFPPRPFP
	Tritrpticin	Pig	ILPWKWPWWPWRR
			VRRFPWWWPFLRR

AMP, antimicrobial peptide; HBD-1, human β-defensin 1; HNP, human neutrophil defensing.

MODE OF ACTION OF AMPs

Enhanced understanding of the mechanism of action (MOA) of AMPs is of great importance to facilitate further development of peptide-based drugs as therapeutic agents. The MOA can be divided into two major classes: direct antimicrobial activity and immune modulation (16). Although it has been thought for many years that membrane destabilization was the sole direct MOA of AMPs against bacteria, additional mechanisms have been described. These MOA embrace non-membrane targeting mechanisms, including inhibition of the cell wall synthesis, intracellular translocation of AMPs, inhibition of protein/nucleic acid synthesis, and disruption of enzymatic/protein activity (20, 26). In both cases, electrostatic interaction is the key factor for the direct antimicrobial activity of cationic AMPs with the negatively charged molecules of the bacterial membrane, enabling further intrusion of the peptides into the inner part of the cell membrane (27). These interactions occur with the anionic phospholipids and phosphate groups of lipopolysaccharides (LPS) in case of Gram-negative bacteria as well with teichoic acids and lipoteichoic acids in case of Gram-positive bacteria (15, 24).

Direct Antibacterial Activity

AMPs exert their direct antibacterial activity by either disrupting bacterial membranes or interfering with intracellular processes following to translocation. The direct antibacterial mechanism of AMPs is schematized in **Figure 2**.

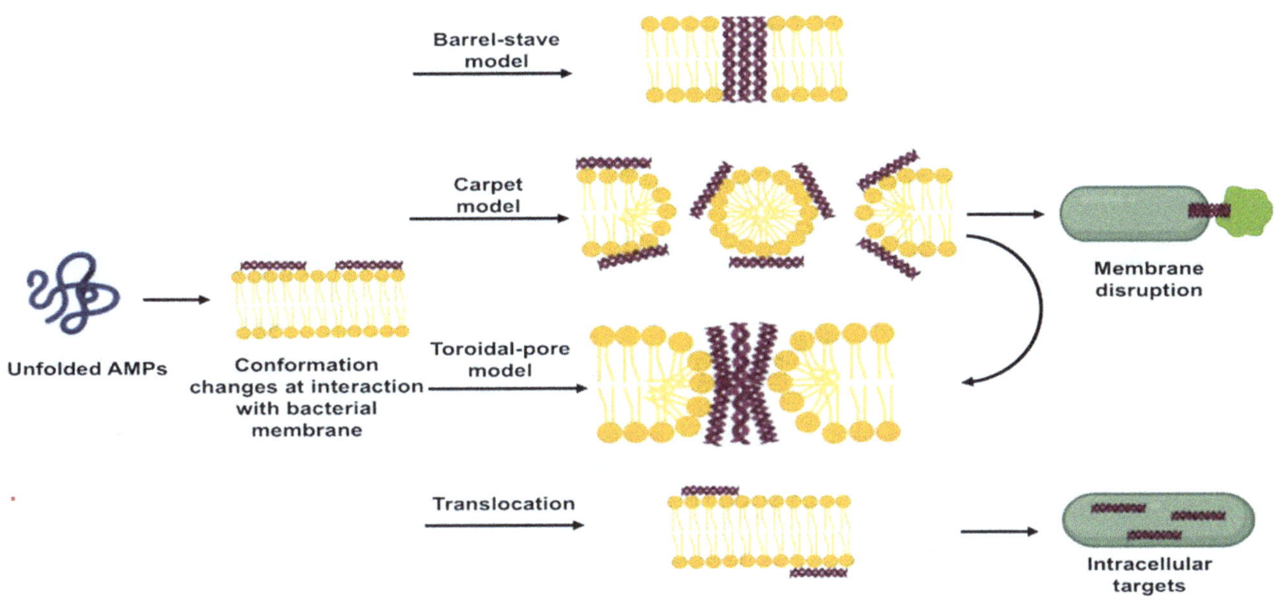

FIGURE 2 | Schematic illustration of direct antibacterial mode of actions of antimicrobial peptides.

Membrane Disruption Mechanism of Action

Upon adsorption into the membrane surface, the AMPs form, if not already present, an amphipathic secondary structure essential for interaction with the cell membrane (28). At this stage, several models have been proposed to describe the next events occurring at the bacterial cytoplasmic membrane, which ultimately lead to a remarkable dose-dependent membrane disruption (26). The three most popular models are the "barrel-stave pore model," "toroidal-pore model," and "carpet model" (10, 20).

In the barrel-stave pore model, when a threshold concentration of the peptides is reached, AMPs insert perpendicularly into the lipid bilayer forming transmembrane pores within the hydrophobic membrane core, in a manner similar to that of membrane protein ion channels. This model is consistent with the MOA of alamethicin, pardaxin, and protegrins (20, 26).

In the toroidal-pore model, once the minimum threshold concentration is reached, the peptides are perpendicularly incorporated into the bilayer membranes, enabling the lipid monolayers to curve around the pore. Consequently, the hydrophobic residues of peptides interact with the hydrophobic region of the membrane, forming pores that are partially bordered by the peptides and partially by the phospholipid head group, allowing the water core to be lined. Magainins and LL-37 adopt this MOA (10, 21).

In the carpet model, AMPs adsorb parallel to the lipid bilayer and cover the surface of the target membrane. Once their concentrations reach a certain threshold, AMPs exert detergent-like effects, which eventually disintegrate the membrane via the formation of micelles and pores. This model explains the MOA of cecropins and some magainins (10, 28). The formed pores act as non-selective channels for ions, toxins, and metabolites, thus preventing the microbe from maintaining vital homeostasis and leading eventually to microbial death (16, 27).

TABLE 2 | Classification of different antimicrobial peptides according to their membrane targeting mechanism of action.

Pore-forming models	Example of AMP	Origin
Barrel-Stave	Ceratotoxin	*Ceratitis capitate* (Mediterranean fruit fly)
	Alamethicin	*Trichoderma viride* (fungus)
	Amphotricin B	*Streptomyces nodosu* (bacteria)
Toroidal	Melittin	*Xenopus Laevis* (African clawed frog)
	LL-37	*Homo sapiens*
	Piscidin	*Morone Saxtilis* (Atlantic striped bass)
	Pardaxin	*Pardarchirus marmoratus* (Finless sole fish)
Carpet-like	Magainin 2	*Xenopus Laevis* (African clawed frog)
	RL-37	*Macaca mulatta* (Rhesus macaque)
	Cecropins	*Hyalophora cecropia* (North American moth)
	Dermaseptins	*Phyllomedusa spp.* (Frogs genus)
	Ovispirin	*Ovis aries* (Sheep)
	Mastoparan X	*Vespa xanthoptera* (Japanese yellow hornet)

AMP, antimicrobial peptide.

The carpet-like model is also called the "detergent-like model," and the toroidal model is called the "wormhole model." **Table 2** shows different AMPs classified based on their membrane disruption mode of action.

Intracellular Targeting Mechanism of Action

Apart from the membrane-targeting MOA, some AMPs may exert other MOA, including the inhibition of extracellular wall synthesis and may have intracellular targets, thus disrupting intracellular processes (26). It has been shown that membrane permeabilization results in AMP translocation into the cytoplasm

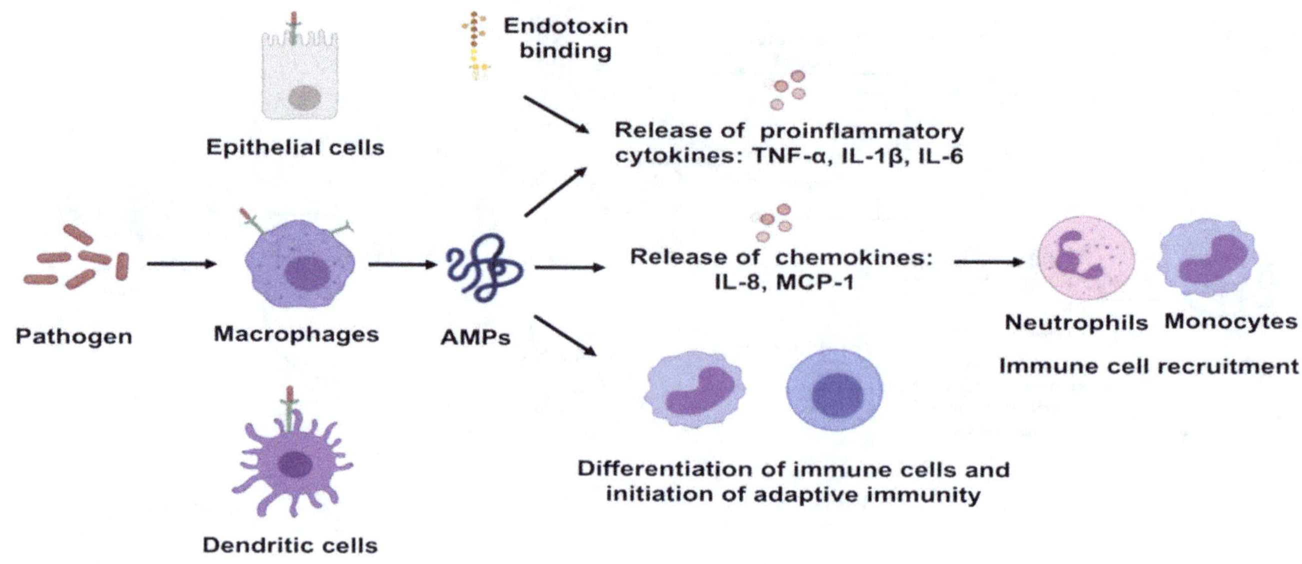

FIGURE 3 | Schematic illustration of immune-regulatory functions of antimicrobial peptides. AMPs, antimicrobial peptides; IL, interleukin; MCP, monocyte chemoattractant protein; TNF-a, tumor necrosis factor alfa.

without disruption of its integrity, allowing binding to the anionic charge present in nucleic acids (DNA/RNA), some intracellular enzymes, and other targets (18, 26). For instance, AMPs, such as defensins, often confer antibacterial activity by interacting with various precursor molecules that are required for cell wall synthesis, such as the highly conserved lipid II (20). Other AMPs, such as indolicidin, interfere with protein synthesis, whereas papiliocin induces the production of oxygen free radicals, which damages both DNA and the cell membrane. Others can inhibit the activity of a few intracellular enzymes crucial for metabolism and proliferation of pathogens (26). Remarkably, it is suggested that AMPs may cause bacterial death via multiple and complementary actions known as a multi-hit mechanism, serving in increasing the efficiency of AMPs and evading resistance development (28).

Immune Modulation

Well-characterized for their antimicrobial activities, AMPs are also known for their immuno-regulatory functions. The expression of these AMPs can be constitutive or can be inducible by infectious and/or inflammatory stimuli, such as proinflammatory cytokines, bacteria, or bacterial molecules that induce innate immunity (29). AMP production constitutes one of the early mechanisms by which the host immune system provides protection against invaders (13). They can recruit and activate immune cells, resulting in enhanced bactericidal activity and/or control of inflammation (20, 28). They act as effective inflammatory modulators by stimulating chemotaxis and angiogenesis, modulation of immune cell differentiation, and initiation of adaptive immunity. The broad range of mechanisms of action exerted by AMPs also includes toxin neutralization in an extremely rapid manner (**Figure 3**) (30). As examples, human neutrophil defensin (HNP)-1, HNP-2, and HNP-3 have been shown to upregulate the production of tumor necrosis factor alfa (TNF-α) and interleukin (IL)-1 by human monocyte activated upon bacterial infection, which, in turn, produces pro-inflammatory cytokines to attract immune cells to fight off the pathogens (31). In addition to that, HBD-2 and HBD-3 promote bacterial clearance of *Pseudomonas aeruginosa* by suppressing macrophage autophagy through downregulation of early growth response gene-1 (EGR1) and proto-oncogene c-FOS (32). Moreover, it has been demonstrated that cathelicidin exerts a direct chemoattractant action on monocytes, neutrophils, and T cells (33) and induces the transcription and release of IL-8 and monocyte chemoattractant protein (MCP)-1 and MCP-3, resulting in the recruitment of different immune cells requisite to remove the invading pathogen (34). LL-37, in addition to its direct MOA, neutralizes the activity of LPS and, thus, helps to protect the tissues from its harmful effects. In addition, it maintains a balance between pro- and anti-inflammatory mediators in the presence of LPS.

ANTIMICROBIAL SPECTRUM OF ACTIVITY

AMPs have broad-spectrum antibacterial activity and may exhibit their effects at minimum inhibitory concentrations (MICs) as low as 1–4 μg/ml (10). In addition to their potent antibacterial impact, some AMPs possess antiviral, antifungal, antiparasitic, and insecticidal properties. For instance, LL-37, the sole human cathelicidin, possesses a broad spectrum of activity against both Gram-positive and Gram-negative bacteria, such as *S. aureus*, *Enterococcus faecalis*, Group A *Streptococcus*, *Escherichia coli*, *P. aeruginosa*, *Klebsiella pneumoniae*, *Proteus mirabilis*, and *Prevotella intermedia* among others, including antibiotic-resistant strains containing methicillin-resistant

TABLE 3 | Example of peptides with their spectrum of activity.

Targeted microbes/PAMP	Examples of AMP
Gram-negative and -positive bacteria	IB-367, protegrin, MSI-78, gramicidin S, indolicidin, CEMA
Gram-negative bacteria	Polymyxin B
Gram-positive bacteria	HNP1, sPLA2-IIA
Fungi	Protegrin, indolicidin, gramicidin S, CEMA, polyphemusin, sPLA2-V
Virus	Indolicidin, protegrin, polyphemusin
Parasite	Magainin II, indolicidin
Endotoxin*	CEMA, polyphemusin variants

AMP, Antimicrobial peptide; PAMP, Pathogen-associated molecular pattern.
**Endotoxin named also LPS, is a PAMP present in the cell wall of Gram-negative bacteria.*

Staphylococcus aureus (MRSA) and vancomycin-resistant *Enterococci* (VRE) (35–37). It has also a preventive action against *S. aureus* biofilm formation (38, 39) and can kill, *in vitro* and *in vivo*, both enveloped and non-enveloped viruses (40). Moreover, this peptide shows toxicity to tripomastigotes of the protozoan parasite *Trypanosama cruzi* at micromolar concentrations (35). On the other hand, magainins exhibit a broad spectrum of antimicrobial activity that includes Gram-positive and Gram-negative bacteria [*E. coli* (41) and *P. aeruginosa* (42)] and fungi, such as *Candida albicans* (43) at concentrations in the range of 1–10 μg/ml (44). The Type-IIA secreted phospholipase A_2 (sPLA2-IIA) kills selectively Gram-positive bacteria (see below) while sPLA2-V contributes to the innate immune response against *C. albicans* by regulating phagocytosis and killing through a mechanism that is likely dependent on phagolysosome fusion (45). Defensins are also active against bacteria, fungi, and some viruses at low concentrations under optimal conditions (37). The antimicrobial activity of defensins is inhibited in the presence of increasing concentrations of salts and plasma proteins (44). Their spectrum of activity includes sexually transmitted infections causing pathogens, such as *Treponema pallidum*, *Chlamydia trachomatis*, human immunodeficiency virus (HIV)-1, and herpes simplex virus (HSV)-2 (43); fungal infections, such as candida species (43); skin infections due to *S. aureus* and *P. aeruginosa*; and other important bacterial pathogens, such as *Salmonella* and *Haemophilus influenzae* (46). Examples of peptides with their spectrum of activity are presented in **Table 3**.

AMPs are generally capable of killing microbes independently. However, they often show enhanced antimicrobial activity when tested in combination with either other AMPs or conventional antibiotics (7, 35). Many previous studies have shown that the use of antibacterial agents in a therapeutic cocktail can reduce the dose of each drug in the combination, limiting the development of resistance *in vitro* (18). For instance, LL-37 and HNP-1 were shown to work synergistically together with a significant enhancement of both their antimicrobial activities and membrane permeabilization effects (35). It has been also demonstrated that the efficacy of conventional antibiotics could be further boosted through combination with AMPs, and some studies revealed synergistic relationships between antibiotics and AMPs (47, 48). For example, Dosler and Mataraci reported the synergistic effect of indolicidin combined to conventional antibiotics daptomycin, teicoplanin, and ciprofloxacin against MRSA biofilm (48). Furthermore, our recent studies showed that the AMP LL-37 potentiated the bactericidal effects of the antibiotics colistin and imipenem on both antibiotic susceptible and multidrug resistant strains of *P. aeruginosa* (49).

TYPE-IIA SECRETED PHOSPHOLIPASE A_2: A PARTICULAR HOST ANTIMICROBIAL PEPTIDE

The type-IIA secreted phospholipase A_2 (sPLA2-IIA) is a member of the super-family of enzymes called sPLA2 originally defined by their ability to catalyze the hydrolysis of phospholipids from both eukaryotic and prokaryotic cell membranes at the *sn*-2 position leading to the generation of lysophospholipids and free fatty acids (50, 51). The sPLA2-IIA can be classified as a member of the AMP family although it kills bacteria via a different MOA (see below) and is larger than most AMPs (120 amino acids). The classifications of $sPLA_2$ in different types is based on the number and position of their disulfide bridges (50, 51). The encoding sequences of some $sPLA_2$ complimentary DNA (cDNA) predicted the presence of the putative signal peptide, thus indicating that these types of $sPLA_2$ are secreted proteins. To date, 10 distinct members of $sPLA_2$s have been identified so far in mammals with around 50% homology among them (50, 51). It becomes clear now that sPLA2-IIA is a major actor in host defense against invading bacteria and is produced by host cells at sufficient levels to ensure this role (52, 53).

Discovery of the Bactericidal Functions of sPLA2-IIA

$sPLA_2$-IIA, the most studied enzyme of the sPLA2 group, is the most abundant in human and animal biological fluids, and it has been initially proposed to play a role in the pathogenesis of various inflammatory diseases (50, 51). However, this notion evolved progressively, and it is now accepted that bacterial killing represents the most physiologically relevant and recognized function of sPLA2-IIA (52, 53). The group of J. Weiss reported for the first time that the potent antistaphylococcal activity present in the inflammatory peritoneal exudate can be attributed mostly to sPLA2-IIA (54). This bactericidal effect is due to the ability of $sPLA_2$-IIA to bind and penetrate the cell wall of Gram-positive bacteria with greater efficiency compared to its Gram-negative effect (52, 53, 55). Subsequent studies report that mouse and human $sPLA_2$ exhibit various bactericidal activities toward two Gram-positive bacteria, *Listeria monocytogenes* and *S. aureus*, and that $sPLA_2$-IIA is, by far, the most bactericidal $sPLA_2$. The concentrations of $sPLA_2$-IIA in biological fluids are sufficient to kill all Gram-positive bacteria that may infect mammals (52, 53). Whereas, the concentrations of $sPLA_2$-IIA in the normal human tear exceed 30 μg/ml, only 1.1 ng/ml of the enzyme is sufficient to achieve the killing of *L. monocytogenes* (56). Concentrations at 15–80 ng/ml of sPLA2-IIA are necessary for *S. aureus* killing. The $sPLA_2$-IIA efficiently kills Gram-positive bacteria due to the high net positive charge of this enzyme compared to that of other $sPLA_2s$, allowing rapid and highly efficient binding of $sPLA_2$-IIA to the negatively charged surface of these bacteria (52, 53). The cell wall bacterial component lipoteichoic acid has been reported to play a key role in the tight binding of sPLA2-IIA to Gram-positive bacteria, such as *S. aureus* (57).

The contribution of sPLA2-IIA to antibacterial host defense is supported by *in vivo* experiments using sPLA2-IIA Tg mice (52, 53). sPLA2-IIA Tg mice were generated in the C57Bl/6 background. This mouse strain contains an inactivating point mutation in murine sPLA2-IIA, making them natural knockouts (58, 59). Therefore, expression of sPLA2-IIA in this strain background is not confounded by the co-expression of murine sPLA2-IIA. Using these mice, it has been established that sPLA2-IIA protects from lethal infections of *S. aureus*, *Bacillus anthracis*, and *Streptococcus pyogenes* (60–64).

AMPs AND DISEASES

The skin or the mucosal surface, such as the respiratory tract, the gastrointestinal tract, and the urogenital tract (11), are classically considered as the primary sites at which a host encounters a pathogen. At these sites, infections are controlled by the innate defense responses that allow the host to maintain its integrity (12). Knockout mice and Tg expression systems have confirmed that AMPs play a central role in limiting microbial proliferation in various host sites, thus preventing spread to the deep tissues where serious infection may occur (14). AMPs are produced by epithelial cells of vertebrates as a first line of defense against microbial invaders and tend to exhibit intrinsic specificity for the encountered pathogens. For instance, HNPs are expressed at high levels in lesions of superficial folliculitis due to skin infection by *S. aureus* (11). As an initial part of the inflammatory response, AMPs are produced by inflammatory cells, such as neutrophils and tissue phagocytes, including macrophages (31). For example, HBD is upregulated in monocytes exposed to bacteria, LPS, or IFNɣ (65). Furthermore, the immunomodulatory activities of AMPs enable the activation of adaptive immune responses. LL-37 represents a classical example of AMPs that binds to LPS leading to repressed LPS-induced responses and targeting the NF-κB pathway. Moreover, studies have shown that a downregulation of AMP expression is associated to an increase in susceptibility to infections by viruses and other microorganisms (13).

AMPs play an integral role in a large number of respiratory diseases [for example, tuberculosis, cystic fibrosis (CF), rhinitis, etc.], gastrointestinal diseases (shigellosis, inflammatory bowel disease, etc.), and cutaneous diseases (atopic dermatitis, psoriasis, wound healing, and rosacea) among others (13, 66). Group B Streptococcus (GBS) is killed by human serum from patients with GBS-related infections in an sPLA2-IIA-mediated manner (63). In healthy patients, sPLA2-IIA is the only sPLA2 isoform that is constitutively present at low ng/ml concentrations in the circulation (67–69). Increased levels of sPLA2-IIA have been observed in biological fluids in various inflammatory and infectious diseases, such as allergic rhinitis, rheumatoid arthritis, pancreatitis, septic shock, acute respiratory distress syndrome (ARDS), or CF, and correlated to symptom severity of these diseases (50, 70). However, it remains unclear whether upregulation of sPLA2-IIA expression is the cause and/or the consequence of inflammation (e.g., increased cytokine production) in these diseases. Elevated sPLA2-IIA levels have also been observed in arterial plasma and in bronchoalveolar lavage fluids of patients with septic shock. These levels have a prognostic value and correlated with the development of pulmonary failure (50). We focus in more detail in the following paragraph, the potential relevance of AMPs in CF.

Cystic Fibrosis

Patients with disruptions in lung immunity or mucosal clearance, such as patients with CF, suffer from bacterial infections that typically don't resolve even with antibiotic treatment (71). CF is a well-characterized, lethal, autosomal, recessive, inherited disorder found predominantly in Caucasians due to mutation in the cystic fibrosis transmembrane conductance regulator (CFTR) gene, characterized by chronic lung bacterial infections (72). These infections are major causes of morbidity and mortality of CF patients. Ultimately, 80 to 95% of patients with CF succumb to respiratory failure brought on by these chronic bacterial infections associated with airway inflammation (73). *P. aeruginosa* is arguably the major colonizing infection for people with CF (74).

The main AMPs detected in lung tissues and secretions of CF patients are neutrophil α-defensins/HNPs, HBDs, LL-37, and sPLA2-IIA that play a major role in lung immunity and protect them against infection with harmful microorganisms (75). The persistence of lung bacterial infection may be partly explained by an acidification of the airway surface liquid (ASL) within the CF lung that exhibits reduced bacterial killing due to the compromised function of AMPs (72, 76). Our recent studies showed that ASL was significantly more acidic in CF than in wild-type (WT) respiratory cells. This was consistent with a defect in bicarbonate secretion involving CFTR and SLC26A4 (pendrin) and a persistent proton secretion by ATP12A. This was associated to a defect in *S. aureus* clearance, which was improved by pH normalization (72).

Abnormal salinity of ASL has also been suggested to impair the bactericidal activity of AMPs, which can form bacterial proliferation within CF airways (77). We recently showed that the defensin BigDefl from the oyster *Crassostrea gigas* exhibits natural salt-stable and broad-range bactericidal activity against various bacterial species. We took advantage of this salt-stability, due to an evolutionary adaptation of oyster defensins to sea environment, to treat bacteria from CF patients. We showed that BigDefl efficiently kills multidrug-resistant clinical isolates of *S. aureus* from CF patients even at high salt concentrations (78).

In the early stages of CF, the airways are mainly colonized by *S. aureus*, whereas in later stages, *P. aeruginosa* is the major pathogen (46). This shift in infection is a characteristic feature of CF. Once it colonizes the CF airways, *P. aeruginosa* induces a robust expression and secretion of sPLA2-IIA by airways epithelial cells via a Krüppel-like transcription factor (KLF)-2-dependent pathway, leading to subsequent and selective killing of *S. aureus* by sPLA2-IIA, a process contributing to the infection shift (16). A similar phenomenon has been reported during periodontal diseases caused by *Porphyromonas gingivalis*. The latter induces sPLA2-IIA production and secretion by oral epithelial cells via activation of the Notch-1 receptor (45). The sPLA2-IIA concentrations reach levels leading to the killing of other oral bacteria much more susceptible to this enzyme sPLA2-IIA compared to *P. gingivalis* (45). This process is a potential cause of dysbiosis associated with periodontal disease. Thus, it is of great importance to examine the role of individual bacterial species within the microbiome in the induction or inhibition of sPLA2-IIA expression at mucosal sites and whether this may contribute to occurrence of dysbiosis at mucosal surfaces in diseases characterized by polymicrobial infections.

ADVANTAGES OF AMPs AND CHALLENGES

As the emergence of super-bacteria is causing a serious concern across the globe, researchers are working on the development of new anti-infective therapies. Among the alternatives to combat antimicrobial resistance, AMPs have garnered much attention over the years (79). AMPs, which are widely expressed in all kind of living organisms and have been preserved in the long evolutionary process, are with no doubt effective natural immunologically active molecules (80). AMPs have excellent *in vitro* antimicrobial activity against a wide range of microbes and, therefore, represent a promising alternative to combat resistance (18). The rapid bactericidal activity of AMPs constitutes a strong advantage to the future of peptide-based antibacterial therapy. In addition, AMPs are active against multidrug-resistant bacteria (49, 81). Furthermore, AMPs possess concomitant broad anti-inflammatory and immunomodulatory activities. Besides, AMPs exhibit synergistic or additive effects upon co-administration with conventional ATBs to treat both susceptible and multidrug-resistant bacteria at non-toxic concentrations (70, 71).

Due to the overlapping MOA of AMPs involving multiple low-affinity targets, unlike the MOA of conventional ATBs characterized by one defined, high-affinity target, the development of bacterial resistance toward AMPs has generally been considered to be improbable (28, 82). In particular, given that the bacterial cell membrane is the primary target of AMPs, it is challenging for microbes to preserve the cell membrane functional and structural integrity while at the same time avoiding the membrane disruption activity of AMPs (28). Because the AMP is composed of amino acids with no specific primary sequence signature, the microbe is unable to synthesize a protease that can cleave the AMP but not its own proteins. Furthermore, our recent study showed that the AMPs LL-37 and CAMA, a derivative of cecropin, were associated with only transient and low levels of induced resistance compared to the induced resistance by the antibiotic gentamicin (49). However, it appears somehow that some bacteria, such as *Serratia marcescens*, present natural resistance to AMPs (83). Moreover, some bacteria exposed to AMPs may evolve under selective pressures to develop resistance mechanisms. Even though the existence of these selective pressures are, evolutionarily speaking, quite old, human AMPs still possess a broad spectrum of effective activity against a diverse range of microorganisms (14).

In the last 30 years, various pharmaceutical companies have tried to develop AMPs as clinically useful antimicrobials. To date, several AMPs are currently undergoing laboratory testing, and a few have already reached clinical trials (19). The review (18) shows a number of AMPs and AMP derivates already at the preclinical stage and in clinical trial.

Although AMPs have very attractive qualities, the challenges for successful development for clinical application are considerable (84). One of the biggest restraints in the large scale of development and commercialization of AMPs may be their high production costs estimated around US$300–$500 per gram, which is several hundred times more expensive than the production of conventional ATBs (17). In addition to that, the excellent antimicrobial activity *in vitro* is rarely translated *in vivo* (41). In most studies in the field, the killing effects of AMPs on bacteria have been examined *in vitro* and in the absence of host cells, which do not reflect real life. Indeed, in human and animal infectious diseases, infecting bacteria multiply within biological fluids and/or in contact with host cells, which may interfere with AMP bactericidal activity. This led us to compare the bactericidal effects of LL-37 on *P. aeruginosa* in a cell-free system and when this strain was added to a bronchial epithelial cell line IB3, isolated from a CF patient, prior to addition of LL-37. These studies show that the presence of IB3 cells markedly reduces the bactericidal effects of LL-37 on *P. aeruginosa*. Although the mechanisms involved in this alteration are still under investigation, we hypothesized that degradation of LL-37 by a protease produced by IB3 cells upon infection by *P. aeruginosa* may explain the alteration of LL-37 bactericidal activity (unpublished data). Thus, most peptides have relatively short circulating plasma half-lives and are cleared primarily by proteolytic degradation and by renal filtration, generally leading to suboptimal pharmacokinetic properties (84). Indeed, the most obvious cause of poor or incomplete *in vivo* activity of AMPs is the lack of stability due to the peptide susceptibility to protease degradation if they are ingested. In regard to drug delivery, oral bioavailability of peptides is often no more than 2% (79). Thus, oral administration of AMPs can lead to proteolytic digestion by enzymes in the digestive tract, such as trypsin and pepsin, making intravenous or subcutaneous injections the only viable routes of administration to treat people. Moreover, systemic administration outcomes with short-half lives *in vivo*, protease degradation, and cytotoxic profiles in blood (20). In addition, the direct antibacterial activity of some of these AMPs is certainly prevented due to the affinity of these AMPs to polyvalent anions, such as glycosaminoglycans (29). AMPs can also bind avidly to host cells, which may reduce their availability to bind to and kill bacteria (unpublished data).

Another key factor to consider is the potential of these peptides to elicit an immunogenic response that can significantly reduce their efficacy and alter their pharmacokinetic profile (84). An additional challenge to overcome is the differences in pH, salt, and serum concentrations *in vivo*, resulting in decreased antimicrobial activity (10). Hence, a number of AMPs have failed approval by the FDA after reaching phase II clinical trials due to their short-half life and their poor physical-chemical properties (17). However, even with limitations, AMPs still possess a broad spectrum of potent antimicrobial activity (14). Another potential issue includes the cytotoxicity to mammalian cells when bactericidal concentrations are high. However, there are very few studies of AMP cytotoxicity on human cells (10).

Methods to overcome these challenges have been evaluated. Scientists and pharmaceutical companies have invested in research and development to overcome the barriers limiting the practical application of AMPs. To circumvent proteolysis, sequence modifications, and half-life, advances in peptide formulation have ended in the development of improved formulas with sufficient plasma exposure using a delivery system (for example, a lipid self-assembly system, inorganic systems, nanoparticles, etc.), chemical modifications of AMPs, and altering structure to have cyclic peptides with strained peptide bonds displaying a resistant profile (41, 85). Another approach is to identify possible molecular cleavage sites followed by substitution of the relevant amino acids (86). The recognized route of administration for therapeutic peptides remains parenteral, in which AMPs pierce the membrane barriers where they are poorly absorbed. Nevertheless, other challenges remain, pre- and post-administration, in achieving both the desired pharmacokinetic profile and high patient compliance (84). Specific cell-penetrating peptide sequences have been identified and can be used to transport AMPs across membranes (79). More tools to increase AMP activity include modifications in charge and hydrophobicity. Among the various methods for peptide optimization, quantitative structure-activity relationship, and the introduction of fluorine atoms or trifluromethyl groups have been recently used (25). Besides, recent studies have focused on designing a sequence of AMP analogs with modified yet improved antibacterial, cytotoxic, and hemolytic activities. Thus, synthetic peptides have been designed to mimic the structure, function, and mode of action of AMPs with enhanced properties, resulting in low cytotoxicity and high resistance to proteolytic degradation, resulting in prolonged half-lives and cost-effective molecules (18). Furthermore, the progress in designing non-immunogenic peptides is rapid, resulting in disarming the immunogenic response, which should increase clinical success (84).

CONCLUSIONS AND PERSPECTIVES

AMPs, owing to their broad spectrum of antibacterial activity and their effectiveness against multidrug-resistant bacteria, are a promising replacement for conventional ATBs, invoking a multi-hit mechanism that cannot be easily overcome by bacteria. However, the future of peptide-based anti-infective drugs is still uncertain. The major barriers that hinder their clinical use are mainly their stability *in vivo*, their non-well-studied toxicity, and their high production costs. Thus, the development of optimal formulations of AMPs at a reasonable cost, finding the preferred route of their administration, and evaluating their cytotoxicity remain the main interest to scientists. Regardless of the field of applications, AMPs constitute the most promising drug candidate in a foreseeable future in overcoming the alarming rise of bacterial resistance.

AUTHOR CONTRIBUTIONS

RG and CM wrote the article. ZX did the figures and tables. LT and DK revised and corrected the manuscript. All authors read and approved the final manuscript. All authors contributed to the article and approved the submitted version.

REFERENCES

1. Fleming A. On a remarkable bacteriolytic element found in tissues and secretions. *Proc R Soc Lond B.* (1922) 93:306–17. doi: 10.1098/rspb.1922.0023
2. Dubos R. Studies on a bactericidal agent extracted from a soil bacillus: I. preparation of the agent. Its acitivity *in vitro. J Exp Med.* (1939) 70:1–10. doi: 10.1084/jem.70.1.1
3. Steiner H, Hultmark D, Engstrom A, Bennich H, Boman H. Sequence and specifity of two antibacterial proteins involved in insect immunity. *Nature.* (1981) 292:246–8. doi: 10.1038/292246a0
4. Zasloff M. Magainins, a class of antimicrobial peptides from Xenopus skin: isolation, characterization of two active forms, and partial cDNA sequence of a precursor. *Proc Natl Acad Sci USA.* (1987) 84:5449–53. doi: 10.1073/pnas.84.15.5449
5. Bulet P, Stöcklin R, Menin L. Anti-microbial peptides: from invertebrates to vertebrates. *Immunol Rev.* (2004) 198:169–84. doi: 10.1111/j.0105-2896.2004.0124.x
6. Skarnes R, Watson D. Antimicrobial factors of normal tissues and fluids. *Bacteriol Rev.* (1957) 21:273–94. doi: 10.1128/MMBR.21.4.273-294.1957
7. Mishra B, Scott R, Zarena D, Wang G. Host defense antimicrobial peptides as antibiotics: design and application strategies. *Curr Opin Chem Biol.* (2017) 38:87–96. doi: 10.1016/j.cbpa.2017.03.014
8. Kang H, Kim C, Seo C, Park Y. The therapeutic applications of antimicrobial peptides (AMPs): a patent review. *J Microbiol.* (2017) 55:1–12. doi: 10.1007/s12275-017-6452-1
9. Baxter AA, Lay FT, Poon IKH, Kvansakul M, Hulett MD. Tumor cell membrane - targeting cationic antimicrobial peptides : novel insights into mechanisms of action and therapeutic prospects. *Cell Mol Life Sci.* (2017) 74:3809–25. doi: 10.1007/s00018-017-2604-z
10. Bastos P, Ferreira R, Vitorino R. Human antimicrobial peptides in bodily fluids : current knowledge and therapeutic perspectives in the postantibiotic era. *Med Res Rev.* (2018) 38:101–46. doi: 10.1002/med.21435
11. Xia X, Cheng L, Zhang S, Wang L, Hu J. The role of natural antimicrobial peptides during infection and chronic inflammation. *Antonie Van Leeuwenhoek.* (2018) 111:5–26. doi: 10.1007/s10482-017-0929-0
12. Si-Tahar M, Touqui L, Chignard M. Innate immunity and inflammation–two facets of the same anti-infectious reaction. *Clin Exp Immunol.* (2009) 156:194–8. doi: 10.1111/j.1365-2249.2009.03893.x
13. Fuente-núñez C De, Silva ON, Lu TK, Luiz O. Antimicrobial peptides : Role in human disease and potential as immunotherapies. *Pharmacol Ther.* (2017) 178:132–40. doi: 10.1016/j.pharmthera.2017.04.002
14. Nizet V. Antimicrobial peptide resistance mechanisms of human bacterial pathogens. *Mol Biol.* (2006) 8:11–26. doi: 10.21775/cimb.008.011

13. Fuente-núñez C De, Silva ON, Lu TK, Luiz O. Antimicrobial peptides : Role in human disease and potential as immunotherapies. *Pharmacol Ther.* (2017) 178:132–40. doi: 10.1016/j.pharmthera.2017.04.002
14. Nizet V. Antimicrobial peptide resistance mechanisms of human bacterial pathogens. *Mol Biol.* (2006) 8:11–26. doi: 10.21775/cimb.008.011
15. Kosikowska P, Lesner A, Kosikowska P, Lesner A. Antimicrobial peptides (AMPs) as drug candidates : a patent review 2003–2015. *Expert Opin Ther Pat.* (2016) 26:689–702. doi: 10.1080/13543776.2016.1176149
16. Rahnamaeian M. Antimicrobial peptides modes of mechanism, modulation of defense responses. *Plant Signal Behav.* (2011) 6:1325–32. doi: 10.4161/psb.6.9.16319
17. da Costa JP, Cova M, Ferreira R, Vitorino R. Antimicrobial peptides: an alternative for innovative medicines? *Appl Microbiol Biotechnol.* (2015) 99:2023–40. doi: 10.1007/s00253-015-6375-x
18. Wang J, Dou X, Song J, Lyu Y, Zhu X, Xu L, et al. Antimicrobial peptides : promising alternatives in the post feeding antibiotic era. *Med Res Rev.* (2019) 39:831–59. doi: 10.1002/med.21542
19. Fry DE. Antimicrobial peptides. *Surg Infect.* (2018) 19:804–11. doi: 10.1089/sur.2018.194
20. Kumar P, Kizhakkedathu JN, Straus SK. Antimicrobial peptides : diversity, mechanism of action and strategies to improve the activity and biocompatibility *in vivo*. *Biomolecules.* (2018) 8:4. doi: 10.3390/biom8010004
21. Xhindoli D, Pacor S, Benincasa M, Scocchi M, Gennaro R, Tossi A. The human cathelicidin LL-37 — a pore-forming antibacterial peptide and host-cell modulator. *Biochim Biophys Acta.* (2016) 1858:546–66. doi: 10.1016/j.bbamem.2015.11.003
22. Fabisiak A, Murawska N, Fichna J. LL-37_ Cathelicidin-related antimicrobial peptide with pleiotropic activity. *Pharmacol Rep.* (2016) 68:802–8. doi: 10.1016/j.pharep.2016.03.015
23. Lee J, Lee DG. Antimicrobial Peptides (AMPs) with dual mechanisms: membrane disruption and apoptosis. *J Microbiol Biotechnol.* (2015) 25:759–64. doi: 10.4014/jmb.1411.11058
24. Ab M, Biomed N, Res T, Naafs MAB. The antimicrobial peptides : ready for clinical trials? *Biomed J Sci Tech Res.* (2018) 5:1–4. doi: 10.26717/BJSTR.2018.07.001536
25. Pasupuleti M, Schmidtchen A, Malmsten M, Pasupuleti M, Schmidtchen A, Malmsten M. Antimicrobial peptides : key components of the innate immune system. *Crit Rev Biotechnol.* (2012) 32:143–71. doi: 10.3109/07388551.2011.594423
26. Sierra JM, Fusté E, Rabanal F, Vinuesa T, Viñas M, Sierra JM, et al. An overview of antimicrobial peptides and the latest advances in their development. *Expert Opin Biol Ther.* (2017) 17:663–76. doi: 10.1080/14712598.2017.1315402
27. Sharma S, Sahoo N, Bhunia A. Antimicrobial peptides and their pore / ion channel properties in neutralization of pathogenic microbes. *Curr Top Med Chem.* (2016) 16:46–53. doi: 10.2174/1568026615666150703115454
28. Mahlapuu M, Håkansson J, Ringstad L, Björn C. Antimicrobial peptides : an emerging category of therapeutic agents. *Front Cell Infect Microbiol.* (2016) 6:194. doi: 10.3389/fcimb.2016.00194
29. Jenssen H, Hamill P, Hancock REW. Peptide antimicrobial agents. *Clin Microbiol Rev.* (2006) 19:491–511. doi: 10.1128/CMR.00056-05
30. Otvos L Jr. Immunomodulatory effects of anti-microbial peptides. *Acta Microbiol Immunol Hung.* (2016) 63:257–77. doi: 10.1556/030.63.2016.005
31. Steinstraesser L, Kraneburg U, Jacobsen F, Al-Benna S. Host defense peptides and their antimicrobial-immunomodulatory duality. *Immunobiology.* (2011) 216:322–33. doi: 10.1016/j.imbio.2010.07.003
32. Wu Y, Li D, Wang Y, Liu X, Zhang Y, Qu W, et al. Beta-Defensin 2 and 3 promote bacterial clearance of pseudomonas aeruginosa by inhibiting macrophage autophagy through downregulation of early growth response gene-1 and c-FOs. *Front Immunol.* (2018) 9:1–14. doi: 10.3389/fimmu.2018.00211
33. De Y, Chen Q, Schimdt A., Anderson G., Wang J., Wooters J, et al. LL-37, the neutrophil granule- and epithelial cell-derived cathelicidn, utilizes formyl peptide receptor-like 1 (FPRL1) as a receptor to chemoattract human peripheral blood neutrophils, monocytes, and T cells. *J Exp Med.* (2000) 192:1069–672. doi: 10.1084/jem.192.7.1069
34. Bowdish D, Davidson D, Lau Y, Lee K, Scott M, Hancock R. Impact of LL-37 on anti-infective immunity. *J Leucoc Biol.* (2005) 77:451–9. doi: 10.1189/jlb.0704380
35. Zanetti M, Gennaro R, Skerlavaj B, Tomasinsig L, Circo R. Cathelicidin peptides as candidates for a novel class of antimicrobials. *Curr Pharm Des.* (2002) 8:779–93. doi: 10.2174/1381612023395457
36. Mallapragada S, Wadhwa A, Agrawal P. Antimicrobial peptides: the miraculous biological molecules. *Indian Soc Periodontol.* (2017) 21:434–8. doi: 10.4103/jisp.jisp_325_16
37. Pach E, Javier S. Perspectives for clinical use of engineered human host defense antimicrobial peptides. *FEMS Microbiol Rev.* (2017) 41:323–42. doi: 10.1093/femsre/fux012
38. Galdiero E, Lombardi L, Falanga A, Libralato G, Guida M, Carotenuto R. Biofilms : novel strategies based on antimicrobial peptides. *Pharmaceutics.* (2019) 11:322. doi: 10.3390/pharmaceutics11070322
39. Shahrour H, Ferrer-espada R, Dandache I, Bárcena-varela S, Sánchez-gómez S, Chokr A, et al. AMPs as anti-biofilm agents for human therapy and prophylaxis. *Antimicrob Pept Adv Exp Med Biol.* (2019) 1117:257–79. doi: 10.1007/978-981-13-3588-4_14
40. Brice D, Diamond G. Antiviral activities of human host defense peptides. *Curr Med Chem.* (2019) 27:1420–43. doi: 10.2174/0929867326666190805151654
41. Hancock R. Review cationic peptides : effectors in innate immunity and novel antimicrobials. *Lancet Infect Dis.* (2001) 1:156–64. doi: 10.1016/S1473-3099(01)00092-5
42. Dosler S, Karaaslan E. Inhibition and destruction of *Pseudomonas aeruginosa* biofilms by antibiotics peptides. *Peptides.* (2014) 62:32–7. doi: 10.1016/j.peptides.2014.09.021
43. Reddy KVR, Yedery RD, Aranha C. Antimicrobial peptides : premises and promises. *Int J Antimicrob Agents.* (2004) 24:536–47. doi: 10.1016/j.ijantimicag.2004.09.005
44. Ganz T. Defensins and other antimicrobial peptides: a historical perspective and an update. *Comb Chem High Throughput Screen.* (2005) 8:209–17. doi: 10.2174/1386207053764594
45. Barbara B, Akiko M, Wei X, Michael HG, Howard, R. Katz Jonathan PA. Group V secretory phospholipase a2 modulates phagosome maturation and regulates the innate immune response against candida albicans. *J Immunol.* (2009) 182:4891–8. doi: 10.4049/jimmunol.0803776
46. Lai Y, Gallo RL. AMPed up immunity : how antimicrobial peptides have multiple roles in immune defense. *Trends Immunol.* (2009) 30:131–41. doi: 10.1016/j.it.2008.12.003
47. Zhang Y, Liu Y, Sun Y, Liu Q, Wang X, Li Z, et al. *In vitro* synergistic activities of antimicrobial peptide brevinin-2CE with five kinds of antibiotics against multidrug-resistant clinical isolates. *Curr Microbiol.* (2014) 68:685–92. doi: 10.1007/s00284-014-0529-4
48. Dosler S, Mataraci E. *In vitro* pharmacokinetics of antimicrobial cationic peptides alone and in combination with antibiotics against methicillin resistant *Staphylococcus aureus* biofilms. *Peptides.* (2013) 49:53–8. doi: 10.1016/j.peptides.2013.08.008
49. Geitani R, Moubareck CA, Touqui L, Sarkis DK. Cationic antimicrobial peptides : alternatives and / or adjuvants to antibiotics active against methicillin-resistant *Staphylococcus aureus* and multidrug-resistant *Pseudomonas aeruginosa*. *BMC Microbiol.* (2019) 19:1–12. doi: 10.1186/s12866-019-1416-8
50. Touqui L, Alaoui-El-Azher M. Mammalian secreted phospholipases A2 and their pathophysiological significance in inflammatory diseases. *Curr Mol Med.* (2001) 1:739–54. doi: 10.2174/1566524013363258
51. Lambeau G, Gelb MH. Biochemistry and physiology of mammalian secreted phospholipases A2. *Annu Rev Biochem.* (2008) 77:495–520. doi: 10.1146/annurev.biochem.76.062405.154007
52. Nevalainen T, Graham G, Scott K. Antibacterial actions of secreted phospholipases A2. *Rev Biochim Biophys Acta.* (2008) 1781:1–9. doi: 10.1016/j.bbalip.2007.12.001
53. Wu Y, Raymond B, Goossens P, Njamkepo E, Guiso N, Paya M, et al. Type-IIA secreted phospholipase A2 is an endogenous antibiotic-like protein of the host. *Biochimie.* (2010) 92:583–7. doi: 10.1016/j.biochi.2010.01.024
54. Weinrauch Y, Abad C, Liang N, Lowry S, Weiss J. Mobilization of potent plasma bactericidal activity during systemic bacterial challenge. role of group IIA phospholipase A2. *J Clin Invest.* (1998) 102:633–8. doi: 10.1172/JCI3121
55. Weiss J. Molecular determinants of bacterial sensitivity and resistance to mammalian Group IIA phospholipase A2. *Biochim Biophys Acta.* (2015) 1848:3072–7. doi: 10.1016/j.bbamem.2015.05.018

56. Qu X, RI L. Secretory phospholipase A2 is the principal bactericide for staphylococci and other gram-positive bacteria in human tears. *Infect Immun.* (1998) 66:2791–7. doi: 10.1128/IAI.66.6.2791-2797.1998
57. Koprivnjak T, Weidenmaier C, Peschel A, Weiss J. Wall teichoic acid deficiency in *Staphylococcus aureus* confers selective resistance to mammalian group IIA phospholipase A(2) and human beta-defensin 3. *Infect Immun.* (2008) 76:2169–76. doi: 10.1128/IAI.01705-07
58. Kennedy BP, Payette P, Vadas P, Pruzanski W, Kwan M, Tang C, et al. A natural disruption of the secretory group II phospholipase A 2 gene in inbred mouse strains a natural disruption of the secretory group II phospholipase A 2 gene in inbred mouse strains*. *J Biol Chem.* (1995) 270:22378–85. doi: 10.1074/jbc.270.38.22378
59. MacPhee M, Chepenik KP, Liddell RA, Nelson KK, Siracusa LD, Buchberg AM. The secretory phospholipase A2 gene is a candidate for the Mom1 locus, a major modifier of ApcMin-induced intestinal neoplasia. *Cell.* (1995) 81:957–66. doi: 10.1016/0092-8674(95)90015-2
60. Piris-Gimenez A, Paya M, Lambeau G, Chignard M, Mock M, Touqui L, et al. *In vivo* protective role of human group IIa phospholipase A2 against experimental anthrax. *J Immunol.* (2005) 175:6786–91. doi: 10.4049/jimmunol.175.10.6786
61. Laine VJO, Grass DS, Nevalainen TJ. Protection by group II phospholipase A2 against *Stapylococcus aureus. J Immunol.* (1999) 162:7402–8.
62. Movert E, Wu Y, Lambeau G, Touqui L, Areschoug T. A novel bacterial resistance mechanism against human group IIA-secreted phospholipase A2: role of *Streptococcus pyogenes* sortase A. *J Immunol.* (2011) 187:6437–46. doi: 10.4049/jimmunol.1100499
63. Movert E, Wu Y, Lambeau G, Kahn F, Touqui L, Areschoug T. Secreted group IIA phospholipase A2 protects humans against the group B streptococcus: experimental and clinical evidence. *J Infect Dis.* (2013) 208:2025–35. doi: 10.1093/infdis/jit359
64. Laine VJO, Grass DS, Nevalainen TJ. Resistance of transgenic mice expressing human group II phospholipase A2 to *Escherichia coli* infection. *Infect Immun.* (2000) 68:87–92. doi: 10.1128/IAI.68.1.87-92.2000
65. Brown KL, Hancock REW. Cationic host defense (antimicrobial) peptides. *Sci Direct.* (2006) 18:24–30. doi: 10.1016/j.coi.2005.11.004
66. Guaní-Guerra E, Santos-Mendoza T, Lugo-Reyes SO, Terán LM. Antimicrobial peptides: general overview and clinical implications in human health and disease. *Clin Immunol.* (2009) 135:1–11. doi: 10.1016/j.clim.2009.12.004
67. Paganelli FL, Leavis HL, He S, van Sorge NM, Payré C, Lambeau G, et al. Group IIA-secreted phospholipase A 2 in human serum kills commensal but not clinical *Enterococcus faecium* isolates. *Infect Immun.* (2018) 86:e00180-18. doi: 10.1128/IAI.00180-18
68. Grönroos JO, Laine VJO, Nevalainen TJ. Bactericidal group IIA phospholipase A2 in serum of patients with bacterial infections. *J Infect Dis.* (2002) 185:1767–72. doi: 10.1086/340821
69. Nevalainen TJ, Eerola LI, Rintala E, Laine VJO, Lambeau G, Gelb MH. Time-resolved fluoroimmunoassays of the complete set of secreted phospholipases A2in human serum. *Biochim Biophys Acta.* (2005) 1733:210–23. doi: 10.1016/j.bbalip.2004.12.012
70. Nakos G, Kitsiouli E, Hatzidaki E, Koulouras V, Touqui L, Lekka M. Phospholipases A2 and platelet-activating-factor acetylhydrolase in patients with acute respiratory distress syndrome. *Crit Care Med.* (2005) 33:772–9. doi: 10.1097/01.CCM.0000158519.80090.74
71. Pragman AA, Berger JP, Williams BJ. Understanding persistent bacterial lung infections: clinical implications informed by the biology of the microbiota and biofilms. *Clin Pulm Med.* (2016) 23:57–66. doi: 10.1097/CPM.0000000000000108
72. Simonin J, Bille E, Crambert G, Noel S, Elise D, Edwards A, et al. Airway surface liquid acidification initiates host defense abnormalities in cystic fibrosis. *Nat Sci Reports.* (2019) 9:1–11. doi: 10.1038/s41598-019-54253-4
73. Lyczak JB, Cannon CL, Pier GB. Lung infections associated with cystic fibrosis. *Antimicrob Agents Chemother.* (2002) 15:194–222. doi: 10.1128/CMR.15.2.194-222.2002
74. Huang YJ, Lipuma JJ, Arbor A, Diseases C, Arbor A. The microbiome in cystic fibrosis. *Clin Chest Med.* (2017) 37:59–67. doi: 10.1016/j.ccm.2015.10.003
75. Hiemstra PS, Amatngalim GD, Does AM Van Der, Taube C. Antimicrobial peptides and innate lung defenses role in infectious and noninfectious lung diseases and therapeutic. *Chest.* (2019) 149:545–51. doi: 10.1378/chest.15-1353
76. Malhotra S, Hayes D, Wozniak DJ. Cystic fibrosis and *Pseudomonas aeruginosa*: the host-microbe interface. *Clin Microbiol Rev.* (2019) 32:e00138-18. doi: 10.1128/CMR.00138-18
77. Bals R, Wang X, Wu Z, Freeman T, Bafna V, Zasloff M, et al. Human beta-defensin 2 is a salt-sensitive peptide antibiotic expressed in human lung. *J Clin Invest.* (1998) 102:874–80. doi: 10.1172/JCI2410
78. Loth K, Vergnes A, Barret C, Da Silva J, Bressan A, Belmadi N, et al. The ancestral N-terminal domain of big defensins drives bacterially triggered assembly into antimicrobial nanonets. *mBio.* (2019) 10:e01821-19. doi: 10.1128/mBio.01821-19
79. Angell Y, Moos WH. Building on success : a bright future for peptide therapeutics. *Protein Pept Lett.* (2018) 25:1044–50. doi: 10.2174/0929866525666181114155542
80. Lau LJ, Dunn KM. Therapeutic peptides_historical perspectives, current development trends, and future directions. *Bioorg Med Chem.* (2018) 26:2700–7. doi: 10.1016/j.bmc.2017.06.052
81. Fedders H, Podschun R, Leippe M. The antimicrobial peptide Ci-MAM-A24 is highly active against multidrug-resistant and anaerobic bacteria pathogenic for humans. *Int J Antimicrob Agents.* (2010) 36:264–6. doi: 10.1016/j.ijantimicag.2010.04.008
82. Zhang L, Parente J, Harris SM, Woods DE, Hancock REW, Falla TJ. Antimicrobial peptide therapeutics for cystic fibrosis. *Antimicrob Agents Chemother.* (2005) 49:2921–7. doi: 10.1128/AAC.49.7.2921-2927.2005
83. Gordon JY, Romanowski EG. A review of antimicrobial peptides and their therapeutic potential as anti-infective drugs. *Curr Eye Res.* (2005) 30:505–15. doi: 10.1080/02713680590968637
84. Henninot A, Collins JC, Nuss JM. The current state of peptide drug discovery: back to the future? *J Med Chem.* (2018) 61:1382–414. doi: 10.1021/acs.jmedchem.7b00318
85. Erak M, Bellman-Sickert K, Els-Heindl S, Beck-Sickinger GA. Peptide chemistry toolbox - transforming natural peptides into peptide therapeutics. *Bioorg Med Chem.* (2018) 26:2759–65. doi: 10.1016/j.bmc.2018.01.012
86. Fosgerau K, Hoffman T. Peptide therapeutics_current status and future directions. *Drug Discov Today.* (2015) 20:122–8. doi: 10.1016/j.drudis.2014.10.003

13

Rhinovirus Infection is Associated with Airway Epithelial Cell Necrosis and Inflammation *via* Interleukin-1 in Young Children with Cystic Fibrosis

Samuel T. Montgomery[1]***, Dario L. Frey***[2,3]***, Marcus A. Mall***[3,4,5]***, Stephen M. Stick***[1,6,7,8] ***and Anthony Kicic***[1,6,7,8,9]****, on behalf of the WA Epithelial Research Program (WAERP)***[6,10] ***and AREST CF***[6,7,11,12]

[1] Faculty of Health and Medical Sciences, School of Biomedical Sciences, The University of Western Australia, Crawley, WA, Australia, [2] Department of Translational Pulmonology, Translational Lung Research Center Heidelberg, University of Heidelberg, Heidelberg, Germany, [3] German Center for Lung Research, Heidelberg, Germany, [4] Department of Pediatric Pulmonology, Immunology and Critical Care Medicine, Charité-Universitätsmedizin Berlin, Berlin, Germany, [5] Berlin Institute of Health, Berlin, Germany, [6] Telethon Kids Institute, The University of Western Australia, Crawley, WA, Australia, [7] Department of Respiratory and Sleep Medicine, Perth Children's Hospital, Nedlands, WA, Australia, [8] Centre for Cell Therapy and Regenerative Medicine, School of Medicine and Pharmacology, The University of Western Australia, Nedlands, WA, Australia, [9] School of Public Health, Curtin University, Bentley, WA, Australia, [10] St John of God Hospital, Subiaco, WA, Australia, [11] Murdoch Children's Research Institute, Melbourne, VIC, Australia, [12] Department of Paediatrics, University of Melbourne, Melbourne, VIC, Australia

***Correspondence:**
Anthony Kicic
anthony.kicic@telethonkids.org.au

Introduction: The responses of cystic fibrosis (CF) airway epithelial cells (AEC) to rhinovirus (RV) infection are likely to contribute to early pathobiology of lung disease with increased neutrophilic inflammation and lower apoptosis reported. Necrosis of AEC resulting in airway inflammation driven by IL-1 signaling is a characteristic finding in CF detectable in airways of young children. Being the most common early-life infection, RV-induced epithelial necrosis may contribute to early neutrophilic inflammation in CF via IL-1 signaling. As little is known about IL-1 and biology of CF lung disease, this study assessed cellular and pro-inflammatory responses of CF and non-CF AEC following RV infection, with the hypothesis that RV infection drives epithelial necrosis and IL-1 driven inflammation.

Methods: Primary AEC obtained from children with ($n = 6$) and without CF ($n = 6$) were infected with RV (MOI 3) for 24 h and viable, necrotic and apoptotic events quantified via flow cytometry using a seven-step gating strategy (% total events). IL-1α, IL-1β, IL-1Ra, IL-8, CXCL10, CCL5, IFN-β, IL-28A, IL-28B, and IL-29 were also measured in cell culture supernatants (pg/mL).

Results: RV infection reduced viable events in non-CF AEC ($p < 0.05$), increased necrotic events in non-CF and CF AEC ($p < 0.05$) and increased apoptotic events in non-CF AEC ($p < 0.05$). Infection induced IL-1α and IL-1β production in both phenotypes ($p < 0.05$) but only correlated with necrosis (IL-1α: $r = 0.80$; IL-1β: $r = 0.77$; $p < 0.0001$) in CF AEC. RV infection also increased IL-1Ra in non-CF and CF AEC ($p < 0.05$), although significantly more in non-CF AEC ($p < 0.05$). Finally, infection stimulated IL-8 production in non-CF and CF AEC ($p < 0.05$) and correlated with IL-1α ($r = 0.63$ & $r = 0.74$ respectively; $p < 0.0001$).

Conclusions: This study found RV infection drives necrotic cell death in CF AEC. Furthermore, RV induced IL-1 strongly correlated with necrotic cell death in these cells. As IL-1R signaling drives airway neutrophilia and mucin production, these observations suggest RV infection early in life may exacerbate inflammation and mucin accumulation driving early CF lung disease. Since IL-1R can be targeted therapeutically with IL-1Ra, these data suggest a new anti-inflammatory therapeutic approach targeting downstream effects of IL-1R signaling to mitigate viral-induced, muco-inflammatory triggers of early lung disease.

Keywords: cystic fibrosis, airway epithelium, rhinovirus, interleukin-1, necrosis

INTRODUCTION

Cystic Fibrosis (CF) lung disease is progressive, evolves within the first months of life, and is characterized by mucus obstruction and inflammation observable on CT even in the absence of clinical symptoms and often in the absence of detectable respiratory infection (1, 2). Neutrophilic inflammation is a key risk factor for airway disease resulting in bronchiectasis and loss of lung function (3). However, the link between mucus obstruction and airway inflammation has not yet been clearly identified.

Recent evidence from the Australian Respiratory Early Surveillance Team for CF (AREST CF) implicates mucin accumulation as the initial trigger of neutrophilic inflammation in the CF airway (4), and suggests respiratory viral infection may trigger the muco-inflammatory phenotype observed in CF since the heterogeneity of early CF lung disease mirrors the heterogeneity of childhood viral infection (5, 6). Human rhinovirus (RV) appears to be able to manipulate host responses switching from apoptotic to necrotic cell death in airway epithelial cells (AEC) (7, 8). Studies investigating non-bacterial inflammation in the CF airway microenvironment have linked interleukin (IL)-1R signaling driven by IL-1α released from necrotic AEC to neutrophilic inflammation (9, 10). As RV is the most common early life viral infection observed in children with CF (11) and IL-1R signaling has already been detected in the airways of young children with mild disease (12), we hypothesize that resultant neutrophilic inflammation may be driven via this signaling pathway triggered by RV-induced AEC necrosis. However, this proposed mechanism has yet to be investigated.

Given our previous observations of defective responses to RV (8) and IL-1 driven inflammatory responses to necrosis in the pediatric CF airway (12), this study aimed to investigate the direct relationship between RV infection, the type of induced cell death, and IL-1R-driven inflammation *in vitro* using primary AEC from infants and young children with CF. We obtained primary AEC from young children with and without CF and assessed viable, necrotic and apoptotic events following RV infection utilizing flow cytometry. Using experimental supernatants; IL-1α, IL-1β, IL-1Ra, sIL-1R2, IL-8, CXCL10, CCL5, IFN-β, IL-28A, IL-28B, and IL-29 were measured and subsequently correlated to viable, necrotic and apoptotic responses.

MATERIALS AND METHODS

Please also refer to the **Supplementary Data** for full details.

Study Population and Establishment of Primary Cell Culture

This study was approved by the relevant institutional Human Ethics Committees with written consent obtained from parents or guardians. This study included samples from six clinically stable infants and children with CF (mean age 2.9 ± 1.8 years old; **Table 1**) participating in the AREST CF early surveillance program (2), and samples from six children without CF (mean age 3.8 ± 1.9 years old; **Table 1**) recruited upon admission to hospital for elective non-respiratory related surgery. Cystic fibrosis transmembrane conductance regulator (CFTR) genotype was determined as part of newborn screening (**Table 1**). Current bacterial infection in CF samples was determined as part of standard clinical practice using gold-standard microbiological screening, with previous infection the presence of a bacterial infection at any previous visit. Prior wheeze was determined by parent-reported wheeze in the three-months prior to recruitment. Children without CF had no respiratory symptoms observed at time of recruitment. Samples were attained by brushing of the tracheal mucosa of children with a single-sheathed nylon bronchial cytology brush as previously described (8, 13). After collection, primary AEC cultures were established as previously described (14).

TABLE 1 | Demographics of the study population.

	Non-CF	CF
Number of subjects	6	6
Age (mean ± standard deviation)	3.52 ± 1.6 years	3.16 ± 0.98 years
Sex (% Male)	66.6%	50%
Prior wheeze status (% Wheeze)	50%	0%
Genotype (% Phe.508del homozygous)	N/A	83.3%
Current bacterial infection	N/A	50%
Previous bacterial infection	N/A	33.3%
Neutrophil elastase presence	N/A	33.3%

Human RV Infection

Human rhinovirus 1b (RV1b) was propagated as previously described (15). To simulate an acute RV infection *in vitro*, primary AEC were infected with $\sim 2.95 \times 10^5$ $TCID_{50}$/mL. To ensure responses were due to actively replicating virus, controls were exposed to an UV-inactivated RV1b at the same $TCID_{50}$ as previously described (16). After 24- and 48-h cells were collected for analysis via flow cytometry and supernatant collected for cytokine measurement. As the peak concentration of RV viral load following infection is observed 24 h post-infection (17, 18), this timepoint was chosen for analysis. Viral load was assessed via qPCR as previously described (19). Infection with RV1b induced typical viral cytokine production from both non-CF and CF AEC (**Table S1**). Data from 48 h of RV1b infection is presented in the **Supplementary Data**.

Flow Cytometry

A flow cytometry methodology to measure cell death and disassembly was adapted for use with AEC (20). Briefly, primary cells were detached from culture surfaces via gentle trypsinization, combined with cells obtained from supernatant following centrifugation, and resuspended at a concentration of 10^6 cells/mL in annexin binding buffer (ThermoFisher Scientific, Scoresby, VIC, Australia). Tubes containing 100 μL of cell suspension were stained for 15 min with 100 μL of Annexin V/AlexaFluor488 (ThermoFisher Scientific, Scoresby, VIC, Australia) (1:40 v/v) and TO-PRO-3 (10 μM final concentration) (ThermoFisher Scientific, Scoresby, VIC, Australia) in annexin binding buffer and flow cytometry performed via a FACSCanto II flow cytometer (BD Biosciences, Franklin Lakes, NJ, USA). A total of 20,000 events were recorded during acquisition for each sample. Analysis was performed using FlowJo software v10.4 (FlowJo LLC, Ashland, OR, USA) using a seven-step gating strategy to separate events into viable, necrotic, A5+ apoptotic, A5- apoptotic, apoptotic bodies and cellular debris as previously described (20) (**Figure S1**). Cutoffs used for positive forward scatter (FSC) and side scatter (SSC) were 50 k. Events were grouped into "viable", "necrotic", and "apoptotic" for further analysis. Data are presented as percentage of total events (% total).

Cytokine Measurement

Interleukin (IL)-1α, IL-1β, and interferon- beta (IFN-β) protein production was determined using commercially available AlphaLISA kits (Perkin Elmer, Waltham, MA, USA) in cell-free culture supernatant. Similarly, IL-8 (BD Biosciences, San Diego, CA, USA), IL-1 receptor antagonist (IL-1Ra), soluble IL-1 receptor 2 (sIL-1R2), C-X-C motif chemokine 10 (CXCL10), Chemokine (C-C motif) ligand 5 (CCL5), IL-28A, IL-28B, and IL-29 protein production (R&D Systems, Minneapolis, MN, USA) were all determined using commercially available ELISA kits performed according to manufacturer's instructions. Samples below the detection range were arbitrarily reported as half the lower limit and included in the analysis with all other samples as previously described (21).

Statistical Analysis

Data were analyzed using GraphPad Prism v7.04 (GraphPad Software, La Jolla, CA, USA). Data were natural log transformed where appropriate. Comparisons between paired data were performed using Wilcoxon matched pairs signed rank test and Friedman's test with Dunn's multiple comparisons test presented as mean ± standard deviation. Comparisons between unpaired data were performed using Mann-Whitney tests presented as mean ± standard deviation. Associations between flow cytometry events and cytokines measured were assessed using Spearman's rank-order correlations. A two tailed P value < 0.05 was considered statistically significant.

RESULTS

Demographic data for the study populations are summarized in **Table 1**. Sex and age were similar between cohorts, with most children with CF homozygous for the p.Phe508del mutation. Infection with RV1b resulted in increased rhinovirus load measured via qPCR compared to UV-inactivated RV1b (31.3 ± 29.8 copy #/ng RNA vs. $2.37 \times 10^7 \pm 1.46 \times 10^7$ copy #/ng RNA; $p < 0.05$), increased typical pro-inflammatory viral cytokines CXCL10 and CCL5 (**Figure S2**), and type I and III interferon responses (**Figures S3, S4**).

Rhinovirus Infection Increases Necrosis but Not Apoptosis in CF AEC

To determine the cellular response to rhinovirus infection, we measured viable, necrotic, and apoptotic events in non-CF ($n = 6$) and CF ($n = 6$) AEC (**Figure 1**). Infection with RV1b resulted in reduced viable events in non-CF AEC (57.6 ± 9.8% vs. 35.4 ± 9.8%; $p < 0.05$) and CF AEC (65.1 ± 17.5% vs. 49.8 ± 19.4%; $p < 0.05$) (**Figure 1A**), and significantly elevated necrotic events in non-CF AEC (8.7 ± 2.3% vs. 12.6 ± 4.9%; $p < 0.05$) and CF AEC (8.5 ± 1.8% vs. 11.8 ± 3.5%; $p < 0.05$) (**Figure 1B**). RV1b infection significantly increased apoptotic events in non-CF AEC (28.8 ± 8.5% vs. 36.9 ± 6.1%; $p < 0.05$), however, this was not observed for CF AEC (23.5 ± 16.6% vs. 26.2 ± 11.9%) (**Figure 1C**). Similarly, infection with RV1b for 48 h decreased viable events, increased necrotic events, and increased apoptotic events in both non-CF and CF AEC (**Figure S5**).

IL-1α and IL-1β Are Increased in Supernatant and Correlate With Cell Death Following Rhinovirus Infection

We next investigated the role of IL-1 signaling in the inflammatory response following rhinovirus-induced cell death *in vitro* by measuring IL-1α and IL-1β protein following RV1b infection and correlated these with viable, necrotic, and apoptotic events in non-CF and CF AEC (**Figure 2**). Infection with RV1b increased IL-1α in non-CF (61.6 ± 31.7 pg/mL vs. 511 ± 252 pg/mL; $p < 0.05$) and CF AEC supernatant compared to controls (46.2 ± 32.7 pg/mL vs. 236 ± 93.1 pg/mL; $p < 0.05$) (**Figure 2A**). IL-1α was higher in supernatant from non-CF AEC when compared to CF AEC ($p < 0.05$). Similarly, IL-1β protein was significantly elevated post infection in both

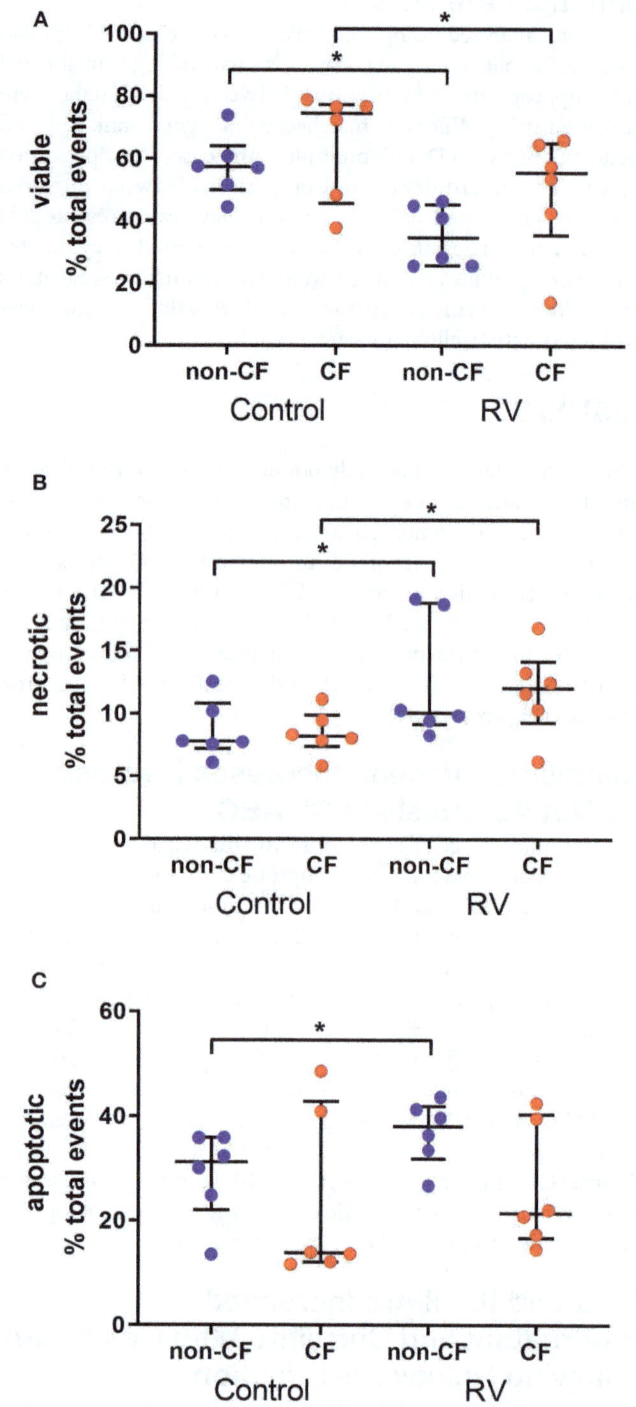

FIGURE 1 | Rhinovirus infection of non-CF and CF AEC decreases viable events, increases necrotic events, and increases apoptotic events in non-CF AEC only. Non-CF ($n = 6$) and CF ($n = 6$) AEC infected with RV1b for 24 h were assessed for changes in viable **(A)**, necrotic **(B)**, and apoptotic **(C)** events measured via flow cytometry. Infection with RV1b for 24 h resulted in **(A)** decreased viable events in non-CF and CF AEC compared to controls, **(B)** increased necrotic events in non-CF and CF AEC compared to controls, and **(C)** increased apoptotic events in non-CF AEC compared to controls. $^*p < 0.05$.

non-CF (4.4 ± 2.3 pg/mL vs. 20.9 ± 9.9 pg/mL; $p < 0.05$) and CF AEC (3.9 ± 3.6 pg/mL vs. 24.2 ± 18.7 pg/mL; $p < 0.05$) (**Figure 2B**) supernatant when compared to controls. Upon analysis, IL-1α was found to be negatively correlated with viable events measured in non-CF AEC only ($r = -0.63$, $p < 0.0001$), positively correlated with necrotic events measured in CF AEC ($r = 0.80$, $p < 0.0001$), as well as apoptotic events measured in non-CF ($r = 0.47$, $p = 0.0011$) (**Figures 3A–C**). Similarly, IL-1β was negatively correlated with viable events measured in non-CF ($r = -0.47$, $p = 0.0029$), strongly positively correlated with necrotic events measured in CF AEC ($r = 0.77$, $p < 0.0001$). A weak correlation was also observed between IL-1β and apoptotic events measured in non-CF AEC only ($r = 0.37$, $p < 0.05$) (**Figures 3D–F**). Infection with RV1b for 48 h produced similar responses, with increased IL-1α and IL-1β following infection (**Figure S6**) significantly associated with necrotic events only in CF AEC, but with apoptotic events in non-CF and CF AEC (**Figure S7**).

IL-1Ra Is Increased in Supernatant Following Rhinovirus Infection

Since we observed differential responses in IL-1 signaling, we next assessed IL-1R regulatory protein expression, namely IL-1Ra and sIL-1R2, by non-CF and CF AEC following infection with RV1b (**Figure 4**). Rhinovirus infection resulted in increased IL-1Ra production from non-CF (1368.2 ± 205.6 pg/mL vs. 8149.0 ± 3013.1 pg/mL; $p < 0.05$) and CF AEC (1930.4 ± 870.4 pg/mL vs. 5334.1 ± 1425.4 pg/mL; $p < 0.05$) compared to control, with significantly higher IL-1Ra observed in non-CF AEC after infection compared to CF AEC ($p < 0.05$) (**Figure 4A**). There was no difference in sIL-1R2 protein production between non-CF or CF AEC, however, sIL-1R2 was significantly induced after infection in CF AEC when compared to non-CF AEC (16.5 ± 2.1 pg/mL vs. 49.8 ± 38.1 pg/mL; $p < 0.05$) (**Figure 4B**). Similarly, infection with RV1b for 48 h increased IL-1Ra but not sIL-1R2 production in both non-CF and CF AEC (**Figure S8**).

IL-8 Is Increased in Supernatant and Associated With IL-1α and Necrotic Events Following Rhinovirus Infection

We next measured inflammation downstream of IL-1R activation by measuring levels of the main neutrophil chemoattractant, IL-8, by non-CF and CF AEC following RV1b infection. Viral infection resulted in a significant increase in IL-8 protein by both non-CF (4890.5 ± 2426.7 pg/mL vs. 15656.4 ± 4102.1 pg/mL; $p < 0.05$) and CF AEC (3915.3 ± 1262.1 pg/mL vs. 8762.8 ± 3919.0 pg/mL; $p < 0.01$) compared to relevant controls (**Figure 4C**), with significantly higher IL-8 produced by non-CF AEC compared to CF AEC ($p < 0.05$). After infection for 48 h, IL-8 was significantly increased in non-CF and CF AEC (**Figure S9A**). When analyzed for associations with IL-1 signaling and cell death, IL-8 was positively correlated with necrotic events in non-CF and CF AEC ($r = 0.35$, $p < 0.05$ and $r = 0.60$, $p = 0.0001$ respectively) (**Figure 4D**), and IL-1α in non-CF and CF AEC ($r = 0.63$ & $r = 0.74$ respectively; $p < 0.0001$) (**Figure 4E**).

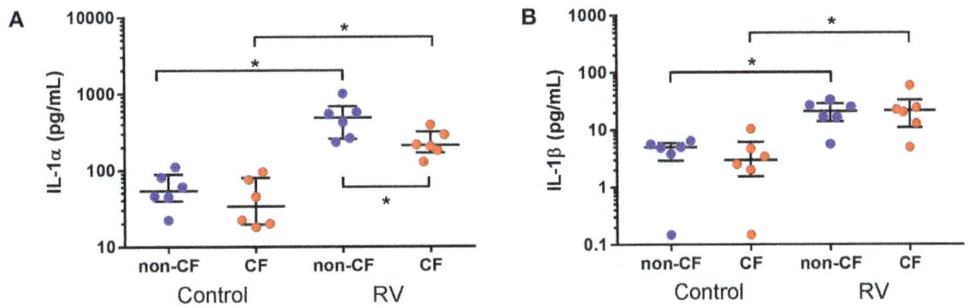

FIGURE 2 | IL-1α and IL-1β is increased in supernatant from non-CF and CF AEC following rhinovirus infection. Supernatant from non-CF ($n = 6$) and CF ($n = 6$) AEC infected with RV1b at for 24 h was assessed for levels of IL-1α and IL-1β protein. Infection with RV1b for 24 h resulted in **(A)** increased IL-1α from non-CF and CF AEC compared to control, with higher levels in non-CF supernatant compared to CF supernatant post-infection, and **(B)** increased IL-1β from non-CF and CF AEC compared to controls. *$p < 0.05$.

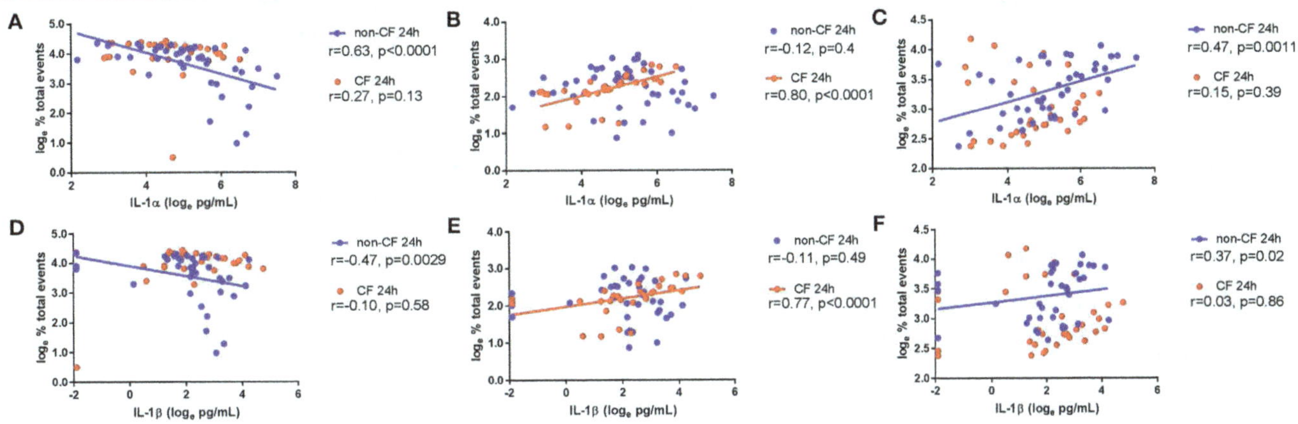

FIGURE 3 | IL-1α and IL-1β in supernatant are associated with necrotic events in CF AEC but not non-CF AEC following 24 h of rhinovirus infection. IL-1α and IL-1β protein in supernatant from non-CF ($n = 44$) and CF ($n = 32$) AEC following RV1b infection for 24 h were assessed for correlations with the corresponding changes in viable, necrotic and apoptotic events measured via flow cytometry. IL-1α protein in supernatant was **(A)** significantly correlated with decreased viable events in non-CF AEC but not CF AEC, **(B)** significantly correlated with increased necrotic events in CF AEC but not non-CF AEC, and **(C)** significantly correlated with increased apoptotic events in non-CF AEC but not CF AEC. Similarly, IL-1β protein in supernatant was **(D)** significantly correlated with decreased viable events in non-CF AEC but not CF AEC, **(E)** significantly correlated with increased necrotic events in CF AEC but not non-CF AEC, and **(F)** significantly correlated with increased apoptotic events in non-CF AEC but not CF AEC.

Similar responses were observed following 48 h of infection, with significant associations between IL-8 and IL-1α and necrotic events in non-CF and CF AEC (**Figures S9B,C**).

DISCUSSION

Our previous work demonstrated a defective response of CF AEC to RV infection (8), and an inflammatory response to epithelial necrosis in CF driven by IL-1R signaling (9) that is already detectable in the airways of infants and children with CF in the absence of bacterial infection (12). In the current study, we add to these earlier findings by conducting a series of *in vitro* experiments on AEC from children with and without CF focusing on the response of the epithelium to RV infection. Utilizing flow cytometry we observed increased necrosis in CF AEC associated with IL-1R signaling, but increased apoptosis in non-CF AEC associated with IL-1R signaling. When we assessed the IL-1 receptor antagonist IL-1Ra, we found that RV induced IL-Ra production in both phenotypes however this was significantly higher in non-CF AEC. This corresponded with increased IL-8 following RV infection that was significantly higher in non-CF AEC. Furthermore, production of IL-8 was associated with IL-1α and epithelial necrosis in non-CF and CF AEC.

This study provides several novel insights into the mechanisms surrounding pro-inflammatory responses and cell death following RV infection in the CF airway. Our data shows RV infection directly increases necrotic events in both non-CF and CF AEC supporting previous data where rhinovirus protease 3C increased necrosis in nasal AEC (7). The lack of apoptosis in CF AEC supports previous work in our laboratory where dampened apoptosis was observed following RV infection (8). This study supports data suggesting RV infection drives lytic cell death (7), potentially responsible for the increased viral load observed in CF (8, 22).

Delayed apoptosis was also observed in CF AEC following RV infection in this study. Defective apoptotic responses have

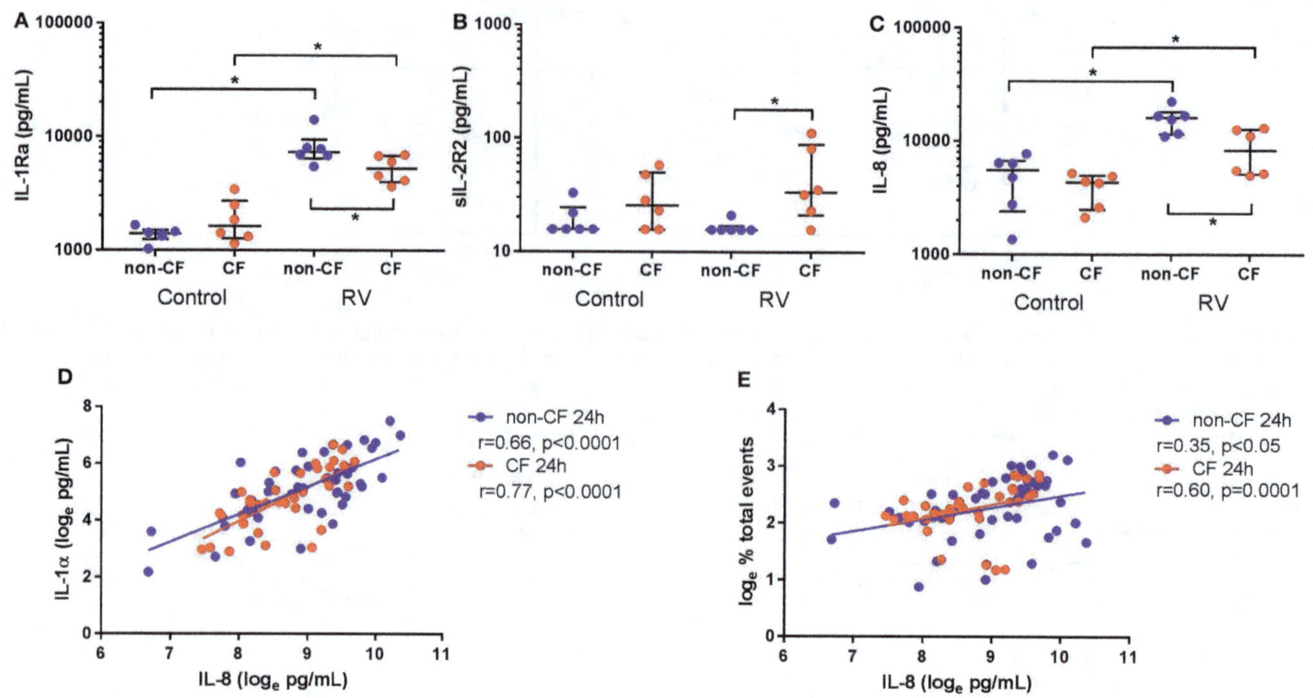

FIGURE 4 | Rhinovirus infection increases IL-1Ra and IL-8 signaling in supernatant from non-CF and CF AEC. Supernatant from non-CF ($n = 6$) and CF ($n = 6$) AEC infected with RV1b for 24 h was assessed for levels of IL-1Ra, sIL-1R2, IL-8 protein, and correlations between IL-8 and IL-1α protein or necrotic events measured via flow cytometry. Infection with RV1b for 24 h resulted in **(A)** increased IL-1Ra from non-CF and CF AEC compared to control, with significantly higher IL-1Ra in supernatant from non-CF AEC compared to CF AEC, **(B)** no change in sIL-1R2 from non-CF and CF AEC compared to control, but significantly higher sIL-1R2 after infection in supernatant from CF AEC compared to non-CF AEC, and **(C)** increased IL-8 in supernatant from non-CF and CF AEC compared to control, with significantly higher IL-8 in supernatant from non-CF AEC compared to CF AEC which **(D)** significantly correlated with IL-1α levels in supernatant from non-CF and CF AEC and **(E)** significantly correlated with increased necrotic events in both non-CF and CF AEC. $^*p < 0.05$.

been observed in AEC and neutrophils in CF (8, 23, 24), we hypothesize reported accumulation of apoptotic cells in the CF airway may be suggestive evidence of defective efferocytosis (25, 26). Cleavage of the phosphatidylserine receptor by neutrophil elastase specifically disrupts phagocytosis of apoptotic cells (26, 27) and as free neutrophil elastase is increased in the CF airway (28, 29), it may explain the reduced apoptotic response and defective efferocytosis observed in the CF airway. Additionally, as suggested by the data in this study, a delayed apoptotic response following RV infection of AEC may also contribute to the defective apoptosis and increased viral load observed in CF (8, 22). The study by Vandivier et al. also found evidence of secondary necrosis following delayed apoptosis, potentially further exacerbating inflammation in the airway via release of DAMPs such as IL-1 signaling (26). As phagocytosis of apoptotic cells can induce anti-inflammatory cytokine production (30, 31), impaired clearance of apoptotic cells may have an additive effect on airway inflammation via reduced anti-inflammatory capacity.

Neutrophilic inflammation is a key risk factor for airway disease resulting in bronchiectasis and loss of lung function (3) which is observed in the absence of detectable bacterial infection (1, 2, 10). It is therefore important to elucidate triggers of early inflammation prior to bacterial colonization of the CF airway. As IL-1R signaling has been investigated as a key pathway driving neutrophilic and eosinophilic inflammation in the airway (9, 12, 32, 33), we next investigated IL-1α and IL-1β signaling following RV infection of AEC. As IL-1α is constitutively active, it can be released directly from necrotic cells in the airway epithelium (9) or actively secreted following activation of the NLRP3 inflammasome and caspase-1 (34, 35) which is required for IL-1β cleavage and release. Activation of the NLRP3 inflammasome has been reported following RV infection resulting from calcium flux resulting from RV ion channel protein 2B activity (36), potassium efflux from lytic cell death such as necrosis or pyroptosis (37), and dysregulated sodium transport due to ENaC upregulation (38). It has also been observed in other inflammatory respiratory diseases with RV associated exacerbations as a hallmark of disease like asthma or COPD, where viral-induced cell death likely contributes to morbidity (36, 39, 40). In this study, we found increased IL-1α and IL-1β alongside increased necrotic cell death suggesting NLRP3 activation could potentially exacerbate the inflammatory cascade following RV infection. This finding supports previously reported data that both IL-1α and IL-1β are released from AEC following RV infection and implicated active secretion via NLRP3 activation (41, 42). Additionally, IL-1α and IL-1β in supernatants of airway mucopurulent secretions have been shown to regulate both MUC5B and MUC5AC through IL-1R (43–45). Release of

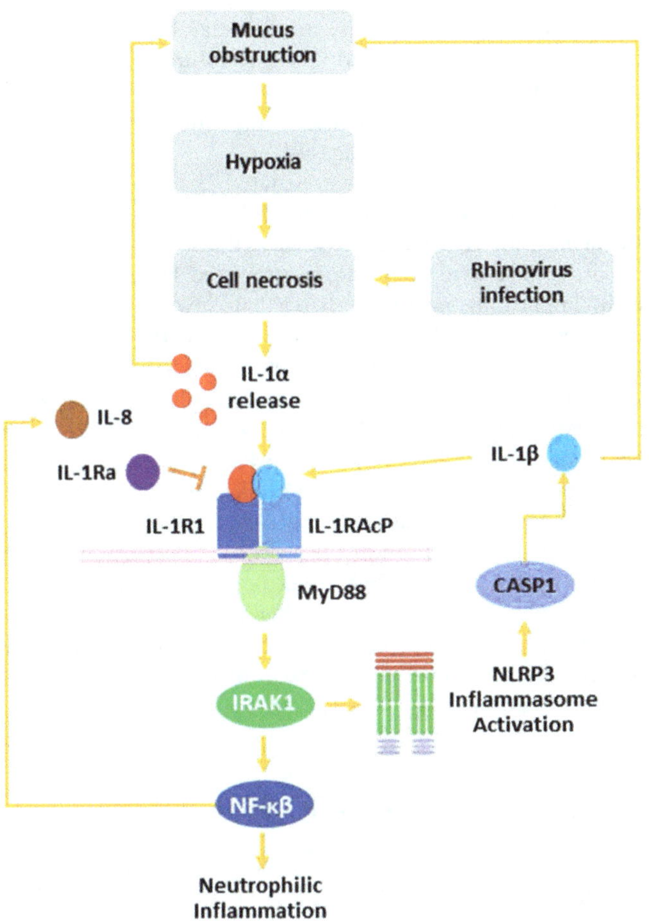

FIGURE 5 | The role of rhinovirus infection in the IL-1 inflammatory response in the CF airway. Mucus obstruction in the CF airway leads to hypoxia of the airway epithelium and epithelial necrosis. Additionally, rhinovirus infection induced necrosis of AEC resulting in release of IL-1α from necrotic cells. Binding of IL-1α to IL-1R recruits MyD88 to the IL-1R:IL-1RAcP complex. Activation of MyD88 leads to IRAK1 activation, which activates the NLRP3 inflammasome leading to CASP1 activation and IL-1β secretion. Additionally, IRAK1 activates NF-κβ, which induces IL-8 release leading to neutrophilic airway inflammation. Both IL-1α and IL-1β induce mucin secretion, which leads to further mucus obstruction creating a positive feedback loop capable of exacerbating CF airway disease. IL-1R activation can be blocked by IL-1Ra to inhibit signaling downstream of IL-1R. IL-1α, interleukin-1 alpha; IL-1β, interleukin-1 beta; IL-1R1, interleukin-1 receptor 1; IL-1Ra, interleukin-1 receptor antagonist IL-1RAcP, interleukin-1 receptor accessory protein; IL-8, interleukin-8; IRAK, interleukin-1 receptor-activated protein kinase; MyD88, myeloid differentiation primary response gene 88; NFκB, nuclear factor kappa beta; NLRP3, nod-like receptor protein 3.

IL-1α is primarily through AEC while IL-1β in the CF lung is mainly released from macrophages and interstitial mononuclear cells (46, 47), potentially explaining the differences between IL-1α and IL-1β levels observed in this study when compared to levels reported in other studies in *ex-vivo* samples (43). This data suggests IL-1α and IL-1β observed following RV-A infection may exacerbate mucus hyperconcentration and obstruction evident in the CF airway (4, 43).

Furthermore, we found IL-1α and IL-1β significantly correlated with necrotic events in CF AEC only, while IL-1α and IL-1β correlated with apoptotic events in non-CF AEC only. Studies utilizing the β-ENaC murine model of CF-like lung disease have observed the presence of mucus obstruction and airway neutrophilia in germ-free conditions (48, 49), with "sterile" inflammation in the CF airway triggered by IL-1α released from necrotic AEC (9, 50). IL-1α is measurable in the airways of young children with CF with mild lung disease and associated with structural lung disease measured via CT in the absence of detectable bacterial infection, suggesting a role for IL-1α in the inflammatory cascade in the CF airway environment in the absence of detectable bacterial infection (12). The current study observed levels of IL-1α higher than measured in BALf in young children with CF, suggesting clinically relevant amounts of IL-1α are released from AEC following RV infection. There was higher IL-1α detected in non-CF AEC compared to CF AEC in response to RV infection suggesting IL-1α release from CF AEC occurs predominantly via necrotic cell death post-infection, and release from non-CF AEC via apoptotic cell death. Additionally, IL-1α is associated with viability of non-CF AEC, suggesting overall cell death had a greater effect on IL-1α release in non-CF AEC. Apoptotic cell death is considered immunologically silent due to efficient phagocytosis (51), however, in an *in vitro* monoculture there is a lack of clearance which results in secondary necrosis and cellular breakdown (52). While epithelial cells can self-phagocytize to reduce inflammatory consequences (53, 54), clearance of apoptotic cells relies on professional phagocytes like macrophages (55) and failure leads to release of immunostimulatory danger associated molecular patterns such as IL-1α (56). Secondary necrosis of AEC *in vitro* may potentially explain the differences in IL-1α detected between phenotypes, likely due to the observed and reported lack of apoptosis in CF AEC following RV infection (8). Defective apoptosis due to cleavage of apoptotic signaling receptors by neutrophil elastase and manipulation of phagocytic ability by *Pseudomonas aeruginosa* in monocytes has been reported in CF (26, 57). As IL-1α is increased in the CF airway during bacterial infection (12), we hypothesize defective apoptotic signaling and efferocytosis may play a role in IL-1R-activated neutrophilic inflammation in the CF airway before and after bacterial colonization of the CF airway.

Several recent studies have shown the potential for anti-inflammatory therapy by blocking of IL-1R via genetic deletion of the receptor or pharmacological inhibition via IL-1Ra to inhibit IL-8 expression and neutrophilic inflammation (9, 43). Deletion of IL-1R and IL-1Ra treatment in the βENaC-transgenic mouse significantly reduced IL-1β, neutrophils present in the airway and levels of keratinocyte chemoattractant—a murine IL-8 ortholog (9). This finding was also observed in primary AEC grown at air-liquid interface after stimulation with supernatants of airway mucopurulent secretions, with IL-1Ra treatment reducing IL-8 mRNA (43). The present study found increased IL-1Ra following RV infection in both non-CF and CF AEC, although IL-1Ra was higher in non-CF AEC when compared to CF AEC. This did not correspond with a reduction in IL-8 signaling likely as a result of the amount measured being dramatically lower than the therapeutic concentrations used in other studies (9, 43). RV infection increased IL-8 in both non-CF and CF AEC, however it was significantly higher in non-CF AEC post-infection. This contrasts with previous data by Sutanto et al. which demonstrated significantly higher IL-8 from CF AEC post-RV infection (8). However, differences in the viral titer used for infection and shorter timepoint may have contributed toward the differences in the observed findings.

There are number of unique strengths to the current study. Firstly, primary AEC from pediatric patients were used for experiments in this study, as most immortalized cell lines that are commonly used in CF research are derived from adult donors and may not accurately recapitulate phenotypic differences observed following RV infection in primary AEC isolated from the pediatric airway (8). Secondly, primary cell cultures were passaged before use in this study to distance *in vitro* cultures from the inflammatory environment from which they were isolated to minimize any pro-inflammatory influences from the *in vivo* airway milieu (58). While using freshly isolated AEC for *in vitro* studies may more accurately recapitulate the environment in the CF airway, it could obfuscate mild and virus-specific inflammatory responses. Finally, the use of a more robust flow cytometry methodology that captures events related to apoptotic cell disassembly to analyze cell death allows us to have greater confidence in data generated (20), as conventional methodologies utilizing propidium iodide staining are suggested to have a false positive rate of up to 40% (59).

For this study, we used a submerged monolayer culture model that doesn't fully represent the physiological features of a differentiated respiratory epithelium (60). However, as the basal cells are epithelial progenitors, they are likely to represent intrinsic properties of the respiratory epithelium. Additionally, since viral replication and pro-inflammatory responses are elevated in air-liquid interface compared to monolayer culture (61) subtle phenotypic and mechanistic differences might be more easily identified in an air-liquid interface system. Rhinovirus species affect viral replication and inflammatory responses differently (17, 62), thus the implications of the findings from this study are limited to RV-A infections. However, RV-A has been reported as the most common strain present in adults with CF and associated with more severe clinical outcomes (63). We used a laboratory strain of RV-A (RV1b) that has been reported to induce cytotoxicity more readily than community-derived strains (8, 64, 65) and therefore future work will focus on corroborating the findings of this study using community RV strains of various serotype in order to determine if all RV induce inflammation via IL-1 signaling (66).

In summary, we have demonstrated that RV-A infection of non-CF and CF AEC drives necrotic cell death specifically associated with IL-1α and IL-1β in CF AEC. Viral infection also drove increased IL-8 release associated with necrotic cell death, implicating necrotic cell death following RV infection as a trigger of IL-1R-mediated neutrophilic inflammation in the CF airway. Collectively, these results suggest a role for RV infection as a trigger of IL-1R-driven neutrophilic inflammation in the early life CF airway (**Figure 5**). Mucin accumulation and hyperconcentration has been identified as the earliest trigger of cystic fibrosis lung disease (4), and linked to IL-1 signaling *in vitro* (43) creating a positive feedback cycle capable of inducing neutrophilic inflammation in the absence of bacterial infection. Previous studies have highlighted the potential translation of IL-1Ra as a novel anti-inflammatory therapy in CF (9, 12, 67, 68), with the aim to prevent further mucus obstruction and viral-induced, muco-inflammatory triggers of early lung disease in young CF children.

AUTHOR CONTRIBUTIONS

SM, MM, SS, and AK contributed conception and design of the study. SM and DF acquired the data and performed the statistical analysis. SM, DF, MM, SS, and AK contributed to data analysis and interpretation. SM wrote the first draft of the manuscript. All authors contributed to manuscript revision, read, and approved the submitted version.

ACKNOWLEDGMENTS

The authors thank the subjects and families for their generous contributions to the AREST CF program.

REFERENCES

1. Sly PD, Brennan S, Gangell C, de Klerk N, Murray C, Mott L, et al. Lung disease at diagnosis in infants with cystic fibrosis detected by newborn screening. *Am J Respir Crit Care Med.* (2009) 180:146–52. doi: 10.1164/rccm.200901-0069OC
2. Stick SM, Brennan S, Murray C, Douglas T, von Ungern-Sternberg BS, Garratt LW, et al. Bronchiectasis in infants and preschool children diagnosed with cystic fibrosis after newborn screening. *J Pediatr.* (2009) 155:623–8 e1. doi: 10.1016/j.jpeds.2009.05.005
3. Sly PD, Gangell CL, Chen L, Ware RS, Ranganathan S, Mott LS, et al. Risk factors for bronchiectasis in children with cystic fibrosis. *N Engl J Med.* (2013) 368:1963–70. doi: 10.1056/NEJMoa1301725
4. Esther CR, Muhlebach MS, Ehre C, Hill DB, Wolfgang MC, Kesimer M, et al. Mucus accumulation in the lungs precedes structural changes and infection in children with cystic fibrosis. *Sci Transl Med.* (2019) 11:eaav3488. doi: 10.1126/scitranslmed.aav3488
5. Meyer KC, Sharma A. Regional variability of lung inflammation in cystic fibrosis. *Am J Respir Crit Care Med.* (1997) 156:1536–40. doi: 10.1164/ajrccm.156.5.9701098
6. Willner D, Haynes MR, Furlan M, Hanson N, Kirby B, Lim YW, et al. Case studies of the spatial heterogeneity of DNA viruses in the cystic fibrosis lung. *Am J Respir Cell Mol Biol.* (2012) 46:127–31. doi: 10.1165/rcmb.2011-0253OC
7. Lötzerich M, Roulin PS, Boucke K, Witte R, Georgiev O, Greber UF. Rhinovirus 3C protease suppresses apoptosis and triggers caspase-independent cell death. *Cell Death Dis.* (2018) 9:272. doi: 10.1038/s41419-018-0306-6
8. Sutanto EN, Kicic A, Foo CJ, Stevens PT, Mullane D, Knight DA, et al. Innate inflammatory responses of pediatric cystic fibrosis airway epithelial cells: effects of nonviral and viral stimulation. *Am J Respir Cell Mol Biol.* (2011) 44:761–7. doi: 10.1165/rcmb.2010-0368OC
9. Fritzsching B, Zhou-Suckow Z, Trojanek JB, Schubert SC, Schatterny J, Hirtz S, et al. Hypoxic epithelial necrosis triggers neutrophilic inflammation via IL-1 receptor signaling in cystic fibrosis lung disease. *Am J Respir Crit Care Med.* (2015) 191:902–13. doi: 10.1164/rccm.201409-1610OC

10. Balazs A, Mall MA. Mucus obstruction and inflammation in early cystic fibrosis lung disease: emerging role of the IL-1 signaling pathway. *Pediatr Pulmonol.* (2019) 54(Suppl. 3):S5–S12. doi: 10.1002/ppul.24462
11. Deschamp AR, Hatch JE, Slaven JE, Gebregziabher N, Storch G, Hall GL, et al. Early respiratory viral infections in infants with cystic fibrosis. *J Cyst Fibros.* (2019) 18:844–50. doi: 10.1016/j.jcf.2019.02.004
12. Montgomery ST, Dittrich AS, Garratt LW, Turkovic L, Frey DL, Stick SM, et al. Interleukin-1 is associated with inflammation and structural lung disease in young children with cystic fibrosis. *J Cyst Fibros.* (2018) 17:715–22. doi: 10.1016/j.jcf.2018.05.006
13. Lane C, Burgess S, Kicic A, Knight D, Stick S. The use of non-bronchoscopic brushings to study the paediatric airway. *Respir Res.* (2005) 6:53–. doi: 10.1186/1465-9921-6-53
14. Martinovich KM, Iosifidis T, Buckley AG, Looi K, Ling K-M, Sutanto EN, et al. Conditionally reprogrammed primary airway epithelial cells maintain morphology, lineage and disease specific functional characteristics. *Sci Rep.* (2017) 7:17971. doi: 10.1038/s41598-017-17952-4
15. Lee W-M, Chen Y, Wang W, Mosser A. Growth of human rhinovirus in H1-HeLa cell suspension culture and purification of virions. In: Jans DA, Ghildyal R, editors. *Rhinoviruses: Methods and Protocols.* New York, NY: Springer New York (2015). p. 49–61. doi: 10.1007/978-1-4939-1571-2_5
16. Kicic A, Stevens PT, Sutanto EN, Kicic-Starcevich E, Ling KM, Looi K, et al. Impaired airway epithelial cell responses from children with asthma to rhinoviral infection. *Clin Exp Allergy.* (2016) 46:1441–55. doi: 10.1111/cea.12767
17. Nakagome K, Bochkov YA, Ashraf S, Brockman-Schneider RA, Evans MD, Pasic TR, et al. Effects of rhinovirus species on viral replication and cytokine production. *J Allergy Clin Immunol.* (2014) 134:332–41. doi: 10.1016/j.jaci.2014.01.029
18. Sykes A, Macintyre J, Edwards MR, del Rosario A, Haas J, Gielen V, et al. Rhinovirus-induced interferon production is not deficient in well controlled asthma. *Thorax.* (2014) 69:240. doi: 10.1136/thoraxjnl-2012-202909
19. Bochkov YA, Palmenberg AC, Lee W-M, Rathe JA, Amineva SP, Sun X, et al. Molecular modeling, organ culture and reverse genetics for a newly identified human rhinovirus C. *Nat Med.* (2011) 17:627–32. doi: 10.1038/nm.2358
20. Jiang L, Tixeira R, Caruso S, Atkin-Smith GK, Baxter AA, Paone S, et al. Monitoring the progression of cell death and the disassembly of dying cells by flow cytometry. *Nat Protoc.* (2016) 11:655. doi: 10.1038/nprot.2016.028
21. Garratt LW, Sutanto EN, Ling KM, Looi K, Iosifidis T, Martinovich KM, et al. Matrix metalloproteinase activation by free neutrophil elastase contributes to bronchiectasis progression in early cystic fibrosis. *Eur Respir J.* (2015) 46:384–94. doi: 10.1183/09031936.00212114
22. Dauletbaev N, Das M, Cammisano M, Chen H, Singh S, Kooi C, et al. Rhinovirus load is high despite preserved interferon-β response in cystic fibrosis bronchial epithelial cells. *PLoS ONE.* (2015) 10:e0143129–e. doi: 10.1371/journal.pone.0143129
23. Gray RD, Hardisty G, Regan KH, Smith M, Robb CT, Duffin R, et al. Delayed neutrophil apoptosis enhances NET formation in cystic fibrosis. *Thorax.* (2018) 73:134–44. doi: 10.1136/thoraxjnl-2017-210134
24. Moriceau S, Lenoir G, Witko-Sarsat V. In cystic fibrosis homozygotes and heterozygotes, neutrophil apoptosis is delayed and modulated by diamide or roscovitine: evidence for an innate neutrophil disturbance. *J Innate Immun.* (2010) 2:260–6. doi: 10.1159/000295791
25. Maiuri L, Raia V, De Marco G, Coletta S, de Ritis G, Londei M, et al. DNA fragmentation is a feature of cystic fibrosis epithelial cells: a disease with inappropriate apoptosis? *FEBS Lett.* (1997) 408:225–31. doi: 10.1016/S0014-5793(97)00347-5
26. Vandivier RW, Fadok VA, Hoffmann PR, Bratton DL, Penvari C, Brown KK, et al. Elastase-mediated phosphatidylserine receptor cleavage impairs apoptotic cell clearance in cystic fibrosis and bronchiectasis. *J Clin Invest.* (2002) 109:661–70. doi: 10.1172/JCI0213572
27. Fadok VA, de Cathelineau A, Daleke DL, Henson PM, Bratton DL. Loss of phospholipid asymmetry and surface exposure of phosphatidylserine is required for phagocytosis of apoptotic cells by macrophages and fibroblasts. *J Biol Chem.* (2001) 276:1071–7. doi: 10.1074/jbc.M003649200
28. Dittrich AS, Kühbandner I, Gehrig S, Rickert-Zacharias V, Twigg M, Wege S, et al. Elastase activity on sputum neutrophils correlates with severity of lung disease in cystic fibrosis. *Eur Respir J.* (2018) 51:1701910. doi: 10.1183/13993003.01910-2017
29. Birrer P, McElvaney NG, Rüdeberg A, Sommer CW, Liechti-Gallati S, Kraemer R, et al. Protease-antiprotease imbalance in the lungs of children with cystic fibrosis. *J Cystic Fibr.* (1994) 150:207–13. doi: 10.1164/ajrccm.150.1.7912987
30. Fadok VA, Bratton DL, Konowal A, Freed PW, Westcott JY, Henson PM. Macrophages that have ingested apoptotic cells *in vitro* inhibit proinflammatory cytokine production through autocrine/paracrine mechanisms involving TGF-beta, PGE2, and PAF. *J Clin Invest.* (1998) 101:890–8. doi: 10.1172/JCI1112
31. McDonald PP, Fadok VA, Bratton D, Henson PM. Transcriptional and translational regulation of inflammatory mediator production by endogenous TGF-beta in macrophages that have ingested apoptotic cells. *J Immunol.* (1999) 163:6164–72.
32. Chen CJ, Kono H, Golenbock D, Reed G, Akira S, Rock KL. Identification of a key pathway required for the sterile inflammatory response triggered by dying cells. *Nat Med.* (2007) 13:851–6. doi: 10.1038/nm1603
33. Brown R, Paulsen M, Schmidt S, Schatterny J, Frank A, Hirtz S, et al. Lack of IL-1 receptor signaling reduces spontaneous airway eosinophilia in juvenile mice with muco-obstructive lung disease. *Am J Respir Cell Mol Biol.* (2019) 62:300–9. doi: 10.1165/rcmb.2018-0359OC
34. Fettelschoss A, Kistowska M, LeibundGut-Landmann S, Beer HD, Johansen P, Senti G, et al. Inflammasome activation and IL-1beta target IL-1alpha for secretion as opposed to surface expression. *Proc Natl Acad Sci USA.* (2011) 108:18055–60. doi: 10.1073/pnas.1109176108
35. Iyer SS, Pulskens WP, Sadler JJ, Butter LM, Teske GJ, Ulland TK, et al. Necrotic cells trigger a sterile inflammatory response through the Nlrp3 inflammasome. *Proc Natl Acad Sci USA.* (2009) 106:20388–93. doi: 10.1073/pnas.0908698106
36. Triantafilou K, Kar S, van Kuppeveld FJ, Triantafilou M. Rhinovirus-induced calcium flux triggers NLRP3 and NLRC5 activation in bronchial cells. *Am J Respir Cell Mol Biol.* (2013) 49:923–34. doi: 10.1165/rcmb.2013-0032OC
37. da Costa LS, Outlioua A, Anginot A, Akarid K, Arnoult D. RNA viruses promote activation of the NLRP3 inflammasome through cytopathogenic effect-induced potassium efflux. *Cell Death Dis.* (2019) 10:346. doi: 10.1038/s41419-019-1579-0
38. Scambler T, Jarosz-Griffiths HH, Lara-Reyna S, Pathak S, Wong C, Holbrook J, et al. ENaC-mediated sodium influx exacerbates NLRP3-dependent inflammation in cystic fibrosis. *eLife.* (2019) 8:e49248. doi: 10.7554/eLife.49248
39. Han M, Bentley JK, Rajput C, Lei J, Ishikawa T, Jarman CR, et al. Inflammasome activation is required for human rhinovirus-induced airway inflammation in naive and allergen-sensitized mice. *Mucosal Immunol.* (2019) 12:958–68. doi: 10.1038/s41385-019-0172-2
40. Radzikowska U, Eljaszewicz A, Wawrzyniak P, Dreher A, Globinska A, Smolinska S, et al. Rhinovirus triggers increased inflammasome activation in human bronchial epithelium in asthma. *Eur Respir J.* (2017) 50(suppl 61):PA996. doi: 10.1183/1393003.congress-2017.PA996
41. Piper SC, Ferguson J, Kay L, Parker LC, Sabroe I, Sleeman MA, et al. The role of interleukin-1 and interleukin-18 in pro-inflammatory and anti-viral responses to rhinovirus in primary bronchial epithelial cells. *PLoS ONE.* (2013) 8:e63365. doi: 10.1371/journal.pone.0063365
42. Shi L, Manthei DM, Guadarrama AG, Lenertz LY, Denlinger LC. Rhinovirus-induced IL-1β release from bronchial epithelial cells is independent of functional P2X7. *Am J Respir Cell Mol Biol.* (2012) 47:363–71. doi: 10.1165/rcmb.2011-0267OC
43. Chen G, Sun L, Kato T, Okuda K, Martino MB, Abzhanova A, et al. IL-1β dominates the promucin secretory cytokine profile in cystic fibrosis. *J Clin Invest.* (2019) 129:10. doi: 10.1172/JCI125669
44. Abdullah LH, Coakley R, Webster MJ, Zhu Y, Tarran R, Radicioni G, et al. Mucin production and hydration responses to mucopurulent materials in normal versus cystic fibrosis airway epithelia. *Am J Respir Crit Care Med.* (2018) 197:481–91. doi: 10.1164/rccm.201706-1139OC
45. Gray T, Coakley R, Hirsh A, Thornton D, Kirkham S, Koo JS, et al. Regulation of MUC5AC mucin secretion and airway surface liquid metabolism by IL-1beta in human bronchial epithelia. *Am J Physiol Lung Cell Mol Physiol.* (2004) 286:L320–30. doi: 10.1152/ajplung.00440.2002
46. Tang A, Sharma A, Jen R, Hirschfeld AF, Chilvers MA, Lavoie PM, et al. Inflammasome-mediated IL-1beta production in humans with cystic fibrosis. *PLoS ONE.* (2012) 7:e37689. doi: 10.1371/journal.pone.0037689

47. Folco EJ, Sukhova GK, Quillard T, Libby P. Moderate hypoxia potentiates interleukin-1beta production in activated human macrophages. *Circ Res.* (2014) 115:875–83. doi: 10.1161/CIRCRESAHA.115.304437
48. Livraghi-Butrico A, Kelly EJ, Klem ER, Dang H, Wolfgang MC, Boucher RC, et al. Mucus clearance, MyD88-dependent and MyD88-independent immunity modulate lung susceptibility to spontaneous bacterial infection and inflammation. *Mucosal Immunol.* (2012) 5:397–408. doi: 10.1038/mi.2012.17
49. Mall M, Grubb BR, Harkema JR, O'Neal WK, Boucher RC. Increased airway epithelial Na+ absorption produces cystic fibrosis-like lung disease in mice. *Nat Med.* (2004) 10:487–93. doi: 10.1038/nm1028
50. Montgomery ST, Mall MA, Kicic A, Stick SM. Hypoxia and sterile inflammation in cystic fibrosis airways: mechanisms and potential therapies. *Eur Respir J.* (2017) 49(1). doi: 10.1183/13993003.00903-2016
51. Szondy Z, Sarang Z, Kiss B, Garabuczi É, Köröskényi K. Anti-inflammatory mechanisms triggered by apoptotic cells during their clearance. *Front Immunol.* (2017) 8:909. doi: 10.3389/fimmu.2017.00909
52. Silva MT. Secondary necrosis: the natural outcome of the complete apoptotic program. *FEBS Lett.* (2010) 584:4491–9. doi: 10.1016/j.febslet.2010.10.046
53. Monks J, Rosner D, Geske FJ, Lehman L, Hanson L, Neville MC, et al. Epithelial cells as phagocytes: apoptotic epithelial cells are engulfed by mammary alveolar epithelial cells and repress inflammatory mediator release. *Cell Death Differ.* (2005) 12:107–14. doi: 10.1038/sj.cdd.4401517
54. Juncadella IJ, Kadl A, Sharma AK, Shim YM, Hochreiter-Hufford A, Borish L, et al. Apoptotic cell clearance by bronchial epithelial cells critically influences airway inflammation. *Nature.* (2013) 493:547–51. doi: 10.1038/nature11714
55. Gordon S, Plüddemann A. Macrophage clearance of apoptotic cells: a critical assessment. *Front Immuno.* (2018) 9:127. doi: 10.3389/fimmu.2018.00127
56. Sachet M, Liang YY, Oehler R. The immune response to secondary necrotic cells. *Apoptosis.* (2017) 22:1189–204. doi: 10.1007/s10495-017-1413-z
57. Bianchi SM, Prince LR, McPhillips K, Allen L, Marriott HM, Taylor GW, et al. Impairment of apoptotic cell engulfment by pyocyanin, a toxic metabolite of Pseudomonas aeruginosa. *Am J Respir Crit Care Med.* (2008) 177:35–43. doi: 10.1164/rccm.200612-1804OC
58. Ribeiro CM, Paradiso AM, Schwab U, Perez-Vilar J, Jones L, O'Neal W, et al. Chronic airway infection/inflammation induces a Ca2+i-dependent hyperinflammatory response in human cystic fibrosis airway epithelia. *J Biol Chem.* (2005) 280:17798–806. doi: 10.1074/jbc.M410618200
59. Rieger AM, Hall BE, Luong LT, Schang LM, Barreda DR. Conventional apoptosis assays using propidium iodide generate a significant number of false positives that prevent accurate assessment of cell death. *J Immunol Methods.* (2010) 358:81–92. doi: 10.1016/j.jim.2010.03.019
60. Schögler A, Blank F, Brügger M, Beyeler S, Tschanz SA, Regamey N, et al. Characterization of pediatric cystic fibrosis airway epithelial cell cultures at the air-liquid interface obtained by non-invasive nasal cytology brush sampling. *Respir Res.* (2017) 18:215. doi: 10.1186/s12931-017-0706-7
61. Ito K, Huang S, Constant S. Comparison of respiratory virus infection between human nasal epithelial cell monolayer and air-liquid interface 3D culture. *Eur Respir J.* (2011) 38(Suppl. 55):p3506.
62. Rajan D, McCracken CE, Kopleman HB, Kyu SY, Lee FE-H, Lu X, et al. Human rhinovirus induced cytokine/chemokine responses in human airway epithelial and immune cells. *PLoS ONE.* (2014) 9:e114322. doi: 10.1371/journal.pone.0114322
63. Flight WG, Bright-Thomas RJ, Tilston P, Mutton KJ, Guiver M, Morris J, et al. Incidence and clinical impact of respiratory viruses in adults with cystic fibrosis. *Thorax.* (2014) 69:247. doi: 10.1136/thoraxjnl-2013-204000
64. Bossios A, Psarras S, Gourgiotis D, Skevaki CL, Constantopoulos AG, Saxoni-Papageorgiou P, et al. Rhinovirus infection induces cytotoxicity and delays wound healing in bronchial epithelial cells. *Respir Res.* (2005) 6:114. doi: 10.1186/1465-9921-6-114
65. Wark PAB, Grissell T, Davies B, See H, Gibson PG. Diversity in the bronchial epithelial cell response to infection with different rhinovirus strains. *Respirology.* (2009) 14:180–6. doi: 10.1111/j.1440-1843.2009.01480.x
66. de Almeida MB, Zerbinati RM, Tateno AF, Oliveira CM, Romão RM, Rodrigues JC, et al. Rhinovirus C and respiratory exacerbations in children with cystic fibrosis. *Emerg Infect Dis.* (2010) 16:996–9. doi: 10.3201/eid1606.100063
67. Iannitti RG, Napolioni V, Oikonomou V, De Luca A, Galosi C, Pariano M, et al. IL-1 receptor antagonist ameliorates inflammasome-dependent inflammation in murine and human cystic fibrosis. *Nat Commun.* (2016) 7:10791. doi: 10.1038/ncomms10791
68. Mall MA, Harkema JR, Trojanek JB, Treis D, Livraghi A, Schubert S, et al. Development of chronic bronchitis and emphysema in beta-epithelial Na+ channel-overexpressing mice. *Am J Respir Crit Care Med.* (2008) 177:730–42. doi: 10.1164/rccm.200708-1233OC

14

Epithelial-Mesenchymal Transition in Asthma Airway Remodeling is Regulated by the IL-33/CD146 Axis

Zhixiao Sun [1†], Ningfei Ji [1†], Qiyun Ma [1], Ranran Zhu [1], Zhongqi Chen [1], Zhengxia Wang [1], Yan Qian [1], Chaojie Wu [1], Fan Hu [2], Mao Huang [1] and Mingshun Zhang [3*]*

[1] Department of Respiratory and Critical Care Medicine, The First Affiliated Hospital of Nanjing Medical University, Nanjing, China, [2] State Key Laboratory of Reproductive Medicine, Nanjing Medical University, Nanjing, China, [3] NHC Key Laboratory of Antibody Technique, Department of Immunology, Nanjing Medical University, Nanjing, China

***Correspondence:**
Mao Huang
hm6114@163.com
Mingshun Zhang
mingshunzhang@njmu.edu.cn

† These authors have contributed equally to this work

Epithelial-mesenchymal transition (EMT) is essential in asthma airway remodeling. IL-33 from epithelial cells is involved in pulmonary fibrosis. CD146 has been extensively explored in cancer-associated EMT. Whether IL-33 regulates CD146 in the EMT process associated with asthma airway remodeling is still largely unknown. We hypothesized that EMT in airway remodeling was regulated by the IL-33/CD146 axis. House dust mite (HDM) extract increased the expression of IL-33 and CD146 in epithelial cells. Increased expression of CD146 in HDM-treated epithelial cells could be blocked with an ST2-neutralizing antibody. Moreover, HDM-induced EMT was dependent on the CD146 and TGF-β/SMAD-3 signaling pathways. IL-33 deficiency decreased CD146 expression and alleviated asthma severity. Similarly, CD146 deficiency mitigated EMT and airway remodeling in a murine model of chronic allergic airway inflammation. Furthermore, CD146 expression was significantly elevated in asthma patients. We concluded that IL-33 from HDM extract-treated alveolar epithelial cells stimulated CD146 expression, promoting EMT in airway remodeling in chronic allergic inflammation.

Keywords: epithelial-mesenchymal transition, IL-33, CD146, asthma, allergy

INTRODUCTION

Asthma is a disease that is characterized by airway inflammation, airway remodeling, and airway hyperresponsiveness (1). Airway remodeling is described as a change in the composition, thickness or volume of airway walls, including subepithelial fibrosis, and increased smooth muscle composition, in asthmatic patients compared to normal individuals (2). Epithelial-mesenchymal transition (EMT) is a pathophysiological process induced by multiple signaling pathways centered on TGF-β and refers to the loss of function of epithelial cells and their transformation to mesenchymal cells, including a decrease in E-cadherin, and an increase in N-cadherin expression (3–5). An increasing number of studies have demonstrated that increased EMT plays an important role in airway remodeling in asthma (5, 6).

CD146 was originally acknowledged as a tumor marker for melanoma (MCAM). As a multifunctional molecule (7), CD146 plays diverse biological roles in tumors, atherosclerosis, systemic sclerosis, and other diseases (8–10). CD146 in macrophages promotes cell adhesion and foam cell formation (8). CD146 in $CD4^+$ T cells is associated with Th17 differentiation in systemic sclerosis (9). CD146 is also associated with pulmonary infections, in which it promotes the adherence of bacteria or viruses to airway epithelial cells (11–14). Increased expression ofCD146 in gastric cancer leads to decreased expression of E-cadherin and increased expression of N-catenin and vimentin (15). CD146 also regulates the EMT process in hepatocellular carcinoma via the MAPK1 signaling pathway, which exacerbates the invasion and metastasis of hepatocellular carcinoma (16). These studies suggest that the EMT process is associated with cancer progression. Increased expression of CD146 in the airway epithelial cells of asthma patients was recently discovered, and IL-13 (a type 2 inflammatory cytokine) regulates the expression and function of CD146 in airway epithelial cells (11, 12). Although the regulation of EMT by CD146 has been extensively reported in studies of tumor metastasis (17), the roles of CD146 in asthma EMT and airway remodeling have not been explored.

Interleukin-33 (IL-33) is a member of the IL-1 cytokine family and is expressed in fibroblasts, endothelial cells, epithelial cells, and other cell types (18, 19). Once bound with the membrane receptor ST2, IL-33 activates the MyD88/NF-κB signaling pathway (20) and induces the type 2 response in $CD4^+$ T cells, which release IL-4, IL-5, and IL-13 (19). Serum IL-33 and the soluble form of ST2 are closely associated with asthma disease progression (21) and exacerbation (22). Moreover, recent studies have shown that IL-33 is involved in asthma airway collagen deposition, suggesting that IL-33 may be involved in the EMT process in the lung (23–25). The regulation of IL-33 signaling related to CD146 expression and the EMT process in asthma, however, remains largely elusive. In the present study, we demonstrated that IL-33 increased the expression of CD146, which promoted the EMT process in asthma.

MATERIALS AND METHODS

Animals and a Murine Model of Asthma

Specific pathogen-free (SPF) female C57BL/J mice aged 6–8 weeks were obtained from the Laboratory Animal Center, Nanjing Medical University (Nanjing, China). CD146 knockout (KO) mice on a C57BL/J background were obtained from Cyagen, Suzhou, China. IL-33 KO mice on a C57BL/J background were obtained from Dr. Hong Zhou (Department of Immunology, Nanjing Medical University). All animal treatments were approved by the Nanjing Medical University Ethics Committee (IACUC 1709011).

To establish a murine model of asthma, the mice were intranasally administered house dust mite (HDM, Greer Laboratories, Lenoir, NC, USA) extract (25 μg of HDM extract dissolved in 40 μL of phosphate-buffered saline) 5 days/week for 5 weeks. All mice were treated with HDM extract under isoflurane anesthesia and were ultimately sacrificed (26).

Cell Culture

The mouse pulmonary epithelial cell lines MLE-12 and A549 were obtained from ATCC (VA, USA) and cultured in DMEM containing 10% fetal bovine serum (FBS), 100 IU/ml penicillin and 100 μg/ml streptomycin in a 5% CO_2 atmosphere at 37°C. MLE-12 or A549 cells were seeded in 6-well plates or 24-well plates overnight and then treated with HDM extract or the cytokine IL-33 for the indicated durations. Primary alveolar epithelial cells from mice were purified using 0.1% collagenase, 0.25% trypsin, and DNase I and were selected with mouse IgG (36111ES60, Yeasen, China) as previously described (27). To exclude the potential effects of lipopolysaccharide (LPS) contamination, HDM extract was treated with the ToxinEraser^{TM} endotoxin removal Kit (L00338, Genscript, China). The purified product was the major constituent of HDM.

TABLE 1 | Antibodies in the study.

Antibody	Brand name	Product code	Source	Dilutability
Anti-CD146 antibody	Abcam	ab75769	Cambridge, UK	1:1000
Anti-IL-33 antibody	Abcam	ab54385	Cambridge, UK	1:1000
Anti-SPD antibody	Abcam	ab220422	Cambridge, UK	1:1000
Anti- E-cadherin antibody	Abcam	ab76055	Cambridge, UK	1:1000
Anti-N-cadherin antibody	Abcam	ab76011	Cambridge, UK	1:5000
Anti-α-SMA antibody	Abcam	ab7817	Cambridge, UK	1:200
AntiTGF-β antibody	Abcam	ab170874	Cambridge, UK	1:1000
Anti- fibronectin antibody	Proteintech	15613-1-AP	Wuhan, Hubei, China	1:1000
Anti-beta-actin antibody	Cell signaling technology	#4970	Beverly, MA	1:1000
Anti-P38 antibody	Cell signaling technology	#8690	Beverly, MA	1:1000
Anti-P38 (phospho-Thr180/Tyr182) antibody	Cell signaling technology	#4511	Beverly, MA	1:1000
Anti-P44/42 antibody	Cell signaling technology	#4695	Beverly, MA	1:1000
Anti- P44/42(phospho-Thr202/Tyr204) antibody	Cell signaling technology	#4370	Beverly, MA	1:1000
Anti-P65 antibody	Cell signaling technology	#8242	Beverly, MA	1:1000
Anti- P65 (phospho-Ser536) antibody	Cell signaling technology	#3033	Beverly, MA	1:1000
Anti-JNK antibody	Cell signaling technology	#9252	Beverly, MA	1:1000
Anti-JNK(phospho-Thr183/Tyr185) antibody	Cell signaling technology	#4668	Beverly, MA	1:1000
Anti-STAT3 antibody	Cell signaling technology	#4904	Beverly, MA	1:1000
Anti-STAT3 (phospho-Tyr705) antibody	Cell signaling technology	#9145	Beverly, MA	1:1000
Anti-SMAD3 antibody	Cell signaling technology	#9523	Beverly, MA	1:1000
Anti-SMAD3 (phospho-Ser423/425) antibody	Cell signaling technology	#9520	Beverly, MA	1:1000

Cell Transfection

MLE-12 cells were seeded and incubated overnight before transfection. The CD146 expression plasmid, an siRNA plasmid, or blank vehicles (Abmgood, China) were mixed with Lipofectamine 2000 (Invitrogen, USA) in DMEM without FBS, penicillin or streptomycin for 25 min and were then transfected into MLE-12 cells at 60–80% density in DMEM for 48 h. The cells were treated with HDM extract or PBS for 24 h before total protein extraction.

Western Blotting

Total protein from the cells or tissues was lysed with RIPA buffer (89900, Thermo, USA) containing protease and phosphatase inhibitors (78443, Thermo, USA) on ice for 20 min. Then, the samples were centrifuged for 10 min, and the supernatants were collected and transferred into new EP tubes. The protein concentrations were measured by a BCA assay (P0012S, Beyotime, China). The proteins were separated by SDS-PAGE and transferred to polyvinylidene difluoride (PVDF) membranes at 300 mA. The PVDF membranes were blocked with 5% skim milk powder for 1 h at room temperature and were then incubated with primary antibodies (**Table 1**) at 4°C overnight. The PVDF membranes were washed with TBST 4 times for 5 min each and were then incubated with goat anti-rabbit HRP IgG (EarthOx Life Sciences) or goat anti-mouse HRP IgG (EarthOx Life Sciences) for 1 h at room temperature. The PVDF membranes were washed with TBST 4 times for 7 min each. The specific antibody-bound proteins were visualized with the Immobilon Western Chemiluminescent HRP Substrate (Millipore, MA, USA) and the G:Box gel doc system (Syngene, UK).

Quantitative Real-Time PCR

Total RNA was extracted from cells using the TaKaRa Universal Total RNA Extraction Kit (Dalian, China) and was then used to synthesize cDNA using PrimeScript RT master mix (TaKaRa). The expression of specific RNAs was quantified by using SYBR Green Universal PCR master mix (TaKaRa) in a StepOnePlus Real-Time PCR System (ABI, USA). The primer sequences used for real-time PCR were synthesized by Genescript. The primer sequences are as follows: CD146 forward, 5′- GGACCTTGAGTTTGAGTGG–3′; CD146 reverse, 5′- CAGTGGTTTGGCTGGAGT–3′; β-actin forward, 5′- GAGAAGCTGTGCTATGTTGCT–3′; and β-actin reverse, 5′- CTCCAGGGAGGAAGAGGATG -3'.

Immunofluorescence

After treatment with HDM extract or PBS for 24 h, the culture medium was removed, and the MLE-12 cells were washed in PBS 3 times. The cells were then fixed in 4% paraformaldehyde at 4°C for 15 min, followed by 3 washes with PBS. Afterwards, the cells were blocked with 5% goat serum for 1 h at room temperature and were incubated with mouse anti-E-cadherin, rabbit anti- N-cadherin or rabbit anti-SPD primary antibody at 4°C overnight. The cells were washed with PBS 3 times and

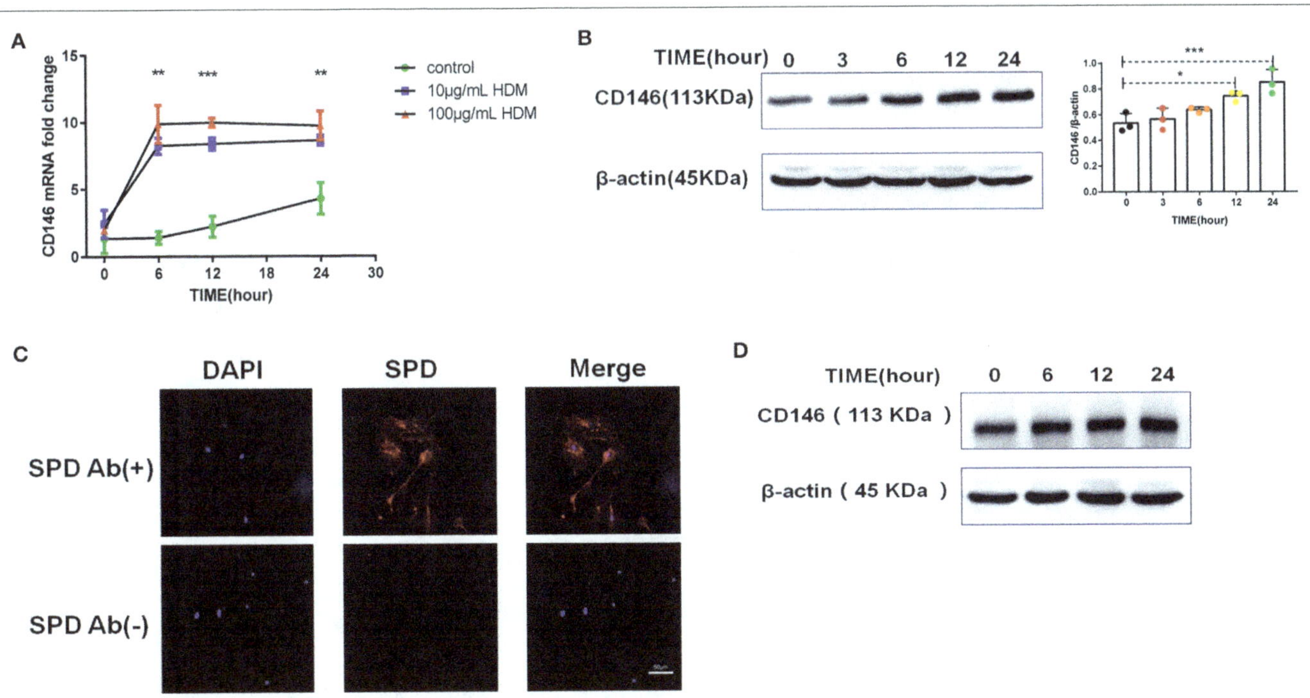

FIGURE 1 | HDM promoted CD146 expression in alveolar epithelial cells. **(A)** CD146 mRNA in HDM-treated MLE-12 cells was measured by qRT-PCR. **(B)** Western blot analysis of CD146 expression in MLE-12 cells treated with HDM extract (100 μg/ml). **(C)** The level of SPD in primary alveolar epithelial cells was measured by immunofluorescence. Ab(+): stained with anti-SPD antibody; Ab(–): stained with isotype antibody **(D)** Western blot analysis of CD146 expression in primary alveolar epithelial cells treated with HDM extract (100 μg/ml). $^{*}P < 0.05$; $^{**}P < 0.01$; $^{***}P < 0.001$.

incubated with Alexa Fluor 555 donkey anti-mouse IgG (H+ L) or Alexa Fluor 647 donkey anti-rabbit IgG (H+L) at 37°C for 1 h in the dark. Next, the cells were washed with PBS and stained with DAPI (4′,6-diamidino-2-phenylindole; Yeasen, China) at 37°C for 10 min in the dark. Images were visualized with a ZEISS LSM710 confocal fluorescence microscope or an Olympus IX73 fluorescence microscope.

Airway Responsiveness

The FinePointe RC System (Buxco Research Systems, Wilmington, NC) was used to measured airway responsiveness. Mice were challenged with aerosolized PBS and methacholine to measure lung resistance. The airway resistance values were recorded for 3 min after each challenge. Then, we calculated the average airway resistance (28).

Differential Counts of Inflammatory Cells in BALF

The bronchoalveolar lavage fluid (BALF) was collected from mice and centrifuged to separate the supernatant and sediment. The sediment was resuspended in PBS and measured with a blood cell analyzer (ADVIA 2120i).

Histological Staining

Lung tissues were fixed in 4% paraformaldehyde and embedded in paraffin. Tissue sections were stained with H&E, PAS, and Sirius red. Images were visualized with a Zeiss Axio Examiner microscope.

Immunohistochemistry

Lung tissues were fixed in 4% paraformaldehyde and embedded in paraffin. Tissue sections were blocked with 5% goat serum for 30 min at 37°C and incubated with mouse anti-E-cadherin at 4°C overnight. Tissue sections were then incubated with horseradish peroxidase-conjugated secondary antibodies for 1 h at room temperature. 3,3-Diaminobenzidine (DAB) was used as a color developer, and hematoxylin was used for counterstaining. Images were visualized with a Zeiss Axio Examiner microscope.

ELISA

Mouse blood was collected and centrifuged to extract the serum. Total IgE was measured with an ELISA kit (432401, Biolegend, USA). The lungs of mice were ground and centrifuged to extract the supernatant. The cytokines IL-4

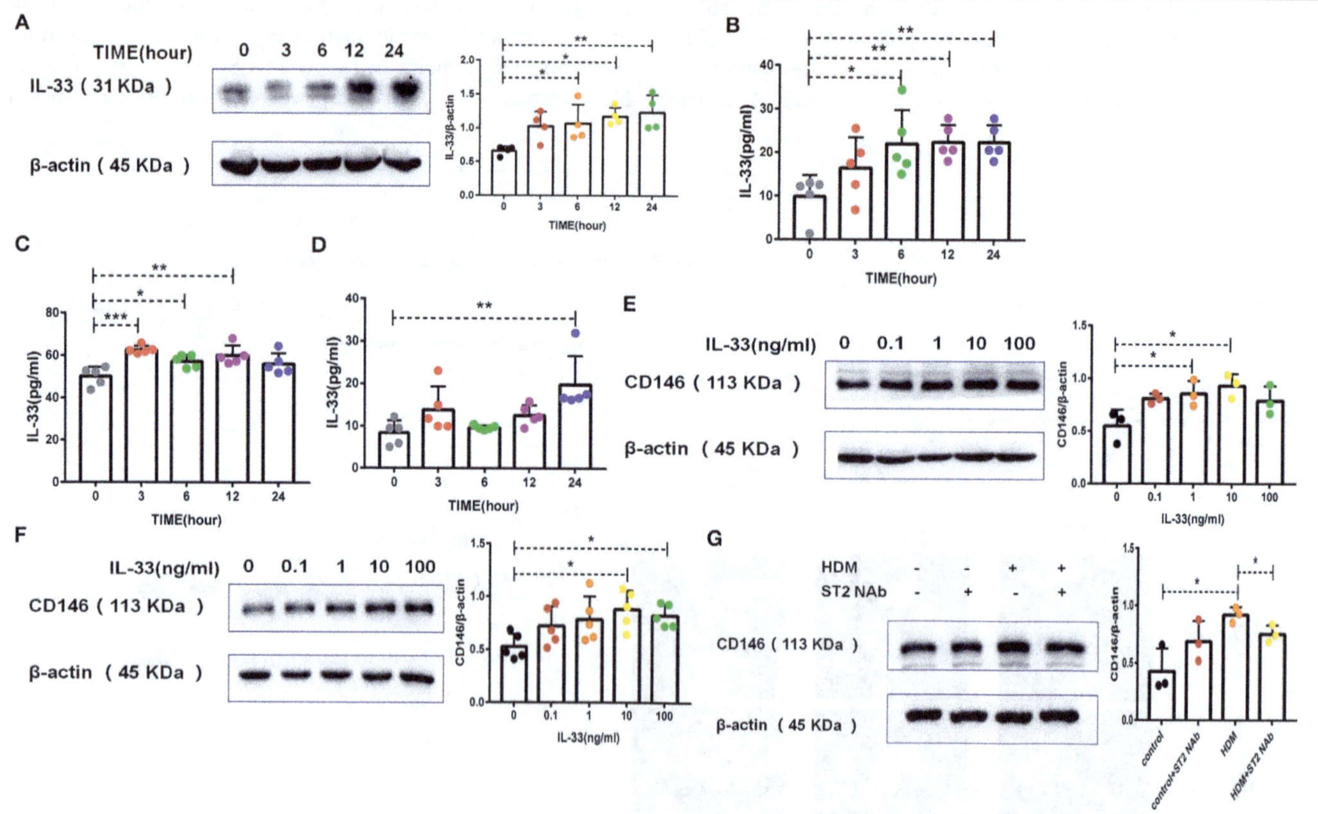

FIGURE 2 | HDM promoted CD146 expression in alveolar epithelial cells via IL-33/ST2 signaling. **(A)** Western blot analysis of IL-33 expression in MLE-12 cells treated with HDM extract (100 μg/ml). **(B)** ELISA analysis of IL-33 levels in the cell culture supernatant of MLE-12 cells treated with HDM extract (100 μg/ml). **(C)** ELISA analysis of IL-33 levels in the cell lysates of MLE-12 cells treated with Derp1 (extracted HDM without LPS). **(D)** ELISA analysis of IL-33 levels in the cell culture supernatant of MLE-12 cells treated with Derp1 (extracted HDM without LPS). **(E)** Western blot analysis of CD146 expression in MLE-12 cells treated with IL-33 for 24 h. **(F)** Western blot analysis of CD146 expression in A549 cells treated with IL-33 for 24 h. **(G)** Western blot analysis of CD146 expression in MLE-12 cells treated with HDM extract (100 μg/ml) with or without an ST2-neutralizing antibody (5 μg/ml). *$P < 0.05$; **$P < 0.01$; ***$P < 0.001$.

(431104, Biolegend, USA), IL-5 (431204, Biolegend, USA), IL-13 (900-K207, PeproTech, USA), IL-33 (88-7333-88, Invitrogen, USA) and IFN-γ (430804, Biolegend, USA) in the supernatants of lung homogenates were measured using an ELISA kit. Collagen I in the lung homogenates was measured using an ELISA kit (E-EL-M0325c, Elabscience, China). Soluble CD146 in human plasma (E-EL-H2403c, Elabscience, China) was measured using commercial ELISA kits. All ELISA experiments were performed according to the instructions provided by the manufacturers.

Statistical Analysis

Statistical analysis was performed using GraphPad Prism 5 (La Jolla, CA), and the data are displayed as the means ± SEM. Images from the Western blotting or immunofluorescence results were analyzed with ImageJ. Student's *t*-test or one-way ANOVA was applied to assess the statistical significance. A value of $P < 0.05$ was considered statistically significant ($^{*}P < 0.05$; $^{**}P < 0.01$; $^{***}P < 0.001$; and $\#P > 0.1$).

RESULTS

HDM Promoted CD146 Expression in Alveolar Epithelial Cells via IL-33/ST2 Signaling

Once inhaled into the respiratory tract, HDMs may directly stimulate alveolar epithelial cells. As shown in **Figure 1A**, HDM extract challenge increased CD146 transcripts in the mouse alveolar epithelial cell line MLE-12, which was further validated in the immunoblotting assay (**Figure 1B**). Primary alveolar epithelial cells purified from the lung were subjected to SPD staining (**Figure 1C**). Similarly, HDM extract increased CD146 expression in primary alveolar epithelial cells (**Figure 1D**). In agreement with a previous study that showed that IL-33 was increased in asthma (29), HDM extract increased IL-33 expression (**Figure 2A**) and secretion (**Figure 2B**) in alveolar epithelial cells. To explore whether HDM-mediated IL-33 induction was associated with the major HDM component Derp or LPS contamination, we removed endotoxin from HDM extract and treated epithelial cells with treated HDM that lacked LPS.

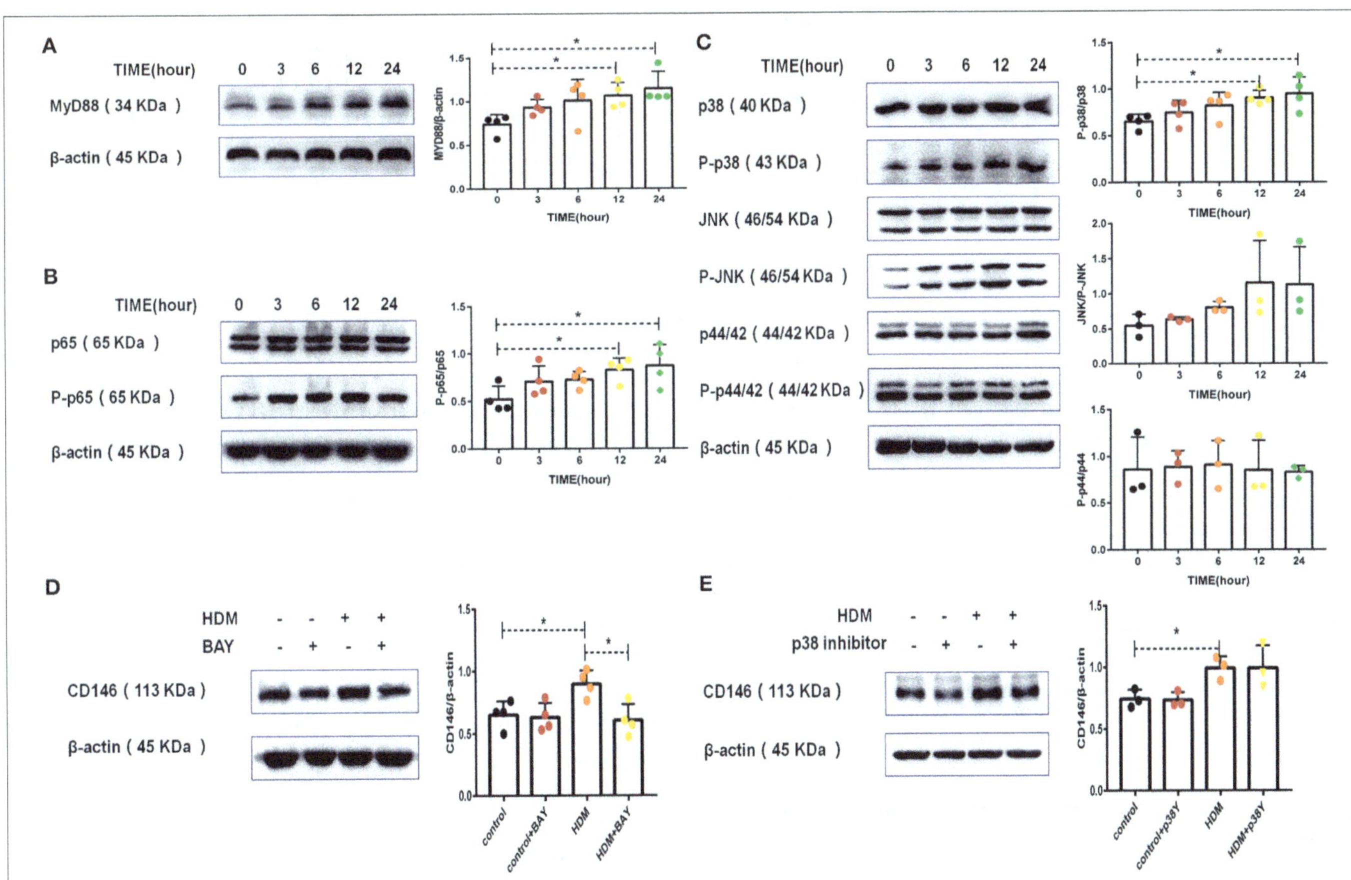

FIGURE 3 | CD146 expression in alveolar epithelial cells was dependent on p65. **(A)** Western blot analysis of MyD88 expression in MLE-12 cells treated with HDM extract (100 μg/ml). **(B)** Western blot analysis of NF-κB p65 expression in MLE-12 cells treated with HDM extract (100 μg/ml). **(C)** Western blot analysis of MAPK expression in MLE-12 cells treated with HDM extract (100 μg/ml). **(D)** Western blot analysis of CD146 expression in MLE-12 cells treated with HDM extract (100 μg/ml) and a p65 inhibitor (BAY, 10 μm) for 24 h. **(E)** Western blot analysis of CD146 expression in MLE-12 cells treated with HDM extract and a p38 inhibitor (SB203580, 10 μm) for 24 h. $^{*}P < 0.05$.

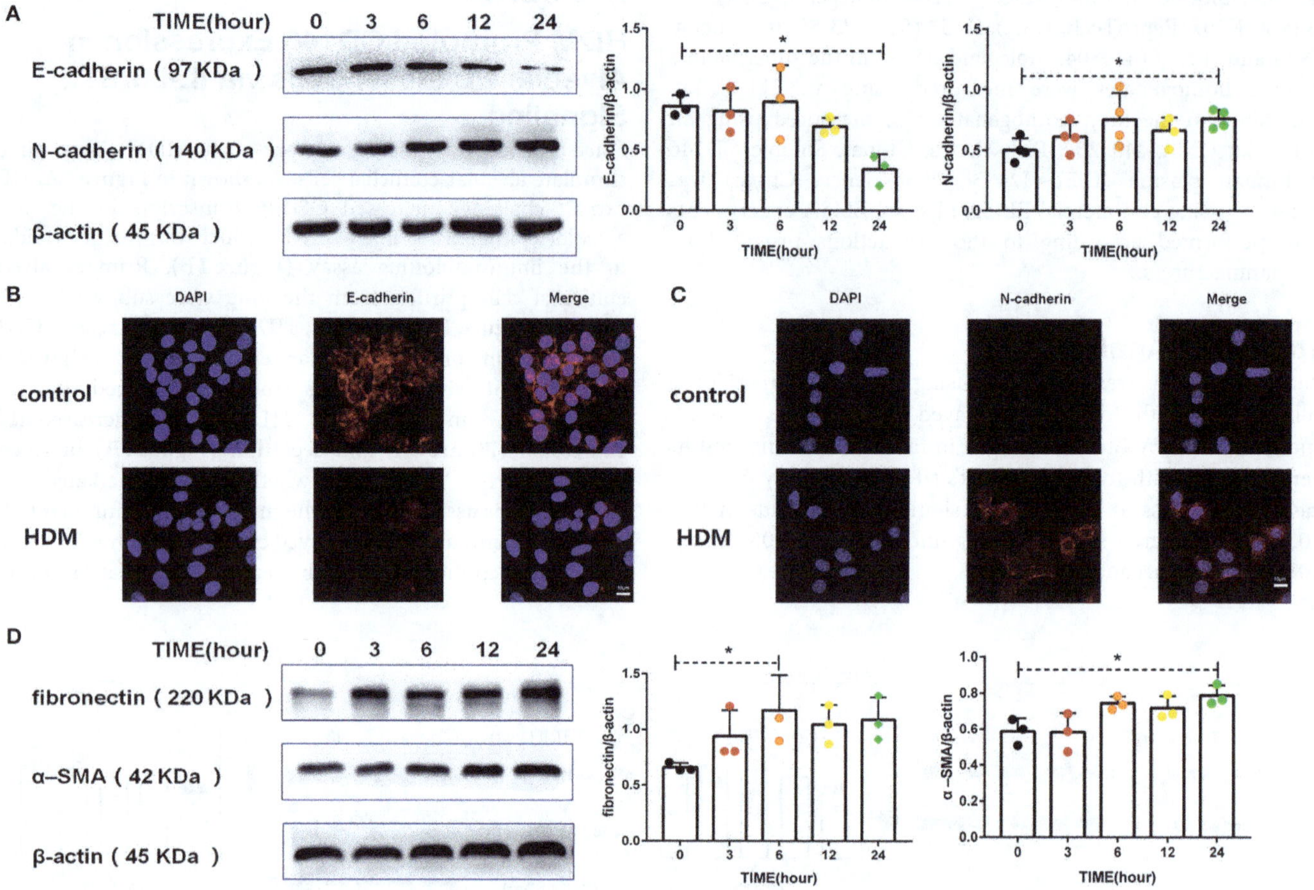

FIGURE 4 | HDM promoted EMT in alveolar epithelial cells. **(A)** Western blot analysis of E-cadherin and N-cadherin expression in MLE-12 cells treated with HDM extract (100 μg/ml). **(B)** Immunofluorescence analysis of E-cadherin expression in MLE-12 cells treated with HDM extract (100 μg/ml) for 24 h. **(C)** Immunofluorescence analysis of N-cadherin expression in MLE-12 cells treated with HDM extract (100 μg/ml) for 24 h. **(D)** Western blot analysis of fibronectin and α-SMA expression in MLE-12 cells treated with HDM extract (100 μg/ml). *$P < 0.05$.

Again, IL-33 was increased in the cell lysate (**Figure 2C**) or culture supernatant (**Figure 2D**) was increased.

To explore whether IL-33 is involved in CD146 expression, we stimulated epithelial cells with IL-33 and found that IL-33 directly promoted CD146 expression in mouse alveolar epithelial MLE-12 cells (**Figure 2E**) and human alveolar epithelial A549 cells (**Figure 2F**). The ST2-neutralizing antibody decreased CD146 expression (**Figure 2G**), suggesting that IL-33/ST2 was required for CD146 expression in HDM-treated epithelial cells. In summary, HDM extract increased the expression of CD146 in alveolar epithelial cells, which was mediated by IL-33 and its receptor ST2.

CD146 Expression in Alveolar Epithelial Cells Was Dependent on p65

IL-33 binding to ST2 on epithelial cells may activate a series of downstream signaling pathways, including the MyD88, NF-κB, and MAPK pathways (30). As shown in **Figure 3A**, HDM extract activated MyD88 in MLE-12 cells. Similarly, HDM extract increased the phosphorylation of NF-κB p65 (**Figure 3B**). In the MAPK signaling pathway, p38 but not JNK, and p42 was activated in MLE-12 cells treated with HDM extract (**Figure 3C**). More importantly, the p65 inhibitor antagonized the HDM-induced upregulation of CD146 (**Figure 3D**), highlighting the importance of NF-κB in CD146 expression. In contrast with the results observed with the p65 inhibitor, the p38 inhibitor showed insignificant effects on the expression of CD146 in MLE-12 cells treated with HDM extract (**Figure 3E**). Therefore, CD146 in HDM-treated alveolar epithelial cells was regulated by NF-κB p65.

HDM Promoted EMT in Alveolar Epithelial Cells via CD146

There is now evidence that asthma patients have more EMT than normal individuals (5, 31). The cadherin switch, which is a fundamental event in EMT, was induced in MLE-12 cells treated with HDM extract. As shown in **Figures 4A–C**, HDM extract decreased the expression of E-cadherin and increased N-cadherin expression. In addition, HDM extract increased fibronectin and α-SMA levels in MLE-12 cells (**Figure 4D**), suggesting that HDM extract promoted EMT in alveolar epithelial cells.

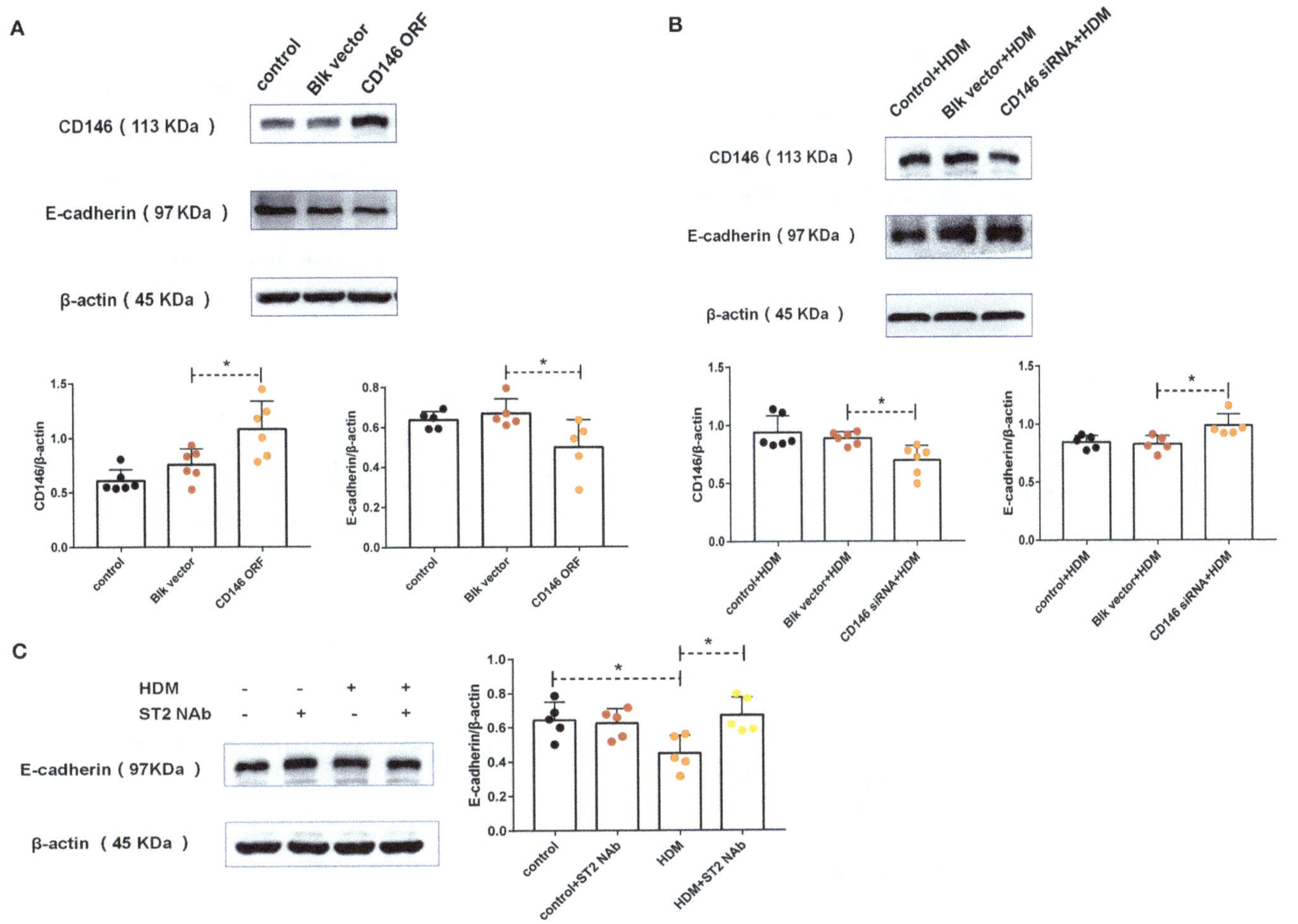

FIGURE 5 | HDM promoted EMT in alveolar epithelial cells via CD146. **(A)** Western blot analysis of CD146 and E-cadherin expression in MLE-12 cells treated with a CD146 expression plasmid (CD146 open reading frame, CD146 ORF) or blank vehicle (Blk vector). **(B)** Western blot analysis of CD146 and E-cadherin expression in MLE-12 cells treated with a CD146 siRNA plasmid and HDM extract (100 μg/ml). **(C)** Western blot analysis of E-cadherin expression in MLE-12 cells treated with HDM extract (100 μg/ml) and an ST2-neutralizing antibody (5 μg/ml). $^{*}P < 0.05$.

To explore the roles of CD146 in HMD-induced EMT, CD146 was either overexpressed via an expression plasmid or silenced with a siRNA plasmid in MLE-12 cells. Accompanied by CD146 elevation, E-cadherin was significantly decreased (**Figure 5A**). In contrast, CD146 silencing caused the increased expression of E-cadherin in epithelial cells (**Figure 5B**). E-cadherin expression was inversely correlated with CD146 expression, suggesting that CD146 may positively regulate EMT in alveolar epithelial cells. Moreover, the ST2-neutralizing antibody rescued E-cadherin expression in epithelial cells treated with HDM extract (**Figure 5C**). Considering that the ST2-neutralizing antibody decreased CD146 expression in epithelial cells treated with HDM extract (**Figure 2G**), we concluded that IL-33/ST2 contributed to CD146-mediated EMT in alveolar epithelial cells treated with HDM extract.

TGF-β and SMAD3 Played Dominant Roles in EMT in Alveolar Epithelial Cells Treated With HDM Extract

TGF-β has been shown to be the most common EMT inducer in asthma (5, 32). Accordingly, HMD extract increased TGF-β levels in alveolar epithelial cells (**Figure 6A**). STAT3 and SMAD3 are downstream molecules of the TGF-β signaling pathway in the EMT process. Administration of HDM extract contributed minimally to STAT3 activation (**Figure 6B**) but resulted in the phosphorylation of SMAD3 (**Figure 6C**) in alveolar epithelial cells. More importantly, a SMAD3 inhibitor (SIS3) partially but significantly increased E-cadherin expression in MLE-12 cells treated with HDM extract (**Figure 6D**), suggesting that TGF-β and SMAD3 regulate EMT in HDM-treated alveolar epithelial cells.

IL-33 Was Essential for CD146 Expression in a Mouse Model of Asthma

To demonstrate the significance of IL-33/ST2 in CD146 expression, we developed an asthma model in wild-type mice and IL-33 KO mice (**Figure 7A**). IL-33 deficiency reduced lung resistance in the murine model of asthma (**Figure 7B**). The number of total cells and eosinophils in BALF were decreased in the IL-33 KO mice treated with HDM extract (**Figures 7C,D**). Similarly, pulmonary tissue sections stained with H&E exhibited more inflammatory infiltration in WT mice than in IL-33 KO

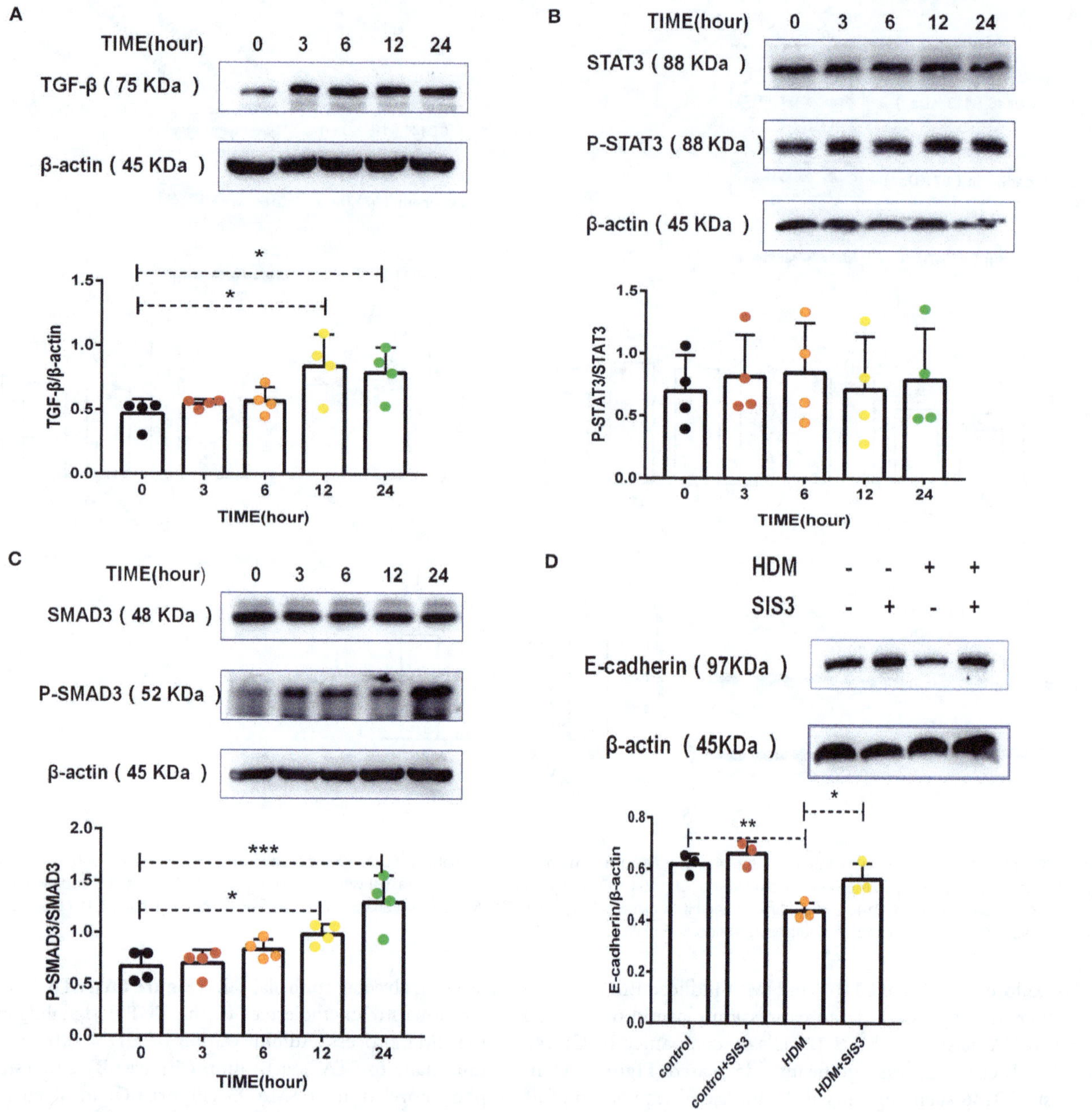

FIGURE 6 | TGF-β and SMAD3 played dominant roles in HDM-treated alveolar epithelial cell EMT. **(A)** Western blot analysis of TGF-β expression in MLE-12 cells treated with HDM extract (100 μg/ml). **(B)** Western blot analysis of STAT3 expression in MLE-12 cells treated with HDM extract (100 μg/ml). **(C)** Western blot analysis of SMAD3 expression in MLE-12 cells treated with HDM extract. **(D)** Western blot analysis of E-cadherin expression in MLE-12 cells treated with HDM extract (100 μg/ml) and a SMAD3 inhibitor (SIS3, 10 μm) for 24 h. $^{*}P < 0.05$; $^{**}P < 0.01$; $^{***}P < 0.001$.

mice (**Figure 7E**). Total IgE in sera was significantly elevated in the HDM-treated mice; however, the IgE concentration was comparable in WT and IL-33 KO mice challenged with HDM extract (**Figure 7F**). The expression of type 2 cytokines, including IL-4, IL-5, and IL-13, was increased in the HDM extract-treated mice. IL-33 deficiency reduced IL-4, IL-5, IL-13, and IFN-γ levels in the lung tissue of the HMD-treated mice (**Figure 7G**). These results suggest that IL-33 deficiency may alleviate asthma disease severity.

To further explore EMT in asthma, collagen I in pulmonary tissue was quantified, and the results showed that the level of collagen I was decreased in IL-33 KO mice compared to WT mice treated with HDM extract (**Figure 8A**). As expected, pulmonary tissue sections stained with PAS (**Figure 8B**) or Sirius red (**Figure 8C**) revealed that collagen deposition and glycogen storage were more pronounced in WT mice than in IL-33 KO mice. Consistent with the previous *in vitro* observations, decreased CD146 (**Figure 8D**) and elevated

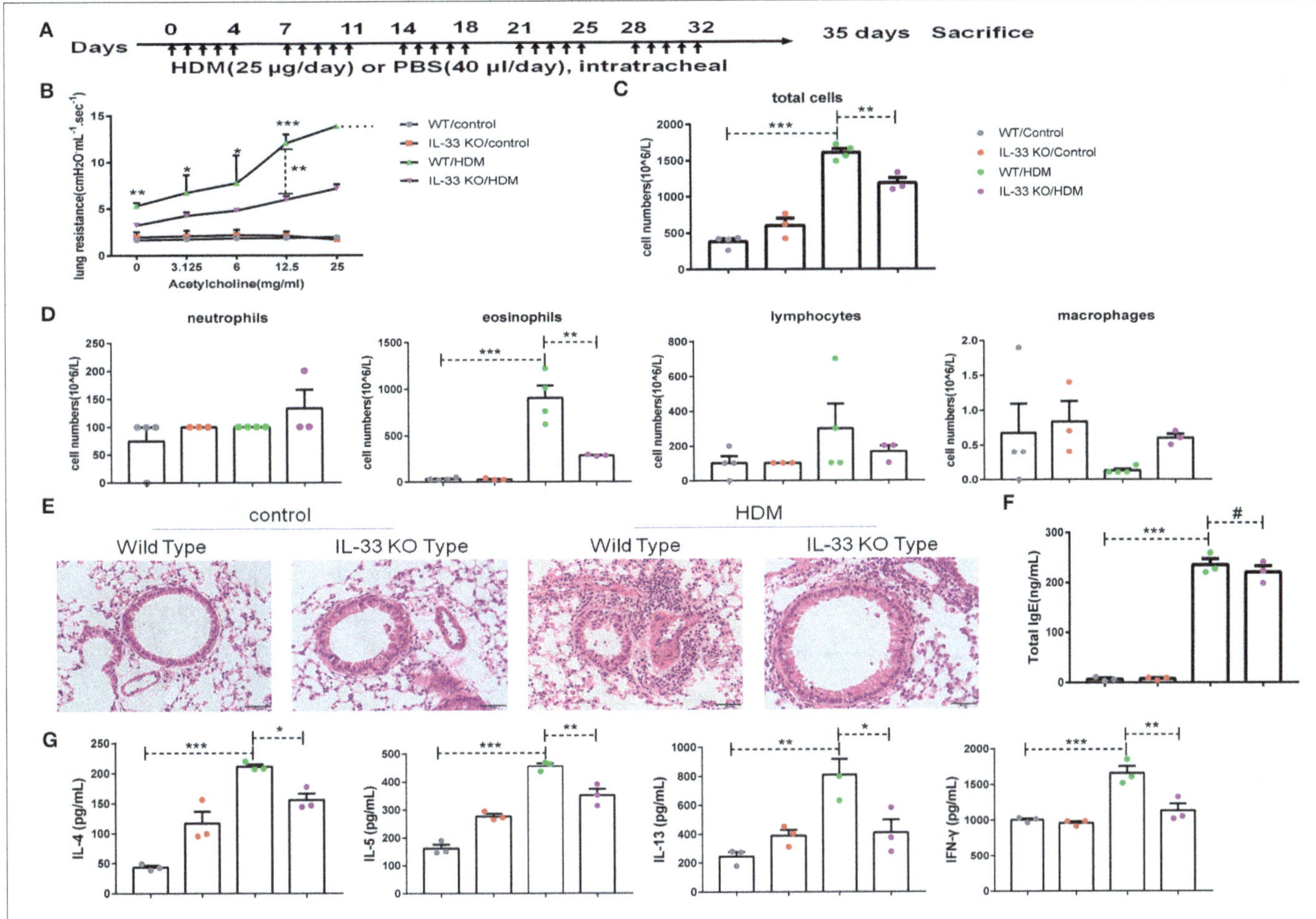

FIGURE 7 | IL-33 played an important role in a mouse model of asthma. **(A)** Flow chart showing the chronic asthma model (5 days/week for 5 weeks). **(B)** Lung resistance in mice was measured with the FinePointe RC System. **(C,D)** The numbers of total cells, eosinophils, neutrophils, and lymphocytes in BALF were quantified. **(E)** Representative images of lung sections stained with H&E. **(F)** ELISA analysis of total IgE levels in sera. **(G)** ELISA analysis of IL-4, IL-5, IL-13, and IFN-γ levels in the supernatants of lung homogenates. $^{*}P < 0.05$; $^{**}P < 0.01$; $^{***}P < 0.001$; $^{\#}P > 0.1$.

E-cadherin (**Figures 8D,E**) levels were observed in IL-33 KO mice compared to WT type mice after HDM treatment. As observed *in vitro*, Myd88, NF-κB, and p38 may be involved in EMT in the mouse model of asthma (**Supplementary Figure 1**). In summary, IL-33 deficiency alleviated disease severity and decreased CD146 expression and EMT in asthma.

CD146 Deficiency Decreased EMT in a Mouse Model of Asthma

To further evaluate the roles of CD146 in the asthma-associated EMT process, we established an asthma model in WT mice and CD146 KO mice. As shown in **Figure 9A**, lung resistance was reduced in CD146 KO mice compared to WT mice treated with HDM extract. The IgE level in the asthmatic WT mice and CD146-deficient mice was comparable (**Figure 9B**). In pulmonary tissues stained with H&E, the inflammatory response was decreased in the CD146 KO murine model of asthma (**Figure 9C**). Pulmonary cytokines, including IL-4, IL-5, IL-13, and IFN-γ, were decreased in CD146 KO mice compared to WT mice after HDM treatment (**Figure 9D**). Of note, IL-33 levels in asthmatic WT or CD146-deficient mice were comparable (**Figure 9E**). Because CD146 regulated EMT in alveolar epithelial cells, the level of collagen I was significantly decreased in the mouse model of asthma with a CD146 KO background (**Figure 10A**). Similarly, collagen deposition and glycogen storage in asthmatic CD146 KO mice were decreased, as evidenced by PAS (**Figure 10B**) and Sirius red staining (**Figure 10C**), respectively. Furthermore, CD146 deficiency caused an increase in E-cadherin in the asthma model (**Figures 10D,E**), suggesting that CD146 may orchestrate EMT in asthma.

Soluble CD146 Was Elevated in the Plasma of Asthma Patients

We demonstrated that CD146 contributed to asthma pathogenesis in a mouse model. CD146 is not only expressed on the cell membrane but could also be released into circulation (33). To demonstrate the clinical significance of the study, we

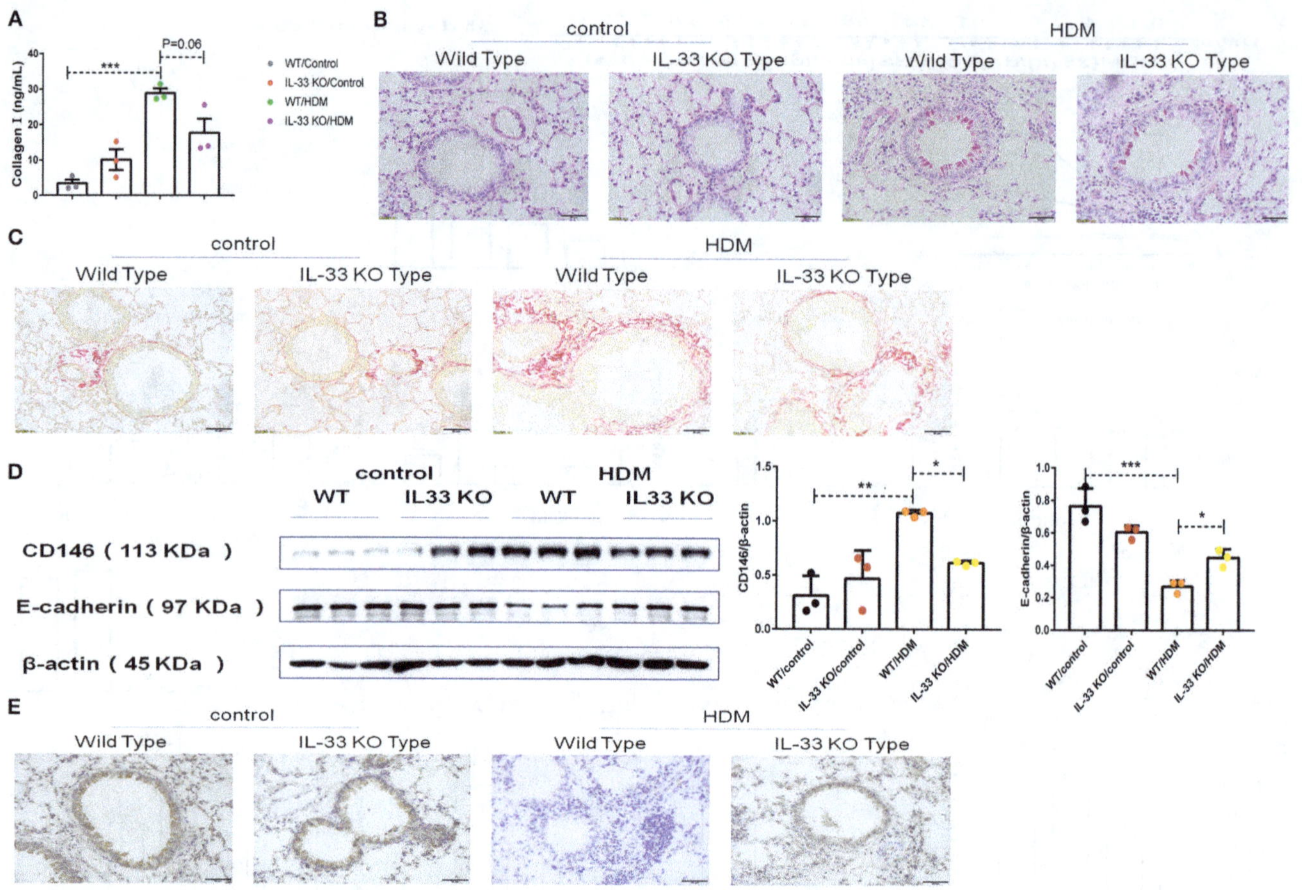

FIGURE 8 | IL-33 was essential for CD146 expression and EMT in a mouse model of asthma. **(A)** ELISA analysis of collagen-I levels in the lung homogenates of mice. **(B)** Representative images of lung sections stained with PAS. **(C)** Representative images of lung sections stained with Sirius red. **(D)** Western blot analysis of CD146 and E-cadherin expression in lung tissues. **(E)** Representative images of immunohistochemical analysis of E-cadherin expression in lung tissues. $^{*}P < 0.05$; $^{**}P < 0.01$; $^{***}P < 0.001$.

measured soluble CD146 (sCD146) levels in the plasma of asthma patients. As shown in **Figure 11**, the level of sCD146 was significantly increased in asthma patients compared to healthy controls. Considering that CD146 was increased in the airway epithelial cells of asthma patients (11, 12), we hypothesized that CD146 may be important in asthma.

DISCUSSION

In the present study, we first demonstrated that HDM extract promoted CD146 expression in alveolar epithelial cells via IL-33, and this effect was blocked with an antibody against the IL-33 receptor ST2. CD146, which was upregulated with an expression plasmid or downregulated with an siRNA plasmid, was found to play essential roles in E-cadherin expression in alveolar epithelial cells, suggesting that CD146 may mediate EMT in asthma. In a chronic asthma model in IL-33-deficient mice, CD146 expression was decreased in the pulmonary tissues, accompanied by increased E-cadherin expression, suggesting that IL-33 is essential in the CD146 expression and airway remodeling observed in asthma. Accordingly, CD146 deficiency in this chronic asthma model caused elevated E-cadherin expression, suggesting that CD146 deficiency reduced EMT in asthma. Moreover, we found that the level of soluble CD146 was increased in asthma patients. Therefore, we hypothesized that CD146 may mediate airway remodeling in chronic asthma in a manner that was dependent on the IL-33 signaling pathway.

In pulmonary epithelial cells, HDM extract stimulated CD146 expression and IL-33 production. As an alarmin molecule (34) and mucosal response amplifier (35), IL-33 binding with its receptor ST2 promoted CD146 expression. It has been demonstrated that IL-33 receptor knockout decreases the airway inflammatory response but induces the persistence of IL-5^{+} IL-13^{+} type 2 innate lymphocytes to maintain certain characteristics of asthma (36). Consistent with the above observation, we observed that IgE levels were comparable in the WT and IL-33 KO murine asthma models. In HDM-treated CD146 KO mice, the IL-33 concentration was similar to that in HDM-treated WT mice and was accompanied by comparable IgE levels in

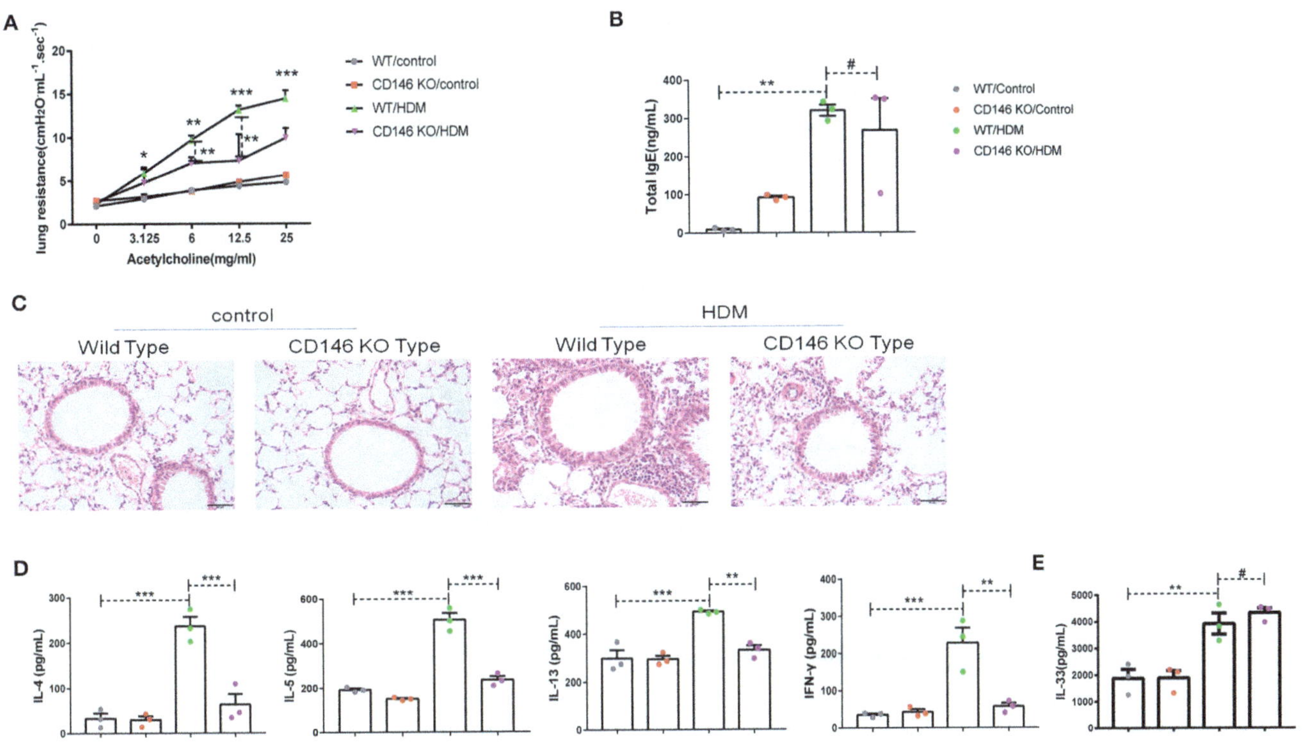

FIGURE 9 | CD146 deficiency mitigated disease severity in a mouse model of asthma. **(A)** Lung resistance in mice was measured with the FinePointe RC System. **(B)** Representative images of lung sections stained with H&E. **(C)** ELISA analysis of total IgE levels in sera. **(D)** ELISA analysis of IL-4, IL-5, IL-13, and IFN-γ levels in the supernatants of lung homogenates. **(E)** ELISA analysis of IL-33 levels in the supernatants of lung homogenates. *$P < 0.05$; **$P < 0.01$; ***$P < 0.001$; #$P > 0.05$.

WT and CD146 KO mice treated with HDM extract. These results suggest that IL-33 was not indispensable for IgE induction in asthma.

EMT has been reported to be intricately involved in airway remodeling in asthma (37, 38). In contrast, inhibition of the EMT process may slow airway remodeling in asthma (39). The increased expression of IL-33 in airway epithelial cells is closely related to the severity of asthma (40), and IL-33 has been shown to not only exacerbate airway inflammation (41) but also promote airway remodeling in asthma (42–44). Downstream signaling molecules of ST2, including MyD88, NF-κB p65, and MAPK, are then activated. However, only NF-κB p65 was indispensable for the CD146 expression observed in alveolar epithelial cells after stimulation with HDM extract. Because CD146 dimerization may activate NF-κB p65 (45), the reciprocal regulatory mechanisms between CD146 and NF-κB p65 warrant further study.

CD146 has been shown to be expressed by diverse cell types with multiple functions (7). In mouse tracheal epithelial cells, CD146 expression was accompanied by IL-13-mediated eotaxin-3 expression, suggesting that CD146 is an enhancer of the IL-13 response (46). In human primary nasal airway epithelial cells stimulated with TLR agonists, the absence of CD146 decreased expression of the inflammatory chemokine IL-8 (47), suggesting that CD146 may amplify inflammation. Consistent with the roles of CD146 in the inflammatory response, IL-4, IL-5, IL-1, and IFN-γ levels were significantly reduced in CD146-deficient mice with chronic asthma. Moreover, CD146 was directly linked to EMT in alveolar epithelial cells, and this relationship was dependent on the TGF-β/Smad-3 signaling pathway.

CD146 has been shown to be expressed on not only epithelial cells but also other cells, including endothelial cells (48), subpopulations of T cells (49), and mesenchymal stromal cells (MSCs) (50). All of these cell types may be involved in asthma pathogenesis and tissue remodeling (51, 52). In addition to epithelial cells, the roles of other $CD146^+$ cells in EMT and airway remodeling in asthma need to be elucidated in the future. Moreover, CD146 is shed from the cell membrane via MMP-3 activity (53). Elevated sCD146 levels in the plasma of asthma patients may enhance the production of vascular endothelial growth factor receptor (VEGFR) and VEGF2 (54). Therefore, we hypothesized that CD146 also regulated neovascularization, which is closely associated with EMT in asthma (55).

In summary, we expanded the role of CD146 in the EMT process from cancer metastasis to airway remodeling in asthma. We proposed that the binding of IL-33 to ST2 on HDM-stimulated airway epithelial cells promoted CD146 expression, which further amplified the inflammatory response, EMT and airway remodeling.

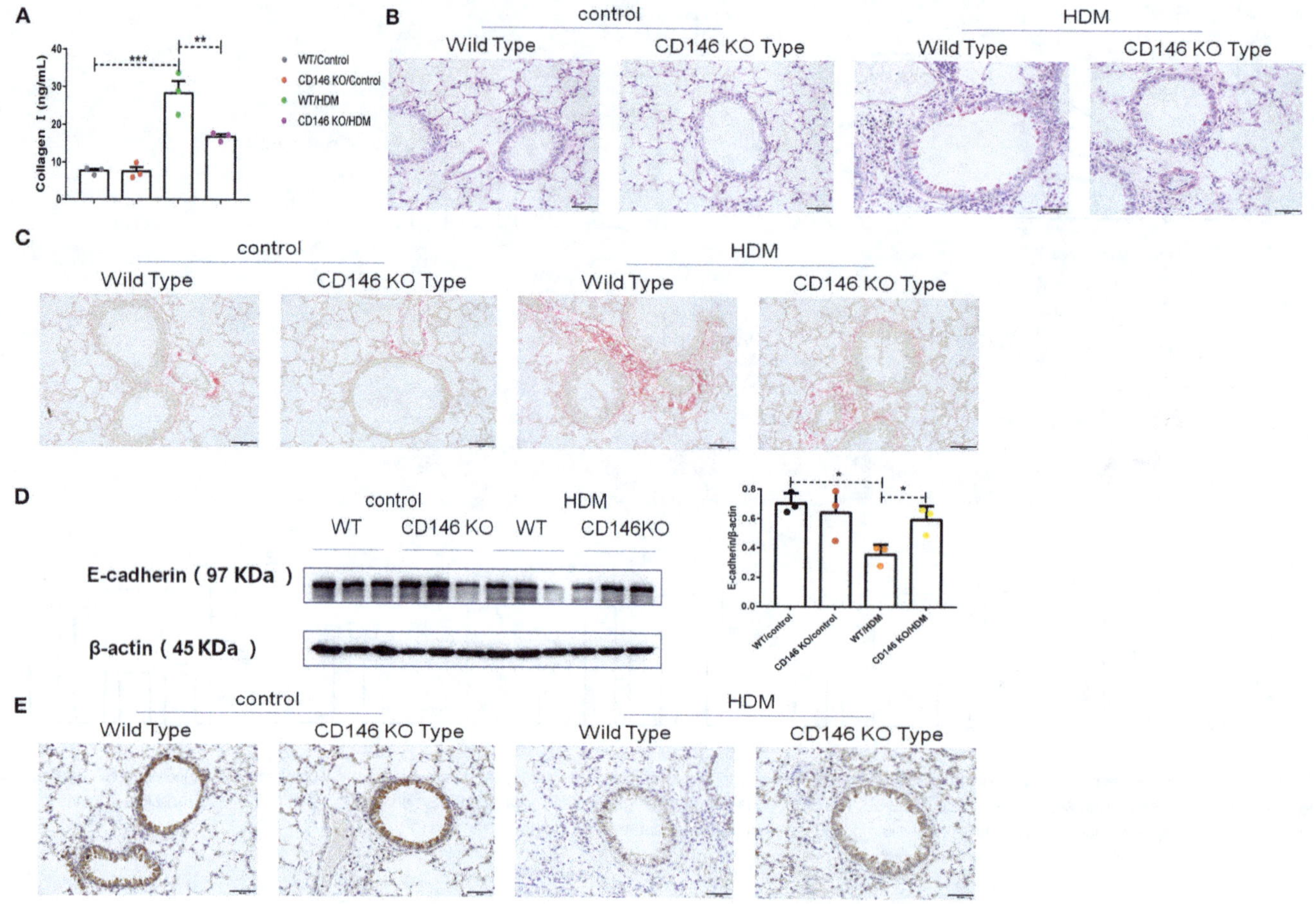

FIGURE 10 | CD146 deficiency decreased EMT in a mouse model of asthma. **(A)** ELISA analysis of collagen-I levels in the supernatants of lung homogenates of WT mice and CD146 KO mice. **(B,C)** Representative images of PAS- or Sirius red-stained lung sections from WT mice and CD146 KO mice. **(D)** Western blot analysis of E-cadherin expression in lung tissues from WT mice and CD146 KO mice. **(E)** Representative images of immunohistochemical analysis of E-cadherin expression in lung tissues from WT mice and CD146 KO mice. *$P < 0.05$; **$P < 0.01$; ***$P < 0.001$.

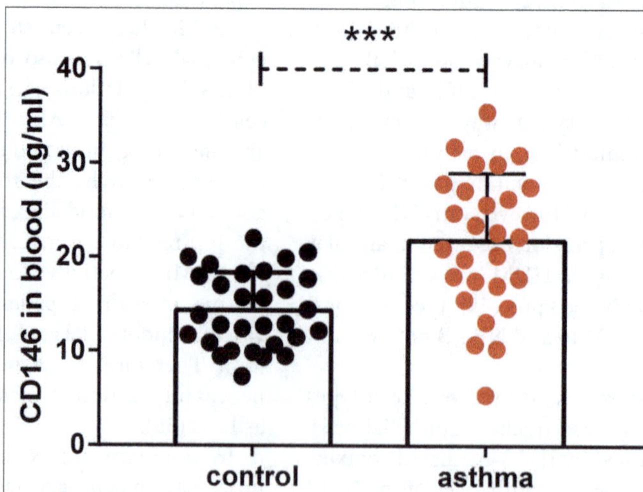

FIGURE 11 | Soluble CD146 was elevated in the plasma of asthma patients. The level of soluble CD146 in the plasma of asthmatic patients and healthy people was measured by ELISA. ***$P < 0.001$.

AUTHOR CONTRIBUTIONS

ZS, MH, and MZ designed the experiments. ZS, QM, RZ, ZC, ZW, and FH performed the experiments and analyzed the data. NJ and CW collected and characterized the clinical samples. MH and MZ conceived and supervised the project. ZS and MZ wrote the manuscript. All authors approved the final version of the manuscript.

REFERENCES

1. Mims JW. Asthma: definitions and pathophysiology. *Int Forum Allergy Rhinol.* (2015) 5(Suppl. 1):S2–6. doi: 10.1002/alr.21609
2. Al-Muhsen S, Johnson JR, Hamid Q. Remodeling in asthma. *J Allergy Clin Immunol.* (2011) 128:451–62. doi: 10.1016/j.jaci.2011.04.047
3. Rout-Pitt N, Farrow N, Parsons D, Donnelley M. Epithelial mesenchymal transition (EMT): a universal process in lung diseases with implications for cystic fibrosis pathophysiology. *Respir Res.* (2018) 19:136. doi: 10.1186/s12931-018-0834-8
4. Hackett TL, Warner SM, Stefanowicz D, Shaheen F, Pechkovsky DV, Murray LA, et al. Induction of epithelial-mesenchymal transition in primary airway epithelial cells from patients with asthma by transforming growth factor-beta1. *Am J Respir Crit Care Med.* (2009) 180:122–33. doi: 10.1164/rccm.200811-1730OC
5. Yang ZC, Qu ZH, Yi MJ, Shan YC, Ran N, Xu L, et al. MiR-448-5p inhibits TGF-beta1-induced epithelial-mesenchymal transition and pulmonary fibrosis by targeting Six1 in asthma. *J Cell Physiol.* (2019) 234:8804–14. doi: 10.1002/jcp.27540
6. Liu T, Liu Y, Miller M, Cao L, Zhao J, Wu J, et al. Autophagy plays a role in FSTL1-induced epithelial mesenchymal transition and airway remodeling in asthma. *Am J Physiol Lung Cell Mol Physiol.* (2017) 313:L27–40. doi: 10.1152/ajplung.00510.2016
7. Wang Z, Yan X. CD146, a multi-functional molecule beyond adhesion. *Cancer Lett.* (2013) 330:150–62. doi: 10.1016/j.canlet.2012.11.049
8. Luo Y, Duan H, Qian Y, Feng L, Wu Z, Wang F, et al. Macrophagic CD146 promotes foam cell formation and retention during atherosclerosis. *Cell Res.* (2017) 27:352–72. doi: 10.1038/cr.2017.8
9. Gabsi A, Heim X, Dlala A, Gati A, Sakhri H, Abidi A, et al. TH17 cells expressing CD146 are significantly increased in patients with systemic sclerosis. *Sci Rep.* (2019) 9:17721. doi: 10.1038/s41598-019-54132-y
10. Piao Y, Guo H, Qu Z, Zheng B, Gao Y. CD146 promotes migration and proliferation in pulmonary large cell neuroendocrine carcinoma cell lines. *Oncol Lett.* (2019) 17:2075–80. doi: 10.3892/ol.2018.9830
11. Simon GC, Martin RJ, Smith S, Thaikoottathil J, Bowler RP, Barenkamp SJ, et al. Up-regulation of MUC18 in airway epithelial cells by IL-13: implications in bacterial adherence. *Am J Respir Cell Mol Biol.* (2011) 44:606–13. doi: 10.1165/rcmb.2010-0384OC
12. Wu Q, Case SR, Minor MN, Jiang D, Martin RJ, Bowler RP, et al. A novel function of MUC18: amplification of lung inflammation during bacterial infection. *Am J Pathol.* (2013) 182:819–27. doi: 10.1016/j.ajpath.2012.11.005
13. Berman R, Jiang D, Wu Q, Stevenson CR, Schaefer NR, Chu HW. MUC18 regulates lung rhinovirus infection and inflammation. *PLoS ONE.* (2016) 11:e0163927. doi: 10.1371/journal.pone.0163927
14. Berman R, Huang C, Jiang D, Finigan JH, Wu Q, Chu HW. MUC18 differentially regulates pro-inflammatory and anti-viral responses in human airway epithelial cells. *J Clin Cell Immunol.* (2014) 5:257. doi: 10.4172/2155-9899.1000257
15. Liu WF, Ji SR, Sun JJ, Zhang Y, Liu ZY, Liang AB, et al. CD146 expression correlates with epithelial-mesenchymal transition markers and a poor prognosis in gastric cancer. *Int J Mol Sci.* (2012) 13:6399–406. doi: 10.3390/ijms13056399
16. Jiang G, Zhang L, Zhu Q, Bai D, Zhang C, Wang X. CD146 promotes metastasis and predicts poor prognosis of hepatocellular carcinoma. *J Exp Clin Cancer Res.* (2016) 35:38. doi: 10.1186/s13046-016-0313-3
17. Stalin J, Nollet M, Dignat-George F, Bardin N, Blot-Chabaud M. Therapeutic and diagnostic antibodies to CD146: thirty years of research on its potential for detection and treatment of tumors. *Antibodies.* (2017) 6:17. doi: 10.3390/antib6040017
18. Pichery M, Mirey E, Mercier P, Lefrancais E, Dujardin A, Ortega N, et al. Endogenous IL-33 is highly expressed in mouse epithelial barrier tissues, lymphoid organs, brain, embryos, and inflamed tissues: *in situ* analysis using a novel Il-33-LacZ gene trap reporter strain. *J Immunol.* (2012) 188:3488–95. doi: 10.4049/jimmunol.1101977
19. Schmitz J, Owyang A, Oldham E, Song Y, Murphy E, McClanahan TK, et al. IL-33, an interleukin-1-like cytokine that signals via the IL-1 receptor-related protein ST2 and induces T helper type 2-associated cytokines. *Immunity.* (2005) 23:479–90. doi: 10.1016/j.immuni.2005.09.015
20. Griesenauer B, Paczesny S. The ST2/IL-33 axis in immune cells during inflammatory diseases. *Front Immunol.* (2017) 8:475. doi: 10.3389/fimmu.2017.00475
21. Li R, Yang G, Yang RQ, Peng XX, Li J. Interleukin-33 and receptor ST2 as indicators in patients with asthma: a meta-analysis. *Int J Clin Exp Med.* (2015) 8:14935–43.
22. Watanabe M, Nakamoto K, Inui T, Sada M, Honda K, Tamura M, et al. Serum sST2 levels predict severe exacerbation of asthma. *Respir Res.* (2018) 19:169. doi: 10.1186/s12931-018-0872-2
23. An G, Zhang X, Wang W, Huang Q, Li Y, Shan S, et al. The effects of interleukin-33 on airways collagen deposition and matrix metalloproteinase expression in a murine surrogate of asthma. *Immunology.* (2018) 154:637–50. doi: 10.1111/imm.12911
24. Tan QY, Cheng ZS. TGFbeta1-Smad signaling pathway participates in interleukin-33 induced epithelial-to-mesenchymal transition of A549 Cells. *Cell Physiol Biochem.* (2018) 50:757–67. doi: 10.1159/000494241
25. Kotsiou OS, Gourgoulianis KI, Zarogiannis SG. IL-33/ST2 axis in organ fibrosis. *Front Immunol.* (2018) 9:2432. doi: 10.3389/fimmu.2018.02432
26. Gregory LG, Causton B, Murdoch JR, Mathie SA, O'Donnell V, Thomas CP, et al. Inhaled house dust mite induces pulmonary T helper 2 cytokine production. *Clin Exp Allergy.* (2009) 39:1597–610. doi: 10.1111/j.1365-2222.2009.03302.x
27. Nabhan AN, Brownfield DG, Harbury PB, Krasnow MA, Desai TJ. Single-cell Wnt signaling niches maintain stemness of alveolar type 2 cells. *Science.* (2018) 359:1118–23. doi: 10.1126/science.aam6603
28. Kerzerho J, Maazi H, Speak AO, Szely N, Lombardi V, Khoo B, et al. Programmed cell death ligand 2 regulates TH9 differentiation and induction of chronic airway hyperreactivity. *J Allergy Clin Immunol.* (2013) 131:1048–57:1057.e1–2. doi: 10.1016/j.jaci.2012.09.027
29. Arae K, Morita H, Unno H, Motomura K, Toyama S, Okada N, et al. Chitin promotes antigen-specific Th2 cell-mediated murine asthma through induction of IL-33-mediated IL-1beta production by DCs. *Sci Rep.* (2018) 8:11721. doi: 10.1038/s41598-018-30259-2
30. Ding W, Zou GL, Zhang W, Lai XN, Chen HW, Xiong LX. Interleukin-33: its emerging role in allergic diseases. *Molecules.* (2018) 23:1665. doi: 10.3390/molecules23071665
31. Gong JH, Cho IH, Shin D, Han SY, Park SH, Kang YH. Inhibition of airway epithelial-to-mesenchymal transition and fibrosis by kaempferol in endotoxin-induced epithelial cells and ovalbumin-sensitized mice. *Lab Invest.* (2014) 94:297–308. doi: 10.1038/labinvest.2013.137
32. Ijaz T, Pazdrak K, Kalita M, Konig R, Choudhary S, Tian B, et al. Systems biology approaches to understanding epithelial mesenchymal transition (EMT) in mucosal remodeling and signaling in asthma. *World Allergy Organ J.* (2014) 7:13. doi: 10.1186/1939-4551-7-13
33. Dufies M, Nollet M, Ambrosetti D, Traboulsi W, Viotti J, Borchiellini D, et al. Soluble CD146 is a predictive marker of pejorative evolution and of sunitinib efficacy in clear cell renal cell carcinoma. *Theranostics.* (2018) 8:2447–58. doi: 10.7150/thno.23002

34. Divekar R, Kita H. Recent advances in epithelium-derived cytokines (IL-33, IL-25, and thymic stromal lymphopoietin) and allergic inflammation. *Curr Opin Allergy Clin Immunol.* (2015) 15:98–103. doi: 10.1097/ACI.0000000000000133
35. Oboki K, Ohno T, Kajiwara N, Arae K, Morita H, Ishii A, et al. IL-33 is a crucial amplifier of innate rather than acquired immunity. *Proc Natl Acad Sci USA.* (2010) 107:18581–6. doi: 10.1073/pnas.1003059107
36. Verma M, Liu S, Michalec L, Sripada A, Gorska MM, Alam R. Experimental asthma persists in IL-33 receptor knockout mice because of the emergence of thymic stromal lymphopoietin-driven IL-9^{+} and IL-13^{+} type 2 innate lymphoid cell subpopulations. *J Allergy Clin Immunol.* (2018) 142:793–803.e8. doi: 10.1016/j.jaci.2017.10.020
37. Heijink IH, Postma DS, Noordhoek JA, Broekema M, Kapus A. House dust mite-promoted epithelial-to-mesenchymal transition in human bronchial epithelium. *Am J Respir Cell Mol Biol.* (2010) 42:69–79. doi: 10.1165/rcmb.2008-0449OC
38. Johnson JR, Roos A, Berg T, Nord M, Fuxe J. Chronic respiratory aeroallergen exposure in mice induces epithelial-mesenchymal transition in the large airways. *PLoS ONE.* (2011) 6:e16175. doi: 10.1371/journal.pone.0016175
39. Pu Y, Liu Y, Liao S, Miao S, Zhou L, Wan L. Azithromycin ameliorates OVA-induced airway remodeling in Balb/c mice via suppression of epithelial-to-mesenchymal transition. *Int Immunopharmacol.* (2018) 58:87–93. doi: 10.1016/j.intimp.2018.03.016
40. Prefontaine D, Nadigel J, Chouiali F, Audusseau S, Semlali A, Chakir J, et al. Increased IL-33 expression by epithelial cells in bronchial asthma. *J Allergy Clin Immunol.* (2010) 125:752–4. doi: 10.1016/j.jaci.2009.12.935
41. Chan BCL, Lam CWK, Tam LS, Wong CK. IL33: roles in allergic inflammation and therapeutic perspectives. *Front Immunol.* (2019) 10:364. doi: 10.3389/fimmu.2019.00364
42. Yao XJ, Liu XF, Wang XD. Potential role of interleukin-25/interleukin-33/thymic stromal lymphopoietin-fibrocyte axis in the pathogenesis of allergic airway diseases. *Chin Med J.* (2018) 131:1983–9. doi: 10.4103/0366-6999.238150
43. Sjoberg LC, Nilsson AZ, Lei Y, Gregory JA, Adner M, Nilsson GP. Interleukin 33 exacerbates antigen driven airway hyperresponsiveness, inflammation and remodeling in a mouse model of asthma. *Sci Rep.* (2017) 7:4219. doi: 10.1038/s41598-017-03674-0
44. Guo Z, Wu J, Zhao J, Liu F, Chen Y, Bi L, et al. IL-33 promotes airway remodeling and is a marker of asthma disease severity. *J Asthma.* (2014) 51:863–9. doi: 10.3109/02770903.2014.921196
45. Zheng CG, Qiu YJ, Zeng QQ, Zhang Y, Lu D, Yang DL, et al. Endothelial CD146 is required for *in vitro* tumor-induced angiogenesis: the role of a disulfide bond in signaling and dimerization. *Int J Biochem Cell B.* (2009) 41:2163–72. doi: 10.1016/j.biocel.2009.03.014
46. Stevenson C, Jiang D, Schaefer N, Ito Y, Berman R, Sanchez A, et al. MUC18 regulates IL-13-mediated airway inflammatory response. *Inflamm Res.* (2017) 66:691–700. doi: 10.1007/s00011-017-1050-6
47. Chu HW, Rios C, Huang C, Wesolowska-Andersen A, Burchard EG, O'Connor BP, et al. CRISPR-Cas9-mediated gene knockout in primary human airway epithelial cells reveals a proinflammatory role for MUC18. *Gene Ther.* (2015) 22:822–9. doi: 10.1038/gt.2015.53
48. Schrage A, Loddenkemper C, Erben U, Lauer U, Hausdorf G, Jungblut PR, et al. Murine CD146 is widely expressed on endothelial cells and is recognized by the monoclonal antibody ME-9F1. *Histochem Cell Biol.* (2008) 129:441–51. doi: 10.1007/s00418-008-0379-x
49. Elshal MF, Khan SS, Takahashi Y, Solomon MA, McCoy JP Jr. CD146 (Mel-CAM), an adhesion marker of endothelial cells, is a novel marker of lymphocyte subset activation in normal peripheral blood. *Blood.* (2005) 106:2923–4. doi: 10.1182/blood-2005-06-2307
50. Sorrentino A, Ferracin M, Castelli G, Biffoni M, Tomaselli G, Baiocchi M, et al. Isolation and characterization of CD146+ multipotent mesenchymal stromal cells. *Exp Hematol.* (2008) 36:1035–46. doi: 10.1016/j.exphem.2008.03.004
51. McDonald DM. Angiogenesis and remodeling of airway vasculature in chronic inflammation. *Am J Respir Crit Care Med.* (2001) 164:S39–45. doi: 10.1164/ajrccm.164.supplement_2.2106065
52. Zanoni M, Cortesi M, Zamagni A, Tesei A. The role of mesenchymal stem cells in radiation-induced lung fibrosis. *Int J Mol Sci.* (2019) 20:3876. doi: 10.3390/ijms20163876
53. Boneberg EM, Illges H, Legler DF, Furstenberger G. Soluble CD146 is generated by ectodomain shedding of membrane CD146 in a calcium-induced, matrix metalloprotease-dependent process. *Microvasc Res.* (2009) 78:325–31. doi: 10.1016/j.mvr.2009.06.012
54. Harhouri K, Kebir A, Guillet B, Foucault-Bertaud A, Voytenko S, Piercecchi-Marti MD, et al. Soluble CD146 displays angiogenic properties and promotes neovascularization in experimental hind-limb ischemia. *Blood.* (2010) 115:3843–51. doi: 10.1182/blood-2009-06-229591
55. Lee CG, Ma B, Takyar S, Ahangari F, Delacruz C, He CH, et al. Studies of vascular endothelial growth factor in asthma and chronic obstructive pulmonary disease. *Proc Am Thorac Soc.* (2011) 8:512–5. doi: 10.1513/pats.201102-018MW

15

Butyrate Attenuates Lung Inflammation by Negatively Modulating Th9 Cells

Raquel de Souza Vieira[1], *Angela Castoldi*[1], *Paulo José Basso*[1], *Meire Ioshie Hiyane*[1], *Niels Olsen Saraiva Câmara*[1,2,3†] *and Rafael Ribeiro Almeida*[1,4*†]

[1] Laboratory of Transplantation Immunobiology, Department of Immunology, Institute of Biomedical Sciences, University of São Paulo, São Paulo, Brazil, [2] Nephrology Division, Department of Medicine, Federal University of São Paulo, São Paulo, Brazil, [3] Renal Pathophysiology Laboratory, Department of Clinical Medicine, University of São Paulo, São Paulo, Brazil, [4] Laboratory of Immunology, Heart Institute (InCor) School of Medicine, University of São Paulo, São Paulo, Brazil

***Correspondence:**
Rafael Ribeiro Almeida
rafaelbio13@usp.br

† These authors share co-senior authorship

Th9 cells orchestrate allergic lung inflammation by promoting recruitment and activation of eosinophils and mast cells, and by stimulating epithelial mucus production, which is known to be mainly dependent on IL-9. These cells share developmental pathways with induced regulatory T cells that may determine the generation of one over the other subset. In fact, the FOXP3 transcription factor has been shown to bind *il9* locus and repress IL-9 production. The microbiota-derived short-chain fatty acids (SCFAs) butyrate and propionate have been described as FOXP3 inducers and are known to have anti-inflammatory properties. While SCFAs attenuate lung inflammation by inducing regulatory T cells and suppressing Th2 responses, their effects on Th9 cells have not been addressed yet. Therefore, we hypothesized that SCFAs would have a protective role in lung inflammation by negatively modulating differentiation and function of Th9 cells. Our results demonstrated that butyrate is more effective than propionate in promoting FOXP3 expression and IL-9 repression. In addition, propionate was found to negatively impact *in vitro* differentiation of IL-13-expressing T cells. Butyrate treatment attenuated lung inflammation and mucus production in OVA-challenged mice, which presented lower frequency of lung-infiltrated Th9 cells and eosinophils. Both Th9 cell adoptive transfer and IL-9 treatment restored lung inflammation in butyrate-treated OVA-challenged mice, indicating that the anti-inflammatory effects of butyrate may rely on suppressing Th9-mediated immune responses.

Keywords: butyrate, Th9 cells, tregs, eosinophils, lung inflammation

INTRODUCTION

Helper T-cell differentiation takes place in secondary lymphoid organs, where the cytokine environment plays a key role in determining the fate of naïve T cells toward many CD4+ T-Cellsubsets. These subsets include effector T helper 1 (Th1), Th2, Th9, and Th17 cells that secrete signature cytokines, and regulatory Foxp3 T (Treg) cells that help hold immune responses in check (1). Interleukin-4 (IL-4) is known to induce the differentiation of Th2 cells, characterized by expressing the transcription factors STAT6 and GATA-3, and by producing the cytokines IL-4, IL-5, and IL-13 (1). These cells are mainly involved in the pathogenesis of allergic diseases, promoting activation of eosinophils and mast cells, mucus production, and triggering antibody class switching to IgE in B cells, which can also be modulated by other T-cell subsets (2).

IL-9-producing T cells, which share developmental pathways with both Th2 and Treg cells, are differentiated in response to IL-4, but only when transforming growth factor-β (TGF-β) is present (3). These cells are characterized by expressing the transcription factors PU.1, STAT6, and IRF4, although other molecules are required for IL-9 production, such as BATF and FOXO1 (4–8). STAT6 is particularly important in cellular polarization as it contributes to repressing TGF-β-mediated expression of FOXP3, known to be an IL-9 suppressor (5). Th9 cells are the main cellular source of IL-9, but also produce other cytokines, such as IL-3, IL-10, and IL-21 (3). While described as important effectors against helminthic infections (9, 10), the role of Th9 cells in many inflammatory diseases, cancer, and allergies has been increasingly studied (11–14).

Th9 cells are found in the draining lymph nodes and respiratory tract, especially during early phases of asthma development (15). The peripheral mononuclear blood cells (PBMC) of atopic infants and adults are featured by a higher frequency of Th9 cells when compared to healthy individuals (15, 16), while single nucleotide polymorphisms (SNPs) in the genes encoding both IL-9 and its receptor (IL9R) have been associated with beneficial outcomes in allergen sensitization (17). Experimental data on the role of Th9 cells in lung inflammation have revealed that it mainly relies on promoting IL-9-dependent eosinophil and mast cell infiltration, mucus production and enhanced release of Th2 cytokines (18). In fact, transgenic expression of IL-9 is sufficient to cause bronchial hyperresponsiveness (19, 20), while antibody-mediated neutralization of this cytokine protects mice from inflammation (8). PU.1, IRF4, and BATF knockout mice present impaired differentiation of Th9 cells and lower inflammation (4, 6, 8). On the other hand, thymic stromal lymphopoietin (TSLP) and nitric oxide-mediated activation of these cells was shown to promote increased IL-9 production and disease exacerbation (21, 22).

Although palliative treatments have reduced the severity of symptoms and death of asthma patients, there is no current therapeutic regimen that can cure the disease. A better understanding of the mechanisms involved in inflammation is likely to provide important cues on how to improve treatment and even cure asthma. In this context, an increasing interest in determining the role of the microbiota and their metabolites during disease development has arisen (23).

Mucosal organs such as gut and lungs harbor a large collection of bacteria and other microorganisms that shape local and distal immune responses (23, 24). Birth mode (vaginal or via cesarean section), diet, use of antibiotics and the surrounding environment represent some of the factors that influence microbiota diversity, which is suggested to play an important role in asthma susceptibility (23). Early life differential colonization may have a determinant role in this process and airway microbial diversity appears to be inversely associated with sensitization to house dust mites in childhood (25, 26).

Experimental data on germ-free (GF) mice have demonstrated that lack of microbiota results in stronger ovalbumin (OVA)-induced type 2 airway inflammation and hypersensitivity, which can be reversed by co-housing GF mice with specific pathogen-free (SPF)-raised animals (27). In line with these observations, it has also been shown that antibiotic-mediated depletion of the microbiota renders mice more susceptible to lung inflammation (28). However, not only the microorganisms but also their metabolites have been indicated as key players in controlling immune responses. In fact, microbiota metabolism of dietary fibers and production of short-chain fatty acids (SCFA), such as propionate and acetate, has been considered a major mechanism by which microorganisms control airway inflammation. Induction of Tregs and dendritic cells with impaired capability of promoting effector Th2 responses were shown to play an important role in attenuating disease (29, 30). Nevertheless, the role of SCFAs on other T-cell subsets that participate in lung inflammation, such as Th9 cells, is yet to be addressed.

Given the well-established role of butyrate and propionate in promoting FOXP3 expression during differentiation of Tregs (31, 32) and that FOXP3 is a potent IL-9 repressor (5, 33), we hypothesized that these SCFAs would have a negative impact on the development and function of Th9 cells. We confirmed previous data by showing that butyrate and propionate promote higher FOXP3 expression in the context of Treg differentiation. We then demonstrated an inverse correlation between IL-9 and FOXP3 expression when CD4+ T cells were exposed *in vitro* to butyrate and propionate early during differentiation into Th9 cells. Butyrate was found to be more efficient than propionate in promoting FOXP3 expression and IL-9 repression. In addition, we demonstrated an opposite effect of butyrate and propionate on Th2 cells. While *in vitro* butyrate treatment was responsible for inducing a small, but significant increase in the frequency of IL-13+ T cells, propionate treatment negatively impacted the same cells. Moreover, we found that butyrate-treated OVA-challenged mice presented lower frequency of lung-infiltrated Th9 cells and attenuated inflammation, represented by lower frequency of lung-infiltrated eosinophils, less inflammatory infiltrates and lower mucus production. Adoptive transfer of OVA-specific Th9 cells and recombinant IL-9 treatment were both sufficient to restore lung inflammation in butyrate-treated mice, indicating that butyrate-mediated effects were likely to be dependent on suppression of Th9 cells.

MATERIALS AND METHODS

Animals and Ethics Statement

Male C57BL/6, FOXP3 GFP, and OT-II mice (6–8 weeks old) were obtained from the animal facility of the Institute of Biomedical Sciences, University of São Paulo. Animals were housed in groups of up to 5 per cage in a light- and temperature-controlled room (12 h light/dark cycles, 21 ± 2°C) with free access to food and water. This study was carried out in accordance with the recommendations of the National Institute of Health, Guide for the Care and Use of Laboratory Animals and the Brazilian National Law (11.794/2008). The protocol was approved by the Institutional Animal Care and Use Committee (CEUA) of the University of São Paulo, under protocol number 2015/006.

OVA-Induced Lung Inflammation

Male C57BL/6 mice were intraperitoneally (IP) injected with 30 μg of ovalbumin (OVA) grade V (Sigma) dissolved in Imject Alum (1.6 mg) (Thermo Fisher), diluted in 200 μl of PBS at days 0 and 7. OVA-sensitized mice were nebulized with an OVA-distillated water solution (3%), using an ultrasonic nebulizer device (Respira Max®) for 15 min at days 14, 15, and 16. Control mice were sensitized as described and nebulized with water only. Mice were euthanized 24 h after the last nebulization (challenge) and lungs were extracted for further analysis.

Butyrate Treatment

Male C57BL/6 mice were IP injected with 250 μl of 1M butyric acid (butyrate) (Sigma) diluted in PBS (pH: 7.2) or PBS only at days 0, 1, 2, 7, 8, and 9 of OVA-sensitization. Mice treated during sensitization also received butyrate (IP) or PBS during the 3 days of OVA-nebulization (challenge).

IL-9 Treatment and T Cell Adoptive Transfer

OVA-sensitized butyrate-treated mice were intraperitoneally injected with 150 ng of recombinant murine IL-9 (R&D Systems) diluted in 200 μl of PBS or PBS only at days 1 and 2 of OVA nebulization. Alternatively, butyrate-treated mice were intraperitoneally injected with 2×10^6 OT-II Th0, Th2, or Th9 cells the day before OVA nebulization. OT-II Th2 and Th9 cells were differentiated *in vitro* as described in T cell differentiation topic.

Lung Digestion and Flow Cytometry

Mice were euthanized and lungs collected, washed in ice-cold PBS, cut in small pieces and incubated in R-10 medium [RPMI-1640 (Thermo Fisher) supplemented with 10% FBS (Thermo Fisher), 2 mM L-glutamine (Thermo Fisher), 1 mM sodium pyruvate (Thermo Fisher), 1% non-essential amino acids (Thermo Fisher), 1% Pen/Strept (Thermo Fisher), 1% vitamin solution (Thermo Fisher), and 5×10^{-5} M 2β-mercaptoetanol (Sigma)] containing 0.5 mg/ml of collagenase IV (Thermo Fisher) and 30 μg/ml of DNAse (Sigma), at 37°C for 45 min and 180 rpm. Digested tissues were passed through 100 μm cell strainers (Sigma) and centrifuged. Pellets were resuspended in 1 ml of ACK buffer (Thermo Fisher) for 2 min, centrifuged and

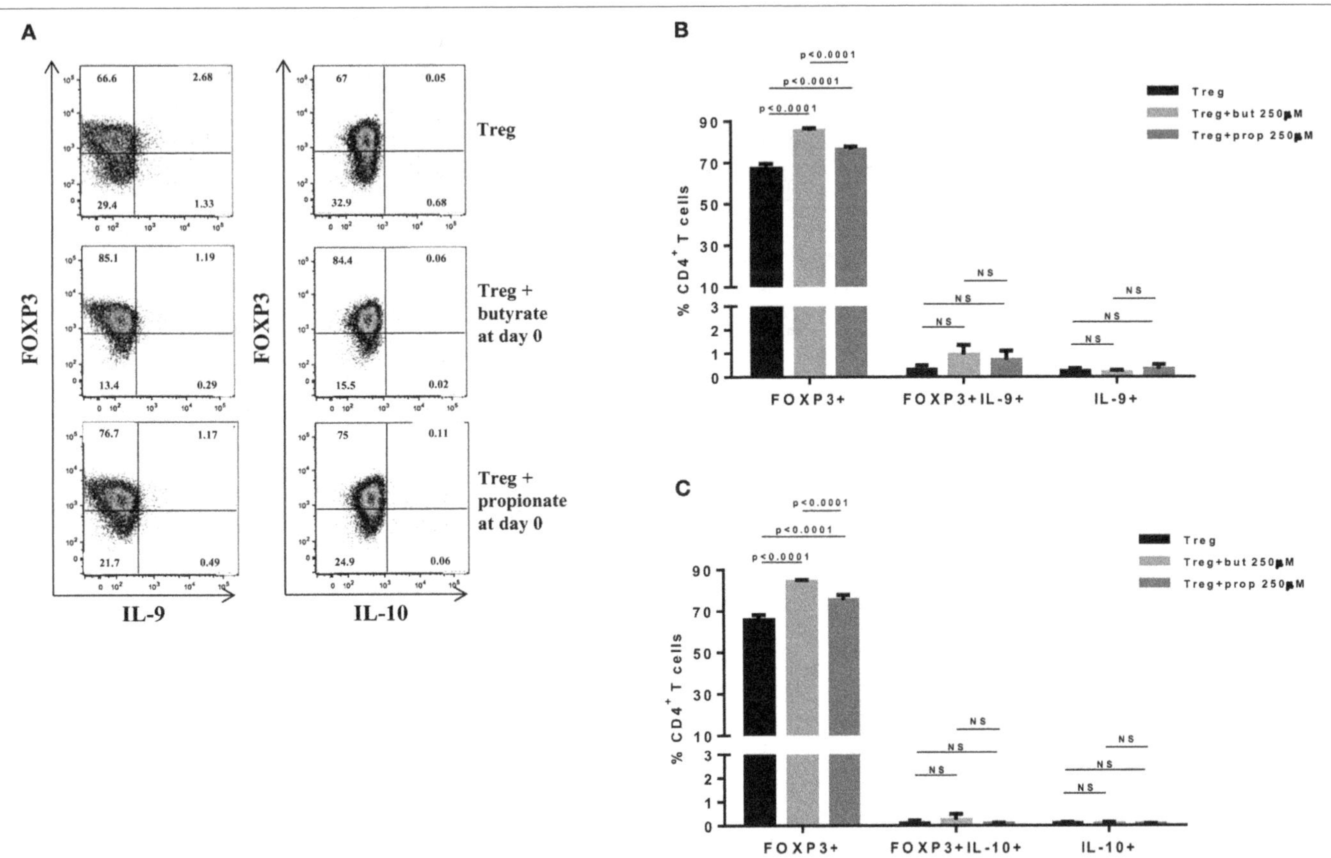

FIGURE 1 | Butyrate and propionate enhances FOXP3 expression in CD4+ T cells differentiated into Tregs. Naïve CD4+ T cells (CD62L+CD44low) were sorted from spleens of FOXP3 GFP mice and cultured in 96-well flat bottom plates with plate bound anti-CD3 (2 μg/ml) and soluble anti-CD28 (0.5 μg/ml) in the presence of Treg (TGF-β 2 ng/ml and IL-2 10 ng/ml) differentiation condition for 4 days. Butyrate and propionate (250 μM) were added in the culture at day 0. At day 4, cells were restimulated with with PMA (50 ng/ml), ionomycin (500 ng/ml), and brefeldin A (5 μg/ml) for 4 h at 37°C and 5% CO_2, and analyzed by flow cytometry **(A)**. The frequencies of FOXP3+ and/or IL-9+ CD4+ T cells **(B)** and FOXP3+ and/or IL-10+ CD4+ T cells **(C)** are represented by bar graphs. Data are shown as mean ± S.D. Linear regression, Two-way ANOVA and Tukey's multiple comparison test were used for statistical analysis. NS, not significant.

resuspended in R-10 medium for further analysis. Cells extracted from lungs were stimulated with PMA (Sigma) 50 ng/ml, ionomycin (Sigma) 500 ng/ml, and brefeldin A (Biolegend) 5 µg/ml for 4 h at 37°C and 5% CO_2. T cell surface staining was performed for 30 min at 4°C using the following antibodies diluted in PBS: anti-CD45 PercP (BD Biosciences), anti-CD4 APCCy7 (Biolegend) and anti-CD8 FITC (Biolegend). Cells were then fixed and permeabilized using the Cytofix/Cytoperm kit (BD Biosciences). Intracellular staining was performed for 30 min at 4°C with the following antibodies diluted in Perm/wash buffer (BD Biosciences): anti-CD3 APC (BD Biosciences), anti-IL-9 PE (Biolegend), and anti-IL-13 PECy7 (Biolegend). To evaluate lung-infiltrated Tregs, cells were surfaced stained for 30 min at 4°C using the following antibodies diluted in PBS: anti-CD45 PercP (BD Biosciences), anti-CD3 APC (BD Biosciences), and anti-CD4 APCCy7 (Biolegend). FOXP3 expression was determined using the FOXP3/Transcription Factor Staining Buffer Set (eBioscience) with anti-FOXP3 PE (Biolegend), according to the manufacturer's instruction. To evaluate lung-infiltrated eosinophils, cells were surfaced stained for 30 min at 4°C using the following antibodies diluted in PBS: anti-CD45 PercP (BD Biosciences), anti-CD11b APCCy7 (Biolegend), anti-CD11c BV421 (Biolegend), anti-CD64 PE (Biolegend), anti-Ly6G FITC (BD Biosciences), and anti-Siglec F Alexa 647 (BD Biosciences). All samples were acquired with a FACS Canto II (BD Biosciences) and analyzed using FlowJo software (version 9.0.2, Tree Star).

T Cell Differentiation

Splenocytes from FOXP3 GFP mice were surfaced stained for 30 min at 4°C using the following antibodies diluted in PBS: anti-CD4 PercP (BD Biosciences), anti-CD44 PECy7

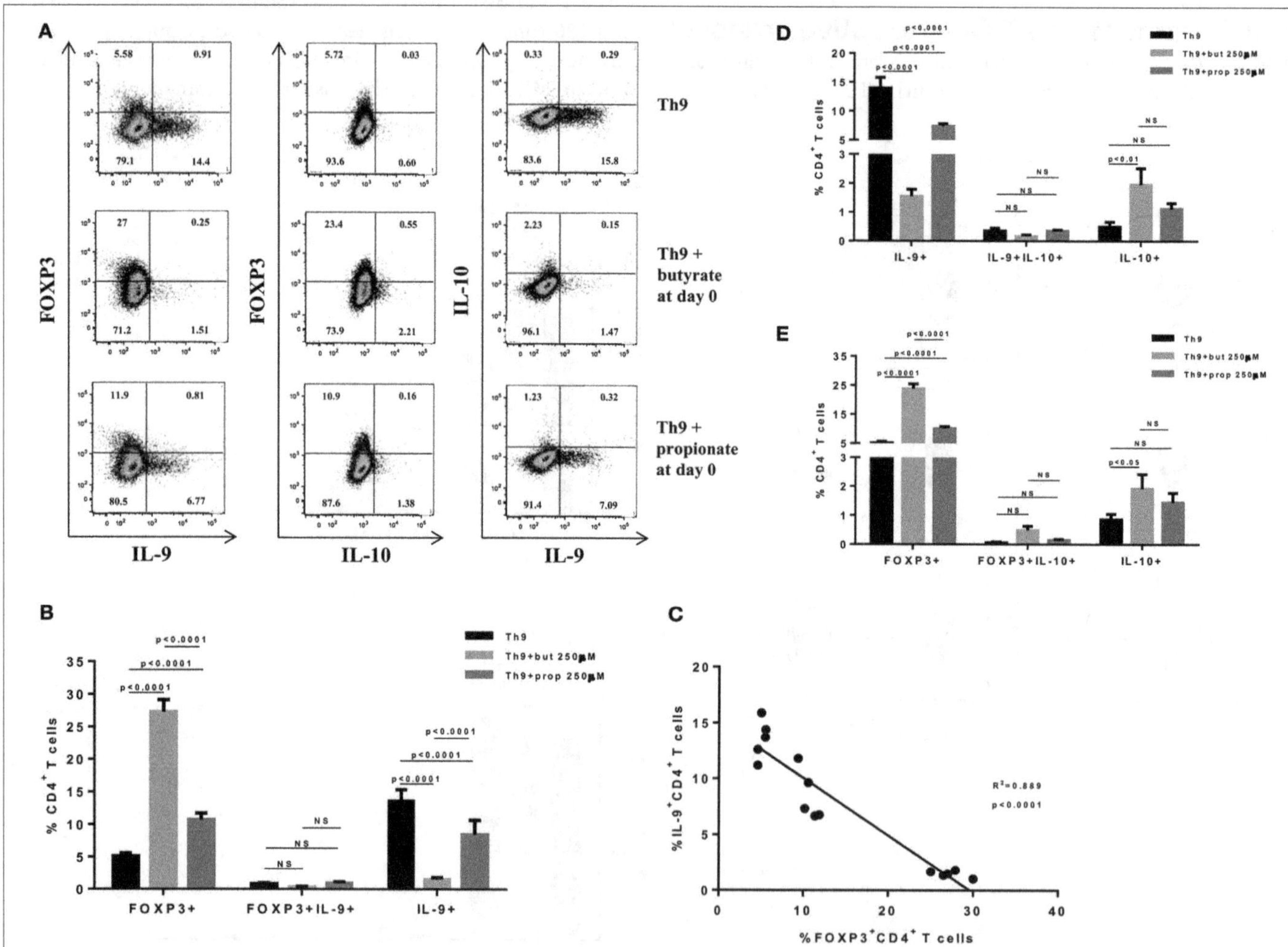

FIGURE 2 | Butyrate enhances FOXP3 expression in CD4+ T cells and impairs the differentiation of Th9 cells. Naïve CD4+ T cells (CD62L+CD44low) were sorted from spleens of FOXP3 GFP mice and cultured in 96-well flat bottom plates with plate bound anti-CD3 (2 µg/ml) and soluble anti-CD28 (0.5 µg/ml) in the presence of Th9 (TGF-β 2 ng/ml, IL-4 10 ng/ml and anti-IFNγ 10 µg/ml) differentiation condition for 4 days. Butyrate and propionate (250 µM) were added in the culture at day 0. At day 4, cells were restimulated with with PMA (50 ng/ml), ionomycin (500 ng/ml), and brefeldin A (5 µg/ml) for 4 h at 37°C and 5% CO_2, and analyzed by flow cytometry **(A)**. The frequencies of FOXP3+ and/or IL-9+ CD4+ T cells are represented by bar graphs **(B)**. A correlation analysis of IL-9 and FOXP3 expression was performed **(C)**. The frequencies of IL-9+ and/or IL-10+ CD4+ T cells **(D)** and FOXP3+ and/or IL-10+ CD4+ T cells **(E)** were determined and are represented by bar graphs. Data are shown as mean ± S.D. Two-way ANOVA and Tukey's multiple comparison test were used for statistical analysis. NS, not significant.

(Biolegend) and anti-CD62L APC (BD Biosciences). Naïve CD4+ T cells (CD62L+CD44^{low}) were sorted using a FACS Aria III (BD Biosciences) and cultured in R-10 medium in 96-well flat bottom plates (Sigma) with plate bound anti-CD3 (2 μg/ml) (BD Biosciences) and soluble anti-CD28 (0.5 μg/ml) (BD Biosciences) in the presence of Th9 [TGF-β 2 ng/ml (R&D Systems), IL-4 10 ng/ml (Peprotech) and anti-IFNγ 10 μg/ml (BD Biosciences)], Th2 [IL-4 10 ng/ml (Peprotech), anti-IL-12 10 μg/ml (BD Biosciences) and anti-IFNγ 10 μg/ml (BD Biosciences)] or Treg [TGF-β 2 ng/ml (R&D Systems) and IL-2 10 ng/ml (Peprotech)] differentiation conditions for 4 days. Butyric and propionic acids (Sigma) diluted in PBS (250 μM–pH: 7.2) were added in the culture at day 0. At day 4, cells were restimulated with PMA (50 ng/ml) (Sigma), ionomycin (500 ng/ml) (Sigma), and brefeldin A (5 μg/ml) (Biolegend) for 4 h at 37°C and 5% CO_2. Alternatively, naïve CD4+ T cells were incubated in the presence of Th9 differentiation condition for 4 days. The supernatants were removed and fresh R-10 medium added to the wells. The cells were incubated for additional 4 days in the presence or absence of butyric acid (Sigma) diluted in PBS (250 μM–pH: 7.2). At day 8, cells were restimulated with PMA (50 ng/ml) (Sigma), ionomycin (500 ng/ml) (Sigma), and brefeldin A (5 μg/ml) (Biolegend) for 4 h at 37°C and 5% CO_2. Cells were then fixed and permeabilized using the Cytofix/Cytoperm kit (BD Biosciences). Intracellular staining was performed for 30 min at 4°C with the following antibodies diluted in Perm/wash buffer (BD Biosciences). Th9 and Treg cells: anti-CD3 APCCy7 (BD Biosciences), anti-IL-9 PE (Biolegend), and anti-IL-10 PercPCy5.5 (Biolegend). Th2 cells: anti-CD3 APCCy7 (BD Biosciences), anti-IL-4 PE (Biolegend), anti-IL-5 APC (Biolegend) and anti-IL-13 PECy7 (Biolegend). Samples were acquired with a FACS Canto II (BD Biosciences) and analyzed using FlowJo software (version 9.0.2, Tree Star).

Histology

Extracted lungs were cut and the left inferior lobes were fixed in 2 ml of 4% buffered formalin at 4°C and embedded into

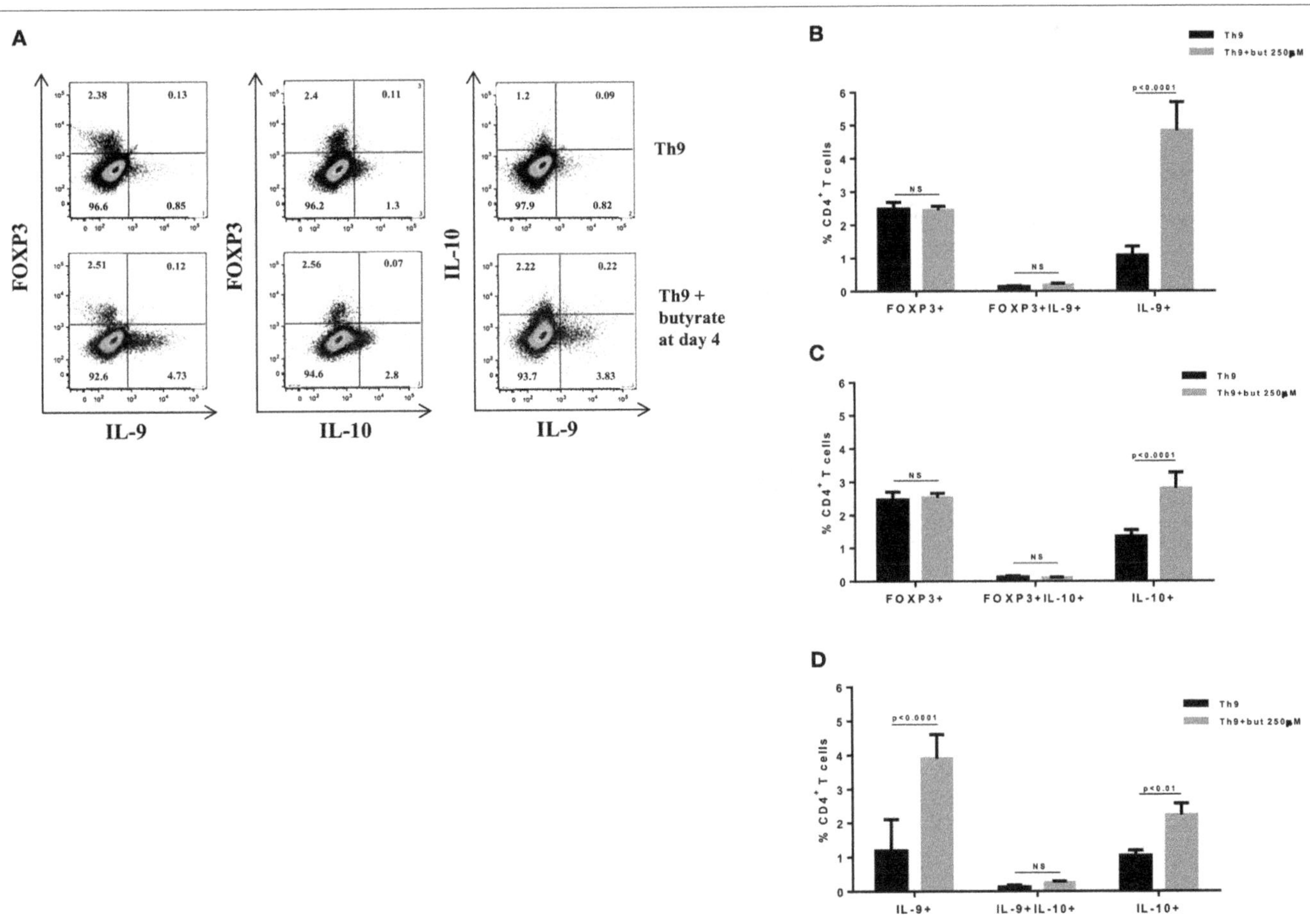

FIGURE 3 | Butyrate sustains cytokine production by differentiated Th9 cells. Naïve CD4+ T cells (CD62L+CD44low) were sorted from spleens of FOXP3 GFP mice and cultured in 96-well flat bottom plates with plate bound anti-CD3 (2 μg/ml) and soluble anti-CD28 (0.5 μg/ml) in the presence of Th9 (TGF-β 2 ng/ml, IL-4 10 ng/ml, and anti-IFNγ 10 μg/ml) differentiation condition for 4 days. At day 4, the medium was replaced by fresh R-10 and butyrate (250 μM) was added in the culture. At day 8, cells were restimulated with with PMA (50 ng/ml), ionomycin (500 ng/ml) and brefeldin A (5 μg/ml) for 4 h at 37°C and 5% CO_2, and analyzed by flow cytometry **(A)**. The frequencies of FOXP3+ and/or IL-9+ CD4+ T cells **(B)**, FOXP3+ and/or IL-10+ CD4+ T cells **(C)** and IL-9+ and/or IL-10+ CD4+ T cells **(D)** are represented by bar graphs. Data are shown as mean ± S.D. Two-way ANOVA and Sidak's multiple comparison test were used for statistical analysis. NS, not significant.

paraffin. Prepared sections (5 μm) were stained with either H&E or PAS reagents using standardized protocols and analyzed with an Eclipse Ti-E microscope (Nikon Instruments Inc.).

Statistical Analysis

Statistical analysis was carried out with Graph Pad Prism 6.0 Software. Two-way ANOVA followed by Dunnett's multiple comparison test or One-way ANOVA followed by Tukey's multiple comparison test were used for statistical analysis, depending on data comparisons. $P < 0.05$ was considered significant.

RESULTS

Butyrate Impairs Th9 Cell Differentiation

SCFAs directly modulate the differentiation of CD4+ T cells into Tregs by promoting FOXP3 expression (31), which has been shown to impair IL-9 production (33). Therefore, we first asked whether the SCFAs butyrate and propionate would have any impact on *in vitro* differentiation of Th9 cells. To address this question, naïve CD4+ T cells were sorted from spleens of FOXP3 GFP mice and differentiated into Th9 cells in the presence or absence of butyrate or propionate. Alternatively, naïve CD4+ T cells were differentiated into Tregs and Th2 cells, also in the presence or absence of butyrate or propionate. We confirmed previous data by showing that butyrate and propionate promote FOXP3 expression in the context of Treg differentiation. As expected, butyrate was found to be more efficient in promoting FOXP3 expression than propionate (**Figures 1A–C**). No significant impact on FOXP3+IL-9+ and FOXP3+IL-10+ T cells was observed (**Figures 1A–C**). We then demonstrated that butyrate added to the culture at day 0 significantly shifted the cellular differentiation from IL-9-expressing to FOXP3-expressing T cells, while propionate was

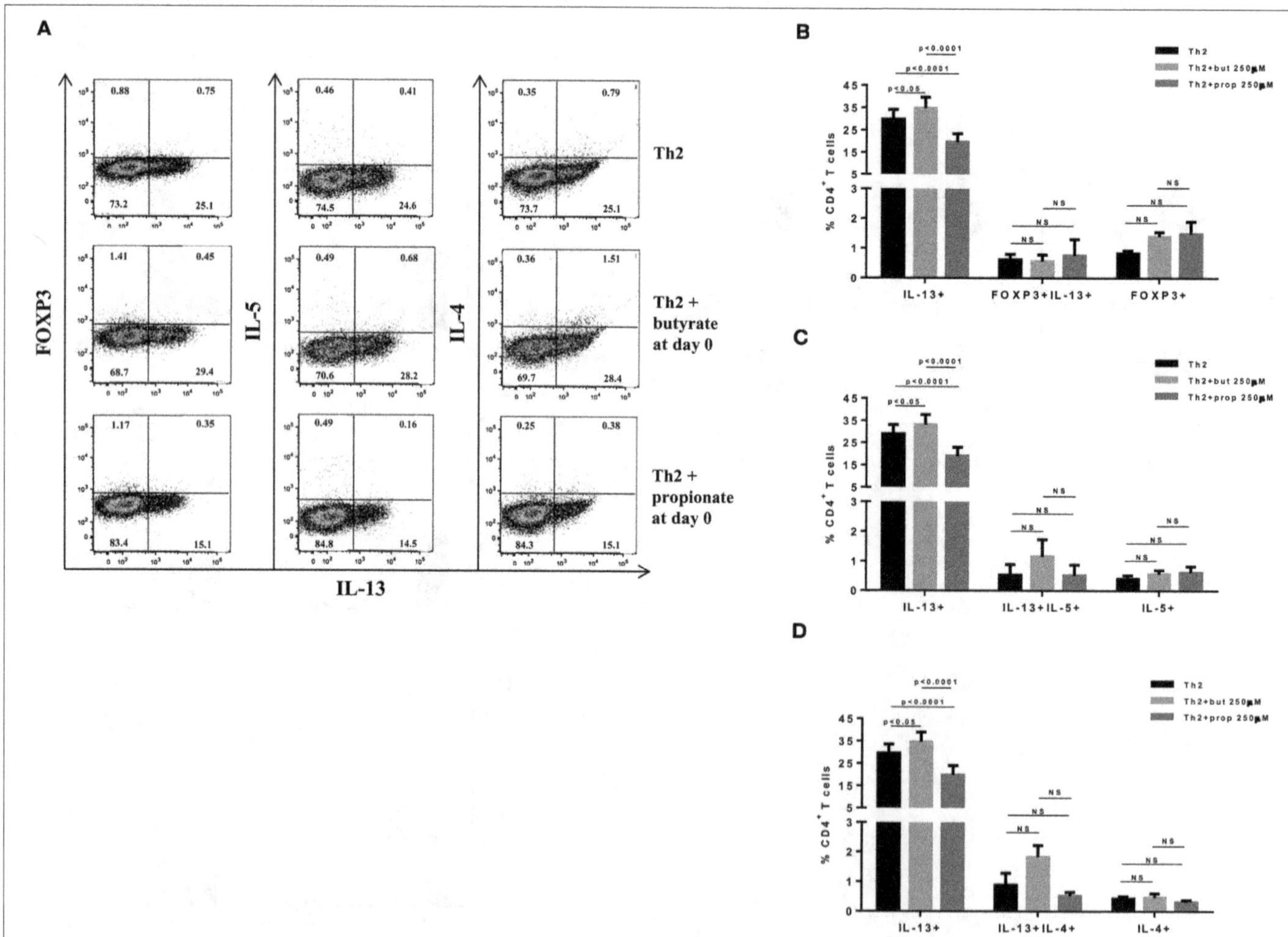

FIGURE 4 | SCFAs have opposite effects on IL-13-expressing T cells. Naïve CD4+ T cells (CD62L+CD44low) were sorted from spleens of FOXP3 GFP mice and cultured in 96-well flat bottom plates with plate bound anti-CD3 (2 μg/ml) and soluble anti-CD28 (0.5 μg/ml) in the presence of Th2 (IL-4 10 ng/ml, anti-IL-12 10 μg/ml, and anti-IFNγ 10 μg/ml) differentiation condition for 4 days. Butyrate and propionate (250 μM) were added in the culture at day 0. At day 4, cells were restimulated with with PMA (50 ng/ml), ionomycin (500 ng/ml), and brefeldin A (5 μg/ml) for 4 h at 37°C and 5% CO_2, and analyzed by flow cytometry **(A)**. The frequencies of FOXP3+ and/or IL-13+ CD4+ T cells **(B)**, IL-13+ and/or IL-5+ CD4+ T cells **(C)** and IL-13+ and/or IL-4+ CD4+ T cells **(D)** are represented by bar graphs. Data are shown as mean ± S.D. Two-way ANOVA and Tukey's multiple comparison test were used for statistical analysis. NS, not significant.

less effective in promoting the same shift (**Figures 2A,B**). We found an inverse correlation between IL-9 and FOXP3 expression when all groups were analyzed together (**Figure 2C**). We also evaluated the impact of butyrate and propionate on IL-10 expression and observed that butyrate treatment resulted in a significantly higher frequency of IL-10-expressing T cells, while IL-10+FOXP3+ and IL-10+IL-9+ T cells were not affected (**Figures 2D,E**). To further characterize the impact of butyrate on IL-9, IL-10, and FOXP3, we differentiated Th9 cells for 4 days and incubated them for additional 4 days in the presence or absence of butyrate. We found that butyrate treatment had no effect on FOXP3 expression when cells were already differentiated (**Figures 3A–C**). Most Th9 cells were not expressing IL-9 after 8 days of culture. However, we observed a less intense decrease in the frequency of IL-9-expressing T cells when differentiated Th9 cells were treated with butyrate (**Figures 3A,B**). No differences were found in FOXP3+IL-9+, FOXP3+IL-10+ and IL-9+IL-10+ T cells (**Figures 3B–D**). In addition, we demonstrated an opposite effect of butyrate and propionate on Th2 cells. While butyrate was responsible for inducing a small, but significant increase in the frequency of IL-13+ T cells, propionate treatment negatively impacted the same cells. In contrast to Th9 cells, no significant impact on FOXP3 expression was observed in the context of Th2 differentiation (**Figures 4A,B**). We also evaluated the impact of butyrate and propionate on the frequency of IL-4 and IL-5-expressing T cells and found no significant differences upon treatment (**Figures 4C,D**). Together, our results demonstrate that

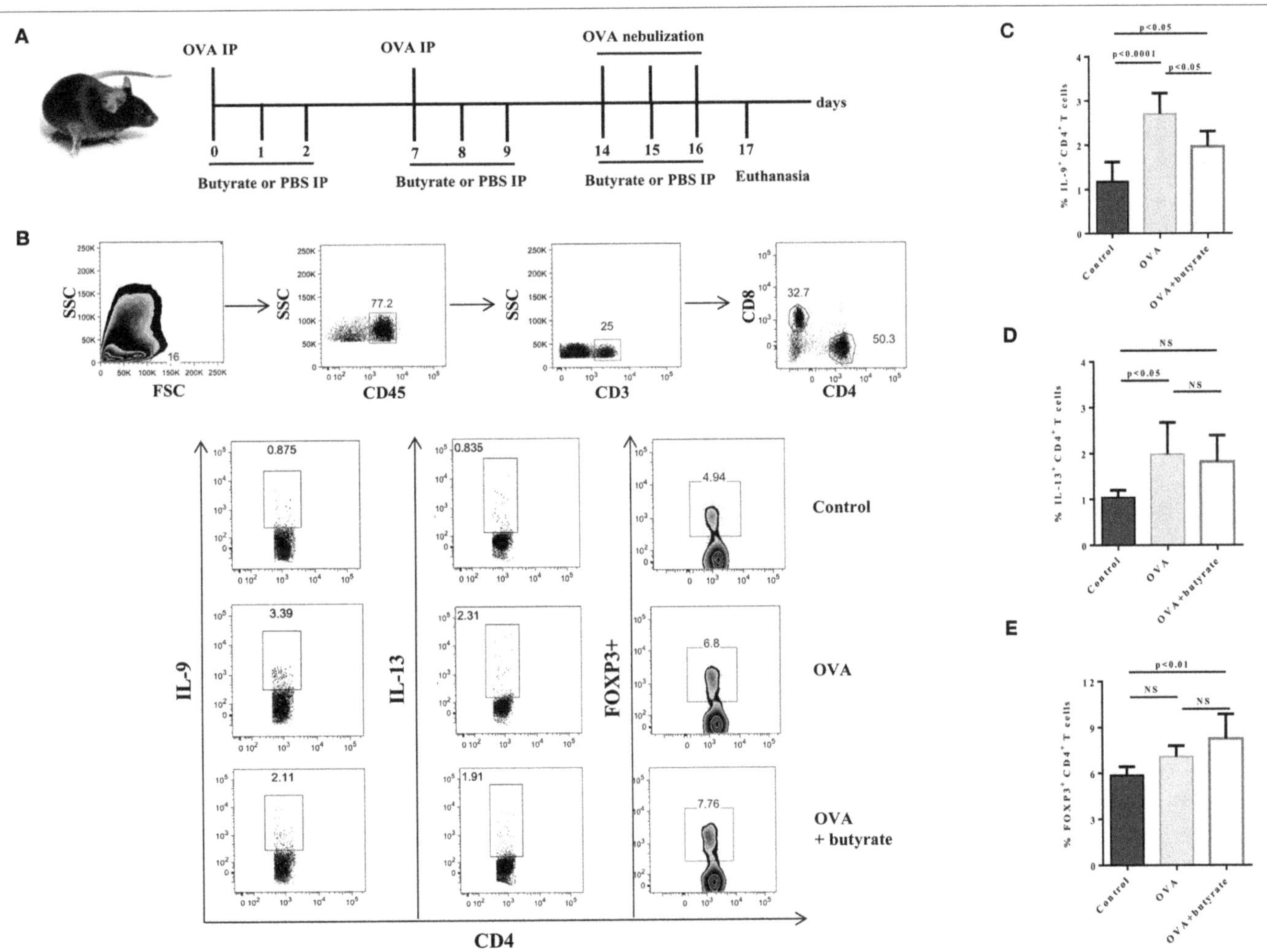

FIGURE 5 | Butyrate treatment negatively impact Th9 cells in the lungs of OVA-challenged mice. Male C57BL/6 mice were intraperitoneally (IP) injected with OVA (30 μg) + Al(OH)3 (1.6 mg) at days 0 and 7. Mice also received 250 μl of either PBS or butyrate (1M) (IP) at days 0, 1, 2, 7, 8, and 9. OVA-sensitized mice were nebulized with an OVA solution (3%) for 15 min at days 14, 15, and 16. The group that received butyrate during sensitization was also treated during challenge. A control group was sensitized and challenged without OVA. Euthanasia was performed 24 h after the last challenge **(A)**. Lungs were digested, cells stimulated with PMA (50 ng/ml), ionomycin (500 ng/ml) and brefeldin A (5 μg/ml) for 4 h at 37°C and 5% CO_2, and stained with monoclonal antibodies to determine the frequencies of IL-9+, IL-13+, and FOXP3+ CD4+ T cells by flow cytometry **(B)**. Bar graphs show the frequencies of IL-9+ **(C)**, IL-13+ **(D)** and FOXP3+ **(E)** CD4+ T cells in the different groups. Data are shown as mean ± SD. One-way ANOVA followed by Tukey's multiple comparison test were used for statistical analysis. n = 5–7 mice per group. NS, not significant.

butyrate and propionate differently modulate the differentiation of Th9, Th2, and Tregs.

Butyrate Treatment Negatively Impacts Th9 Cells and Attenuates Lung Inflammation

Given the *in vitro* effect of butyrate on Th9 cells, we next sought to determine whether it would also have an *in vivo* impact on these cells. To address this question, we induced OVA-mediated lung inflammation in C57BL/6 mice treated or not with butyrate (**Figure 5A**) and evaluated the frequencies of lung-infiltrated Th9, Th2, and Treg cells by flow cytometry (**Figure 5B**). We found that butyrate-treated animals presented a significantly lower frequency of lung-infiltrated Th9 cells (**Figure 5C**) while no difference was observed for IL-13-expressing Th2 cells (**Figure 5D**). Butyrate-treated OVA-challenged mice had significantly higher lung-infiltrated Treg cells when compared to control, but no statistical significance was found when compared to OVA-challenged mice (**Figure 5E**). Considering the pre-established role of IL-9 in promoting the recruitment of eosinophils to the lungs and supporting inflammation (34), we further analyzed animal lungs for the presence of eosinophils (CD45+CD64-Ly6G-CD11b+Siglec-F+CD11c-) (**Figure 6A**) and found a significantly higher frequency of these cells infiltrated in the lungs of OVA-challenged mice when compared to both control and butyrate-treated OVA-challenged mice (**Figure 6B**). Higher inflammation and mucus production were also observed in OVA-challenged mice when compared to the other groups (**Figure 6C**). Therefore, our results indicate that butyrate may protect mice from

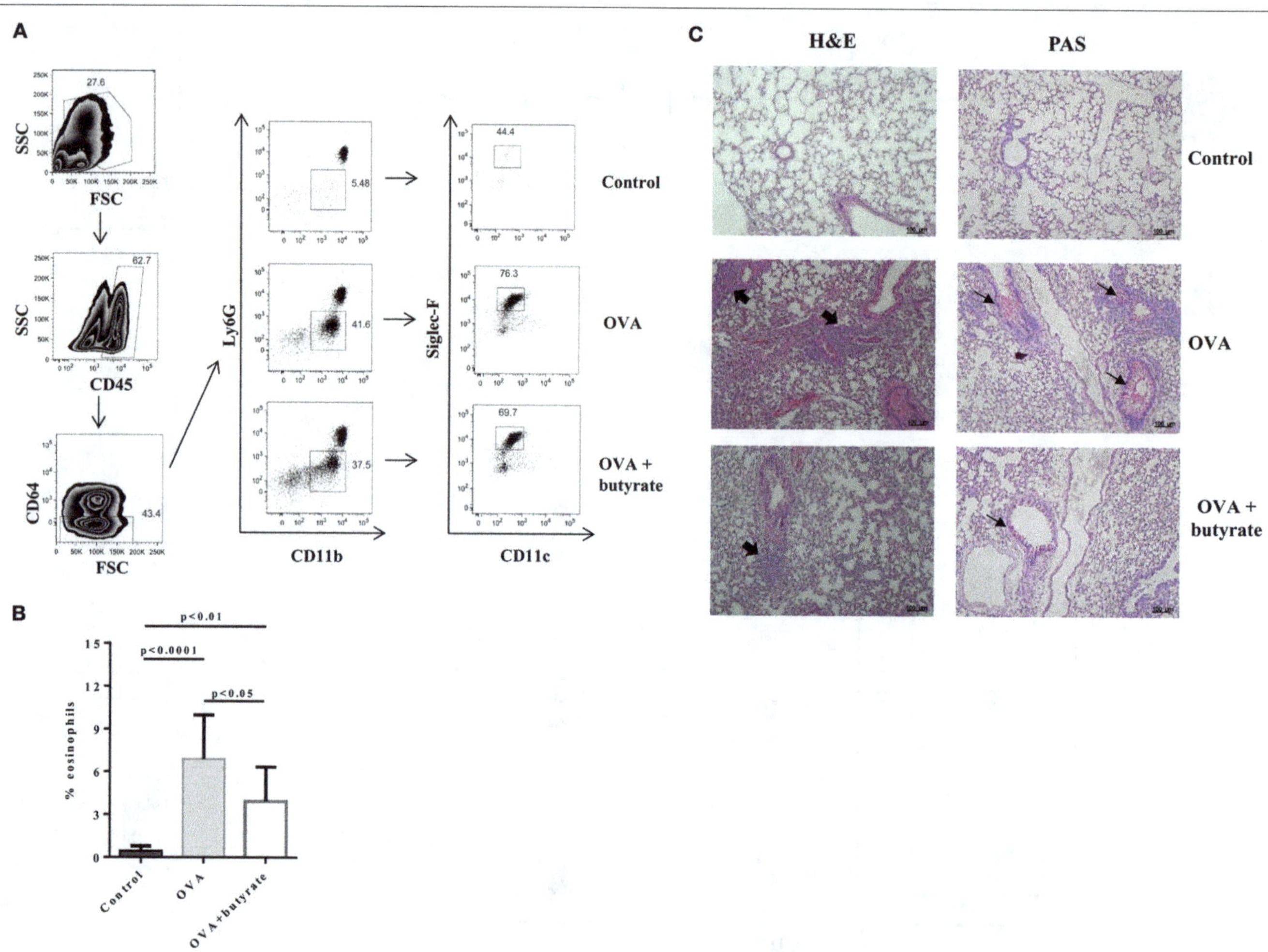

FIGURE 6 | Butyrate treatment protects OVA-challenged mice from lung inflammation. Male C57BL/6 mice were intraperitoneally (IP) injected with OVA (30 μg) + Al(OH)3 (1.6 mg) at days 0 and 7. Mice also received 250 μl of either PBS or butyrate (1 M) (IP) at days 0, 1, 2, 7, 8, and 9. OVA-sensitized mice were nebulized with an OVA solution (3%) for 15 min at days 14, 15, and 16. The group that received butyrate during sensitization was also treated during challenge. A control group was sensitized and challenged without OVA. Euthanasia was performed 24 h after the last challenge. Lungs were digested and cells stained with monoclonal antibodies to determine the frequency of eosinophils (CD45+CD64-Ly6G-CD11b+Siglec-F+CD11c-) by flow cytometry **(A)**. Bar graph shows the frequency of eosinophils in the different groups **(B)**. Lung tissues were also stained with hematoxylin/eosin (H&E) and periodic acid–Schiff (PAS), scale bars: 100 μm. Thick and thin arrows indicate inflammatory infiltrates and mucus production, respectively **(C)**. Data are shown as mean ± SD. One-way ANOVA followed by Tukey's multiple comparison test were used for statistical analysis. $n = 5$–7 mice per group.

lung inflammation by impairing the differentiation of Th9 cells.

Adoptive Transfer of Th9 Cells Reverses Butyrate Effects on Lung Inflammation

To confirm that butyrate treatment protected mice from lung inflammation by negatively modulating the differentiation of Th9 cells, we performed OVA-challenge experiments as previously described, in which butyrate-treated mice also received an adoptive transfer of either naïve OT-II Th0 cells or *in vitro*-differentiated OT-II Th2 or Th9 cells one day before initiating OVA-challenge (**Figure 7A**). We observed that adoptive transfer of Th9 cells restored the frequency of lung-infiltrated eosinophils in butyrate-treated OVA-challenged mice to the same level of mice not treated with butyrate (**Figure 7B**). Th2 adoptive transfer resulted in a higher frequency of lung-infiltrated eosinophils, although it was not statistically significant (**Figure 7B**). We also demonstrated that the frequency of lung-infiltrated Th9 cells was restored in animals that received these cells (**Figure 7C**). Th2 adoptive transfer resulted in a small increase in the frequency of these cells into the lungs of butyrate-treated OVA-challenged mice (**Figure 7D**). Lung inflammation and mucus production were also higher in animals that received adoptive transfer of Th9 cells, and in a lesser extent in those that received Th2 cells, when compared to butyrate-treated Th0-injected mice (**Figure 7E**). Taken together, these results reinforce our hypothesis that butyrate treatment attenuates lung inflammation by negatively modulating Th9 cells.

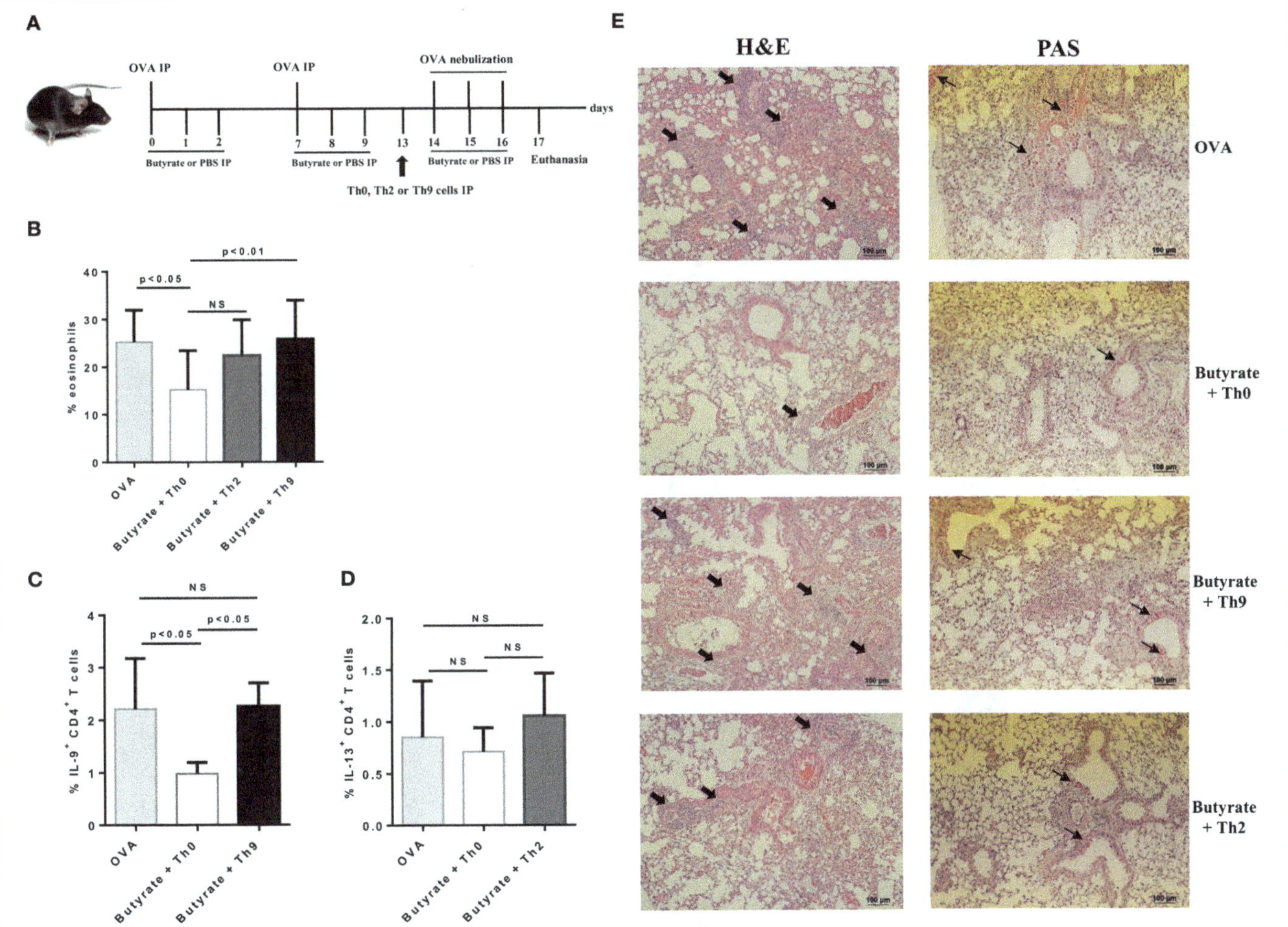

FIGURE 7 | Adoptive transfer of Th9 cells restores lung inflammation in butyrate-treated OVA-challenged mice. Male C57BL/6 mice were intraperitoneally (IP) injected with OVA (30 μg) + Al(OH)3 (1.6 mg) at days 0 and 7. Mice also received 250 μl of either PBS or butyrate (1 M) (IP) at days 0, 1, 2, 7, 8, and 9. OVA-sensitized mice were nebulized with an OVA solution (3%) for 15 min at days 14, 15, and 16. The groups that received butyrate during sensitization were treated during challenge. Butyrate-treated mice also received an adoptive transfer (IP) of OT-II Th0, Th2, or Th9 cells 24 h before challenge initiation. Euthanasia was performed 24 h after the last challenge **(A)**. Lungs were digested and cells stained with monoclonal antibodies to determine the frequency of eosinophils as shown by the bar graph **(B)**. Alternatively, cells were stimulated with PMA (50 ng/ml), ionomycin (500 ng/ml), and brefeldin A (5 μg/ml) for 4 h at 37°C and 5% CO_2, and stained with monoclonal antibodies to determine the frequency of IL-9+CD4+ and IL-13+CD4+ T cells as shown by the bar graphs **(C,D)**, respectively. Lung tissues were also stained with hematoxylin/eosin (H&E) and periodic acid–Schiff (PAS), scale bars: 100 μm. Thick and thin arrows indicate inflammatory infiltrates and mucus production, respectively **(E)**. Data are shown as mean ± SD. One-way ANOVA followed by Tukey's multiple comparison test were used for statistical analysis. $n = 5$–7 mice per group. NS, not significant.

IL-9 Treatment Counteracts Butyrate Effects on Lung Inflammation

To address the question whether butyrate treatment was attenuating lung inflammation by decreasing IL-9 effects, we performed OVA-challenge experiments as previously described, but including a new group of butyrate-treated mice that also received recombinant IL-9 (**Figure 8A**). We demonstrated that intraperitoneal treatment with IL-9 during OVA-challenge was sufficient to restore the frequency of lung-infiltrated eosinophils in butyrate-treated mice to a similar level of OVA-challenged mice (**Figure 8B**). We also observed that IL-9 treatment promoted higher inflammation and mucus production in butyrate-treated mice when compared to animals not treated with IL-9 (**Figure 8C**). We then looked at the frequencies of lung-infiltrated Th9, Th2, and Treg cells and found that IL-9 treatment had no effect on these cells (**Figures 9A–C**, respectively). Thus, these results indicate that butyrate may exert an anti-inflammatory impact on OVA-challenged mice by reducing IL-9 effects.

DISCUSSION

In this study, we demonstrate that butyrate is more effective than propionate in promoting FOXP3 expression and IL-9 repression. In addition, we show that propionate negatively impact *in vitro* differentiation of IL-13-expressing T cells. Butyrate treatment attenuated lung inflammation and mucus production in OVA-challenged mice, which presented lower frequency of lung-infiltrated Th9 cells and eosinophils. Both Th9 cell adoptive transfer and IL-9 treatment restored lung inflammation in

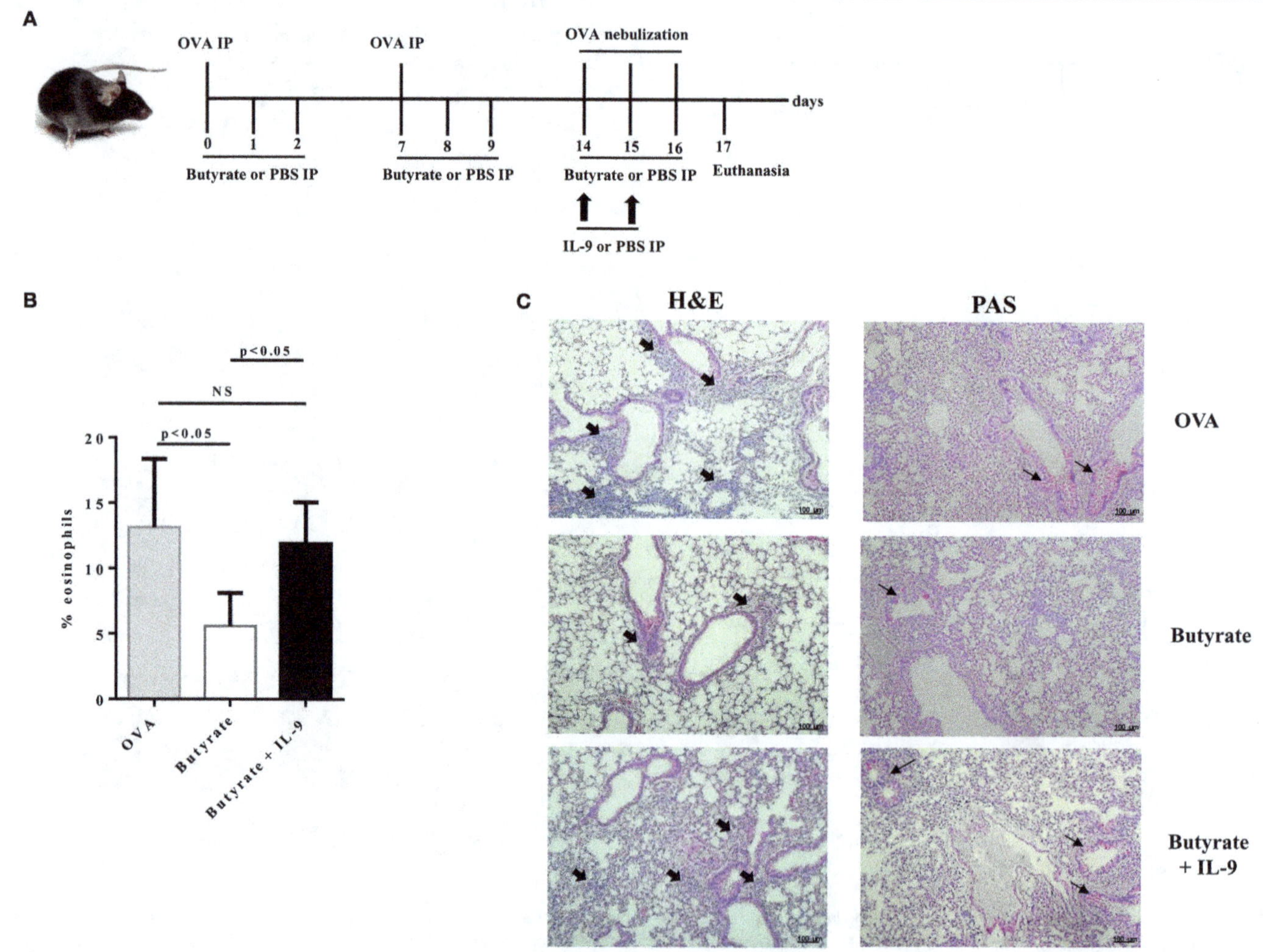

FIGURE 8 | IL-9 treatment restores lung inflammation in butyrate-treated OVA-challenged mice. Male C57BL/6 mice were intraperitoneally (IP) injected with OVA (30 μg) + Al(OH)3 (1.6 mg) at days 0 and 7. Mice also received 250 μl of either PBS or butyrate (1M) (IP) at days 0, 1, 2, 7, 8, and 9. OVA-sensitized mice were nebulized with an OVA solution (3%) for 15 min at days 14, 15, and 16. The groups that received butyrate during sensitization were also treated during challenge. Butyrate-treated mice also received either PBS or recombinant IL-9 (IP) at days 14 and 15. Euthanasia was performed 24 h after the last challenge **(A)**. Lungs were digested and cells stained with monoclonal antibodies to determine the frequency of eosinophils as shown by the bar graph **(B)**. Lung tissues were also stained with hematoxylin/eosin (H&E) and periodic acid–Schiff (PAS), scale bars: 100 μm. Thick and thin arrows indicate inflammatory infiltrates and mucus production, respectively **(C)**. Data are shown as mean ± SD. One-way ANOVA followed by Tukey's multiple comparison test were used for statistical analysis. $n = 5–7$ mice per group. NS, not significant.

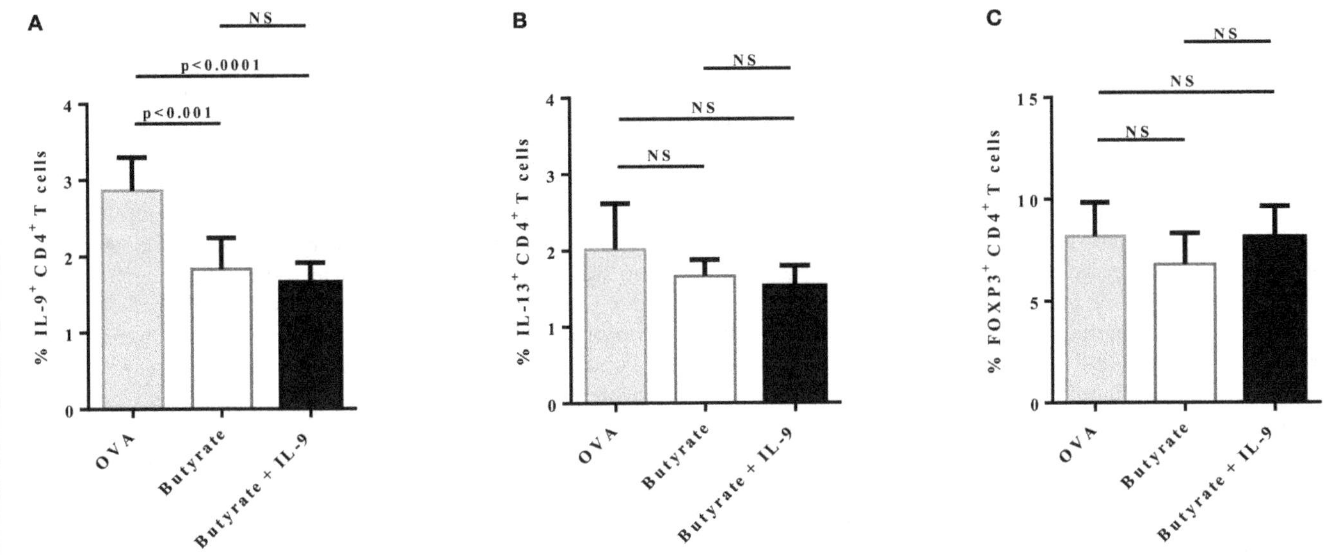

FIGURE 9 | IL-9 treatment has no impact on IL-9+, IL-13+, and FOXP3+ CD4+ T cells in the lungs of butyrate-treated OVA-challenged mice. Male C57BL/6 mice were intraperitoneally (IP) injected with OVA (30 μg) + Al(OH)3 (1.6 mg) at days 0 and 7. Mice also received 250 μl of either PBS or butyrate (1 M) (IP) at days 0, 1, 2, 7, 8, and 9. OVA-sensitized mice were nebulized with an OVA solution (3%) for 15 min at days 14, 15, and 16. The groups that received butyrate during sensitization were also treated during challenge. Butyrate-treated mice also received either PBS or recombinant IL-9 (IP) at days 14 and 15. Euthanasia was performed 24 h after the last challenge. Lungs were digested, cells stimulated with PMA (50 ng/ml), ionomycin (500 ng/ml), and brefeldin A (5 μg/ml) for 4 h at 37°C and 5% CO_2, and stained with monoclonal antibodies to determine the frequencies of IL-9+ **(A)**, IL-13+ **(B)**, and FOXP3+ **(C)** CD4+ T cells in the different groups. Data are shown as mean ± SD. One-way ANOVA followed by Tukey's multiple comparison test were used for statistical analysis. $n = 5–7$ mice per group. NS, not significant.

butyrate-treated OVA-challenged mice, indicating that the anti-inflammatory effects of butyrate may rely on suppressing Th9-mediated immune responses.

Given the increasing evidence that microbiota-derived metabolites contribute to modulating inflammatory diseases such as asthma, colitis and arthritis (29, 30, 35–37), we sought to evaluate whether the SCFAs butyrate and propionate would have an impact on the differentiation of Th9 cells, key players in inflammation (3). We demonstrated that butyrate added to the culture at day 0 significantly shifted the cellular differentiation from IL-9-expressing to FOXP3-expressing T cells, while propionate was less effective in promoting the same shift. A strong inverse correlation between IL-9 and FOXP3 expression was found when all groups were analyzed together. Additional analysis showed that butyrate treatment led to higher frequency of IL-10-expressing T cells that were not expressing either FOXP3 or IL-9. Although we cannot assume that the cells generated by the exposition to butyrate or propionate under Th9 differentiation were converted to induced regulatory T cells (iTregs), we were still able to demonstrate the negative impact of these SCFAs on Th9 cells.

To further characterize the impacts of butyrate on Th9 cells, we treated differentiated cells and found no impact on FOXP3 expression. We found that most Th9 cells were not expressing IL-9 after 8 days of culture, when compared to cells stimulated with PMA after 4 days of differentiation. Surprisingly, we observed a less intense decrease in the frequency of IL-9-expressing T cells when differentiated Th9 cells were treated with butyrate, suggesting that this SCFA may have opposite effects on naïve CD4+ T cells and differentiated Th9 cells. A higher frequency of IL-10-expressing T cells was also found when differentiated Th9 cells were exposed to butyrate. A recent study demonstrated that butyrate promotes IL-10 expression by differentiated Th1 cells through interaction with the GPR43 receptor (38), supporting our findings. Although we also observed higher frequency of IL-9-expressing T cells when Th9 cells were treated with butyrate, no impact on IFN-γ-expressing T cells was demonstrated in the previous report, suggesting that the effector cytokines produced by Th9 and Th1 cells are differentially affected by butyrate.

The effects of butyrate and other SCFAs on FOXP3 expression in CD4+ T cells differentiated into iTregs have been previously demonstrated (31, 32), as we have also shown here. It is known that Th9 cells and iTregs share key transcription factors and common induction pathways that may determine the generation of one over the other subset. While GITR engagement was shown to subvert iTregs differentiation by favoring Th9 cells, FOXP3-mediated repression of the *Il9* locus contributed to blocking the differentiation of Th9 cells (33). Therefore, we believe that the negative impact of butyrate on Th9 cells are likely to be dependent on FOXP3-mediated repression of IL-9 early during differentiation, as we have not found the same effect when exposing differentiated cells to butyrate. This SCFA could also be acting through epigenetic remodeling of the *Il9* locus (39) or by breaking down signal pathways involved in IL-9 expression. Studies with FOXP3-deficient cells could be performed to further confirm the role of FOXP3 in mediating butyrate-induced IL-9 repression.

To further investigate the effects of butyrate on Th9 cells, we established an OVA-induced lung inflammation model and demonstrated that butyrate treatment resulted in lower frequency of lung-infiltrated Th9 cells, while no impact on Th2 cells was observed. Higher frequency of lung-infiltrated FOXP3+ T cells was found in butyrate-treated OVA-challenged mice when compared to control animals, but no significant differences were found when compared to OVA-challenged mice. Acetate-mediated protection against house dust mite extract (HDM)-induced lung inflammation has been previously reported, indicating that SCFAs may act through induction of iTregs to inhibit inflammation. However, a 3 week-treatment period was necessary for the observed results (30). In our experiments, animals were treated for a much shorter period, which could explain the lack of significant difference in terms of lung-infiltrated FOXP3+ T cells between OVA-challenged groups. As regulatory T cells naturally migrate to inflamed tissues to suppress inflammation (40), it is possible that butyrate-mediated induction of iTregs was masked in OVA-challenged mice due to the increased influx of these cells into the lungs, independently of their origin. On the other hand, iTregs generated in the gut upon intraperitoneal butyrate treatment may have not appropriately responded to the lung OVA challenge, resulting in less lung infiltration than expected. The *in vivo* instability of iTregs (41) could also be an explanation for not having a significant increase in lung infiltration upon butyrate treatment. These cells may have lost FOXP3 expression during the sensitization period. Therefore, it is unlikely that induction of iTregs played a major role in our study, although our *in vitro* experiments suggest an inverse correlation of FOXP3 and IL-9 expression upon treatment with SCFAs.

Lung-infiltrated eosinophils were used as a parameter to evaluate Th9-mediated immune responses in our model, given the well-established role of IL-9 in promoting eotaxin/CCL11 expression and influx of these cells into different body tissues, including lungs (34, 42, 43). We found that butyrate-treated OVA-challenged mice presented lower frequency of lung-infiltrated eosinophils, attenuated inflammatory infiltrates and mucus production, indicating that Th9-mediated immune responses were suppressed. In line with our observations, a previous study has demonstrated that dietary fiber and the SCFA propionate protected mice from lung inflammation and asthma symptoms. However, the effects of propionate relied on promoting dendritic cells with impaired capability of inducing effector Th2 cells in an HDM-mediated model. Significant differences in the immunological parameters of propionate-treated mice were observed 5–6 days after the last challenge (29). In our study, we have found a more acute effect of butyrate, with significant differences 24 h after the last challenge, suggesting that these SCFAs may have different impacts on the immune system in the context of lung inflammation.

Although we have demonstrated that *in vitro* butyrate treatment induced a small, but significant increase in the frequency of IL-13-expressing T cells, no *in vivo* effects on these cells were observed, indicating that Th9-mediated immune responses were likely to be the most affected in our model. As we have not found a significant *in vitro* impact of butyrate on the frequency of IL-4 and IL-5-expressing T cells, these cytokines were not evaluated in our *in vivo* experiments. However, to further characterize the effects of SCFAs on Th2 cells, we also treated naïve CD4+ T cells with propionate and demonstrated that it partially impaired the differentiation of IL-13-expressig T cells while not affecting IL-4 and IL-5. We understand that more studies are still necessary to unveil the mechanisms involved in this phenomenon, but conceive that our results complement the previous report on the impact of propionate on Th2 cells.

To confirm that butyrate was attenuating lung inflammation by suppressing Th9 cells, we performed either adoptive transfer of OVA-specific OT-II Th9 cells or recombinant IL-9 treatment and found that both strategies were sufficient to restore lung inflammation in butyrate-treated OVA-challenged mice. Adoptive transfer of OT-II Th2 cells also increased lung inflammation, but to a lesser extent than that observed with Th9 transfer. Although it has been shown that IL-9 may promote IL-13-mediated lung inflammation and mucus production (20), we found no difference in the frequency of lung-infiltrated IL-13-expressing Th2 cells in IL-9-treated mice, suggesting that other cells may have mediated the inflammatory process. In fact, type II innate lymphoid cells (ILC2) are known to produce IL-13 and to play a role in experimental and clinical asthma pathology (44, 45). A synergistically effect of ILC2 and Th9 cells in lung inflammation has also been described (46, 47), suggesting that ILC2 may have a role in our model. On the other hand, our results could be partially explained by the fact that IL-9 exerts a direct effect on lung epithelial cells and promotes mucus production (48). We cannot rule out the possibility that butyrate directly impacted ILC2 and even other cell populations, as recently reported (49). However, our data strongly suggest that Th9/IL-9 played a major role in our model. Further studies are still necessary to mechanistically confirm our hypothesis.

Our findings bring new insights on the mechanisms by which microbiota-derived metabolites regulate diseases, suggesting that butyrate attenuates lung inflammation most likely through a negative modulation of Th9 cell-mediated immune responses. Therefore, butyrate should be clinically considered in the treatment of inflammatory diseases in which suppression of Th9 cells is necessary.

AUTHOR CONTRIBUTIONS

RA and RV conceived and designed the experiments. RV, AC, and PB performed and analyzed experiments. RA and RV prepared figures and wrote the manuscript. RA and NC performed final review of the manuscript. NC provided structure and reagents. All authors read and approved the final article.

FUNDING

This research was supported by Fundação de Amparo à Pesquisa do Estado de São Paulo (FAPESP 2017/02564-7), Conselho Nacional de Desenvolvimento Científico e Tecnológico (CNPq) and Coordenação de Aperfeiçoamento de Pessoal de Nível Superior (CAPES). RA, RV, AC, and PB are recipients of FAPESP scholarships: 2015/13817-0, 2016/03532-1, 2017/00721-0 and 2015/26682-6, respectively.

ACKNOWLEDGMENTS

We would like to thank the animal facility of the Biomedical Science Institute for proving all animals used in this study, and Paulo Albe for experimental support. We also thank Centro de Facilidades de Apoio à Pesquisa (CEFAP-USP) for flow cytometry support.

REFERENCES

1. DuPage M, Bluestone JA. Harnessing the plasticity of CD4(+) T cells to treat immune-mediated disease. *Nat Rev Immunol.* (2016) 16:149–63. doi: 10.1038/nri.2015.18
2. Lloyd CM, Hessel EM. Functions of T cells in asthma: more than just T(H)2 cells. *Nat Rev Immunol.* (2010) 10:838–48. doi: 10.1038/nri2870
3. Kaplan MH, Hufford MM, Olson MR. The development and *in vivo* function of T helper 9 cells. *Nat Rev Immunol.* (2015) 15:295–307. doi: 10.1038/nri3824
4. Chang HC, Sehra S, Goswami R, Yao W, Yu Q, Stritesky GL, et al. The transcription factor PU.1 is required for the development of IL-9-producing T cells and allergic inflammation. *Nat Immunol.* (2010) 11:527–34. doi: 10.1038/ni.1867
5. Goswami R, Jabeen R, Yagi R, Duy P, Zhu J, Goenka S, et al. STAT6-dependent regulation of Th9 development. *J Immunol.* (2012) 188:968–75. doi: 10.4049/jimmunol.1102840
6. Jabeen R, Goswami R, Awe O, Kulkarni A, Nguyen ET, Attenasio A, et al. Th9 cell development requires a BATF-regulated transcriptional network. *J Clin Invest.* (2013) 123:4641–53. doi: 10.1172/JCI 69489
7. Malik S, Sadhu S, Elesela S, Pandey RP, Chawla AS, Sharma D, et al. Transcription factor Foxo1 is essential for IL-9 induction in T helper cells. *Nat Commun.* (2017) 8:815. doi: 10.1038/s41467-017-00674-6
8. Staudt V, Bothur E, Klein M, Lingnau K, Reuter S, Grebe N, et al. Interferon-regulatory factor 4 is essential for the developmental program of T helper 9 cells. *Immunity* (2010) 33:192–202. doi: 10.1016/j.immuni.2010.07.014
9. Licona-Limon P, Henao-Mejia J, Temann AU, Gagliani N, Licona-Limon I, Ishigame H, et al. Th9 cells drive host immunity against gastrointestinal worm infection. *Immunity* (2013) 39:744–57. doi: 10.1016/j.immuni.2013.07.020
10. Turner JE, Morrison PJ, Wilhelm C, Wilson M, Ahlfors H, Renauld JC, et al. IL-9-mediated survival of type 2 innate lymphoid cells promotes damage control in helminth-induced lung inflammation. *J Exp Med.* (2013) 210:2951–65. doi: 10.1084/jem.20130071
11. Lu Y, Hong S, Li H, Park J, Hong B, Wang L, et al. Th9 cells promote antitumor immune responses *in vivo*. *J Clin Invest.* (2012) 122:4160–71. doi: 10.1172/JCI65459
12. Purwar R, Schlapbach C, Xiao S, Kang HS, Elyaman W, Jiang X, et al. Robust tumor immunity to melanoma mediated by interleukin-9-producing T cells. *Nat Med.* (2012) 18:1248–53. doi: 10.1038/nm.2856
13. Gerlach K, Hwang YY, Nikolaev A, Atreya R, Dornhoff H, Steiner S, et al. T(H)9 cells that express the transcription factor PU.1 drive T cell-mediated colitis via IL-9 receptor signaling in intestinal epithelial cells. *Nat Immunol.* (2014) 15:676–86. doi: 10.1038/ni.2920
14. Ciccia F, Guggino G, Rizzo A, Manzo A, Vitolo B, La Manna MP, et al. Potential involvement of IL-9 and Th9 cells in the pathogenesis of rheumatoid arthritis. *Rheumatology* (2015) 54:2264–72. doi: 10.1093/rheumatology/kev252
15. Jones CP, Gregory LG, Causton B, Campbell GA, Lloyd CM. Activin A and TGF-beta promote T(H)9 cell-mediated pulmonary allergic pathology. *J Allergy Clin Immunol.* (2012) 129:1000–10.e3. doi: 10.1016/j.jaci.2011.12.965
16. Jia L, Wang Y, Li JP, Li S, Zhang YN, Shen J, et al. Detection of IL-9 producing T cells in the PBMCs of allergic asthmatic patients. *BMC Immunol.* (2017) 18:38. doi: 10.1186/s12865-017-0220-1
17. Namkung JH, Lee JE, Kim E, Park GT, Yang HS, Jang HY, et al. An association between IL-9 and IL-9 receptor gene polymorphisms and atopic dermatitis in a Korean population. *J Dermatol Sci.* (2011) 62:16–21. doi: 10.1016/j.jdermsci.2011.01.007
18. Koch S, Sopel N, Finotto S. Th9 and other IL-9-producing cells in allergic asthma. *Semin Immunopathol.* (2017) 39:55–68. doi: 10.1007/s00281-016-0601-1
19. Temann UA, Geba GP, Rankin JA, Flavell RA. Expression of interleukin 9 in the lungs of transgenic mice causes airway inflammation, mast cell hyperplasia, and bronchial hyperresponsiveness. *J Exp Med.* (1998) 188:1307–20. doi: 10.1084/jem.188.7.1307
20. Temann UA, Ray P, Flavell RA. Pulmonary overexpression of IL-9 induces Th2 cytokine expression, leading to immune pathology. *J Clin Invest.* (2002) 109:29–39. doi: 10.1172/JCI0213696
21. Niedbala W, Besnard AG, Nascimento DC, Donate PB, Sonego F, Yip E, et al. Nitric oxide enhances Th9 cell differentiation and airway inflammation. *Nat Commun.* (2014) 5:4575. doi: 10.1038/ncomms5575
22. Yao WG, Zhang YL, Jabeen R, Nguyen ET, Wilkes DS, Tepper RS, et al. Interleukin-9 is required for allergic airway inflammation mediated by the cytokine TSLP. *Immunity* (2013) 38:360–72. doi: 10.1016/j.immuni.2013.01.007
23. Sokolowska M, Frei R, Lunjani N, Akdis CA, O'Mahony L. Microbiome and asthma. *Asthma Res Pract.* (2018) 4:1. doi: 10.1186/s40733-017-0037-y
24. Ignacio A, Morales CI, Saraiva Camara NO, Almeida RR. Innate sensing of the gut microbiota: modulation of inflammatory and autoimmune diseases. *Front Immunol.* (2016) 7:54. doi: 10.3389/fimmu.2016.00054
25. Abrahamsson TR, Jakobsson HE, Andersson AF, Bjorksten B, Engstrand L, Jenmalm MC. Low gut microbiota diversity in early infancy precedes asthma at school age. *Clin Exp Allergy* (2014) 44:842–50. doi: 10.1111/cea.12253
26. Arrieta MC, Stiemsma LT, Dimitriu PA, Thorson L, Russell S, Yurist-Doutsch S, et al. Early infancy microbial and metabolic alterations affect risk of childhood asthma. *Sci Transl Med.* (2015) 7:307ra152. doi: 10.1126/scitranslmed.aab2271
27. Herbst T, Sichelstiel A, Schar C, Yadava K, Burki K, Cahenzli J, et al. Dysregulation of allergic airway inflammation in the absence of microbial colonization. *Am J Respir Crit Care Med.* (2011) 184:198–205. doi: 10.1164/rccm.201010-1574OC
28. Sudo N, Yu XN, Aiba Y, Oyama N, Sonoda J, Koga Y, et al. An oral introduction of intestinal bacteria prevents the development of a long-term Th2-skewed immunological memory induced by neonatal antibiotic treatment in mice. *Clin Exp Allergy* (2002) 32:1112–6. doi: 10.1046/j.1365-2222.2002.01430.x
29. Trompette A, Gollwitzer ES, Yadava K, Sichelstiel AK, Sprenger N, Ngom-Bru C, et al. Gut microbiota metabolism of dietary fiber influences allergic airway disease and hematopoiesis. *Nat Med.* (2014) 20:159–66. doi: 10.1038/nm.3444
30. Thorburn N, McKenzie CI, Shen S, Stanley D, Macia L, Mason LJ, et al. Evidence that asthma is a developmental origin disease influenced by maternal diet and bacterial metabolites. *Nat Commun.* (2015) 6:7320. doi: 10.1038/ncomms8320
31. Arpaia N, Campbell C, Fan X, Dikiy S, van der Veeken J, deRoos P, et al. Metabolites produced by commensal bacteria promote peripheral regulatory T-cell generation. *Nature* (2013) 504:451–5. doi: 10.1038/nature12726
32. Furusawa Y, Obata Y, Fukuda S, Endo TA, Nakato G, Takahashi D, et al. Commensal microbe-derived butyrate induces the differentiation of colonic regulatory T cells. *Nature* (2013) 504:446–50. doi: 10.1038/nature12721
33. Xiao X, Shi X, Fan Y, Zhang X, Wu M, Lan P, et al. GITR subverts Foxp3(+) Tregs to boost Th9 immunity through regulation of histone acetylation. *Nat Commun.* (2015) 6:8266. doi: 10.1038/ncomms9266
34. Dong Q, Louahed J, Vink A, Sullivan CD, Messler CJ, Zhou YH, et al. IL-9 induces chemokine expression in lung epithelial cells and baseline airway eosinophilia in transgenic mice. *Eur J Immunol.* (1999) 29:2130–9. doi: 10.1002/(SICI)1521-4141(199907)29:07<2130::AID-IMMU2130>3.0.CO;2-S

35. Halnes I, Baines KJ, Berthon BS, MacDonald-Wicks LK, Gibson PG, Wood LG. Soluble fibre meal challenge reduces airway inflammation and expression of GPR43 and GPR41 in asthma. *Nutrients* (2017) 9:317–27. doi: 10.3390/nu9010057
36. Maslowski M, Vieira AT, Ng A, Kranich J, Sierro F, Yu D, et al. Regulation of inflammatory responses by gut microbiota and chemoattractant receptor GPR43. *Nature* (2009) 461:1282–6. doi: 10.1038/nature 08530
37. Singh N, Gurav A, Sivaprakasam S, Brady E, Padia R, Shi H, et al. Activation of Gpr109a, receptor for niacin and the commensal metabolite butyrate, suppresses colonic inflammation and carcinogenesis. *Immunity* (2014) 40:128–39. doi: 10.1016/j.immuni.2013.12.007
38. Sun MM, Wu W, Chen L, Yang WJ, Huang XS, Ma CY, et al. Microbiota-derived short-chain fatty acids promote Th1 cell IL-10 production to maintain intestinal homeostasis. *Nat Commun.* (2018) 9:3555. doi: 10.1038/s41467-018-05901-2
39. Canani RB, Di Costanzo M, Leone L. The epigenetic effects of butyrate: potential therapeutic implications for clinical practice. *Clin Epigenetics* (2012) 4:4. doi: 10.1186/1868-7083-4-4
40. Campbell DJ. Control of regulatory T cell migration, function, and homeostasis. *J Immunol.* (2015) 195:2507–13. doi: 10.4049/jimmunol.1500801
41. Kanamori M, Nakatsukasa H, Okada M, Lu QJ, Yoshimura A. Induced regulatory T cells: their development, stability, and applications. *Trends Immunol.* (2016) 37:803–11. doi: 10.1016/j.it.2016. 08.012
42. Louahed J, Zhou YH, Maloy WL, Rani PU, Weiss C, Tomer Y, et al. Interleukin 9 promotes influx and local maturation of eosinophils. *Blood* (2001) 97:1035–42. doi: 10.1182/blood.V97. 4.1035
43. Gounni S, Hamid Q, Rahman SM, Hoeck J, Yang J, Shan LY. IL-9-mediated induction of eotaxin1/CCL11 in human airway smooth muscle cells. *J Immunol.* (2004) 173:2771–9. doi: 10.4049/jimmunol.173.4.2771
44. Jia Y, Fang X, Zhu XH, Bai CX, Zhu L, Jin ML, et al. IL-13(+) Type 2 innate lymphoid cells correlate with asthma control status and treatment response. *Am J Respir Cell Mol Biol.* (2016) 55:675–83. doi: 10.1165/rcmb.2016-0099OC
45. Wolterink R, KleinJan A, van Nimwegen M, Bergen I, de Bruijn M, Levani Y, et al. Pulmonary innate lymphoid cells are major producers of IL-5 and IL-13 in murine models of allergic asthma. *Eur J Immunol.* (2012) 42:1106–16. doi: 10.1002/eji.201142018
46. Moretti S, Renga G, Oikonomou V, Galosi C, Pariano M, Iannitti R, et al. A mast cell-ILC2-Th9 pathway promotes lung inflammation in cystic fibrosis. *Nat Commun.* (2017) 8:14017. doi: 10.1038/ncomms14017
47. Ying XY, Su ZL, Bie QL, Zhang P, Yang HJ, Wu YM, et al. Synergistically increased ILC2 and Th9 cells in lung tissue jointly promote the pathological process of asthma in mice. *Mol Med Rep.* (2016) 13:5230–40. doi: 10.3892/mmr.2016.5174
48. Louahed J, Toda M, Jen J, Hamid Q, Renauld JC, Levitt RC, et al. Interleukin-9 upregulates mucus expression in the airways. *Am J Respir Cell Mol Biol.* (2000) 22:649–56. doi: 10.1165/ajrcmb.22.6.3927
49. Thio CL, Chi PY, Lai AC, Chang YJ. Regulation of type 2 innate lymphoid cell–dependent airway hyperreactivity by butyrate. *J Allergy Clin Immunol.* (2018) 142:1867–83.e12 doi: 10.1016/j.jaci.2018.02.032

16

Cigarette Smoke-Induced Pulmonary Inflammation Becomes Systemic by Circulating Extracellular Vesicles Containing Wnt5a and Inflammatory Cytokines

*Diana Feller[1,2,3], Jozsef Kun[2,3], Istvan Ruzsics[4], Judit Rapp[1,3], Veronika Sarosi[4], Krisztian Kvell[1,3], Zsuzsanna Helyes[2,3] and Judit E. Pongracz[1,3]**

[1] Department of Pharmaceutical Biotechnology, School of Pharmacy, University of Pecs, Pecs, Hungary, [2] Department of Pharmacology and Pharmacotherapy, Medical School, University of Pecs, Pecs, Hungary, [3] Szentagothai Research Center, University of Pecs, Pecs, Hungary, [4] Department of Internal Medicine, Clinical Centre and Medical School, University of Pecs, Pecs, Hungary

***Correspondence:**
Judit E. Pongracz
pongracz.e.judit@pte.hu

Chronic obstructive pulmonary disease (COPD) is a devastating, irreversible pathology affecting millions of people worldwide. Clinical studies show that currently available therapies are insufficient, have no or little effect on elevated comorbidities and on systemic inflammation. To develop alternative therapeutic options, a better understanding of the molecular background of COPD is essential. In the present study, we show that non-canonical and pro-inflammatory Wnt5a is up-regulated by cigarette smoking with parallel up-regulation of pro-inflammatory cytokines in both mouse and human model systems. Wnt5a is not only a pro-inflammatory Wnt ligand but can also inhibit the anti-inflammatory peroxisome proliferator-activated receptor gamma transcription and affect M1/M2 macrophage polarization. Both Wnt5a and pro-inflammatory cytokines can be transported in lipid bilayer sealed extracellular vesicles that reach and deliver their contents to every organ measured in the blood of COPD patients, therefore, demonstrating a potential mechanism for the systemic nature of this crippling disease.

Keywords: chronic obstructive pulmonary disease, Wnt5a, extracellular vesicles, peroxisome proliferator-activated receptor gamma, inflammatory cytokines

INTRODUCTION

Chronic obstructive pulmonary disease (COPD) is an irreversible condition of airflow limitation characterized by inflammation and impaired respiratory gas exchange (1). The prevalence of COPD is approximately 10% among individuals older than 40 years of age (2). Furthermore, based on recent statistics, COPD is the seventh and fourth highest cause of disability and death worldwide, respectively (3). The main cause of COPD is tobacco smoking, but other factors, such as air pollution, occupational hazards, and infections can also initiate the disease (4, 5). Despite all the therapeutic efforts, COPD is not just irreversible but is also progressive in nature (6). Although COPD is recognized primarily as a lung disease, it has systemic manifestations and the comorbidities affect the heart, pancreas, skeletal muscle, and other organs (7). To suppress systemic inflammation, glucocorticoid therapy is used to treat acute exacerbations of the disease (8–10). Unfortunately, apart from the limited efficacy, unwanted side effects occur including histone deacetylase regulated resistance to corticosteroids (11, 12).

To find a permanent cure for COPD, more research is required into both drug target identification and disease pathomechanism. In recent years, peroxisome proliferator-activated receptor (PPAR)-gamma was identified as a central molecule in inflammation (13, 14). PPAR gamma, a member of the ligand-activated nuclear hormone receptor super family, controls gene transcriptions associated with lipid metabolism, adipogenesis, inflammation, and metabolic homeostasis (15, 16), making PPAR gamma an emerging anti-inflammatory and anti-oxidative target gene (13, 17). PPAR gamma agonists exert strong anti-atherogenic, anti-inflammatory (18–21), and anti-oxidant effects by inhibiting several inflammatory mediators (22–25).

Regulation of PPAR gamma, however, is essentially Wnt signaling dependent (26). Mostly, if the canonical or beta-catenin-dependent Wnt pathway is up-regulated, PPAR gamma is down-regulated (27–29). Additionally, PPAR gamma is also a non-canonical Wnt pathway target and is involved in the regulation of blood vessel growth *via* a non-canonical Wnt5a-dependent mechanism (30). Interestingly, Wnt5a is also a strong pro-inflammatory molecule that has been reported as a potent activator of cigarette smoke-induced inflammatory cytokine expression (30–32) and is characteristically up-regulated in squamous cell carcinomas (30). Cigarette smoke (CS) is also the initial trigger of macrophage activation (33) and macrophage polarization toward the classical M1 and the alternative M2 lineages (34). The anti-inflammatory activity of PPAR gamma is associated with inflammatory disorders of the lung leading to the hypothesis that treatment with PPAR gamma agonists can suppress inflammation (35, 36) and reverse CS-induced emphysema (37). Such theories have been substantiated by studies where PPAR gamma-deficient macrophages contributed toward spontaneous lung inflammation (38) and that PPAR gamma agonists promoted differentiation of the immune suppressive M2 macrophage phenotype (39). It is accepted that macrophage polarization is a multifactorial process and is associated with PPAR gamma in COPD. Based on the literature and our previous studies we hypothesized that although both canonical and non-canonical Wnt signaling regulate PPAR gamma, the non-canonical Wnt signaling pathway turns into dominant upon CS exposure. We also theorized that CS exposure induced local lung inflammation which becomes systemic *via* delivery of inflammatory messages in extracellular vesicles. To investigate our hypotheses, first, mice were exposed to CS. Then, mRNA and protein expressions of the most characteristic, pro-inflammatory Wnt ligand—Wnt5a—was measured. Next, expression of Wnt signaling, PPAR gamma and pro-inflammatory cytokines were investigated in aggregate cultures of primary human lung cell types and monocyte-derived macrophages. Finally, extracellular vesicles (EV-s) were isolated from sera of control volunteers and COPD patients to measure pro-inflammatory molecules.

MATERIALS AND METHODS

Materials

Cigarette smoke extract (CSE) was diluted in cell culture media to a final concentration of 0.5%. Recombinant human Wnt5a (rhWnt5a) (Chinese Hamster Ovary Cell Line, CHO-derived Gln38-Lys380) protein was obtained from R&D Systems (Minneapolis, MN, USA) and used at a concentration of 1 μg/ml. PPAR gamma agonist, rosiglitazone (RSG), and antagonist GW9662 were purchased from Sigma-Aldrich (St. Louis, USA) and used at 10 μM concentrations each.

Collection of Human Serum Samples

Human blood samples were collected from the Division of Pulmonology, 1st Department of Internal Medicine, Medical School, University of Pecs. A total of 5 COPD patients and 5 age-matched control samples were collected in blood collection tubes (BD Vacutainer, SST: BD SST™ Tubes with Silica Clot Activator and Polymer Gel, Franklin Lakes, NJ, USA). Blood samples were clotted for 30 min at room temperature. Samples were then centrifuged at 1,500 rpm for 10 min. Serum samples were stored at −80°C until used for further analysis.

Animals

CS Exposure of Mouse Lungs

C57BL/6 male mice (20–25 g; n = 4–5/group) were housed in the animal facility of the Department of Pharmacology and Pharmacotherapy at the University of Pecs. Water and food was supplied *ad libitum*. Mice were exposed to CS in a whole-body smoke exposure system using 3R4F research cigarettes (College of Agriculture, University of Kentucky; Lexington, KY, USA). Passive smoking was performed in a manual smoking system (TE2; Teague Enterprises, Woodland, CA, USA). The exposures were performed 2 × 30 min/day with two cigarettes per occasion. The average concentration of the total suspended particles in the chamber was 70 mg/m^3.

Microvesicle/Exosome Homing Study

BALB/C mice (20–25 g; n = 3/group) were housed in the animal facility of the Department of Immunology and Biotechnology at the University of Pecs. Water and food was supplied *ad libitum*. Microvesicles/exosomes were isolated from supernatants of Wnt5a-A549 cell lines and were fluorescently labeled with DiI (see below in detail). Native and fluorescently labeled microvesicles/exosomes were resuspended in 200 μl of phosphate-buffered saline (PBS) and injected into the tail veins of BALB/C mice. Control mice were injected with non-fluorescent exosomes.

Mouse Lung Cell Isolation

Mice were anesthetized intraperitoneally with ketamine-xylazine (5 mg/kg), sacrificed by cervical dislocation, and their lungs were excised. Lung tissues were divided into three groups and were stored in RNA-later (Qiagen; Hilden, Germany) for molecular biological studies, in 1 ml lysis buffer for Western blot analysis or in 4% buffered formaldehyde (Szkarabeusz Ltd., Pecs, Hungary) for immunohistochemical examinations.

For the cell sorting procedure, 3 mice/group were anesthetized. Abdominal aorta was intersected, and mice were perfused with 10 ml of PBS through right ventricle to reduce blood content of the lung. To initiate the fine digestion 3 ml trypsin was applied, 10 ml PBS was used to wash out trypsin thereafter. 3 ml collagenase-dispase 3 mg/ml collagenase (Sigma-Aldrich, St. Louis, USA), 1 mg/ml dispase (Roche F. Hoffmann-LaRoche Ltd., Basel, Switzerland), and 1 u/μl DNase I (Sigma-Aldrich,

St. Louis, USA) were used to fill up the lungs through the trachea. Pulmonary lobes were dissected into smaller pieces and digested in 10 ml collagenase-dispase for 50 min with continuous stirring. Digested lung cells were filtered with 70 μm cell-strainer (BD Becton, Dickinson and Company, Franklin Lakes, NJ, USA).

Cell Sorting

Single cell suspensions of mouse lungs were labeled with anti-mouse CD45-FITC produced at the University of Pecs, Department of Immunology and Biotechnology and anti-mouse EpCAM1 (G8.8 anti-rat-PE) (40). Cell sorting was performed in a FACSAria III (BD Biosciences, San Jose, CA, USA) cell sorter. The following populations were collected: $EpCAM^-CD45^-$, $EpCAM^+CD45^-$, $EpCAM^+CD45^+$, and $EpCAM^+CD45^-$. The purity of sorting was above 99%.

Preparation of CSE

Cigarette smoke extract solution was prepared using a modification of the method described earlier (41). CS of two 3R4F research grade cigarettes (Kentucky Tobacco Research and Development Center at the University of Kentucky, Lexington, KY, USA) were bubbled into 10 ml of RPMI without FBS (Lonza, Basel, Switzerland) using a Harvard peristaltic pump (Harvard Apparatus, P-1500, Holliston, USA) at a 550 ml/min flow rate for approximately 3 min. CSE solution was filtered through a 0.22 μm filter (TPP, Trasadingen, Switzerland). This solution was considered as 100% stock and diluted with culture media to 0.5% for further experiments. The pH of each CSE solution was measured as a mean pH 7.28. The prepared CSE solution was used within 30 min of preparation. The OD of the inner particles of the CSE was measured spectrophotometrically at the wavelength of 360 nm and compared to the control media.

Cell Lines and Primary Cells

Human adenocarcinoma A549 cell line was obtained from American Type Culture Collection (Rockville, MD, USA). Transgenic Wnt5a overexpressing-A549 (Wnt5a-A549) cell line was created in our laboratory using lentiviral transgenesis (42). A549 cell lines were cultured in complete Dulbecco's Modified Eagle Medium (DMEM) supplemented with 10% FBS. Primary human small airway epithelial cells (SAEC), normal human lung fibroblast cells (NHLF), and normal human lung microvascular endothelial cells (HMVEC-L) were cultured according to the manufacturers' recommendations (Lonza, Basel, Switzerland). Cells were cultured in small airway epithelial cell growth medium (SAGM), fibroblast growth medium, and endothelial growth medium, respectively. All the above cell cultures were incubated at 37°C in humidified atmosphere containing 5% CO_2.

Isolation of Primary Human Monocytes

Macrophages were obtained from healthy blood donors (Hungarian National Blood Transfusion Service of Pecs, Pecs, Hungary). Peripheral blood mononuclear cells (PBMCs) were isolated from heparinized whole peripheral blood by standard density Ficoll-Paque (GE Healthcare, Sigma-Aldrich, St. Louis, USA) gradient centrifugation. Positive selection of monocytes was performed using $CD14^+$ MACS colloidal superparamagnetic microbeads (Miltenyi Biotec, GmbH, Bergisch Gladbach, Germany) conjugated with monoclonal anti-human CD14 antibodies. Cell suspensions were mixed with the beads then $CD14^+$ cells were separated by high gradient magnetic separation using MACS MultiStand, OctoMACS (Miltenyi Biotec GmbH, Bergisch Gladbach, Germany). Monocyte purity was regularly >85%. Macrophage differentiation was induced by incubation with 10 nM PMA, for 5 h, at 37°C in humidified atmosphere containing 5% CO_2.

Three-Dimensional (3D) Human Lung Aggregates

Three-dimensional lung aggregate tissues were generated as described in previous studies (30, 43, 44). Briefly, NHLF, SAEC, and HMVEC-L all purchased from Lonza (Lonza, Basel, Switzerland) were mixed (40% NHLF, 30% SAEC, and 30% HMVEC-L) in the absence or presence of peripheral monocyte-derived macrophages (30% NHLF, 25% SAEC, 25% HMVEC-L, and 20% macrophages) as described, then the cell suspensions were dispensed onto a low attachment 96-well U-bottom plate (Corning, New York, USA) and were centrifuged at 600 *g* for 10 min at room temperature. Tissue aggregates were maintained in 2:2:1 ratio of endothelial cell growth medium, SAGM, and fibroblasts growth medium. In the various experiments, aggregates were treated with 0.5% CSE or 1 μg/ml recombinant human Wnt5a (R&D Systems, Minneapolis, USA) for 48 h.

RNA Isolation, cDNA Synthesis, and Quantitative RT-PCR

Total RNA was prepared from 3D cell cultures using NucleoSpin RNAII kit (Macherey-Nagel, Düren, Germany) with on-column DNase digestion. Random hexamer primers of the high capacity RNA to cDNA kit (Thermo Fisher Scientific, Waltham, MA, USA) was applied. For cDNA synthesis, 1 μg of total RNA was used according to the manufacturers' protocol. For gene expression analysis, quantitative RT-PCR was performed using SensiFAST SYBR Green reagent (BioLine, London, UK) on ABI StepOne and StepOnePlus instruments (Thermo Fisher Scientific, Waltham, MA, USA). Data were analyzed using StepOne software and expression changes were normalized to beta-actin housekeeping gene.

TaqMan Array

Total RNA was isolated from human monocytes then cDNA was synthesized. TaqMan master mix was combined with the cDNA samples then the mixed solutions were loaded onto the Human WNT Pathway, Fast 96-well TaqMan Array (Thermo Fisher Scientific, Waltham, MA, USA) plate. Gene expression was analyzed using ABI StepOnePlus instrument (Thermo Fisher Scientific, Waltham, MA, USA).

Immunohistochemistry and Fluorescent Staining

Mice were anesthetized with ketamine-xylazine and their lungs were excised. After a formaldehyde fixation of the lung tissue, paraffin embedded sections were made using a microtome.

Before proceeding with the staining protocol, the slides had to be deparaffinized by xylene and rehydrated. Antigen retrieval was performed in citrate buffer (10 mM citric acid, 0.05% Tween 20, pH 6.0). Fluorescent staining was performed using rat anti-human Wnt5a (1:100, Clone 442625, R&D Systems, Minneapolis, USA) monoclonal antibody as primary, then Alexa Fluor 488 donkey anti-rat IgG polyclonal antibody (1:200, Thermo Fisher Scientific, Waltham, MA, USA) as secondary antibodies.

The 3D human lung tissue aggregates were carefully removed from the 96-well plate and embedded into Cryomount (Histolab, Finland) embedding medium then immediately frozen to −80°C. Sections were made using a Leica CM1950 cryostat (Leica, Wetzlar, Germany). After a drying step, sections were fixed in cold acetone (Molar Chemicals Kft., Hungary) for 10 min. Fixed slides were blocked in PBS containing 5% BSA (Sigma Aldrich, St. Louis, USA) for 20 min. Wnt5a protein expression was detected by rat anti-human Wnt5a (1:100, Clone 442625, R&D Systems, Minneapolis, USA) monoclonal antibody as primary antibody. The secondary antibody was Alexa Fluor 488 donkey anti-rat IgG antibody (1:200, Thermo Fisher Scientific, Waltham, USA). Nuclei were counterstained with DAPI (1:1000, Serva, Heidelberg, Germany). Fluorescent images were captured using Olympus IX81 fluorescence microscope (Shinjuku, Tokyo, Japan) equipped with CCD camera and analysis software. Images were processed and analyzed with ImageJ.

Flow Cytometric Bead Array (CBA) Cytokine Assay

Production of pro-inflammatory cytokines IL-6 and IL-8 were measured in cell culture medium using the multiplexed flow CBA Human Inflammatory Cytokines Kit (BD Biosciences, San Jose, CA, USA). For this assay, 50 µl culture medium/each sample of 3D aggregate cell cultures were collected at 48 h time points. The CBA kits were used according to the manufacturer's instructions. The collected samples were diluted four times in the kit's assay buffer. Diluted samples (50 µl) were added to equal amounts of fluorescent cytokine capture bead suspension (50 µl), and human inflammatory cytokine-phycoerythrin detection reagent (50 µl). Samples were then incubated for 3 h at room temperature. Labeled beads were measured using FACS Canto II flow cytometer (BD Immunocytometry Systems, Erembodegen, Belgium) with BD FACS DIVA software V6 and data were analyzed by FCS Express V3 software.

EV Isolation From Human Serum Samples

Extracellular vesicles were isolated from human serum samples of 5 COPD patients and 5 healthy controls using the Total Exosome Isolation kit (from serum) (Invitrogen, Thermo Fisher Scientific, Waltham, MA, USA) following the manufacturer's protocol. Frozen serum samples were thawed at room temperature. Samples were then centrifuged at 300 × *g* for 30 min at 4°C to remove cells and cell debris. Then the supernatant was centrifuged with 2,000 × *g* for 30 min at 4°C to collect megasomes/oncosomes in the pellet. The supernatant was then mixed with total exosome isolation reagent and vortexed. Samples were incubated at 2–8°C for 30 min, then centrifuged at 14,000 × *g* for 10 min at room temperature. The pellets containing EV-s (microvesicles/oncosomes) were collected and resuspended in cold EV resuspension buffer and stored at −80°C until further analysis.

EV Isolation From A549 and Wnt5a-A549 Cell Lines

Extracellular vesicles were isolated from cell culture media following the protocol of the total exosome isolation (from cell culture media) kit (Invitrogen, Cat. number: 4478359). A549 and Wnt5a-A549 cell lines were cultured in DMEM supplemented with 10% FBS at 37°C in humidified atmosphere containing 5% CO_2 until confluent. The medium was then removed, the cell layer washed in PBS, and FBS-free medium was added to the cultures. After 2 days at 37°C, 5% CO_2, the FBS-free culture medium was harvested and centrifuged at 300 × *g* for 10 min at 4°C to remove cells and cell debris. Then the supernatant was centrifuged with 2,000 × *g* for 30 min at 4°C to collect megasomes/oncosomes in the pellet. Finally, total exosome isolation (for cell culture media) reagent was added in 0.5 volumes. Samples were incubated at 4°C overnight, and then centrifuged at 10,000 × *g* for 1 h at 4°C. The pellets containing EV-s were collected after centrifugation and resuspended in cold PBS until further analysis. Isolated EV-s were stored at −80°C.

Staining of EV-s (Microvesicles or Exosomes)

Isolated microvesicles (exosomes) were centrifuged for 1 h at 4°C. Pellets were resuspended in PBS containing DiI (Molecular Probes, Thermo Fisher Scientific, Waltham, MA, USA) (dilution 1:10,000). Samples were incubated for 30 min at 37°C, then centrifuged with 10,000 × *g* for 1 h at 4°C. Supernatant was then removed and the pellet was resuspended in PBS.

Fluorescence Analysis of Microvesicle (Exosome) Localization

Balb/c mice were injected with equal amount of stained or unstained exosome suspension in 200 µl of PBS. Mice were sacrificed after 20 h of exosome injection. Lung, liver, thymus, and the spleen were removed for fluorescence imaging of extracellular vesicle accumulations in mouse organs by the IVIS Lumina III *In Vivo* Imaging System using the Living Image Software (IVIS Imaging Systems) (PerkinElmer, Waltham, MA, USA). Fluorescence intensity was compared to fluorescence intensity of unstained control organs.

Electron Microscopic Detection of Microvesicles (Exosomes)

Microvesicles isolated from cell lines were visualized by electron microscopy. First, microvesicles were resuspended in PBS and then fixed in 2.5% glutaraldehyde aqueous solution. 5 µl of fixed exosomes were embedded in the EM grid, which was flushed by water and blown dry for 24 h. Samples were treated with 5% uranyl-acetate at pH 7 for 5 min. The grid was examined using Morgagni 268D transmission electron microscope at 80 kV. Images were acquired using an integrated MegaView III digital camera (Olympus Soft Imaging Solutions GmbH; Munster, Germany).

Sandwich Enzyme-Linked Immunosorbent Assay (ELISA)

Mega EV (oncosome) and micro EV (exosome) samples were resuspended in PBS containing 0.5% Tween 20. 100 µl of each sample was loaded to wells in the Aviva Systems Biology WNT5A ELISA Kit (Human) (OKEH00723). The plate was pre-coated with a Wnt5a-specific antibody (96-well plate, 12 × 8 well strips) and blocked. Standards were also provided by the manufacturer. Samples were incubated for 2 h at 37°C, then the wells were washed and incubated further with a biotinylated Wnt5a-specific detector antibody for further 1 h at 37°C. After a washing step, incubation continued with Avidin-HRP conjugate for 1 h at 37°C. The wells were then washed and TMB (3,3′,5,5′-Tetramethylbenzidine) substrate was added for 15 min at 37°C in the dark. The reaction was then stopped and the color reaction was measured at 450 nm absorbance. Results were calculated against the standard curve.

Statistical Analysis

Statistical analysis was performed with GraphPad version 6 software. Data are presented as mean ± SEM, and statistical analysis was performed using the independent samples *t*-test and one-way ANOVA with Bonferroni correction. $p < 0.05$ was considered as significant.

RESULTS

CS and CSE Trigger Wnt5a Up-Regulation in Both Mouse and Human Lung Tissues

To investigate the effects of CS as a systemic inducer of inflammation, *in vivo* and *in vitro* studies were performed. First, C57BL/6 mice were exposed to CS for 2 × 30 min each day over 2 months. The test animals developed emphysema-like tissue damage (**Figure 1A**) that correlated with decreased epithelial cell number (**Figure 1B**). Epithelial cells were also separated from the $CD45^+$ leukocyte population (**Figure 1B**). Both the epithelial cell enriched and the $CD45^+$ cell populations had elevated Wnt5a mRNA levels (**Figure 1C**). Wnt5a protein expression levels were also increased (**Figures 1D,E**). Different isoforms of CD45 are expressed in many leukocyte populations including T and B lymphocytes and antigen-presenting cells, no effect of these immune cells, except macrophages, were investigated further. To test whether CSE can trigger Wnt5a up-regulation in human lung tissues, *in vitro* human lung aggregate cultures were used. The aggregate cultures contained SAEC, mesenchyme (NHLF), and endothelial cells (HMVEC-L) in the presence or absence of human blood monocyte-derived macrophages and were treated with CSE for a maximum of 48 h. The CSE treated aggregates have shown increased levels of Wnt5a both at mRNA and protein levels but only if monocytes were present in the aggregate tissues (**Figures 2A–D**) (45, 46).

Increased Inflammatory Cytokine Production in the Lung After CS Exposure Is Associated With the Presence of Macrophages

After the recruitment of immune cells to help in eliminating foreign materials and to aid tissue repair after damage or infection, immune reactions are resolved and the tissue homeostasis is normalized. Macrophages are involved in self-limiting, regulated resolution of inflammatory processes at different levels. Tissue-resident macrophages and activated monocytes can adopt different activation status, and although the process is still not fully characterized, M1 and M2 type polarization can provide an outline of how macrophage activity can change during inflammation. To test the effects of CS on the human lung, aggregate cultures of primary human lung cell types were exposed to CSE for 48 h and pro-inflammatory cytokine gene expressions were measured. Both in the presence or absence of macrophages, significant increase of IL6 peptide levels were detected compared to untreated controls (**Figure 3A**). If the human lung aggregate cultures were exposed to rhWnt5a (1 µg/ml, for 48 h) then both IL-6 and IL-8 peptide levels increased significantly in the monocyte containing tissue cultures indicating a sequential activation of pro-inflammatory cytokine and pro-inflammatory Wnt5a production (**Figure 3B**). To attempt to dissect such a dynamic process, blood monocytes were exposed to CSE, then, Wnt signaling TaqMan Array was performed (**Figures 3C,D**). Compared to untreated controls, up-regulation of characteristic non-canonical Wnt signaling molecules were detected, including Wnt5a, Wnt5b, Wnt11 as ligands and an inhibitor of the canonical Wnt pathway, Dickkopf 2 (DKK-2) (**Figures 3C,D**). In addition to specific molecules of the Wnt pathway, increased transcription of CXXC4—a member of the zinc finger domain-containing protein family—was detected. Up-regulation of CXXC4 that functions as an antagonist of the canonical Wnt/integrated signaling pathway indicates active suppression of the canonical Wnt pathway. Furthermore, increased mRNA levels of CSNKD1 a casein kinase I gene family member, transducin-like enhancer of split 4 (TLE4), and Wnt10a were also detected. While CSNKD1 is an essential serine/threonine-protein kinase and regulator of diverse cellular growth and survival; TLE4 is a transcriptional corepressor. Overexpression of the Wnt10a gene may be of particular interest as Wnt10a can play key roles in carcinogenesis through activation of the Wnt-beta-catenin-TCF signaling pathway. Simultaneously, reduced transcription of Axin2 that plays an important role in the regulation of beta-catenin stability and a characteristic canonical Wnt ligand, Wnt1, were down-regulated. Reduced transcription of TLE2 and secreted frizzled-related protein 5 was also observed, demonstrating deregulation of Wnt signaling in macrophages as a direct effect of CS exposure. Deregulation of either the canonical or the non-canonical Wnt signaling results in modification of PPAR gamma expression and activity (31). To investigate how such changes in the Wnt signaling pathway can affect the dynamic polarization of macrophages, pro-inflammatory cytokines characteristic to the pro-inflammatory M1, and the anti-inflammatory but pro-tumorigenic M2 phenotypes (47) were measured in association with PPAR gamma expression and activity. To study how PPAR gamma is involved in the CS induced Wnt5a up-regulation as well as consequent pro-inflammatory cytokine production, human lung aggregate cultures were exposed to Wnt5a and CSE in the presence or absence of PPAR gamma agonist, rosiglitazone (RSG), and inhibitor (GW9662) (**Figures 4A,B**). The M1 phenotype is mostly characterized by pro-inflammatory cytokines IL-6, IL-8, IL-23, and IL-1β, while M2 by anti-inflammatory cytokines IL-10 and TGF-beta (34). In the studied time frame, inhibition

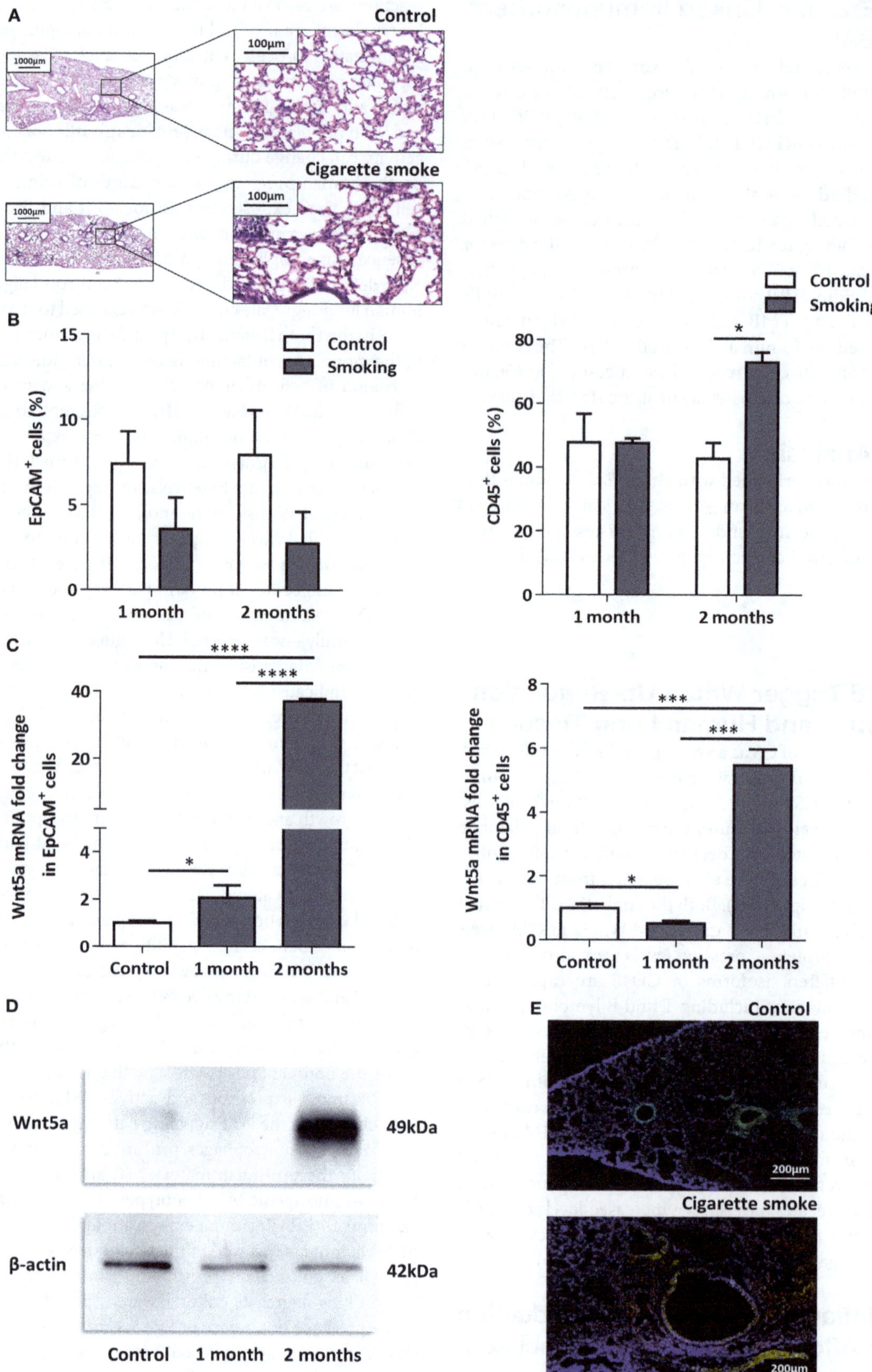

FIGURE 1 | Continued

FIGURE 1 | Effects of cigarette smoke (CS) on C57BL/6 mouse lungs. **(A)** Hematoxylin-eosin staining of paraffin embedded sections of healthy control and CS exposed lungs. Mice were exposed to CS for 1 h/day for 2 months. (Scale bars, 100 μm.) **(B)** Changes in EpCAM⁺ and CD45⁺ cell populations in control and CS exposed lungs determined by flow cytometry. **(C)** Wnt5a mRNA expression changes in sorted EpCAM⁺ and CD45⁺cells following 1 and 2 months of CS exposure (*n* = 3). **(D)** Western blot analysis of Wnt5a protein expression in control and CS exposed lung tissue extracts. **(E)** Detection of Wnt5a protein expression in control and CS exposed lung tissue sections [EpCAM⁺ (green)/Wnt5a (red)/Nucleus (blue), Scale bars, 200 μm].

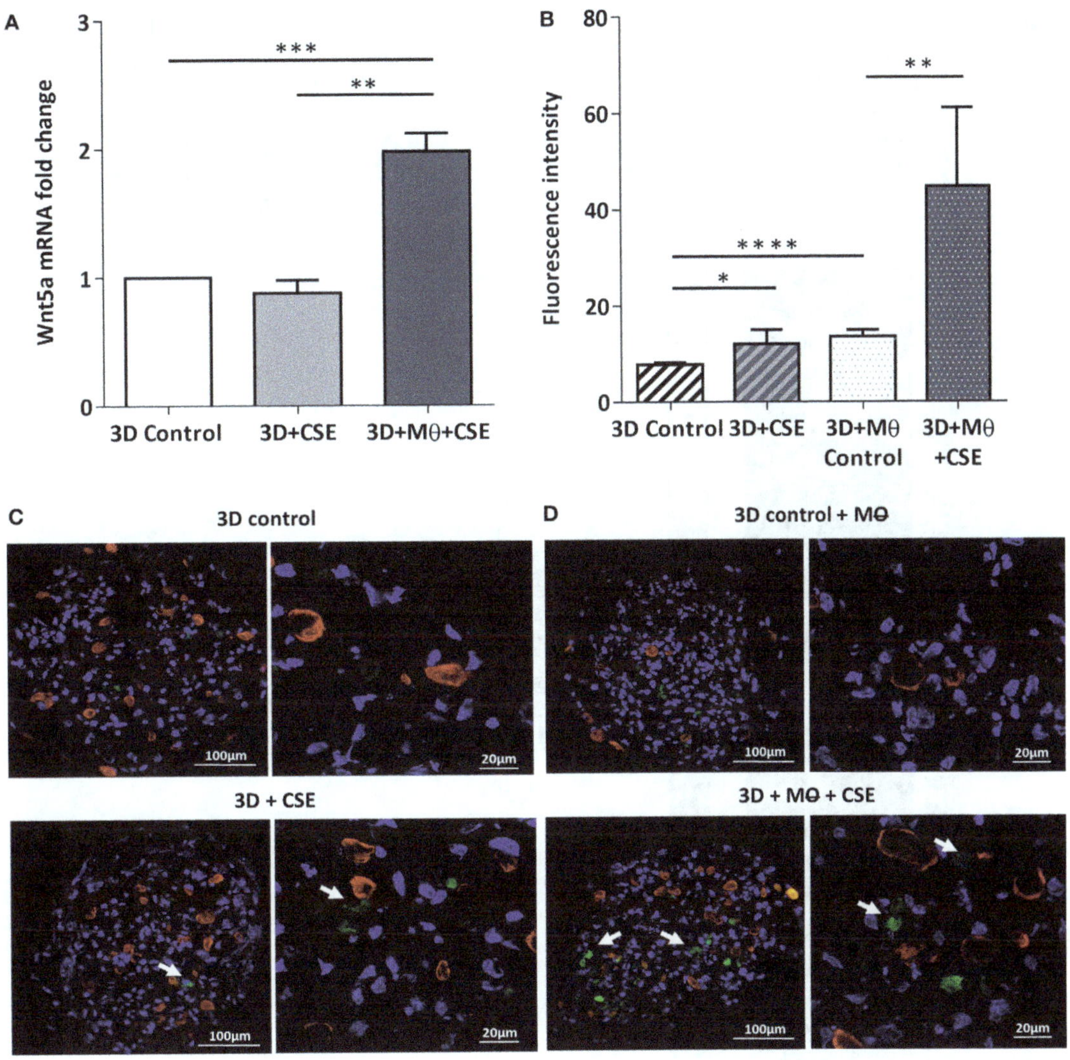

FIGURE 2 | Effects of cigarette smoke extracts (CSE) on primary human 3D lung aggregate cultures. **(A)** Wnt5a mRNA was measured by qRT-PCR in control and CSE treated (48 h) aggregate cultures containing and not containing macrophages (M). **(B)** Fluorescence intensity of Wnt5a protein was analyzed by ImageJ. **(C)** Immunofluorescence staining of Wnt5a (green) and Cytokeratin7 (red) proteins in frozen sections of control aggregates and CSE (48 h) exposed aggregates not containing M. **(D)** Immunofluorescence staining of Wnt5a (green) and Cytokeratin7 (red) proteins in frozen sections of control aggregates and CSE (48 h) exposed aggregates containing M. Nuclei were stained by TO-PRO-3 Iodide (1:1,000, pseudo-blue). [Scale bars: 100 μm (magnification, 20x), 20 μm (magnification, 63x)].

of the anti-inflammatory PPAR gamma by GW9662 reduced the gene expression of IL-10—the characteristic cytokine marker of the anti-inflammatory M2 phenotype (**Figure 4B**). Cytokine production, however, is a dynamic process. In order to investigate it, human blood monocyte-derived macrophages were exposed to CSE for two different time points 3 and 48 h, then PPAR gamma transcription was measured. Interestingly, at the 3 h time point the anti-inflammatory PPAR gamma transcription significantly increased, but by 48 h the transcript level reduced to control levels (**Figure 4C**) indicating that expression of the anti-inflammatory PPAR gamma would not keep up with the prolonged inflammatory stimuli.

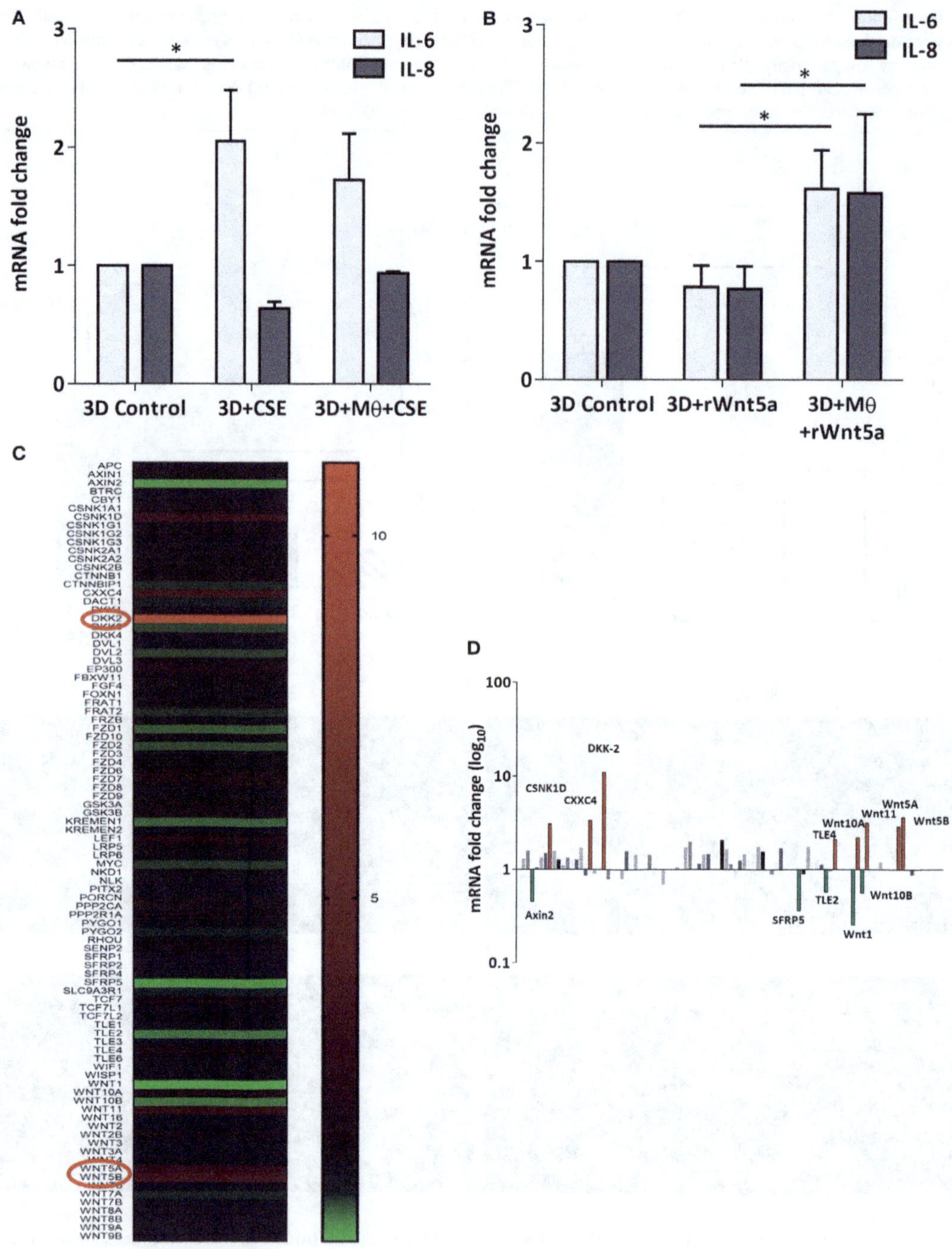

FIGURE 3 | Inflammatory cytokine and Wnt mRNA levels in primary human 3D lung aggregate cultures and human macrophages (M) after cigarette smoke extracts (CSE) exposure. **(A)** IL-6 and IL-8 inflammatory cytokine mRNA levels in control and CSE exposed (48 h) lung aggregate cultures, containing and not containing M. **(B)** IL-6 and IL-8 inflammatory cytokine mRNA levels in control and rWnt5a (1 µg/ml) treated lung aggregate cultures, containing and not containing M. **(C)** Taqman array heat map analysis of pooled (n = 4) cDNA of human M compared with control. M were treated with CSE for 3 h. **(D)** Changes in mRNA levels of Wnt signaling pathway genes measured by Taqman Array analysis using pooled (n = 4) cDNA samples of human M compared with control.

Chronic CS Exposure Increases Wnt5a Protein Levels in EV-s of COPD Patients' Sera

The lipo-glycoprotein Wnt ligands are highly hydrophobic (48), therefore, their transport in aqueous body fluids is facilitated by EV-s (49). EV-s (both megasomes/oncosomes or microsomes/exosomes) are now widely accepted as a novel route of cellular communication that can influence the long-range Wnt signal gradients (50, 51). Based on the above, we hypothesized that Wnt5a and low serum levels of pro-inflammatory cytokines can be measured in EV-s isolated from human sera (52, 53).

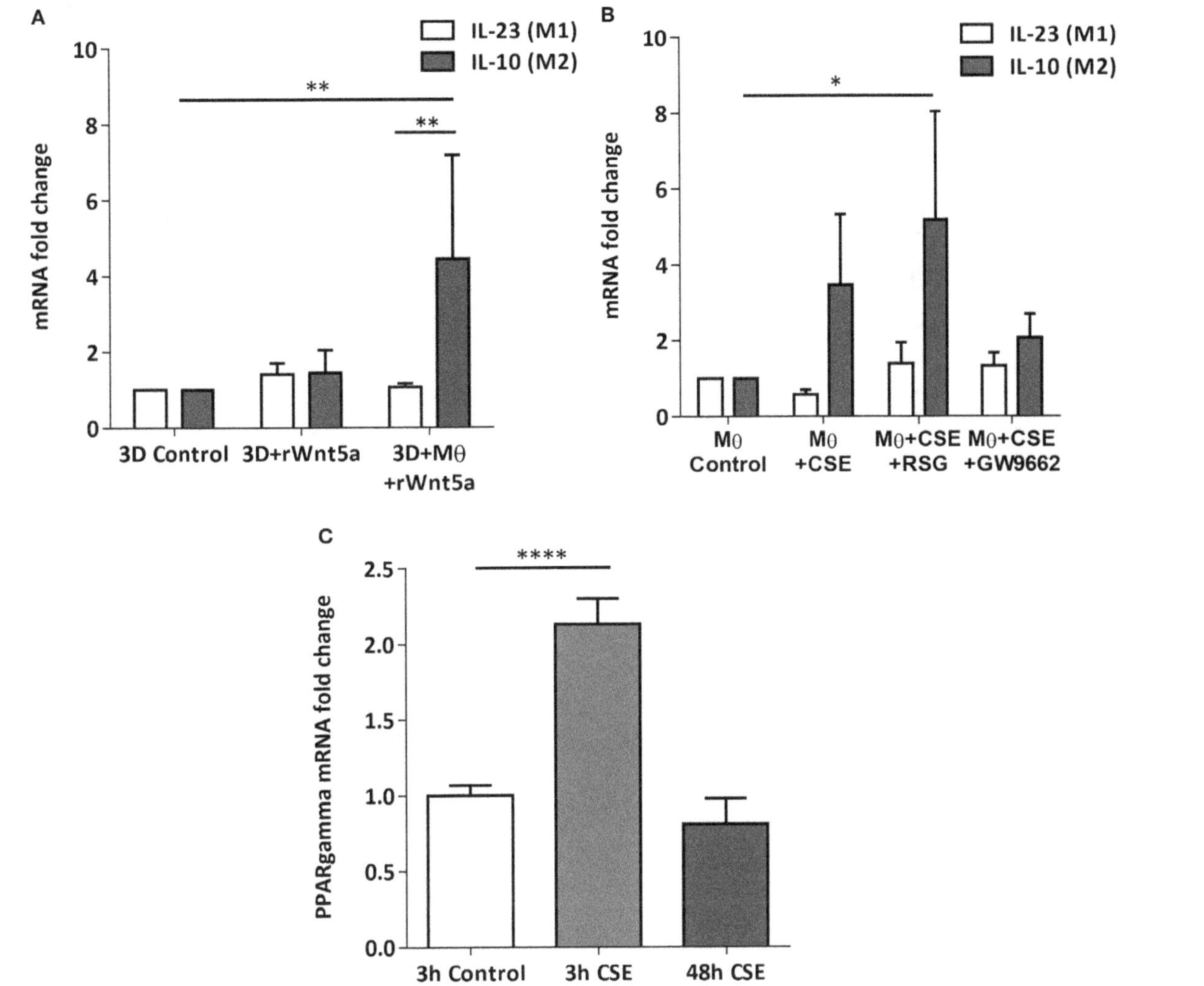

FIGURE 4 | Changes of peroxisome proliferator-activated receptor (PPAR) gamma mRNA levels in M1 and M2 M type differentiation in primary human 3D lung aggregate cultures and M monocultures. **(A)** qRT-PCR analysis of M1 (differentiation marker IL-23) and M2 (differentiation marker IL-10) after human rWnt5a (1 µg/ml) treatment for 48 h. **(B)** Effects of cigarette smoke extracts (CSE), PPAR gamma agonist (RSG), and antagonist (GW9662) treatment on expression of M1 (IL-23) and M2 (IL-10) differentiation markers. CSE treatment (48 h) and also CSE + RSG (10 µM) and CSE + GW9662 (10 µM) treatment on human M. **(C)** PPAR gamma mRNA levels in CSE treated human macrophage cultures after 3 and 48 h of CSE treatment compared with controls.

If EV-s can travel from the organ of origin and reach any cells and organs of the human body safely delivering their contents, such transport system would explain the systemic nature of COPD. To test our theory, the larger megavesicles/oncosomes and the smaller microvesicles/exosomes were isolated from sera of COPD patients as well as age-matched healthy controls. The non-small cell carcinoma cell line A549 and its engineered Wnt5a overexpressing sister cell line Wnt5a-A549 were used as positive controls. Wnt5a was measured by ELISA (**Figure 5A**), whereas pro-inflammatory cytokines were measured by a bead assay using flow cytometry (**Figures 5B,C**). While Wnt5a was not detectable in sera of neither COPD patients nor age-matched healthy volunteers, megavesicles/oncosomes isolated from sera of COPD patients contained similar levels of Wnt5a as measured in the Wnt5a overexpressing Wnt5a-A549 cell line (**Figure 5A**). Similarly, while many pro-inflammatory cytokines remained undetectable in pure human sera (data not shown), exosomes contained high levels of such cytokines (**Figure 5C**) with an extremely high level detected for IL-8 (**Figure 5C**).

To investigate whether these concentrated "cellular messages" can reach other organs, extracellular vesicles were isolated from the supernatant of the Wnt5a-A549 cell line and the lipid bilayer was stained with a DiI fluorescent dye to be injected into the tail veins of Balb/c mice. Mice were sacrificed after 20 h and the organs were removed to detect fluorescence. The experiments provided evidence that inflammatory cytokine containing microvesicles/exosomes can reach and become concentrated in the liver, lungs, spleen, and thymus of test animals (**Figures 5D–F**).

DISCUSSION

Cigarette smoke induced chronic lung inflammation, PPAR gamma activity, Wnt signaling deregulation and increased overall risk of carcinogenesis are all interconnected (54, 55). Our report

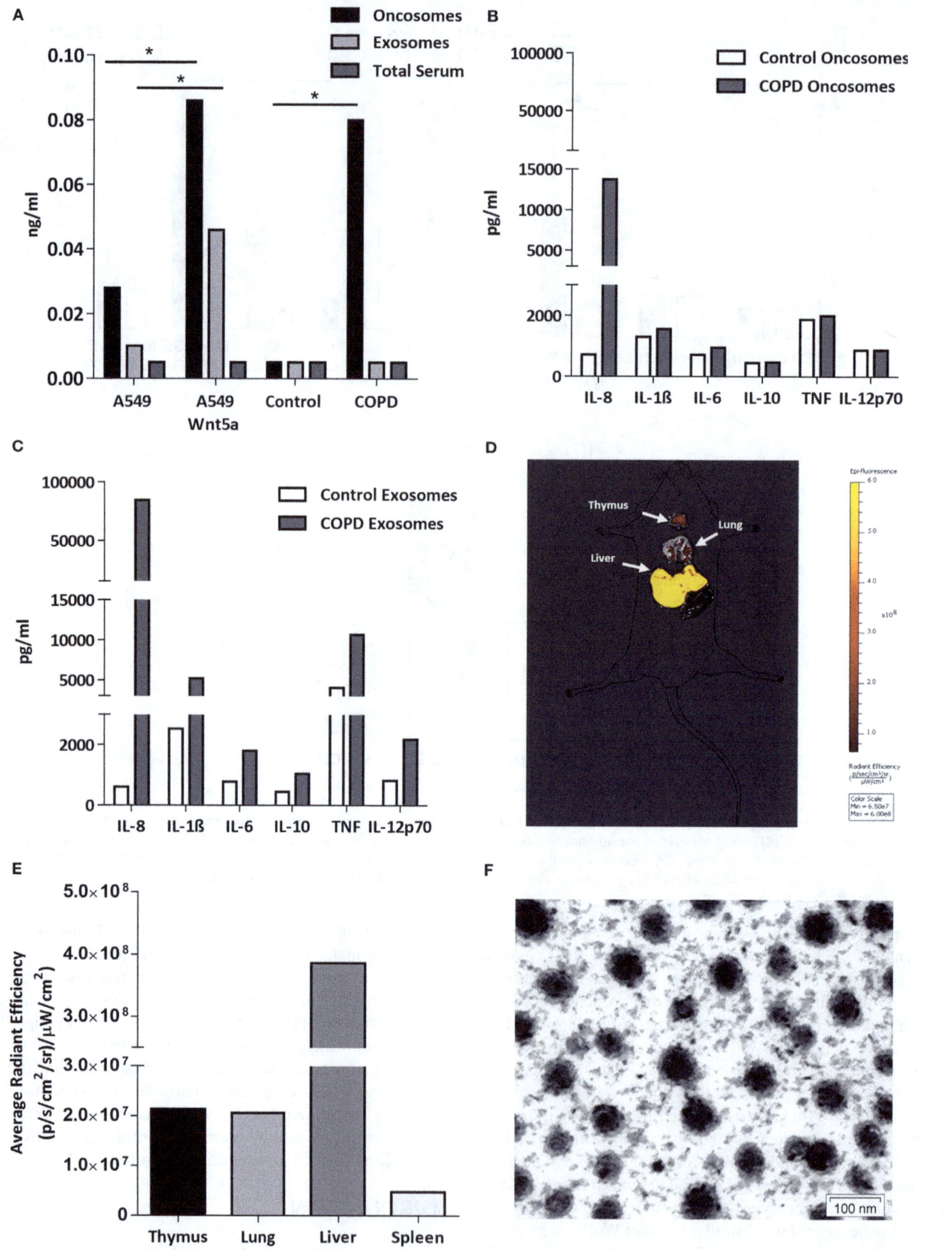

FIGURE 5 | Continued

FIGURE 5 | Wnt5a and proinflammatory cytokine levels in extracellular vesicles (EV-s). **(A)** Wnt5a protein levels were measured in EV-s in sera of healthy donors and chronic obstructive pulmonary disease (COPD) patients as well as EV-s of A549 and Wnt5a-A549 cell lines as controls using a Wnt5a-specific enzyme-linked immunosorbent assay kit. **(B)** Inflammatory cytokine levels were measured in pooled megavesicles/oncosome samples of five healthy and five COPD patients isolated from human sera measured by cytometric bead array Flex kit using flow cytometry. **(C)** Inflammatory cytokine proteins were detected in pooled microvesicle/exosome samples of five healthy and five COPD patients isolated from human sera. **(D)** Fluorescent staining (DiI) labeled Wnt5a-containing EV-s are detectable in various organs (representative image of $n = 3$). **(E)** Fluorescence intensity of Wnt5a containing EV-s in various organs (representative data of $n = 3$). **(F)** Electron microscopic image of purified EV-s (microvesicle/exosome population) purified from the Wnt5a-A549 cell line. Scale bar is 100 nm.

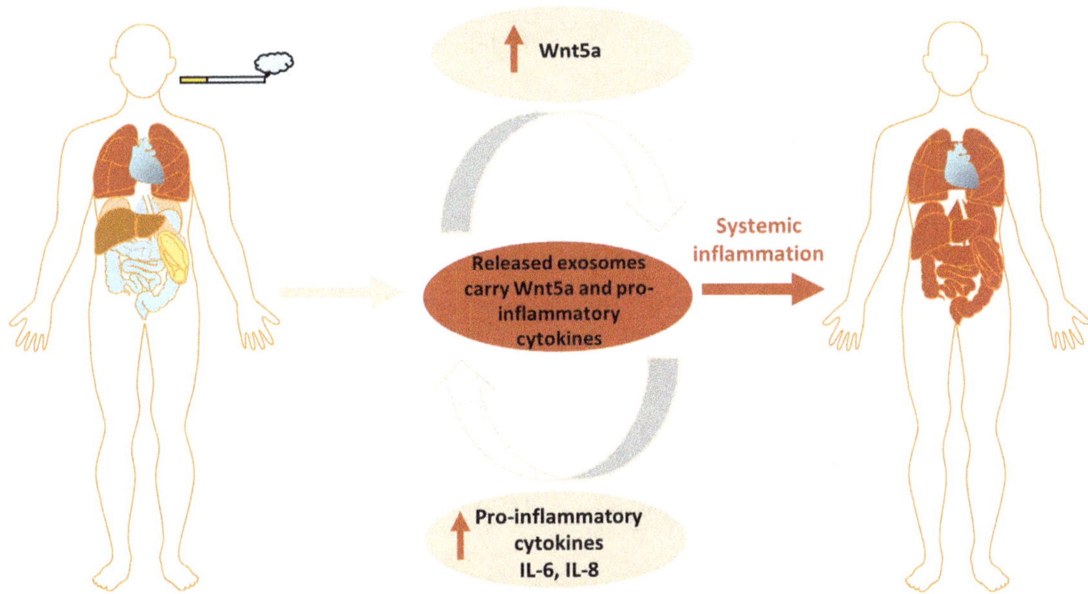

FIGURE 6 | Summary figure of cigarette smoke induced local inflammation becoming systemic by the contribution of Wnt5a and inflammatory cytokines.

is the first to shed light on a potential mechanism. We have shown that CS induces the expression of molecules of the non-canonical Wnt signaling pathway that simultaneously suppress the canonical Wnt pathway. This observation is significant as the canonical Wnt signaling is essential to maintain stem cell niches in the lung (56). In fact, CS creates a tissue microenvironment that is similar to the ones observed during aging (43). Similarly to smokers, the aging microenvironment is associated with a significant decrease of the EpCAM$^+$ epithelial cell layer that correlates with emphysema and decreased gas exchange surface (43). In parallel, inflammatory environment is present marked by the increased number of the CD45$^+$ leukocyte population of immune cells in the tissue of the lung and up-regulated non-canonical Wnt signaling (43). While the lung is young and healthy, inflammatory respiratory diseases are kept in check by dynamic polarization of macrophages into the anti-inflammatory M2 subsets that suppress the pro-inflammatory M1 macrophage phenotype (57). PPAR gamma plays an important and similarly dynamic anti-inflammatory role by inducing M2 type polarization (39, 58). Prolonged exposure to CS, however, re-enforces the "aging" process by reducing PPAR gamma expression. Repeated exposure to CS also alters the lung tissue homeostasis and the Wnt microenvironment that closely interacts with PPAR gamma (59). Although the precise molecular regulation remains largely unclear, PPAR gamma (60, 61) and the Wnt signaling pathways (62) have been suspected to somehow regulate the systemic nature of COPD. The non-canonical Wnt5a that is associated with aging (43), carcinogenesis (30), as well as with activation of pro-inflammatory processes during M1 phenotype macrophage differentiation and pro-inflammatory cytokine production (63–65) was up-regulated upon CS exposure and was found in megavesicles/oncosomes of COPD patients. Wnt5a can also suppress levels of the anti-inflammatory PPAR gamma *via* increasing miR27b that binds to the PPAR gamma promoter and blocks its transcription (31). As both pro-inflammatory cytokines and Wnt5a can be wrapped and protected by the lipid bilayer of EV-s then not just the inflammation can become systemic but also the inhibition of the anti-inflammatory activity of PPAR gamma (**Figure 6**). Although previous studies hypothesized that PPAR gamma agonist treatments can modulate and suppress inflammation (35, 66) or even reverse CS-induced emphysema (37), our experiments have highlighted the difficulty of achieving such anti-inflammatory therapy targeting solely PPAR gamma. Furthermore, as PPAR gamma agonists can promote M2 phenotype differentiation of macrophages (39), such PPAR gamma agonist therapy can even lead to unintended promotion of carcinogenesis.

In summary, in the present study we demonstrated that during cigarette smoking the inflammation inducer and PPAR gamma inhibitor Wnt5a as well as pro-inflammatory cytokines can be carried to every organ in the human body in various types of extracellular vesicles triggering systemic inflammation and making COPD a complex disease that is hard to control. Further studies are needed to investigate how to utilize our discovery in identification of differential diagnostic and prognostic markers as well as application of extracellular vesicles in targeted therapy.

AUTHOR CONTRIBUTIONS

JP, DF, KK, and ZH contributed conception and design of the study. DF, JR, and JK performed experimental work. DF and JR performed the statistical analysis. IR and VS designed and selected patients, collected sera, and advised on clinical aspects. JP wrote the first draft of the manuscript. DF wrote sections of the manuscript. All authors contributed to manuscript revision, read and approved the submitted version.

ACKNOWLEDGMENTS

The authors are grateful for technical assistance to Ms. Anikó Perkecz in microtome sectioning and to Tamás Kiss for IVIS Lumina III Imaging (Department of Pharmacology and Pharmacotherapy, Medical School and Szentagothai Research Centre, University of Pecs).

REFERENCES

1. Hillas G, Perlikos F, Tsiligianni I, Tzanakis N. Managing comorbidities in COPD. *Int J Chron Obstruct Pulmon Dis* (2015) 10:95–109. doi:10.2147/COPD.S54473
2. Halbert RJ, Natoli JL, Gano A, Badamgarav E, Buist AS, Mannino DM. Global burden of COPD: systematic review and meta-analysis. *Eur Respir J* (2006) 28:523–32. doi:10.1183/09031936.06.00124605
3. Mannino DM, Buist AS. Global burden of COPD: risk factors, prevalence, and future trends. *Lancet* (2007) 370:765–73. doi:10.1016/S0140-6736(07)61380-4
4. Eisner MD, Anthonisen N, Coultas D, Kuenzli N, Perez-Padilla R, Postma D, et al. An official American Thoracic Society public policy statement: novel risk factors and the global burden of chronic obstructive pulmonary disease. *Am J Respir Crit Care Med* (2010) 182:693–718. doi:10.1164/rccm.200811-1757ST
5. Tashkin DP, Murray RP. Smoking cessation in chronic obstructive pulmonary disease. *Respir Med* (2009) 103:963–74. doi:10.1016/j.rmed.2009.02.013
6. D'Armiento JM, Scharf SM, Roth MD, Connett JE, Ghio A, Sternberg D, et al. Eosinophil and T cell markers predict functional decline in COPD patients. *Respir Res* (2009) 10:113. doi:10.1186/1465-9921-10-113
7. Cazzola M, Matera MG, Rogliani P, Page C. Treating systemic effects of COPD. *Trends Pharmacol Sci* (2007) 28:544–50. doi:10.1016/j.tips.2007.09.006
8. Leuppi JD, Schuetz P, Bingisser R, Bodmer M, Briel M, Drescher T, et al. Short-term vs conventional glucocorticoid therapy in acute exacerbations of chronic obstructive pulmonary disease: the REDUCE randomized clinical trial. *JAMA* (2013) 309:2223–31. doi:10.1001/jama.2013.5023
9. Schuetz P, Leuppi JD, Tamm M, Briel M, Bingisser R, Durring U, et al. Short versus conventional term glucocorticoid therapy in acute exacerbation of chronic obstructive pulmonary disease. *Swiss Med Wkly* (2010) 140:w13109. doi:10.4414/smw.2010.13109
10. Sethi S, Nag N. A 5-day course of systemic corticosteroids is adequate to treat acute exacerbations of chronic obstructive pulmonary disease. *Evid Based Med* (2014) 19:57. doi:10.1136/eb-2013-101475
11. Hakim A, Adcock IM, Usmani OS. Corticosteroid resistance and novel anti-inflammatory therapies in chronic obstructive pulmonary disease: current evidence and future direction. *Drugs* (2012) 72:1299–312. doi:10.2165/11634350-000000000-00000
12. Barnes PJ. Mechanisms of allergic diseases Corticosteroid resistance in patients with asthma and chronic obstructive pulmonary disease. *J Allergy Clin Immunol* (2013) 131:636–45. doi:10.1016/j.jaci.2012.12.1564
13. Daynes RA, Jones DC. Emerging roles of PPARs in inflammation and immunity. *Nat Rev Immunol* (2002) 2:748–59. doi:10.1038/nri912
14. Lakshmi SP, Reddy AT, Zhang Y, Sciurba FC, Mallampalli RK, Duncan SR, et al. Down-regulated peroxisome proliferator-activated receptor γ (PPARγ) in lung epithelial cells promotes a PPARγ agonist-reversible proinflammatory phenotype in chronic obstructive pulmonary disease (COPD). *J Biol Chem* (2014) 289:6383–93. doi:10.1074/jbc.M113.536805
15. de sá PM, Richard AJ, Hang H, Stephens JM. Transcriptional regulation of adipogenesis. *Compr Physiol* (2017) 7:635–74. doi:10.1002/cphy.c160022
16. Tomas J, Mulet C, Saffarian A, Cavin J-B, Ducroc R, Regnault B, et al. High-fat diet modifies the PPAR-γ pathway leading to disruption of microbial and physiological ecosystem in murine small intestine. *Proc Natl Acad Sci U S A* (2016) 113:E5934–43. doi:10.1073/pnas.1612559113
17. Mazzei JC, Zhou H, Brayfield BP, Hontecillas R, Bassaganya-Riera J, Schmelz EM. Suppression of intestinal inflammation and inflammation-driven colon cancer in mice by dietary sphingomyelin: importance of peroxisome proliferator-activated receptor γ expression. *J Nutr Biochem* (2011) 22:1160–71. doi:10.1016/j.jnutbio.2010.09.017
18. Huang THW, Razmovski-Naumovski V, Kota BP, Lin DSH, Roufogalis BD. The pathophysiological function of peroxisome proliferator-activated receptor-γ in lung-related diseases. *Respir Res* (2005) 6:102. doi:10.1186/1465-9921-6-102
19. Huang W, Glass CK. Nuclear receptors and inflammation control: molecular mechanisms and pathophysiological relevance. *Arterioscler Thromb Vasc Biol* (2010) 30:1542–9. doi:10.1161/ATVBAHA.109.191189
20. Pascual G, Fong AL, Ogawa S, Gamliel A, Li AC, Perissi V, et al. A SUMOylation-dependent pathway mediates transrepression of inflammatory response genes by PPAR-gamma. *Nature* (2005) 437:759–63. doi:10.1038/nature03988
21. Wahli W, Michalik L. PPARs at the crossroads of lipid signaling and inflammation. *Trends Endocrinol Metab* (2012) 23:351–63. doi:10.1016/j.tem.2012.05.001
22. Cabrero A, Laguna JC, Vazquez M. Peroxisome proliferator-activated receptors and the control of inflammation. *Curr Drug Targets Inflamm Allergy* (2002) 1:243–8. doi:10.2174/1568010023344616
23. Polvani S, Tarocchi M, Galli A. PPARgamma and oxidative stress: Con(beta) catenating NRF2 and FOXO. *PPAR Res* (2012) 2012:641087. doi:10.1155/2012/641087
24. Staels B, Fruchart JC. Therapeutic roles of peroxisome proliferator-activated receptor agonists. *Diabetes* (2005) 54:2460–70. doi:10.2337/diabetes.54.8.2460
25. Chung SS, Kim M, Youn B-S, Lee NS, Park JW, Lee IK, et al. Glutathione peroxidase 3 mediates the antioxidant effect of peroxisome proliferator-activated receptor gamma in human skeletal muscle cells. *Mol Cell Biol* (2009) 29:20–30. doi:10.1128/MCB.00544-08
26. Takada I, Mihara M, Suzawa M, Ohtake F, Kobayashi S, Igarashi M, et al. A histone lysine methyltransferase activated by non-canonical Wnt signalling suppresses PPAR-γ transactivation. *Nat Cell Biol* (2007) 9:1273–85. doi:10.1038/ncb1647
27. Liu J, Wang H, Zuo Y, Farmer SR. Functional interaction between peroxisome proliferator-activated receptor gamma and beta-catenin. *Mol Cell Biol* 26:5827–37. doi:10.1128/MCB.00441-06 (2006)

28. Lecarpentier Y, Claes V, Vallée A, Hébert J-L. Thermodynamics in cancers: opposing interactions between PPAR gamma and the canonical WNT/beta-catenin pathway. *Clin Transl Med* (2017) 6:14. doi:10.1186/s40169-017-0144-7
29. Pongracz JE, Stockley RA. Wnt signalling in lung development and diseases. *Respir Res* (2006) 7:15. doi:10.1186/1465-9921-7-15
30. Rapp J, Kiss E, Meggyes M, Szabo-Meleg E, Feller D, Smuk G, et al. Increased Wnt5a in squamous cell lung carcinoma inhibits endothelial cell motility. *BMC Cancer* (2016) 16:915. doi:10.1186/s12885-016-2943-4
31. Rauner M, Stein N, Winzer M, Goettsch C, Zwerina J, Schett G, et al. WNT5A is induced by inflammatory mediators in bone marrow stromal cells and regulates cytokine and chemokine production. *J Bone Miner Res* (2012) 27(3): 575–85. doi:10.1002/jbmr.1488
32. Whang YM, Jo U, Sung JS, Ju HJ, Kim HK, Park KH, et al. Wnt5a is associated with cigarette smoke-related lung carcinogenesis via protein kinase C. *PLoS One* (2013) 8:e53012. doi:10.1371/journal.pone.0053012
33. Yang S-R, Chida AS, Bauter MR, Shafiq N, Seweryniak K, Maggirwar SB, et al. Cigarette smoke induces proinflammatory cytokine release by activation of NF-kappaB and posttranslational modifications of histone deacetylase in macrophages. *Am J Physiol Lung Cell Mol Physiol* (2006) 291:L46–57. doi:10.1152/ajplung.00241.2005
34. Wojtan P, Mierzejewski M, Osińska I, Domagała-Kulawik J. Macrophage polarization in interstitial lung diseases. *Cent Eur J Immunol* (2016) 41(2): 159–64. doi:10.5114/ceji.2016.60990
35. Yin Y, Hou G, Li E, Wang Q, Kang J. PPAR Gamma agonists regulate tobacco smoke-induced toll like receptor 4 expression in alveolar macrophages. *Respir Res* (2014) 15:28. doi:10.1186/1465-9921-15-28
36. Belvisi MG, Hele DJ, Birrell MA. Peroxisome proliferator-activated receptor gamma agonists as therapy for chronic airway inflammation. *Eur J Pharmacol* (2006) 533:101–9. doi:10.1016/j.ejphar.2005.12.048
37. Shan M, You R, Yuan X, Frazier MV, Porter P, Seryshev A, et al. Agonistic induction of PPARγ reverses cigarette smoke-induced emphysema. *J Clin Invest* (2014) 124:1371–81. doi:10.1172/JCI70587
38. Malur A, Mccoy AJ, Arce S, Barna BP, Kavuru MS, Malur AG, et al. Deletion of PPAR in alveolar macrophages is associated with a Th-1 pulmonary inflammatory response. *J Immunol* (2009) 182:5816–22. doi:10.4049/jimmunol.0803504
39. Bouhlel MA, Derudas B, Rigamonti E, Dièvart R, Brozek J, Haulon S, et al. PPARγ activation primes human monocytes into alternative M2 macrophages with anti-inflammatory properties. *Cell Metab* (2007) 6(2):137–43. doi:10.1016/j.cmet.2007.06.010
40. Balogh P, Bebök Z, Németh P. Cellular enzyme-linked immunocircle assay. A rapid assay of hybridomas produced against cell surface antigens. *J Immunol Methods* (1992) 153:141–9. doi:10.1016/0022-1759(92)90316-L
41. Kode A, Yang S-R, Rahman I. Differential effects of cigarette smoke on oxidative stress and proinflammatory cytokine release in primary human airway epithelial cells and in a variety of transformed alveolar epithelial cells. *Respir Res* (2008) 9:6. doi:10.1186/1465-9921-9-6
42. Bartis D, Csongei V, Weich A, Kiss E, Barko S, Kovacs T, et al. Down-regulation of canonical and up-regulation of non-canonical wnt signalling in the carcinogenic process of squamous cell lung carcinoma. *PLoS One* (2013) 8:e57393. doi:10.1371/journal.pone.0057393
43. Kovacs T, Csongei V, Feller D, Ernszt D, Smuk G, Sarosi V, et al. Alteration in the Wnt microenvironment directly regulates molecular events leading to pulmonary senescence. *Aging Cell* (2014) 13:838–49. doi:10.1111/acel.12240
44. Vesel M, Rapp J, Feller D, Kiss E, Jaromi L, Meggyes M, et al. ABCB1 and ABCG2 drug transporters are differentially expressed in non-small cell lung cancers (NSCLC) and expression is modified by cisplatin treatment via altered Wnt signaling. *Respir Res* (2017) 18. doi:10.1186/s12931-017-0537-6
45. Demirjian L, Abboud RT, Li H, Duronio V. Acute effect of cigarette smoke on TNF-α release by macrophages mediated through the erk1/2 pathway. *Biochim Biophys Acta* (2006) 1762:592–7. doi:10.1016/j.bbadis.2006.04.004
46. Hodge S, Matthews G, Mukaro V, Ahern J, Shivam A, Hodge G, et al. Cigarette smoke-induced changes to alveolar macrophage phenotype and function are improved by treatment with procysteine. *Am J Respir Cell Mol Biol* (2011) 44:673–81. doi:10.1165/rcmb.2009-0459OC
47. Chanmee T, Ontong P, Konno K, Itano N. Tumor-associated macrophages as major players in the tumor microenvironment. *Cancers (Basel)* (2014) 6:1670–90. doi:10.3390/cancers6031670
48. Willert K, Brown JD, Danenberg E, Duncan AW, Weissman IL, Reya T, et al. Wnt proteins are lipid-modified and can act as stem cell growth factors. *Nature* (2003) 423:448–52. doi:10.1038/nature01611
49. Korkut C, Ataman B, Ramachandran P, Ashley J, Barria R, Gherbesi N, et al. Trans-synaptic transmission of vesicular Wnt signals through Evi/Wntless. *Cell* (2009) 139:393–404. doi:10.1016/j.cell.2009.07.051
50. Gangoda L, Boukouris S, Liem M, Kalra H, Mathivanan S. Extracellular vesicles including exosomes are mediators of signal transduction: are they protective or pathogenic? *Proteomics* (2015) 15:260–71. doi:10.1002/pmic.201400234
51. Luga V, Zhang L, Viloria-Petit AM, Ogunjimi AA, Inanlou MR, Chiu E, et al. Exosomes mediate stromal mobilization of autocrine Wnt-PCP signaling in breast cancer cell migration. *Cell* (2012) 151:1542–56. doi:10.1016/j.cell.2012.11.024
52. Gallo A, Tandon M, Alevizos I, Illei GG. The majority of microRNAs detectable in serum and saliva is concentrated in exosomes. *PLoS One* (2012) 7:e30679. doi:10.1371/journal.pone.0030679
53. Mathivanan S, Simpson RJ. ExoCarta: a compendium of exosomal proteins and RNA. *Proteomics* (2009) 9:4997–5000. doi:10.1002/pmic.200900351
54. Sakurai R, Cerny LM, Torday JS, Rehan VK. Mechanism for nicotine-induced up-regulation of Wnt signaling in human alveolar interstitial fibroblasts. *Exp Lung Res* (2011) 37:144–54. doi:10.3109/01902148.2010.490288
55. Rapp J, Jaromi L, Kvell K, Miskei G, Pongracz JE. WNT signaling – lung cancer is no exception. *Respir Res* (2017) 18(1):167. doi:10.1186/s12931-017-0650-6
56. Nabhan A, Brownfield DG, Harbury PB, Krasnow MA, Desai TJ. Single-cell Wnt signaling niches maintain stemness of alveolar type 2 cells. *Science* (2018) 359(6380):1118–23. doi:10.1126/science.aam6603
57. Yuan A, Hsiao YJ, Chen HY, Chen HW, Ho CC, Chen YY, et al. Opposite effects of M1 and M2 macrophage subtypes on lung cancer progression. *Sci Rep* (2015) 5:14273. doi:10.1038/srep14273
58. Lea S, Plumb J, Metcalfe H, Spicer D, Woodman P, Fox JC, et al. The effect of peroxisome proliferator-activated receptor-γ ligands on in vitro and in vivo models of COPD. *Eur Respir J* (2014) 43:409–20. doi:10.1183/09031936.00187812
59. Ikemura S, Aramaki N, Fujii S, Kirita K, Umemura S, Matsumoto S, et al. Changes in the tumor microenvironment during lymphatic metastasis of lung squamous cell carcinoma. *Cancer Sci* (2017) 108(1):136–42. doi:10.1111/cas.13110
60. Hammad H, de Heer HJ, Soullie T, Angeli V, Trottein F, Hoogsteden HC, et al. Activation of peroxisome proliferator-activated receptor-gamma in dendritic cells inhibits the development of eosinophilic airway inflammation in a mouse model of asthma. *Am J Pathol* (2004) 164(1):263–71. doi:10.1016/S0002-9440(10)63116-1
61. Solleti SK, Simon DM, Srisuma S, Arikan MC, Bhattacharya S, Rangasamy T, et al. Airway epithelial cell PPARγ modulates cigarette smoke-induced chemokine expression and emphysema susceptibility in mice. *Am J Physiol Lung Cell Mol Physiol* (2015) 309:L293–304. doi:10.1152/ajplung.00287.2014
62. Suryawanshi A, Tadagavadi RK, Swafford D, Manicassamy S. Modulation of inflammatory responses by Wnt/β-catenin signaling in dendritic cells: a novel immunotherapy target for autoimmunity and cancer. *Front Immunol* (2016) 7:460. doi:10.3389/fimmu.2016.00460
63. Bergenfelz C, Medrek C, Ekström E, Jirström K, Janols H, Wullt M, et al. Leandersson K. Wnt5a induces a tolerogenic phenotype of macrophages in sepsis and breast cancer patients. *J Immunol* (2012) 188(11):5448–58. doi:10.4049/jimmunol.1103378
64. Zhao Y, Wang C-L, Li R-M, Hui T-Q, Su Y-Y, Yuan Q, et al. Wnt5a promotes inflammatory responses via nuclear factor κB (NF-κB) and mitogen-activated protein kinase (MAPK) pathways in human dental pulp cells. *J Biol Chem* (2014) 289:21028–39. doi:10.1074/jbc.M113.546523
65. Yu CH, Nguyen TTK, Irvine KM, Sweet MJ, Frazer IH, Blumenthal A. Recombinant Wnt3a and Wnt5a elicit macrophage cytokine production and tolerization to microbial stimulation via toll-like receptor 4. *Eur J Immunol* (2014) 44:1480–90. doi:10.1002/eji.201343959

17

Bleomycin Aggravates Atopic Dermatitis *via* Lung Inflammation in 2,4-Dinitrochlorobenzene-Induced NC/Nga Mice

Yoon-Young Sung[1], Seung-Hyung Kim[2], Won-Kyung Yang[2], Yang-Chun Park[2] and Ho Kyoung Kim[1]**

[1] Herbal Medicine Research Division, Korea Institute of Oriental Medicine, Daejeon, South Korea, [2] Institute of Traditional Medicine and Bioscience, Daejeon University, Daejeon, South Korea

***Correspondence:**
Yang-Chun Park
omdpyc@dju.kr
Ho Kyoung Kim
hkkim@kiom.re.kr

Atopic dermatitis (AD) is a chronic inflammatory skin disease. Bleomycin (BLM) contributes to the induction of pulmonary inflammation and fibrosis in animals. Although skin and lung tissue inflammation is closely related in the pathogenesis of allergic diseases, a proper animal model for investigating the relationship between skin and lung inflammation is lacking. Therefore, we developed a mouse model of AD with relapsing dermatitis and pulmonary fibrosis caused by the administration of allergen and BLM. The present study determined whether lung injury caused by the bronchial application of BLM would exacerbate AD-like allergic inflammation induced by 2, 4-dinitrochlorobenzene (DNCB) in NC/Nga mice. NC/Nga mice treated with BLM and DNCB had increased severity of clinical symptoms and airway hyperresponsiveness as well as increased inflammatory cell infiltration and collagen deposition in the dorsal skin and lung. Compared to normal mice, interleukin (IL)-6 and tumor necrosis factor (TNF)-α production in bronchoalveolar lavage fluid were increased in NC/Nga mice treated with both DNCB and BLM and in animals treated with DNCB alone. Administration of BLM and DNCB increased the levels of IL-4 and IL-13 production in spleen cells and eotaxin-2 mRNA expression in dorsal skin, compared to NC/Nga mice treated with DNCB alone. The total cell numbers in axillary lymph node, bronchoalveolar lavage, and thymus were increased in DNCB-BLM mice compared to those in mice treated with DNCB alone. Administration of BLM and DNCB increased the numbers of cluster of differentiation 4 (CD4)+ T cells and CD11b+granulocyte-differentiation antigen-1 (Gr-1)+ cells among peripheral blood mononuclear cells, CD4+ cells in bronchoalveolar lavage, CD4+ and B220+CD23+ B cells in the axillary lymph node, and CD4+ cells in thymus, compared to DNCB-treated mice. The number of total, CD4+, and CD11b+Gr-1+ cells in the lung were increased in both DNCB and DNCB-BLM mice. These results demonstrate that BLM aggravates allergic skin inflammation and promotes airway hyperreactivity and lung inflammation when combined with DNCB in NC/Nga mice.

Keywords: bleomycin, CD4+ cells, dinitrochlorobenzene, hyperresponsiveness, lung, pulmonary fibrosis

INTRODUCTION

Atopic dermatitis (AD) is a chronic inflammatory skin disease that has a high prevalence among infants and children (Han et al., 2011). The pathogenesis of AD is strongly influenced by both genetic and environmental factors (Bantz et al., 2014). The skin, located on the outermost body surface, is an important interface between the host and its environment, and the skin is believed, in Oriental medicine, to be influenced by the physiological function of the lung on the body (Im et al., 2002; Glick, 2005). In Asia, AD is called 'skin asthma,' because so many infants and children with AD already have, or will develop, asthma (Glick, 2005). Development of AD in infancy, and the subsequent development of other allergic respiratory diseases such as asthma in later childhood is referred to as the atopic march (Spergel and Paller, 2003; Zheng et al., 2011). Some studies have developed animal models with localized AD induced by repeated epicutaneous sensitization with ovalbumin, and airway hyperresponsiveness to methacholine after challenge with aerosolized ovalbumin, to study the progression from AD to asthma (Spergel et al., 1998). Recently, Han et al. (2017) reported that neonatal capsaicin treatment induced chronically relapsing pruritic dermatitis and asthmatic airway changes in rats (Han et al., 2017). However, a proper animal model for investigating the relationship among skin and lung inflammation in AD is still lacking.

Bleomycin (BLM) administration is a widely used method for inducing local skin and pulmonary inflammation and fibrosis in animals (Liang et al., 2015). Intratracheal instillation of BLM in mice causes bronchial fibrotic changes, acute interstitial and intra-alveolar inflammation, and upregulation of alveolar inflammatory cells (Della Latta et al., 2015). C57BL/6 mice, which are more susceptible than Balb/c mice to BLM-induced fibrosis, are used in most studies, and only few researchers employ other strains such as 129, CBA, Balb/c, and ICR (Della Latta et al., 2015). We developed a mouse model of AD with relapsing dermatitis and pulmonary fibrosis by the administration of BLM and allergen. The present study determined whether lung injury induced by the bronchial application of BLM would exacerbate the AD-like allergic inflammation induced by 2, 4-dinitrochlorobenzene (DNCB) in NC/Nga mice, an inbred animal model for human AD (Choi et al., 2012; Kim et al., 2014). It has been reported that repeated applications of DNCB to the skin of NC/Nga mice induced AD-like skin lesions, which is associated with an increase in serum immunoglobulin (Ig) E and T-helper (Th) 2 cytokines such as interleukin (IL)-4, IL-5, and IL-13 at the chronic dorsal skin lesions (Choi et al., 2012). In addition, NC/Nga mice showed high airway hyperresponsiveness to acetylcholine and marked enhancement of airway resistance after a single intranasal challenge with ovalbumin or mite allergen *Dermatophagoides farinae*, thus suggesting that NC/Nga mice are a useful animal model to investigate the pathogenesis of allergic asthma and AD (Iwasaki et al., 2001; Shibamori et al., 2006).

Therefore, the purpose of this study was to develop an animal model for studying AD in mice using timely administration of BLM and DNCB. We induced AD by repeated topical application of DNCB to the skin after induction of lung fibrosis by bronchial injection of BLM in NC/Nga mice. In the present study, we have demonstrated, using a murine model of AD, that bleomycin, when administered in combination with allergens, has an additive and synergistic effect in driving cutaneous eczematoide skin changes, and promotes airway hyperreactivity and lung inflammation upon allergen challenge.

MATERIALS AND METHODS

Animals

Five-week-old male NC/Nga and C57BL/6 mice were obtained from Central Lab Animal Inc. (Seoul, South Korea). All animal experiments and procedures were approved by the Committee for Animal Welfare at the Daejeon University (DJUARB2016-036). All animal procedures were conducted in accordance with the guidelines of the Animal Care and Use Committee of the South Korea Research Institute of Bioscience and Biotechnology (Daejeon, South Korea) and the US guidelines (NIH publication number 85-23. Revised 1996). All animals were housed in air-conditioned animal room at a temperature of 21 ± 2°C and humidity of 50 ± 5% under a 12:12-h light/dark cycle and had *ad libitum* access to food and water for 1 week.

Induction of Lung Fibrosis

The mice were divided into four groups ($n = 4$): group 1, C57BL/6 (vehicle)-Normal; group 2, NC/Nga (vehicle)-Normal; group 3, NC/Nga (DNCB)-Control; group 4, NC/Nga (DNCB-BLM). As previously described (Della Latta et al., 2015), the NC/Nga mice were administered a single-dose intratracheal instillation of bleomycin (BLM-treated group, 0.125 U/100 g; Sigma) or vehicle (normal and control group, saline) using bronchial tubes. Normal C57BL/6 mice received vehicle only.

Induction of AD

The back hair of mice was shaved with electric clippers a day before BLM administration. AD was induced in C57BL/6 and NC/Nga mice 7 days after BLM or vehicle administration (Park et al., 2014; Saba et al., 2016). For the sensitization process, 200 µl of a 1% DNCB solution (acetone: olive oil = 3:1) was applied dermally to the shaved back area twice per week for 1 week using 1 × 1 cm patches. At 1 week after the first DNCB sensitization, the back skin was challenged with 150 µl of a 0.4% DNCB solution three times per week for 3 weeks. At the end of the experiment, mice were sacrificed by intraperitoneal (i.p.) injection of urethane (2.5 mg/kg), and samples were collected. The schematic diagram of the experimental protocol is shown in **Figure 1A**.

Collection of Bronchoalveolar Lavage Fluid (BALF)

After the mice were sacrificed by i.p. injection of urethane (2.5 mg/kg), BALF was collected by washing the airway lamina by tracheal cannulation. The fluid collected from airway lavage was defined as BALF, centrifuged, and the supernatant collected and stored at −25°C for determination of cytokine levels. The cell pellets were suspended in 1 ml PBS and the total cell number was counted using a hemocytometer.

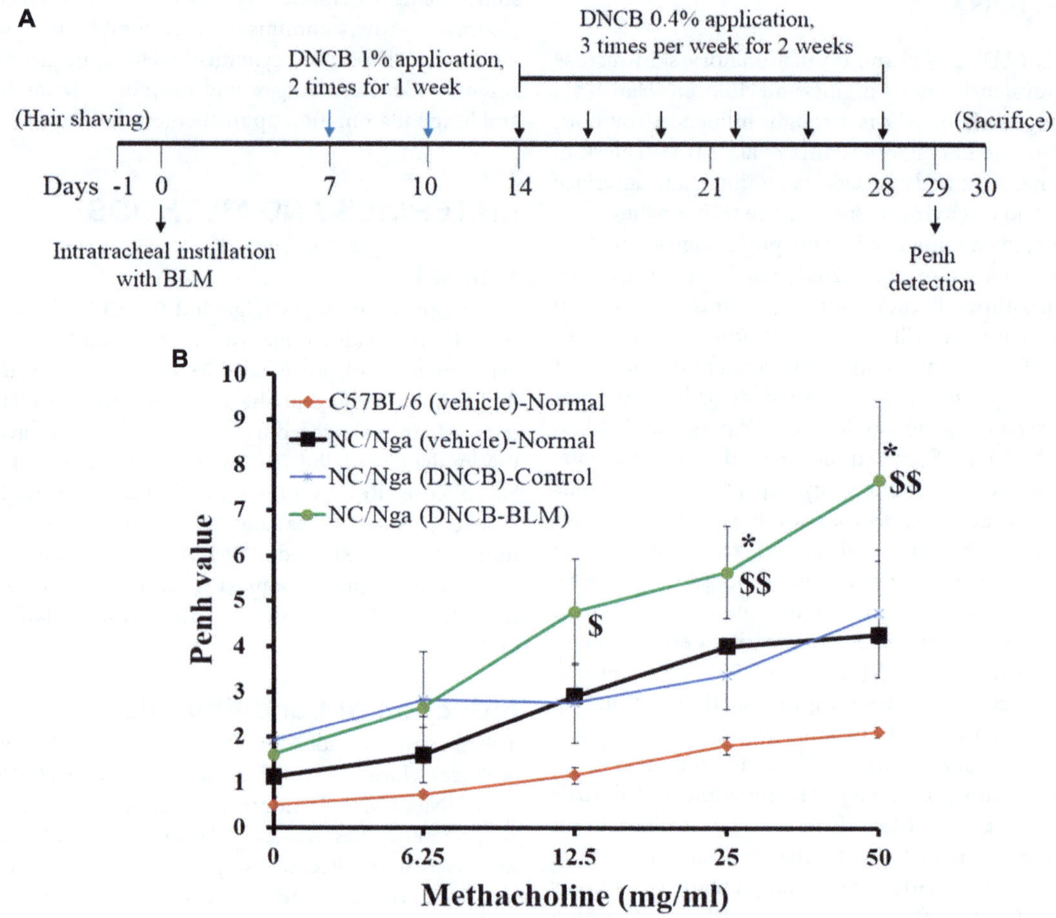

FIGURE 1 | Effect of BLM on airway hyperresponsiveness. **(A)** Schematic diagram of the treatment protocol. **(B)** Airway resistance was measured after exposure to increasing doses of aerosolized methacholine (6.25, 12.5, 25, and 50 mg/ml). The mice were divided into four groups (n = 4); C57BL/6 (vehicle)-Normal, NC/Nga (vehicle)-Normal, NC/Nga (DNCB)-Control, and NC/Nga (DNCB-BLM). Values are expressed as the mean ± standard error of mean (SEM) (n = 4). $^{\$}p < 0.05$, $^{\$\$}p < 0.01$ [compared with C57BL/6 (vehicle)-Normal], and $^{*}p < 0.05$ [compared with NC/Nga (DNCB)-Control] as determined by one-way ANOVA followed by multiple comparison tests.

Determination of Airway Hyperresponsiveness (AHR)

Airway hyperresponsiveness in mice was measured using non-invasive whole-body plethysmography Buxco system (Biosystems XA; DSI Inc., MN, United States) as previously described (Kim et al., 2011). Each chamber was equipped with a pneumotachograph (Halcyon, Buxco) to measure airflow, and this information was transmitted to analysis software (Biosystem XA for windows, Buxco). The software uses various algorithms to calculate several flow-derived parameters, including respiratory rate, lung volume, peak flow, and time intervals. The software reported data as 'enhanced pause' (Penh), an index of airway hyperreactivity derived from the equation: Penh is equal to Pause × PEF/PIF, where Pause = (Te−Tr)/Tr (PIF, peak inspiratory flow; PEF, peak expiratory flow; Te, expiratory time; Tr, relaxation time). One day after the final DNCB treatment, the mice were placed in Buxco chamber and were given aerosolized normal saline, followed by increasing doses (6.25, 12.5, 25, and 50 mg/ml) of aerosolized methacholine (Sigma-Aldrich Korea, Seoul, South Korea). Airway reactivity was then monitored for 30 min and respiratory curves were converted into enhanced pause (Penh) values.

Measurement of Clinical Skin Severity Score

Dermatitis skin scores of AD-like skin lesions were evaluated as described previously (Suto et al., 1999). The severity of dermatitis was assessed according to four symptoms: (1) erythema/hemorrhage, (2) scarring/dryness, (3) edema, and (4) excoriation/erosion. Each symptom was scored from 0 to 3 (none, 0; mild, 1; moderate, 2; severe, 3). Clinical skin severity score was defined as the sum of the individual scores, ranging from 0 to 12.

Enzyme-Linked Immunosorbent Assay (ELISA)

The levels of IgE in the serum were determined using a mouse ELISA kit (R&D Systems, Minneapolis, MN, United States). Interleukin (IL)-6 and TNF-α secretion in BALF were determined by ELISA (R&D systems) according to the manufacturer's instructions.

IL-4, IL-5, IL-13, and IFN-γ production was detected in spleen cells suspended in RPMI 1640 medium supplemented with 2 mM L-glutamine and 5% FBS. Spleen cells were cultured in 96-well plates for 48 h at a concentration of 1×10^5 cells/well with plate-bound anti-CD3 antibody (0.5 μg/ml) in a humidified atmosphere of 5% CO_2 at 37°C. The culture supernatants were then collected and IL-4, IL-5, IL-13, and IFN-γ levels in the supernatants were measured using an ELISA kit (R&D systems).

The limits of detection (sensitivity) were 1.8 pg/ml of IL-6, 7.21 pg/ml of TNF-α, 2 pg/ml of IL-4, 7.0 pg/ml of IL-5, 1.5 pg/ml of IL-13, and 2 pg/ml of IFN-γ. According to the certificate of analysis supplied by the manufacturer of the commercial assay, the intra-assay coefficient of variation (CV) of the IL-4 ELISA system was 4.7% and the inter-assay CV was 5.2%. The intra- and inter-assay CV of IL-5 was 5.2 and 4.4%, respectively. The intra- and inter-assay CV of IL-13 was 2.8 and 6.7%, respectively. The intra-and inter-assay CV of IFN-γ was 3.6 and 9.3%, respectively. The intra- and inter-assay CV of IL-6 was 4.7 and 7.5%, respectively. The intra- and inter-assay CV of TNF-α was 3.2 and 7.7%, respectively.

Sample Collection and Cell Preparations

Peripheral blood mononuclear cells (PBMCs) were isolated from the heparinized blood of mice by Percoll density-gradient centrifugation. Cell suspensions were prepared from fresh tissues processed in RPMI 1640 medium. Single cell suspensions from tissues and BALF were isolated by mechanical disruption in RPMI 1640 medium supplemented with 2 mM L-glutamine, 100 U/mL penicillin, 100 μg/mL streptomycin, 50 μM 2-mercaptoethanol, 20 mM HEPES, and 2% heat-inactivated fetal bovine serum (FBS, GIBCO, Grand Island, NY, United States). Briefly, the tissues (axillary lymph node, thymus, dorsal skin, and lung) were removed from the mice, minced using scalpels, and then incubated in PBS containing 1 mg/mL collagenase IV (Sigma-C5138, Sigma, St. Louis, MO, United States) at 37°C. After incubation for 40 min, each tissue was vigorously pipetted up and down to further dissociate the remaining tissue clumps. The cell suspension was filtered using a 70-μm pore size nylon cell strainer (BD Falcon, Bedford, MA, United States) and then centrifuged for 20 min at 450 g. The cell pellet was collected, and the cells were washed twice. Total cell number was determined using a hemocytometer chamber (Thermo Fisher Scientific, Grand Island, NY, United States). The cells obtained were stained immediately with various antibodies for flow cytometry analysis.

Flow Cytometry Analysis

Prior to flow cytometry analysis, samples abundant with RBCs were treated with ammonium-chloride-potassium (ACK) lysis buffer for 2 min at room temperature. PBMCs, as well as cells from the axillary lymph node (ALN), BAL, thymus, dorsal skin, and lung tissue were stained with the indicated antibodies in staining solution (PBS containing 1% FBS and 0.01% NaN3) for 10 min on ice. After the samples were stained, the stained cells were assessed on a fluorescence-activated cell sorter flow cytometry system (FACS Calibur; BD Biosciences, Mountain View, CA, United States) and the data were analyzed with CellQuest software (BD Biosciences). All antibodies, including anti-CD4, anti-B220, anti-CD11b, anti-Gr-1, anti-CD25, and anti-CD23 were purchased from BD PharMingen (San Diego, CA, United States). The absolute number of each cell subtype was calculated from the subtype percent and the total number of cells in the tissues of each individual mouse.

Hematoxylin-Eosin (H&E), Masson's Trichrome (MT), and Toluidine Blue (TB) Staining

Dorsal skin and lung tissue were removed and subjected to histological analysis using a previously published protocol (Kim et al., 2011; Sung et al., 2014). Tissues was fixed in 10% (v/v) neutral-buffered formalin, embedded in paraffin, and then cut into 3-μm thick sections. Dorsal skin and lung sections were stained with H&E to assess the infiltration of inflammatory cells and epidermal hyperplasia. To determine the degree of pathologic changes (epidermal and dermal hypertrophy and inflammation), index counts extent of epidermal/dermal thickness and inflammatory cells in the dorsal skin lesions were blindly quantified with subjective scores of 0 (none), 1 (mild), 2 (moderate), and 3 (severe) for each of the four symptoms using a previously published protocol with modification (Kang et al., 2015). Other sections were stained with TB to evaluate the infiltration of mast cells in the dorsal skin, and with MT solution (Sigma-Aldrich Korea) to determine collagen deposition in the lung. At least three different sections of each tissue were evaluated under light microscopy.

Quantitative Real-Time Polymerase Chain Reaction (RT-qPCR)

Dorsal skin tissues from the mice were removed and immediately frozen by immersion in liquid nitrogen for subsequent RNA isolation. Total RNA from the dorsal skin was extracted using RNAzol B (Tel-Test, Austin, TX, United States) according to the manufacturer's instructions. The cDNA was synthesized from 3 μg of total RNA using a ReverTra Ace-a-cDNA Synthesis kit (Toyobo, Osaka, Japan). The cDNA template was mixed with SYBR Green PCR Master Mix (Applied Biosystems, Grand Island, NY, United States) and 200 nM primers. Glyceraldehyde-3-phosphate dehydrogenase (GAPDH) was used as an internal control. Quantitative real-time RT-PCR was performed in triplicate using the Applied Biosystems 7500 Fast Real-Time PCR system (Applied Biosystems) and analyzed according to the manual (threshold: 0.05, baseline: 6–15 cycles). PCR was performed under the following set of conditions: 2 min at 50°C, 10 min at 94°C, 40 cycles of 1 min at 94°C, and 1 min at 60°C. The cycle number at which the emission intensity of the sample rose above baseline was defined as the relative quantity (RQ) and was proportional to the target concentration. The RQ in target gene expression relative to control mice was normalized to the internal control, glyceraldehyde 3-phosphate dehydrogenase (GAPDH), using the $2^{-\Delta\Delta Ct}$ method. The primer sequences were as follows: GAPDH, sense 5′-TGAAG CAGGCATCTGAGGG-3′, antisense 5′-CGAAGGTGGAAGA

GTGGGAG-3′; IL-31R, sense 5′-ATGCCCAACAAAGCAGAGAC-3′, antisense 5′-TGAGAGAACCAGGGAGCTGT-3′; and eotaxin-2, sense 5′- CTGTGACCATCCCCTCATCT-3′, antisense 5′-CTTATGGCCCTTCTTGGTGA-3′.

Statistical Analysis

Results were expressed as mean ± standard error of the mean (SEM). Statistical analyses of the results were performed by one-way ANOVA followed by Tukey's or Duncan's multiple comparison tests using the SigmaPlot 13.0 software. Significance level was set at $p < 0.05$.

RESULTS

Induction of Airway Hyperresponsiveness by Bleomycin

To determine the effects of BLM on lung fibrosis and function, we analyzed airway resistance in response to methacholine (doses of 6.25, 12.5, 25, and 50 mg/kg) by non-invasive WBP (**Figure 1B**). Pehn values for NC/Nga (vehicle) and NC/Nga (DNCB) mice were similar. However, Pehn values showed a greater increase in NC/Nga mice treated with both DNCB and BLM (DNCB-BLM) than in NC/Nga mice treated with DNCB alone (DNCB-Control) at doses of 25 (F-value = 5.470 and p = 0.017) and 50 mg/kg methacholine (F-value = 4.012 and p = 0.041).

DNCB-Induced AD-Like Symptoms

To determine whether BLM treatment in the lung exacerbates AD-like symptoms in DNCB-induced NC/Nga mice, we treated mice with DNCB and BLM. AD-like symptoms were evaluated by dermatitis skin score (Method 2.6) and the skin clinical score significantly increased in both DNCB-Control and DNCB-BLM mice when compared to NC/Nga-Normal mice (F-value = 19.696 and $p \leq 0.01$) (**Figure 2A**). Consistent with previous reports (Choi et al., 2017), the overall clinical symptoms of AD, including erythema, hemorrhage, edema, scarring, excoriation, and lichenification, were induced by the repeated application

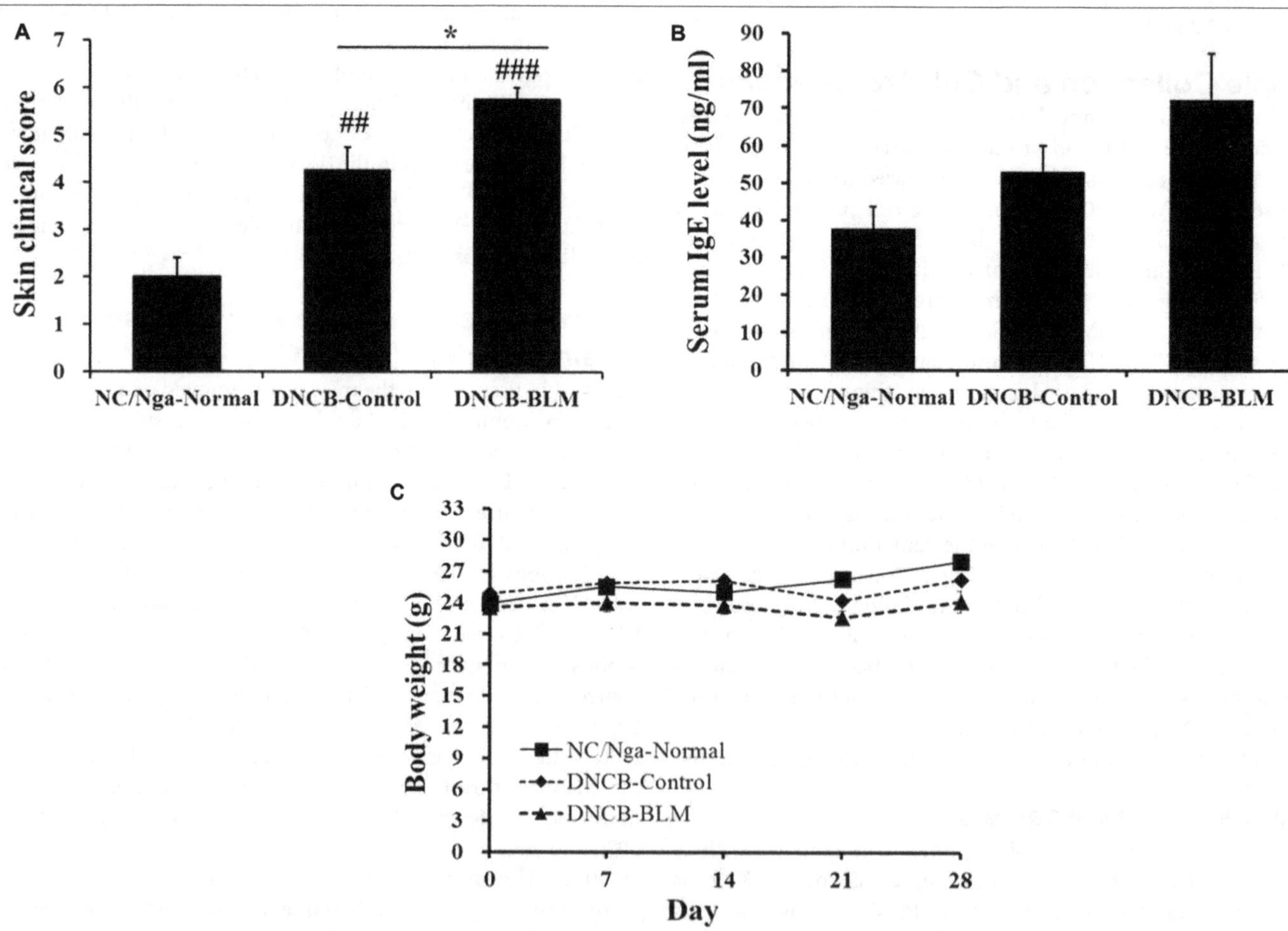

FIGURE 2 | Effect of BLM on AD-like symptoms, serum IgE level, and body weight. **(A)** The severity of clinical symptoms of the skin lesions was evaluated macroscopically and calculated as the sum of the individual scores for the following four AD signs and symptoms: erythema/hemorrhage, edema, excoriation/erosion, and scaling/dryness. **(B)** Total IgE levels in serum were determined by ELISA. **(C)** Body weight were measured once a week. Values are expressed as the mean ± standard error of mean (SEM) (n = 4). $^{\#\#}p < 0.01$, $^{\#\#\#}p < 0.001$ (compared with NC/Nga-Normal), and $^{*}p < 0.05$ (compared with DNCB-Control) as determined by one-way analysis of variance (ANOVA) followed by multiple comparison tests.

of DNCB to the back skin of the NC/Nga mice for 2 weeks (p = 0.003). More importantly, BLM administered to the lung dramatically increased the skin clinical severity score of AD in DNCB-treated mice ($p \leq 0.001$, compared to NC/Nga-Normal mice; p = 0.049, compared to DNCB-Control mice) (**Figure 2A**). In addition, although it did not achieve significance, the serum IgE concentration showed a greater increase in mice treated with DNCB and BLM than in mice treated with DNCB alone (**Figure 2B**). The body weight, in accordance with the worsening of AD symptoms, showed a tendency to decline in DNCB-treated or DNCB-BLM-treated mice; however, this reduction was not statistically significant (**Figure 2C**).

Total Leukocyte Cell Numbers From the ALN, Dorsal Skin, BALF, Thymus, and Lung

Next, we investigated whether BLM treatment in the lung in AD mice altered the total number of leukocytes in ALN, dorsal skin, BAL, thymus, and lung. Total ALN cells were significantly higher in DNCB-BLM-treated mice than in the NC/Nga-Normal (F = 8.842 and p = 0.015) and DNCB-control groups (p = 0.040) (**Figure 3A**). Total BAL cells were significantly higher in DNCB-BLM-treated mice than in the NC/Nga-Normal (F = 3.54 and p = 0.005) and DNCB-control groups (p = 0.011) (**Figure 3C**). Total thymus cells were significantly higher in DNCB-BLM-treated mice than in the NC/Nga-Normal (F-value = 5.521 and p = 0.036) and DNCB-control groups ($p < 0.05$) (**Figure 3D**). Our analysis demonstrated a statistically significant increase in total cell numbers of dorsal skin in both DNCB-Control (F-value = 9.6 and $p \leq 0.05$) and DNCB-BLM mice ($p < 0.01$) when compared to NC/Ng-Normal mice (**Figure 3B**). Total lung cells were significantly higher in DNCB-Control and DNCB-BLM mice compared to NC/Nga mice (F-value = 22.403 and $p \leq 0.05$, **Figure 3E**); the values in dorsal skin and lung cells were significantly higher in the DNCB-BLM-treated mice than in NC/Nga-Normal mice ($p < 0.05$), but there was no significant difference between DNCB-Control and DNCB-BLM-treated mice (**Figures 3B,E**).

Absolute Number of Immune Cell Subtypes

To confirm whether the AHR and inflammatory changes observed in mice subjected to various treatments were reflected in altered T cell subtypes and B cell distributions in PBMCs, BAL, ALN, dorsal skin, thymus, and lung, flow cytometry analysis was performed (**Figure 4**).

The DNCB-BLM-treated mice displayed a statistically significant higher number of CD4+ helper T cells in PBMCs (F-value = 4.872 and p = 0.047), BAL (F-value = 4.823 and p = 0.048), ALN (F-value = 7.286 and p = 0.002), thymus (F-value = 10.93 and p = 0.044), and lung (F-value = 15.61 and p = 0.003) compared to NC/Nga-Normal mice. In addition, CD4+ helper T cells in the PBMCs, BALF, ALN, and thymus were significantly increased in the DNCB-BLM-treated mice when compared to DNCB-Control mice ($p < 0.05$). IgE-producing B220+CD23+ B cells in the ALN were higher in DNCB-BLM-treated mice than in NC/Nga-Normal (F-value = 8.000 and p = 0.002) and DNCB-Control (p = 0.022) mice, but were unchanged in PBMCs. In PBMC, CD11b+Gr-1+ granulocytes showed a statistically significant increase (F-value = 4.120 and $p \leq 0.05$) in the

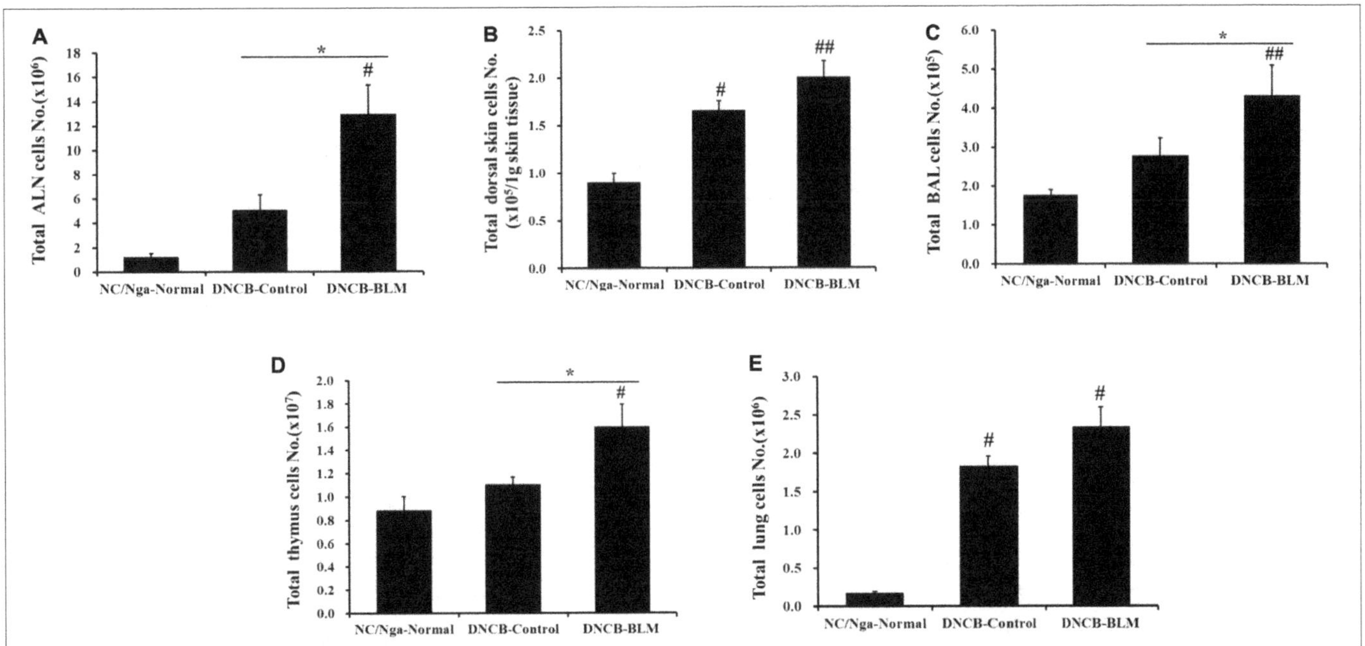

FIGURE 3 | Effect of BLM on total cell numbers in the **(A)** ALN, **(B)** dorsal skin, **(C)** BAL, **(D)** thymus, and **(E)** lung. Values are expressed as the mean ± standard error of mean (SEM) (n = 4). $^{\#}p < 0.05$, $^{\#\#}p < 0.01$ (compared with NC/Nga-Normal), and $^{*}p < 0.05$ (compared with DNCB-Control) as determined by one-way analysis of variance (ANOVA) followed by multiple comparison tests.

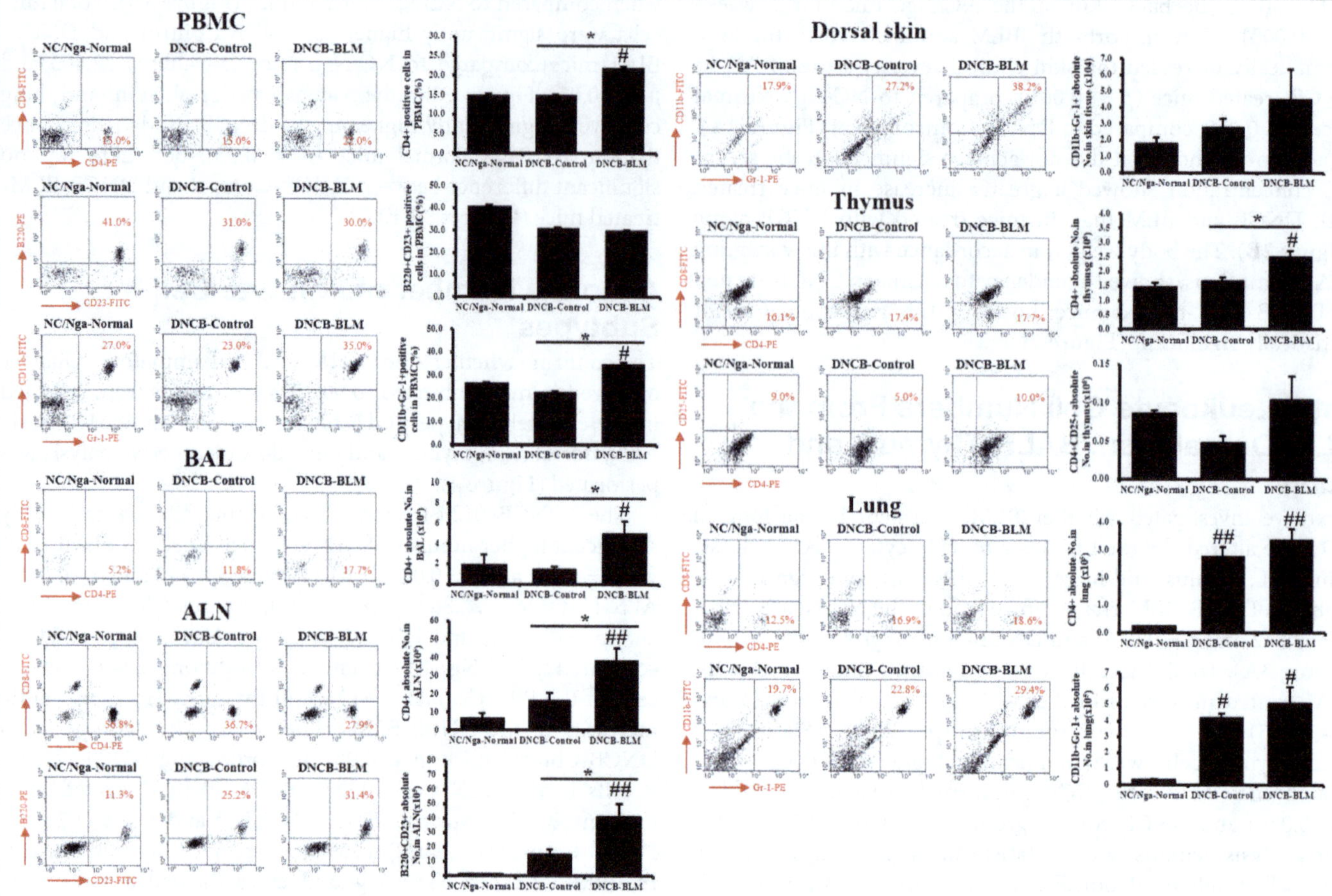

FIGURE 4 | Immune cell subtypes in PBMCs, BAL, ALN, dorsal skin, thymus, and lung. The cell subtypes were analyzed by fluorescence-activated cell sorting analysis (FACS). Red numbers on the scatter plots indicate the percentage of each cell type in the total immune cell population. The absolute number of each cell type was calculated from the specific cell type percentage and total cell number counted in the tissues of each individual mouse. Values are expressed as the mean ± standard error of mean (SEM) ($n = 4$). #$p < 0.05$, ##$p < 0.01$ (compared with NC/Nga-Normal), and *$p < 0.05$ (compared with DNCB-Control) as determined by one-way analysis of variance (ANOVA) followed by multiple comparison tests.

DNCB-BLM-treated mice when compared to NC/Nga-Normal mice. Further, the number of CD11b+Gr-1+ granulocytes in the PBMC were significantly elevated in the DNCB-BLM-treated mice when compared to DNCB-Control ($p = 0.04$). In lung, CD11b+Gr-1+ granulocytes showed a statistically significant increase (F-value = 8.364 and $p < 0.05$) in the DNCB-Control and DNCB-BLM-treated mice when compared to NC/Nga-Normal mice. In the dorsal skin, CD11b+Gr-1+ cells were increased in the DNCB-BLM mice, but the differences were not significant among the groups. CD4+CD25+ regulatory T cells in the thymus also showed no significant differences among the three groups.

Increase in Cytokine Production in BALF and Splenocyte Culture Supernatant

To investigate whether BLM influenced pro-inflammatory cytokine secretion in BALF, the levels of IL-6 and TNF-α were measured by ELISA. The differences in IL-6 levels in BALF between the groups were statistically significant (F-value = 24.351 and $p \leq 0.001$). As shown in **Figure 5A**, IL-6 levels were significantly increased in the DNCB-Control ($p = 0.002$) and DNCB-BLM-treated mice ($p < 0.001$) when compared to the NC/Nga-Normal mice. TNF-α levels in BALF were increased in the DNCB-Control and DNCB-BLM-treated mice, but this difference was not statistically significant across the groups. The differences in IL-4 (F-value = 10.113 and $p \leq 0.001$), IL-5 ($p \leq 0.001$), IL-13 ($F = 11.731$ and $p =\leq 0.001$), and IFN-γ ($p = 0.033$) levels in spleen cell culture supernatants between the groups were statistically significant. Our data indicate that DNCB-BLM treatment resulted in a dramatic increase in the Th1 cytokine IFN-γ ($p < 0.05$), as well as in the Th2 cytokines IL-4 ($p < 0.001$), IL-5 ($p < 0.001$), and IL-13 ($p < 0.001$) compared to NC/Nga-Normal mice. These levels in DNCB-BLM mice were higher than those observed in DNCB-Control mice ($p < 0.05$ for IL-4 and $p < 0.01$ for IL-13) (**Figure 5B**).

Histopathological Analysis of Dorsal Skin and Lung Tissues

To investigate the effects of BLM on histopathological changes in the DNCB-induced AD model, dorsal skin tissues were

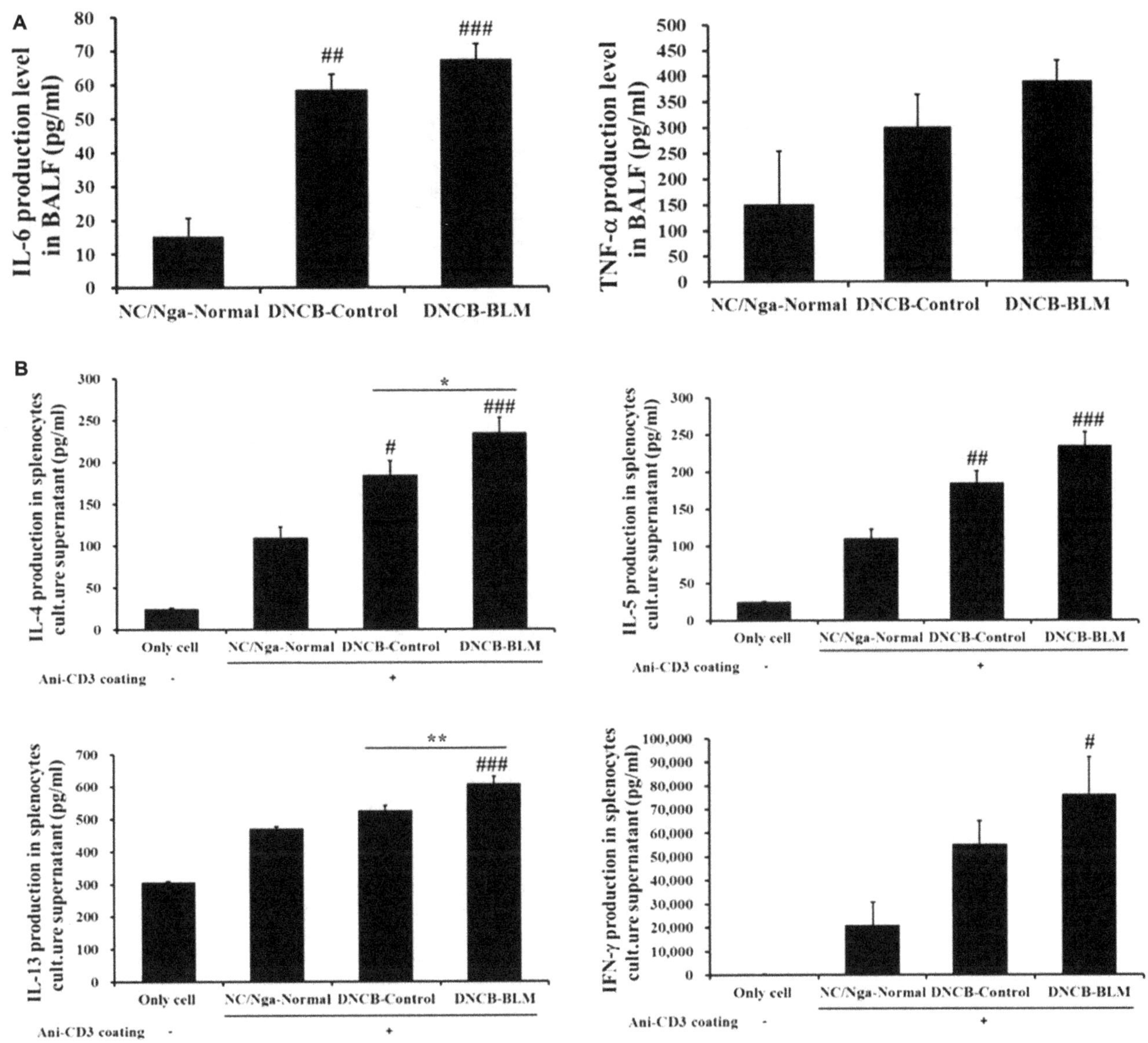

FIGURE 5 | Effect of BLM on the production of pro-inflammatory cytokines (IL-6 and TNF-α) in BALF **(A)**, and Th2 cytokines (IL-4, IL-5, and IL-13) and Th1 cytokines (IFN-γ) production in spleen cells **(B)**. Spleen cells were cultured for 48 h at a concentration of 1×10^5 cells/well using anti-CD3 coated 96-well plates. The 'Only cell' group represents the negative control (i.e., no exposure to anti-CD3 antibody). Cytokine production was measured by ELISA. Values are expressed as the mean ± standard error of mean (SEM) ($n = 4$). $^{\#}p < 0.05$, $^{\#\#}p < 0.01$, $^{\#\#\#}p < 0.001$ (compared with NC/Nga-Normal), $^{*}p < 0.05$, $^{**}p < 0.01$ (compared with DNCB-Control) as determined by one-way analysis of variance (ANOVA) followed by multiple comparison tests.

stained with H&E and TB staining solution. **Figures 6A,B** demonstrate the differences among the groups, which were also found to be statistically significant (F-value = 28.886 and $p = \leq 0.001$). The staining results showed that the dorsal skin of DNCB-Control mice exhibited epidermal hypertrophy, inflammatory cell infiltration ($p = 0.003$), and increased mast cell numbers ($p < 0.05$). These inflammatory and mast cell number changes were worse in the DNCB-BLM mice ($p < 0.05$).

In addition, we performed H&E and MT staining of lung tissue sections to evaluate lung inflammation and collagen identification. Collagen content has been used as a measure of the degree of fibrosis in the lung (McAnulty and Laurent, 1995); these measurements were made in the lungs of DNCB- or DNCB-BLM-treated mice. BLM increased inflammatory infiltrate and collagen deposition in the peribronchial and perivascular areas of DNCB-BLM mice ($F = 73.4$, $p < 0.001$ compared with NC/Nga-Normal mice, $p = 0.006$ compared with DNCB-Control mice; **Figures 6C,D**).

Increase of Eotaxin-2 and IL-31R mRNA in Dorsal Skin Tissues

To determine the effects of BLM on the gene expression levels of allergy-related biomarkers in dorsal skin tissue, we measured

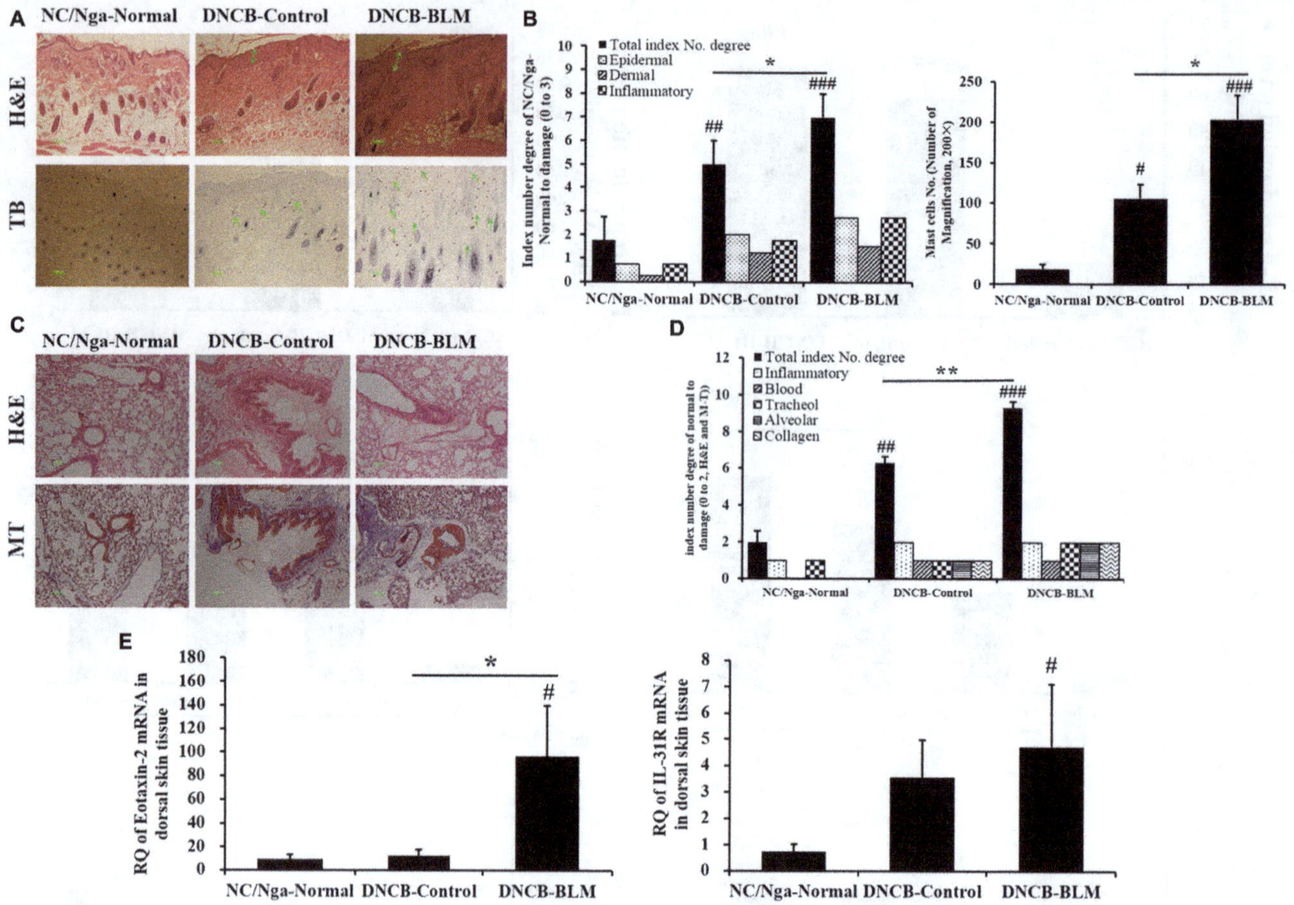

FIGURE 6 | Histopathological changes in dorsal skin and lung tissues, and expression of eotaxin-2 and IL-31R mRNA in dorsal skin. **(A)** Skin sections were stained with H&E and TB. **(B)** Total index number and mast cell number in the dorsal skin were quantitated. **(C)** Lung sections were stained with H&E and MT. **(D)** Total index number of degree in the lung was quantified. **(E)** Expression levels of eotaxin2 and IL-31R mRNA in dorsal skin tissue were analyzed by real-time RT-PCR. The results are expressed as RQ to control. H&E, hematoxylin-eosin stain; TB, toluidine blue stain; MT, Masson trichrome stain; RQ, relative quantity. Values are expressed as the mean ± standard error of mean (SEM) (n = 4). $^{\#}p < 0.05$, $^{\#\#}p < 0.01$, $^{\#\#\#}p < 0.001$ (compared with NC/Nga-Normal), $^{*}p < 0.05$, $^{**}p < 0.01$ (compared with DNCB-Control) as determined by one-way analysis of variance (ANOVA) followed by multiple comparison tests.

the expression of eotaxin-2 and IL-31R mRNA by real-time RT-PCR. The results showed that mRNA expression of eotaxin-2 was dramatically increased in the DNCB-BLM mice compared to that in NC/Nga-Normal and DNCB-Control mice ($p < 0.05$, **Figure 6E**). Expression of IL-31R mRNA was significantly higher in DNCB-BLM mice compared to that in NC/Nga mice ($p < 0.05$), and the levels were not significantly different between DNCB-Control and DNCB-BLM mice (**Figure 6E**).

DISCUSSION

We developed a mouse model of AD induced by DNCB-BLM treatment. In the present study, we showed in NC/Nga mice that, when combined with allergens DNCB, BLM has an additive effect on driving AD-like symptoms and promotes asthmatic changes such as airway hyperreactivity and allergic lung inflammation. Taken together, this model could be useful for studying the pathogenesis and progression of allergic atopic diseases. Mice that received both DNCB and BLM showed AD-like symptoms including erythema, edema, hemorrhage, scarring, and excoriation. DNCB and BLM treatment increased the protein production of Th2 cytokines (such as IL-4, IL-5, and IL-13) and IFN-γ in spleen cells, and of IL-6 and TNF-α in BALF. Th2 lymphocytes play a prominent role in the initiation and progression of allergic disease, including asthma and AD, by releasing IL-4, IL-5, and IL-13, which promote IgE-mediated allergic inflammation, and IFN-γ, a Th1 cytokine secreted by Th1 cells, acts in conjunction with Th2 cytokines in maintaining the chronic inflammatory response in allergic disease, particularly in asthmatic airways (Ngoc et al., 2005). IL-4 causes a switch to IgE production by differentiating B cells, and elevated eosinophilic inflammation is under the control of IL-5 and TNF-α (Deo et al., 2010). IL-13 directly induces mucus hypersecretion and airway hyperresponsiveness (Kim et al., 2011). Furthermore, changes of cytokines in BALF reflect the immunological reaction of the lung in asthma and other inflammatory pulmonary diseases.

Together with TNF-α, IL-6 as a pro-inflammatory cytokine plays a major role in dictating the immune response against allergens, as well as in specific pathological features of allergic airway inflammation such as mucus production (Neveu et al., 2009).

Eotaxin-1, −2, and −3 are potent and specific eosinophil chemoattractants involved in the activation and recruitment of eosinophils through binding to their CC chemokine receptor 3. Thus, eotaxins might contribute to increasing blood and tissue eosinophils in allergic inflammation responses (Kaplan, 2001). Eotaxin-1 is an important mediator involved in the early phase of allergic inflammation via allergen-induced recruitment of eosinophils to sites of allergic inflammation, and eotaxin-2 and eotaxin-3 play a prominent role in the subsequent persistence of allergen-induced skin or bronchial eosinophilia (Ravensberg et al., 2005). Eotaxin-2 and eotaxin-3 are produced by bronchial epithelial cells in response to Th2 cytokines such as IL-4 and IL-13 (Komiya et al., 2003), which might suggest that these chemokines could be secreted at sites of Th2-dominant allergic inflammation. Studies demonstrate that the levels of eotaxin and IL-5 in skin of patients with AD were higher than those of healthy controls, and that these molecules are involved in the proliferation, recruitment, activation, and survival of eosinophils in AD (Park et al., 2005). The present study demonstrated that mRNA expression levels of eotaxin-2 are increased in dorsal skin lesions of mice that received both DNCB and BLM. The results indicate that increased eotaxin-2 and IL-5 expression in mice that received both DNCB and BLM contribute to eosinophil-mediated inflammation in AD.

IL-31 is a cytokine produced mainly by activated CD4+ Th2 cells or by mast cells, and is involved in the development of AD-induced skin inflammation and pruritus (Saito et al., 2017). IL-31, a pruritogenic cytokine, signals via a heterodimeric receptor composed of IL-31 receptor A and oncostatin M receptor β' which is expressed by a number of cell types, including epidermal keratinocytes, epithelial cells, mast cell, eosinophils, and activated monocytes and macrophages (Cheung et al., 2010). The IL-31 receptor (IL-31R) was expressed at higher levels on epidermal keratinocytes in skin biopsy specimens from AD patients, compared to those from healthy individuals (Bilsborough et al.' 2006). The anti-IL-31 receptor α subunit neutralizing antibody reduced ear swelling and dermatitis score in a chronic AD model in BALB/c mice (Kasutani et al., 2014). The present study showed that expression of IL-31R mRNA was increased in dorsal skin lesions of mice that received both DNCB and BLM compared to those of normal mice. But, IL-31R mRNA levels were not significantly different between DNCB-Control and DNCB-BLM mice. These results indicate that increased IL-31R expression by DNCB-BLM treatment might contribute to the development of AD-induced skin inflammation and pruritus.

The present study showed that DNCB-BLM treatment induced an increase in total leukocytes and specific CD4+ helper T cells in the ALN, BALF, and thymus of the mice. The CD4+ T cell is a dominant activated T cell subtype in clinical allergic asthma and in animal models of asthma, an mainly contributes to AHR development and allergic inflammation by secreting Th2 cytokines such as IL-4, IL-5, and IL-13 (Serre et al., 2010; Raemdonck et al., 2016). Moreover, B220+CD23+ B cells were increased in the ALN of DNCB-BLM-treated mice. CD23 is a low-affinity receptor for IgE (FcεRII) which is expressed on B cells, monocytes, T cells, dendritic cells, and neutrophils, and the CD23 surface density on antigen-presenting B cells is associated with IgE levels as well as the activation of allergen-specific T cells (Selb et al., 2017). DNCB-BLM treatment increased B cell-dependent production of total IgE in serum by approximately twofold compared to that in normal mice, albeit without statistical significance; this finding correlates with the observation of increased B220+CD23+ B cells in the ALN of mice that received both DNCB and BLM. CD11b is a cell surface molecule that is highly expressed in eosinophils, and its expression on the eosinophil surface is increased in allergic diseases including bronchial asthma and AD (Yachie et al., 1993). Gr-1 is a granulocytic marker that is related to the differentiation and maturation of granulocytes including eosinophils, basophils, and neutrophils (Fleming et al., 1993). Eosinophils are one of the cell types known to express Gr-1; therefore, eosinophils may constitute a substantial portion of the CD11b+Gr-1+ population (Kim et al., 2011). Our results showed that CD11b+Gr-1+ cells were increased in PBMCs and in the lungs of DNCB-BLM-treated mice; this increase in CD11b+Gr-1+ cells may contribute to development of allergic inflammation.

CONCLUSION

The present study demonstrated the development of an animal model for studying AD in mice using timely administration of bleomycin and DNCB. This study demonstrates that bleomycin, when administrated in combination with DNCB, aggravates allergic skin inflammation and promotes airway hyperreactivity and lung inflammation, in NC/Nga mice. These findings indicate that this bioassay has potential as a tool to use in furthering our understanding of AD, as well as a screen for irritants and treatments in future studies.

AUTHOR CONTRIBUTIONS

Y-CP and HK contributed to the conceptualization and design of the work. S-HK performed the animal experiment. W-KY carried out the analysis of animal samples. Y-YS contributed the analysis and interpretation of data. Y-YS wrote the manuscript. All authors approved the final version to be published.

REFERENCES

1. Bantz, S. K., Zhu, Z., and Zheng, T. (2014). The atopic march: progression from atopic dermatitis to allergic rhinitis and asthma. *J. Clin. Cell. Immunol.* 5:202. doi: 10.4172/2155-9899.1000202
2. Bilsborough, J., Leung, D. Y., Maurer, M., Howell, M., Boguniewicz, M., Yao, L., et al. (2006). IL-31 is associated with cutaneous lymphocyte antigen-positive skin homing T cells in patients with atopic dermatitis. *J. Allergy Clin. Immunol.* 117, 418–425.
3. Cheung, P. F., Wong, C. K., Ho, A. W., Hu, S., Chen, D. P., and Lam, C. W. (2010). Activation of human eosinophils and epidermal keratinocytes by Th2 cytokine IL-31: implication for the immunopathogenesis of atopic dermatitis. *Int. Immunol.* 22, 453–467. doi: 10.1093/intimm/ dxq027
4. Choi, J. H., Park, B. H., Kim, H. G., Hwang, Y. P., Han, E. H., Jin, S. W., et al. (2012). Inhibitory effect of *Psidium guajava* water extract in the development of 2,4-dinitrochlorobenzene-induced atopic dermatitis in NC/Nga mice. *Food Chem. Toxicol.* 50, 2923–2929. doi: 10.1016/j.fct.2012. 04.044
5. Choi, J. H., Song, Y. S., Lee, H. J., Kim, G. C., and Hong, J. W. (2017). The topical application of low-temperature argon plasma enhances the anti-inflammatory effect of Jaun-ointment on DNCB-induced NC/Nga mice. *BMC Complement. Altern. Med.* 17:340. doi: 10.1186/s12906-017- 1850-9
6. Della Latta, V., Cecchettini, A., Del Ry, S., and Morales, M. A. (2015). Bleomycin in the setting of lung fibrosis induction: from biological mechanisms to counteractions. *Pharmacol. Res.* 97, 122–130. doi: 10.1016/j.phrs.2015. 04.012
7. Deo, S. S., Mistry, K. J., Kakade, A. M., and Niphadkar, P. V. (2010). Role played by Th2 type cytokines in IgE mediated allergy and asthma. *Lung India* 27, 66–71. doi: 10.4103/0970-2113.63609
8. Fleming, T. J., Fleming, M. L., and Malek, T. R. (1993). Selective expression of Ly-6G on myeloid lineage cells in mouse bone marrow. RB6-8C5 mAb to granulocyte-differentiation antigen (Gr-1) detects members of the Ly-6 family. *J. Immunol.* 151, 2399–2408.
9. Glick, S. (2005). Treating childhood eczema with acupuncture and Chinese herbs. *Acupunct. Today* 6, 1–8.
10. Han, N. R., Kim, H. M., and Jeong, H. J. (2011). Kanamycin activates caspase-1 in NC/Nga mice. *Exp. Dermatol.* 20, 659–663. doi: 10.1111/j.1600-0625.2011. 01291.x
11. Han, R. T., Kim, S., Choi, K., Jwa, H., Lee, J., Kim, H. Y., et al. (2017). Asthma-like airway inflammation and responses in a rat model of atopic dermatitis induced by neonatal capsaicin treatment. *J. Asthma Allergy* 10, 181–189. doi: 10.2147/JAA.S124902
12. Im, G. M., Jeong, H. W., Kim, H. S., and Heong, W. Y. (2002). Oriental medical approach on the allergic disease. *Korean J. Orient. Physiol. Pathol.* 16, 831–839.
13. Iwasaki, T., Tanaka, A., Itakura, A., Yamashita, N., Ohta, K., Matsuda, H., et al. (2001). Atopic NC/Nga mice as a model for allergic asthma: severe allergic responses by single intranasal challenge with protein antigen. *J. Vet. Med. Sci.* 63, 413–419.
14. Kang, H., Lee, C. H., Kim, J. R., Kwon, J. Y., Seo, S. G., Han, J. G., et al. (2015). Chlorella vulgaris attenuates dermatophagoides farinae-induced atopic dermatitis-like symptoms in NC/Nga mice. *Int. J. Mol. Sci.* 16, 21021–21034. doi: 10.3390/ijms160921021
15. Kaplan, A. P. (2001). Chemokines, chemokine receptors and allergy. *Int. Arch. Allergy Immunol.* 124, 423–431.
16. Kasutani, K., Fujii, E., Ohyama, S., Adachi, H., Hasegawa, M., Kitamura, H., et al. (2014). Anti-IL-31 receptor antibody is shown to be a potential therapeutic option for treating itch and dermatitis in mice. *Br. J. Pharmacol.* 171, 5049–5058. doi: 10.1111/bph.12823
17. Kim, H., Kim, J. R., Kang, H., Choi, J., Yang, H., Lee, P., et al. (2014). 7,8,4[1] -Trihydroxyisoflavone attenuates DNCB-induced atopic dermatitis-like symptoms in NC/Nga mice. *PLoS One* 9:e104938. doi: 10.1371/journal.pone.01 04938
18. Kim, S. H., Kim, B. K., and Lee, Y. C. (2011). Antiasthmatic effects of hesperidin, a potential Th2 cytokine antagonist, in a mouse model of allergic asthma. *Mediators Inflamm.* 2011:485402. doi: 10.1155/2011/48 5402
19. Komiya, A., Nagase, H., Yamada, H., Sekiya, T., Yamaguchi, M., Sano, Y., et al. (2003). Concerted expression of eotaxin-1, eotaxin-2, and eotaxin-3 in human bronchial epithelial cells. *Cell. Immunol.* 225, 91–100.
20. Liang, M., Lv, J., Zou, L., Yang, W., Xiong, Y., Chen, X., et al. (2015). A modified murine model of systemic sclerosis: bleomycin given by pump infusion induced skin and pulmonary inflammation and fibrosis. *Lab. Invest.* 95, 342–350. doi: 10.1038/labinvest.2014.145
21. McAnulty, R. J., and Laurent, G. J. (1995). "Collagen and its regulation in pulmonary fibrosis," in *Pulmonary Fibrosis*, eds S. H. Phan and R. S. Thrall (New York, NY: Marcel Dekker Inc), 135–171.
22. Neveu, W. A., Allard, J. B., Dienz, O., Wargo, M. J., Ciliberto, G., Whittaker, L. A., et al. (2009). IL-6 is required for airway mucus production induced by inhaled fungal allergens. *J. Immunol.* 183, 1732–1738. doi: 10.4049/ jimmunol.080 2923
23. Ngoc, P. L., Gold, D. R., Tzianabos, A. O., Weiss, S. T., and Celedón, J. C. (2005). Cytokines, allergy, and asthma. *Curr. Opin. Allergy Clin. Immunol.* 5, 161–166.
24. Park, B. K., Park, Y. C., Jung, I. C., Kim, S. H., Choi, J. E., Park, S., et al. (2014). Oral administration of SSC201, a medicinal herbal formula, suppresses atopic dermatitis-like skin lesions. *J. Med. Food* 17, 496–504. doi: 10.1089/jmf.2013. 2941
25. Park, C. W., Lee, B. H., Han, H. J., Lee, C. H., and Ahn, H. K. (2005). Tacrolimus decreases the expression of eotaxin, CCR3, RANTES and interleukin-5 in atopic dermatitis. *Br. J. Dermatol.* 152, 1173–1181 doi: 10.1111/j.1365-2133. 2005.06474.x
26. Raemdonck, K., Baker, K., Dale, N., Dubuis, E., Shala, F., Belvisi, M. G., et al. (2016). CD4+ and CD8+ T cells play a central role in a HDM driven model of allergic asthma. *Respir. Res.* 17:45. doi: 10.1186/s12931-016- 0359-y
27. Ravensberg, A. J., Ricciardolo, F. L., van Schadewijk, A., Rabe, K. F., Sterk, P. J., Hiemstra, P. S., et al. (2005). Eotaxin-2 and eotaxin-3 expression is associated with persistent eosinophilic bronchial inflammation in patients with asthma after allergen challenge. *J. Allergy Clin. Immunol.* 115, 779–785.
28. Saba, E., Lee, C. H., Jeong da, H., Lee, K., Kim, T. H., Roh, S. S., et al. (2016). Fermented rice bran prevents atopic dermatitis in DNCB-treated NC/Nga mice. *J. Biomed. Res.* 30, 334–343. doi: 10.7555/JBR.30.2016K 0001
29. Saito, S., Aoki, A., Arai, I., Takaishi, S., Ito, H., Akiyama, N., et al. (2017). Regulation of Th2 responses by different cell types expressing the interleukin-31 receptor. *Allergy Asthma Clin. Immunol.* 13:23. doi: 10.1186/s13223-017-0194-9
30. Selb, R., Eckl-Dorna, J., Neunkirchner, A., Schmetterer, K., Marth, K., Gamper, J., et al. (2017). CD23 surface density on B cells is associated with IgE levels and determines IgE-facilitated allergen uptake, as well as activation of allergen-specific T cells. *J. Allergy Clin. Immunol.* 139, 290.e–299.e. doi: 10.1016/j.jaci. 2016.03.042
31. Serre, K., Mohr, E., Gaspal, F., Lane, P. J., Bird, R., Cunningham, A. F., et al. (2010). IL-4 directs both CD4 and CD8 T cells to produce Th2 cytokines *in vitro*, but only CD4 T cells produce these cytokines in response to alum-precipitated protein *in vivo*. *Mol. Immunol.* 47, 1914–1922. doi: 10.1016/j. molimm.2010. 03.010
32. Shibamori, M., Ogino, K., Kambayashi, Y., and Ishiyama, H. (2006). Intranasal mite allergen induces allergic asthma-like responses in NC/Nga mice. *Life Sci.* 78, 987–994. doi: 10.1016/j.lfs.2005.06.020
33. Spergel, J. M., Mizoguchi, E., Brewer, J. P., Martin, T. R., Bhan, A. K., and Geha, R. S. (1998). Epicutaneous sensitization with protein antigen induces localized allergic dermatitis and hyperresponsiveness to methacholine after single exposure to aerosolized antigen in mice. *J. Clin. Invest.* 101, 1614–1622.
34. Spergel, J. M., and Paller, A. S. (2003). Atopic dermatitis and the atopic march. *J. Allergy Clin. Immunol.* 112, S118–S127.
35. Sung, Y. Y., Lee, A. Y., and Kim, H. K. (2014). The *Gardenia jasminoides* extract and its constituent, geniposide, elicit anti-allergic effects on atopic dermatitis by inhibiting histamine *in vitro* and *in vivo*. *J. Ethnopharmacol.* 156, 33–40. doi: 10.1016/j.jep.2014.07.060
36. Suto, H., Matsuda, H., Mitsuishi, K., Hira, K., Uchida, T., Unno, T., et al. (1999). NC/Nga mice: a mouse model for atopic dermatitis. *Int. Arch. Allergy Immunol.* 129, 70–75.
37. Yachie, A., Toma, T., Miyawaki, T., and Taniguchi, N. (1993). Expression of surface CD11b antigen and eosinophil activation. *Nippon Rinsho* 51, 593–597.
38. Zheng, T., Yu, J., Oh, M.H., and Zhu, Z. (2011). The atopic march: progression from atopic dermatitis to allergic rhinitis and asthma. *Allergy Asthma Immunol. Res.* 3, 67–73. doi: 10.4168/aair.2011.3.2.67

18

SARS-CoV-2 Nsp5 Protein Causes Acute Lung Inflammation: A Dynamical Mathematical Model

Antonio Bensussen[1], Elena R. Álvarez-Buylla[2,3] and José Díaz[1]**

[1]Laboratorio de Dinámica de Redes Genéticas, Centro de Investigación en Dinámica Celular, Universidad Autónoma del Estado de Morelos, Cuernavaca, Mexico, [2]Centro de Ciencias de la Complejidad (C3), Universidad Nacional Autónoma de México, Ciudad de México, Mexico, [3]Laboratorio de Genética Molecular, Epigenética, Desarrollo y Evolución de Plantas, Instituto de Ecología, Universidad Nacional Autónoma de México, Ciudad de México, Mexico

***Correspondence:**
José Díaz
biofisica@yahoo.com
Elena R. Álvarez Buylla
elenabuylla@protonmail.com

In the present work we propose a dynamical mathematical model of the lung cells inflammation process in response to SARS-CoV-2 infection. In this scenario the main protease Nsp5 enhances the inflammatory process, increasing the levels of NF kB, IL-6, Cox2, and PGE2 with respect to a reference state without the virus. In presence of the virus the translation rates of NF kB and IkB arise to a high constant value, and when the translation rate of IL-6 also increases above the threshold value of 7 pg mL^{-1} s^{-1} the model predicts a persistent over stimulated immune state with high levels of the cytokine IL-6. Our model shows how such over stimulated immune state becomes autonomous of the signals from other immune cells such as macrophages and lymphocytes, and does not shut down by itself. We also show that in the context of the dynamical model presented here, Dexamethasone or Nimesulide have little effect on such inflammation state of the infected lung cell, and the only form to suppress it is with the inhibition of the activity of the viral protein Nsp5. To that end, our model suggest that drugs like Saquinavir may be useful. In this form, our model suggests that Nsp5 is effectively a central node underlying the severe acute lung inflammation during SARS-CoV-2 infection. The persistent production of IL-6 by lung cells can be one of the causes of the cytokine storm observed in critical patients with COVID19. Nsp5 seems to be the switch to start inflammation, the consequent overproduction of the ACE2 receptor, and an important underlying cause of the most severe cases of COVID19.

Keywords: SARS-CoV-2 infection, interleukin 6, NFKB, NSP5, COX2, SARS-CoV-2 interactome, nonlinear dynamics of inflammation

INTRODUCTION

Severe Acute Respiratory Syndrome Coronavirus 2 (SARS-CoV-2) virus is an intracellular infectious agent whose replication cycle depends on the host's cell structures and functions. In particular, it uses the translational apparatus of different types of infected cells to express its proteins (Nakagawa et al., 2016). SARS-CoV-2 causes the Coronavirus Disease 2019 (COVID19) that has infected over 241, 000, 000 persons and killed over 4,900,000 worldwide since the end of 2019. No specific and effective therapeutic drugs to defeat SARS-CoV-2 infection have been developed yet (Díaz, 2020a), although several effective vaccines have been developed and are being applied. Therefore, it is necessary to continue the search for effective therapeutic agents that complement the use of vaccines, to minimize the risk of death from COVID19.

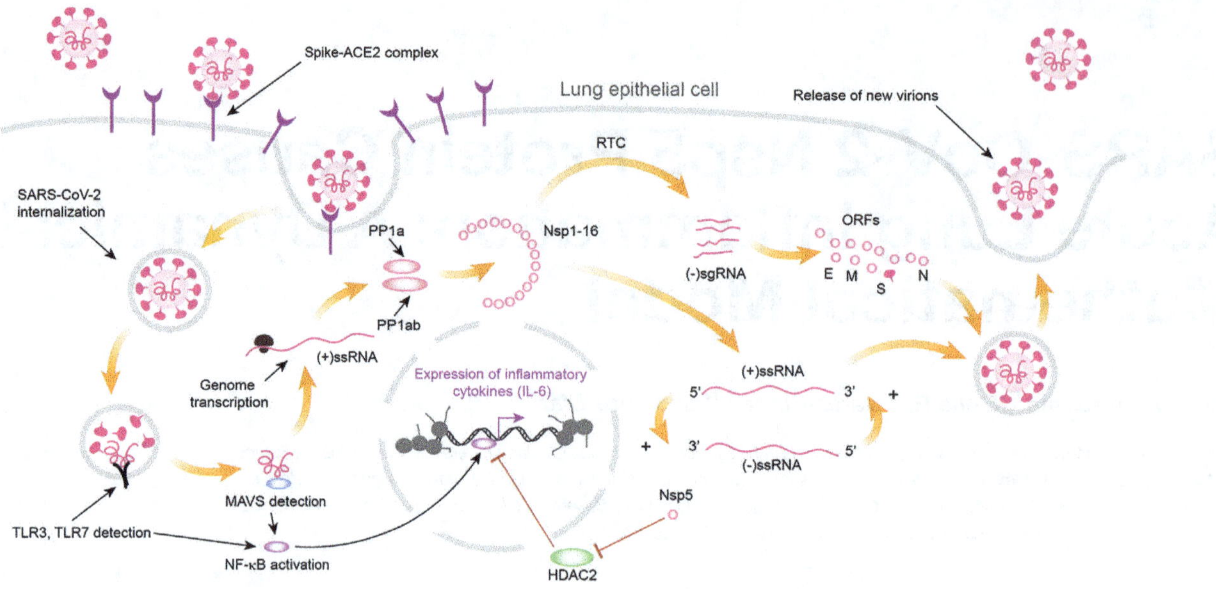

FIGURE 1 | Process of infection of lung cells by SARS-CoV-2. Infection begins when the protein S of the virion binds with high affinity to the cells surface receptor ACE2 (Angiotensin-Converting Enzyme 2) that is highly abundant in the lung alveolar type II cells. The formation of the complex S-ACE2 initiates the process of fusion between the virion envelope and the cells membrane leading to the liberation of the nucleocapside with the viral genome into the cytoplasm. SARS-CoV-2 genome consists of a positive-sense nonsegmented single stranded mRNA [(+)ssRNA] of ~30 kb. The open reading frames 1a (orf1a) and 1b (orf1b) are located near the 5′UTR of the (+)ssRNA and they code for the polyproteins pp1a and pp1ab. Maturation of these polyproteins results in 11 nonstructural proteins (Nsp) from the orf1a segment (Nsp1 to Nsp11) and 5 nonstructural proteins from the orf1b segment (Nsp12 to Nsp16). Nsp proteins form the replication-transcription complex (RTC) a set of nested subgenomic minus-strands of RNA [(−)sgRNA] are synthesized in a process of discontinuous transcription. These (− sgRNAs serve as the templates for the production of subgenomic mRNAs from which the structural proteins E, M, N and S, together with the accessory proteins orf 3a, orf6, orf7a, orf7b, orf8, orf9b, orf9c and orf10 are synthesized. The presence of viral (+)ssRNA initiates the TLR3 and TLR4 mediated immune response, which increases the concentration of free NF κB in cytoplasm. Cytoplasmic NF κB enters the nucleus where promotes the transcription of a series of target genes. Viral protein Nsp5 inhibits the inhibition exerted by HDAC2 on nuclear NF κB transcription factor, enhancing the synthesis of inflammatory cytokines like IL-6.

SARS-CoV-2 virion is formed by four proteins: spike (S), envelope (E), membrane (M) and nucleocapside (N) that enclose the virus genome (McBride and Fielding, 2012), which consists of a positive-sense nonsegmented single stranded mRNA [(+) ssRNA] of 30 kb. The open reading frames 1a (orf1a) and 1b (orf1b) are located near the untranslated 5′ region (5′UTR) of the positive single stranded RNA [(+)ssRNA] and they encode for the polyproteins pp1a and pp1ab.

When SARS-CoV-2 virion infects the organism, S protein binds with high affinity to the surface receptor Angiotensin-Converting Enzyme 2 (ACE2), highly abundant in the lung alveolar type II cells and other cell types (Hamming et al., 2004; Gordon et al., 2020), and forms a molecular complex that begins the process of fusion of the virion envelope with the host cell membrane. Finally, viral (+)ssRNA is released into the host cytoplasm (Letko et al., 2020) (**Figure 1**).

The process of translation occurs in the cytoplasm and produces a set of viral polyproteins whose maturation results in 11 nonstructural proteins (Nsp) from the orf1a segment (Nsp1 to Nsp11) and 5 nonstructural proteins from the orf1b segment (Nsp12 to Nsp16). Nsp proteins form the replication-transcription complex (RTC) in a double-membrane vesicle where a set of nested subgenomic minus-strands of RNA ((-) sgRNA) are synthesized in a process of discontinuous transcription. These (-) sgRNAs serve as the templates for the production of subgenomic mRNAs from which the structural proteins E, M, N and S, together with the accessory proteins orf 3a, orf6, orf7a, orf7b, orf8, orf9b, orf9c and orf10 are synthesized (Sevajol et al., 2014; Díaz, 2020a; Dongwan et al., 2020). SARS-CoV-2 uses the host translational machinery to redirect it to viral protein synthesis and replication, while host mRNA translation is inhibited (Nakagawa et al., 2016). SARS-CoV and SARS-CoV-2 genomes have ~79% of homology (Forster et al., 2020), and most of the set of structural and nonstructural proteins are practically the same. However, the virus species differ in the accessory proteins orf8, orf8a, orf 8b, orf9c and orf10 (Bartlam et al., 2005; Gordon et al., 2020).

Viral proteins are inserted into the host molecular machinery to modify and redirect a great number of host cell functions towards the production of additional viral particles (Masters, 2006; Wu et al., 2020). Experimental analysis of the interaction of viral and host proteins, or *interactome*, by Gordon and collaborators (Gordon et al., 2020) has been a fundamental contribution to understand the form in which SARS-CoV-2 virus takes control of the host molecular network to produce new virions and propagate the infection (Hekman et al., 2020). Gordon and collaborators (2020) cloned, tagged and expressed 26 viral proteins in human cells using affinity-purification mass spectrometry to identify the human proteins physically associated with each other. They found around 332 SARS-CoV-2-human protein-protein interactions that constitute the virus interactome. From these results, the construction of the network representation of the interactome is possible. In the particular case of the Gordon interactome, the analysis of its undirected network model indicates a modular free-scale hierarchical type of structure in which proteins orf8, N and Nsp7 are the main hubs (Díaz, 2020a).

Despite all the molecular knowledge rapidly accumulated on SARS-CoV-2 itself and the infection or inflammation processes in which it is involved in human cells, we still lack dynamical models to understand which are the key nodes underlying severe inflammation processes in some cases. Mathematical and computational dynamic network models are useful tools to integrate data, find experimental holes and also propose or understand the underlying dynamics mechanisms involved in the complex viral/human networks involved during SARS-CoV-2 infection (Breitling, 2010; Díaz, 2020a; Enciso et al., 2020; Weinstein et al., 2020). The number of nodes, the number of connections of each node to its neighbours, and the distribution of these connections in the network determine its complexity, structure and dynamical properties (Kumar et al., 2020).

In this network, the viral main protease Nsp5 is the main protease (Mpro) involved in the assembly of the polyprotein cluster that translates viral RNA, and in the post-translational modification of viral proteins through its ADP ribose phosphatase activity (Nakagawa et al., 2016). SARS-CoV-2 Nsp5 has 96% sequence homology with its SARS-CoV counterpart, and its level of phylogenetic conservation by sequence and structure is high having high homogeneity in its volume and electrostatic profile throughout the Coronaviridae family. Interest in elucidating the functional structure of this protease has resulted in new reports of 3D structures showing that Nsp5 is a complex formed by two equal protomers (A and B) each consisting of 306 residues structured in three domains: I Chymotrypsin-like domain (residues 8–101), Picornavirus 3C protease-like domain II (residues 102–184), and Globular Cluster domain III (residues 201–303). Domains I and II have an antiparallel β-barrel structure and associate with their counterparts to form a dimer, which loop residues 185–200 connect to domain III made up of five α-helixes. The substrate binding site is found in the antiparallel β-barrels located between domains I and II, forming a catalytic pocket composed of four subsites (S1, S2, S3 and S4) that exhibit charged residues that include the nucleophilic sulphur atom of Cys145, which forms a dyad with the imidazole ring of His 41. Therefore, the blocking one of these residues with a small molecule could inhibit the enzymatic activity of Nsp5 (Mukherjee et al., 2011; Pillaiyar et al., 2016; Konwar and Sarma, 2021).

There are several crystallographic structures of Mpro with peptidomimetic inhibitors that show interactions with the enzyme at S3-S4 subsites in SARS-CoV-2, SARS-CoV and MERS. This type of inhibitor incorporates an imidazole ring of cyclic ketoamides with five-components that binds covalently to Cys145 or its equivalent in the different isoforms of the enzyme. Although these types of molecules are not optimal for

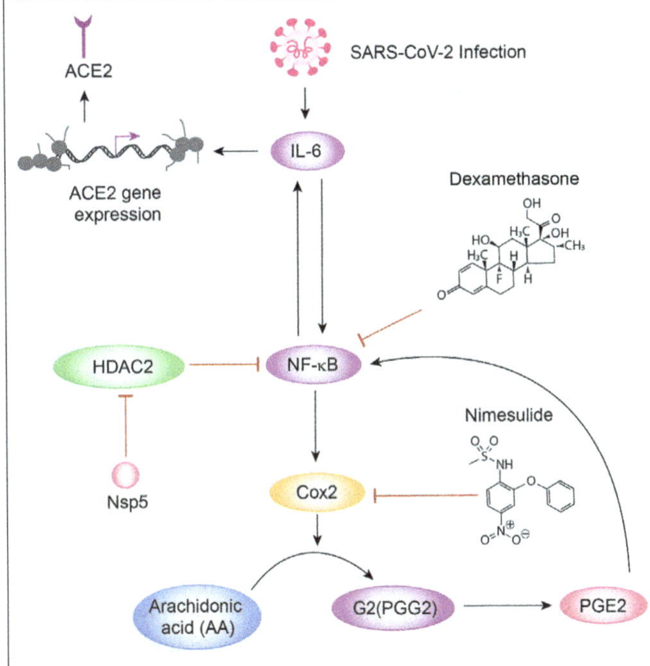

FIGURE 2 | Circuit representation of inflammation. IL-6, NF κB, Cox2, and PGE2 are the basic nodes of the circuit that represents the basic features of inflammation of lung cells during SARS-CoV-2 infection. In this circuit the arrows represent activation and the bars inhibition. In the figure are shown two positive feedback loops between IL-6 and NF κB, and between NF κB and Cox2. IL-6 also induces the expression of the ACE2 receptor in the lung cell membrane. NF κB is inhibited by HDAC2, which in turn is inhibited by the viral protein Nsp5. The circuit has two targets for the anti-inflammatory drugs Nimesulide and Dexamethasone.

drug development, due to proteolytic degradation, they have made possible to describe the dynamics of the enzymatic mechanism of this active site for the search and development of molecules with better pharmacodynamic parameters. An example of viable candidates for clinical implementation is boceprevir and telaprevir, whose mechanism of action consists of blocking the catalytic dyad through the covalent binding to the sulphur atom of Cys145 (Pan et al., 2012).

In the SARS-CoV-2 molecular network, Nsp5 has a special role in lung inflammation process through its link with Histone Deacetylase 2 (HDAC2) (Díaz, 2020a; Gordon et al., 2020; Hekman et al., 2020) (**Figures 1, 2**); suggesting that Nsp5 represses HDAC2 inhibitory action on NF κB (**Figure 1**), and thus enhances the transcription of the pro-inflammatory genes targeted by the Nuclear Factor κB (NF κB) (**Figures 1, 2**) (Wagner et al., 2015). Such role distinguishes SARS-CoV and SARS-CoV-2. The SARS-CoV virus uses N protein to promote the sustained transcription of the Cyclooxygenase 2 (Cox2) enzyme by binding directly to the NF-κB transcriptional regulatory elements, and to the CCAAT/enhancer binding proteins of the gene *Cox2* (Yan et al., 2006). Hence, SARS-CoV and SARS-CoV-2 produce severe acute respiratory syndrome through different molecular mechanisms.

The change from a hub (N protein in SARS-CoV) to a poor connected protein (Nsp5 in SARS-CoV-2) as the underlying

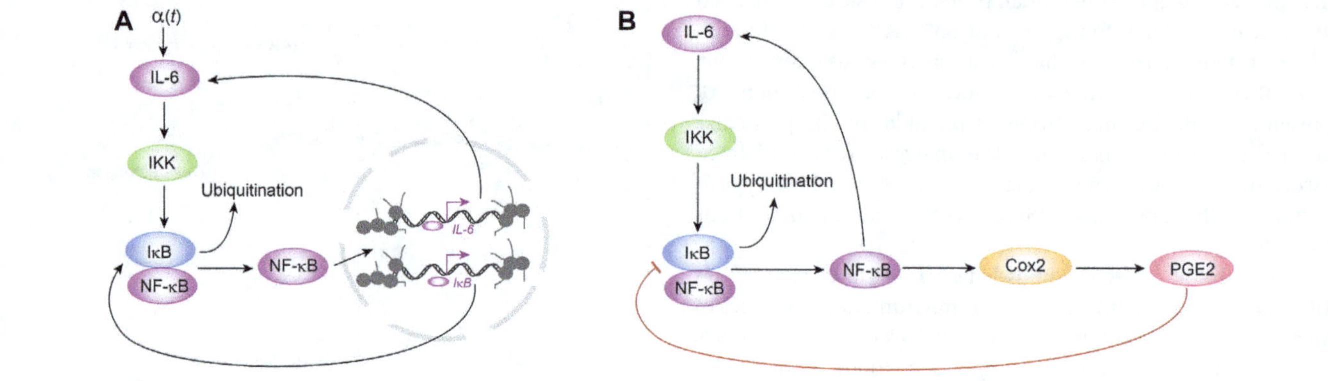

FIGURE 3 | Feedback loops of the model of inflammation. The mathematical model proposed in this work is based on the dynamical features of three feedback loops: **(A)** two positive feedback loops between IL-6 and NF κB, and NF κB and IκB; **(B)** a negative feedback loop between PGE2 and IκB. In Figure A, α (t) is a external signal that represents the amount of IL-6 produced by immune cells like monocytes and lymphocytes, among others.

cause of severe acute respiratory syndrome could be an adaptation that made SARS-CoV-2 more pathogenic (8,098 people worldwide became sick with SARS during the 2003 outbreak against 241, 000, 000 during the 2020–2021 SARS-Cov-2 outbreak). Nsp5 is also the main protease that cleavages the SARS-CoV-2 polyprotein at 11 conserved sites, and its malfunction or deletion could stop the viral replication cycle and lung inflammation (Cohen et al., 2000; Xun et al., 2020). Thus, Nsp5 is a molecular switch that shows a low rate of mutation (Vilar and Isom, 2020), and its malfunctioning can decrease the strength of inflammation and the persistence of ACE2 in the lung epithelial cells giving rise to a less intense inflammatory response (Cohen et al., 2000; Xun et al., 2020).

Activation of the NF κB family of proteins (p65/RelA, p105/p50, p100/p52, RelB, and c-Rel) is mediated by the phosphorylation of the inhibitor of NF κB proteins (IκBs) by IκB kinases (IKKs) and the posterior ubiquitinylation and degradation of the phosphorylated IκBs (**Figure 1**). The released NF κB proteins enter the nucleus to activate specific genes (Wagner et al., 2015). In the nucleus, HDAC2 blocks the transcriptional activity of NF κB, inhibiting the production and release of the cytokine Interleukin 6 (IL-6) and IκB, and interfering with the functioning of the positive feedback circuit between IL-6 and NF κB (Rahman, and MacNee, 1998) (**Figure 3A**). As we mentioned before, the sustained inactivation of HDAC2 by Nsp5 produces a sustained increase in the transcriptional activity of NF κB (**Figures 1, 2**) that leads to a high production of IL-6 in the lung epithelium cells. Release of this excess of IL-6 to the vascular system contributes to the "cytokines storm" observed in critical patients (Leisman et al., 2020; Magro, 2020), although the average serum concentration of IL-6 in critical COVID19 patients are lower with respect to other respiratory syndromes (Leisman et al., 2020). However, the uninterrupted production of IL-6 is closely associated to a persistent presence of the ACE2 receptor in the alveolar type 2 cells due to enhanced ACE2 gene expression mediated by the JAK-STAT and PI3K/Akt pathways (Zegeye et al., 2018; Hennighausen and Lee, 2020; Mokuda et al., 2020) (**Figure 2**).

NF κB also promotes transcription of the *Cox2* gene leading to the expression and increased enzymatic activity of Cox2 enzyme (**Figures 2, 3B**). However, NF κB, Cox2 and IL-6 also form a positive feedback circuit in which NF κB promotes Cox2 enzymatic activity that catalyses the conversion of Arachidonic acid (AA) into Prostaglandin G2 (PGG2), which is in turn modified by the peroxidase moiety of the Cox2 enzyme to produce prostaglandin H2 (PGH2) that is converted to prostaglandin E2 (PGE2) (Alexanian and Sorokin, 2017). PGE2 is then released to the vascular system, binds to its membrane EP2 and EP4 prostanoid receptors and promotes the cleavage of the IκB-NF κB complex increasing the amount of free NF κB, which increases the production of IL-6 (**Figure 3B**) (Cho et al., 2014; Bouffi et al., 2010). IL-6, in turn, increases NF κB activity (Wang et al., 2003) (**Figure 2**). These regulatory circuits has three therapeutic targets: IL-6 production (Tocilizumab) (Magro 2020), Cox2 (Nimesulide) (Alexanian and Sorokin, 2017) and NF κB (Dexamethasone) (Newton et al., 1998; Aghai et al., 2006). However, none of these have shown to be really effective for preventing or reverting acute inflammatory cases after SARS-CoV-2 infection.

In this work, we propose a dynamical mathematical model that suggests that the three feedback loops mentioned above constitute a minimal circuit for the inflammatory process in the epithelial lung cells during SARS-CoV-2 infection (**Figure 2**), and we use an ordinary differential equations (ODEs) continuous model to explore the effect of Nsp5 in the qualitative dynamics of this circuit in which this viral protein acts as an enhancing perturbation in the phase space of this dynamical system (Díaz, 2020b) (**Figure 2**). For the model of the circuit, we chose as main molecular components the proteins NF κB, IκB, IL-6, Cox2, and PGE2. In this model, Nsp5 prevents the movement of HDAC2 into the nucleus allowing an increase in NF κB transcriptional activity. The input that turns *on* the circuit in lung cells is a signal from monocytes, lymphocytes, and other immune cells that activates IL-6 production. We propose that this model represents the basic set of interactions that settles *on* the inflammation reaction to the invasion of the lung cells by

SARS-CoV-2, and that it is a first approximation to understand the main dynamical features of this response.

Our hypothesis is that Nsp5 leads to the sustained overproduction of IL-6, Cox2, PGE2, and NF κB, in the epithelial lung cells, which is *a necessary but not a sufficient condition* for a cytokine storm. In the particular case of epithelial lung cells, we found that the computational and mathematical analysis of the model supports our hypothesis, and that Nsp5 effectively enhances NF κB, IL-6, Cox2 and PGE2 production during the time that remains bounded to HDAC2. Furthermore, the model predicts the existence of an over stimulated immune state (OSIS) in which the amount of IL-6 produced by the infected lung cells is high, and such state becomes autonomous and robust, independent of any stimulus from external sources like monocytes, and lymphocytes. Hence this OSIS *cannot be completely shut down* by classical anti-inflammatory drugs like Nimesulide and Dexamethasone, and can be possibly beaten only with specific inhibitors of Nsp5 (Xun et al., 2020).

MODEL

Immune response to infections involves complex spatio-temporal processes involving multiple molecular components, non-linear interactions and cell-cell interactions. In consequence, the immune response to infections is a multidimensional, multiscale and multilevel dynamical process in which innate and acquired immunity mechanisms are involved to protect the organism against pathogens (Eftimie et al., 2016). In this scenario, the number of variables that become both sufficient and necessary for a detailed enough description of the spatio-temporal dynamics of the immune system is tremendously high. Some computational integrative efforts have been made in this direction (Danos et al., 2007), but imply very large systems that cannot be modeled with continuous quantitative models that are, in turn, necessary if we want to understand which are key nodes driving the system towards the OSIS. The lack of quantitative experimental data and knowledge of the values of most of the model parameters are additional challenges to achieve such dynamic models of the immune system in response to specific infectious diseases. Thus, most models of the immune system have been qualitative (Eftimie et al., 2016; Martinez-Sanchez et al., 2018).

A possible approach implies the use of ordinary differential equations (ODEs) qualitative modeling that is oriented to determine all the possible trajectories of a dynamical system along its n-dimensional phase space (with $n > 0$), when the system is subject to a set of initial conditions and parameters values. High dimensional nonlinear dynamical systems can exhibit a variety of coexisting dynamical behaviors that determine the structure of their phase space (Strogatz, 2015). However, the structure of the phase space of biological nonlinear dynamical systems is highly dependent on the set of parameters values. Variations in the value of one or more parameters can drive a drastic change in phase space generating a different qualitative dynamics of the system. This process is known as bifurcation, and it is important to find the possible bifurcations in the system and to identify which parameter or parameters are the responsible of these changes (Strogatz, 2015) (**Supplementary Material S1**).

In order to avoid the problem due to the high dimensionality and complexity of the immune response to SARS-CoV-2 infection, and to use the minimum number of parameters in the model that we are proposing in this work, we assume that the interaction between nodes IL-6, NF κB, IκB, Cox2 and PGE2 settles on the main dynamical features of the inflammation process in lung epithelial cells due to the presence of the Nsp5 viral protein. In the proposed circuit shown in **Figure 2**, IL-6, NF κB, Cox2 and PGE2 define three feedback loops (**Figures 3A,B**): a positive feedback loop between NF κB and IL-6 (**Figure 3A**); a positive feedback loop between NF κB and IκB (**Figure 3A**); and a negative feedback loop between PGE2 and IκB (**Figure 3B**).

These feedback loops are distributed between three compartments:

1) IL-6 is secreted into the extracellular medium where it acts in paracrine and exocrine form. IL-6 binds to its receptor IL6R at the cell surface. Once the complex IL6-IL6R is formed, it activates IKK in the cytoplasm (Wang et al., 2003). PGE2 is also secreted into this compartment where it binds to EP2 and EP4 receptors at the cell surface, activating Protein Kinase B (Akt) in the cytoplasm (Cho et al., 2014).
2) IKK, free NF κB, and the complex IκB-NF κB are located in the cytoplasm, where IκB is degraded by ubiquitination. Protein Cox2 is located in the endoplasmic reticulum (ER).
3) Free NF κB enters the nucleus where induce the transcription of IL6, Cox2, IKB and NF κB genes. Transcriptional activity of nuclear NF κB is inhibited by HDAC2, and enhanced by Nsp5.

In this form, the model cell consists of three compartments: extracellular medium, cytoplasm and nucleus. We assume that the ratio of the cytoplasmatic volume to external volume (V_{cyt}/V_{out}) is one, and that the radio of the cytoplasmatic volume to the nuclear volume (V_{cyt}/V_{nuc}) is 2. In each compartment the concentration of the molecules are measured in pg mL^{-1}.

In the circuit of **Figure 2**, the rate of production of free cytoplasmic NF κB depends on the rate of its release from the IκB-NF κB complex, which is proportional to the product of the concentrations of IκB and IKK (**Figure 3A**), its own rate of production due to nuclear NF κB transcriptional activity inhibited by HDAC2 (**Figures 1, 3A**), the rate at which is recaptured by IκB (**Figure 3A**), and the rate of transport into the nucleus:

$$\frac{d(nf)}{dt} = V_{nf}^{\max} p_{nf}^{on}(t) + k_a ikk \cdot i\kappa bnf - k_4 nf \cdot i\kappa b - D \cdot nf \quad (1)$$

where nf is the concentration of free cytoplasmic NF κB, $V_{nf}^{\max}$ is the maximum rate of translation of the NF κB gene, $p_{nf}^{on}(t)$is the probability that the NF κB gene is in its active state (on), ikk is the concentration of IKK, $i\kappa bnf$ is the concentration of IκB-NF κB complex, k_a and k_2 are rate constants and D is the transport constant (**Table 1**).

We assume that the concentration of IKK activated by IL-6 is proportional to the external concentration of the cytokine:

TABLE 1 | Equations and parameters of the basic model of inflammation.

Basic inflammation circuit	**Parameters**
$d(nf)/dt = V_{nf}^{max} p_{nf}^{on}(t) + k_1 \cdot il6 \cdot i\kappa bnf + k_{11} pge2 \cdot i\kappa bnf - k_4 i\kappa b \cdot nf - D \cdot nf$ $i\kappa bnf = I\kappa B - NF\kappa B$ molecular complex	$k_1 = 0.5$ pg $ml^{-1}s^{-1}$; $k_4 = 5$ pg $ml^{-1}s^{-1}$; $D = 1\ s^{-1}$
$\frac{d(nf*)}{dt} = D(\frac{V_{cyt}}{V_{nuc}})nf - k_{deg} nf*$ $nf*$ = nuclear concentration of $NF\kappa B$	$k_{deg} = 2\ s^{-1}$; $(\frac{Vcyt}{Vnuc}) = 2$
$\frac{d(i\kappa bnf)}{dt} = k_4 nf \cdot i\kappa b - k_5 il6 \cdot i\kappa bnf - k_{11} pge2 \cdot i\kappa bnf$ $i\kappa bnf = I\kappa B - NF\kappa B$ molecular complex $pge2$ = amount of PGE2	$k_4 = 5$ pg $ml^{-1}s^{-1}$; $k_5 = 0.5$ pg $ml^{-1}s^{-1}$
$\frac{dp_{IL6}^{on}(t)}{dt} = k_2 \frac{nf*}{hd* + 1} p_{IL6}^{off}(t) - k_{-2} p_{IL6}^{on}(t)$ $p_{IL6}^{on}(t)$ = probability of $IL6$ activation at time t $hd*$ = amount of HDAC2 in nucleus	$k_2 = 0.1$ (Number of Molecules)$^{-1}s^{-1}$; $k_{\_2} = 0.035\ s^{-1}$
$\frac{dp_{I\kappa B}^{on}(t)}{dt} = k_3 \frac{nf*}{hd* + 1}(1 - p_{I\kappa B}^{on}(t)) - k_{-3} p_{I\kappa B}^{on}(t)$ $p_{I\kappa B}^{on}(t)$ = probability of $I\kappa B$ activation at time t	$k_3 = 0.1$ (Number of Molecules)$^{-1}s^{-1}$; $k_{\_3} = 0.035\ s^{-1}$
$\frac{dp_{Cox2}^{on}(t)}{dt} = k_7 \frac{nf*}{hd* + 1}(1 - p_{Cox2}^{on}(t)) - k_{-7} p_{Cox2}^{on}(t)$ $p_{Cox2}^{on}(t)$ = probability of $Cox2$ activation at time t	$k_7 = 0.1$ (Number of Molecules)$^{-1}s^{-1}$; $k_{\_7} = 0.035\ s^{-1}$
$\frac{dp_{NF\kappa B}^{on}(t)}{dt} = k_{15} \frac{nf*}{hd* + 1}(1 - p_{NF\kappa B}^{on}(t)) - k_{-15} p_{NF\kappa B}^{on}(t)$ $p_{NF\kappa B}^{on}(t)$ = probability of $NF\kappa B$ activation at time t	$k_{15} = 0.1$ (Num of Molecules)$^{-1}s^{-1}$; $k_{\_15} = 0.035\ s^{-1}$
$\frac{d(nsp5)}{dt} = \phi - k_{18} nsp5$ $nsp5$ = amount of viral Nsp5 in cell ϕ = rate of Nsp5 production	$k_{18} = 0.7\ s^{-1}$; $\phi = 14$ pg $ml^{-1}s^{-1}$
$\frac{d(hd)}{dt} = \frac{r}{nsp5 + 1} - D_2 \cdot hd$ hd = amount of HDAC2 in cytoplasm D_2 = transport constant of HDAC2	$r = 30$ pg $ml^{-1}s^{-1}$; $D_2 = 2\ s^{-1}$; $\eta = 1$ pg ml^{-1}
$\frac{d(hd*)}{dt} = D_2(\frac{V_{cyt}}{V_n})hd - k_{deg2} hd*$	$D_2 = 2\ s^{-1}$ $k_{deg2} = 2\ s^{-1}$; $(\frac{Vcyt}{Vnuc}) = 2$
$\frac{d(il6)}{dt} = \alpha(t) + V_{IL6}^{max} p_{IL6}^{on}(t) - k_5 \cdot il6 \cdot i\kappa bnf - k_6 il6$	$k_5 = 0.5$ pg $ml^{-1}s^{-1}$; $k_6 = 0.5\ s^{-1}$; $\alpha(t) = 10$ pg $ml^{-1}s^{-1}$
$\frac{d(i\kappa b)}{dt} = V_{I\kappa B}^{max} p_{I\kappa B}^{on}(t) - k_4 i\kappa b \cdot nf$	$k_4 = 5$ pg $ml^{-1}s^{-1}$
$\frac{d(cox2)}{dt} = V_{Cox2}^{max} p_{Cox2}^{on}(t) - k_{10} cox2$	$k_{10} = 0.4\ s^{-1}$
$\frac{d(pge2)}{dt} = k_{17} cox2 - k_{11} pge2 \cdot i\kappa bnf - k_{12} pge2$	$k_{17} = 0.8\ s^{-1}$; $k_{11} = 0.8$ pg $ml^{-1}s^{-1}$; $k_{12} = 3\ s^{-1}$

In the reference state the translation velocities are: $V_{nf}^{max} = V_{Cox2}^{max} = V_{IL6}^{max} = V_{I\kappa B}^{max} = 2\ pg\ mL^{-1}s^{-1}$

$ikk = \gamma_1 \cdot il6$, where γ_1 is a constant of proportionality. In a similar form, PGE2 increases the rate of cleavage of the complex IκB-NF κB by phosphorylation of the IKKα subunit by Akt (Bai et al., 2009) (**Figure 3B**). Thus, we assume that the concentration of Akt is proportional to the external concentration of PGE2: $akt = \gamma_2 \cdot pge2$. Substituting both expressions in **Eq. 1** we finally obtain:

$$\frac{d(nf)}{dt} = V_{max\,nf} P_{nf}^{on}(t) + k_1 il6 \cdot i\kappa bnf + k_{11} pge2 \cdot i\kappa bnf - k_4 nf \cdot i\kappa b - D \cdot nf \quad (2)$$

where k_1 and k_{11} are the new rate constants (**Table 1**).

The rate at which the complex IκB-NF κB is broken in presence of IKK depends on the rate at which IKK and Akt remove IκB from the complex under the action of IL-6 and PGE2, and the rate at which the complex is formed again:

$$\frac{d(i\kappa bnf)}{dt} = k_4 nf \cdot i\kappa b - k_5 il6 \cdot i\kappa bnf - k_{11} pge2 \cdot i\kappa bnf \quad (3)$$

where *iκbnf* is the concentration of the complex IκB-NF κB, and k_4 and k_5 are rate constants (**Table 1**).

The rate at which NF κB enter the nucleus depends on the rate of transport of the molecule into de nucleus, adjusted for the change in volume between the cytoplasmic and nuclear compartments, and on the rate of inhibition of nuclear NK κB by its inhibitors:

$$\frac{dnf*}{dt} = D\left(\frac{V_{cyt}}{V_{nuc}}\right)nf - k_{deg} nf* \quad (4)$$

where nf^* is the nuclear concentration of NF κB and k_{deg} is a rate constant.

The probabilities of activation of genes *IL6*, *Cox2*, *IκB* and *NF κB* (**Figures 3A,B**) are given by:

$$\frac{dp_{IL6}^{on}(t)}{dt} = k_2\left(\frac{nf*}{hd*+1}\right)(1 - p_{IL6}^{on}(t)) - k_{-2}p_{IL6}^{on}(t) \quad (5)$$

$$\frac{dp_{I\kappa B}^{on}(t)}{dt} = k_3\left(\frac{nf*}{hd*+1}\right)(1 - p_{I\kappa B}^{on}(t)) - k_{-3}p_{I\kappa B}^{on}(t) \quad (6)$$

$$\frac{dp_{Cox2}^{on}(t)}{dt} = k_7\left(\frac{nf*}{hd*+1}\right)(1 - p_{Cox2}^{on}(t)) - k_{-7}p_{Cox2}^{on}(t) \quad (7)$$

$$\frac{dp_{NF\kappa B}^{on}(t)}{dt} = k_{15}\left(\frac{nf*}{hd*+1}\right)\cdot(1 - p_{NF\kappa B}^{on}(t)) - k_{-15}p_{NF\kappa B}^{on}(t) \quad (8)$$

Supplementary Material S2 for the mathematical deduction of these equations. For **Eqs (5)–(7)**, the variable $p_i^{on}(t)$, with $i \in \{\text{IL}-6, \text{I}\kappa\text{B}, \text{Cox2}, \text{NF}\,\kappa\text{B}\}$, is the probability that the gene i is expressed at time t, hd^* is the amount of HDCA2 in nucleus, and k_2, k_{-2}, k_3, k_{-3}, k_7, k_{-7}, k_{15}, k_{-15} are rate constants (**Table 1**).

We assume that free cytoplasmic HDAC2 is produced according to the rate equation:

$$\frac{d(hd)}{dt} = \frac{r}{\eta(nsp5+1)} - D_2\cdot hd \quad (9)$$

where hd is the amount of free cytoplasmic HDAC2 that is produced at a constant rate r, D_2 is the rate of transport of free HDAC2 into the nucleus. In this equation, $nsp5$ is the amount of Nsp5 in the infected cell that sequester HDAC2 in cytoplasm (El Baba & Herbein, 2020), and η is a constant (**Table 1**). Free cytoplasmic HDCA2 enters the nucleus according to the equation:

$$\frac{d(hd*)}{dt} = D_2\left(\frac{V_{cyt}}{V_n}\right)hd - k_{deg2}hd* \quad (10)$$

where hd^* is the amount of HDAC2 in the nucleus, and k_{deg2} is a rate constant (**Table 1**).

Nsp5 is a protein with only one link in the virus interactome (Gordon et al., 2020; Díaz. 2020a; Hekman et al., 2020), which is an input to the circuit of **Figure 2**. However, the real kinetic mechanism of production of this viral protein is unknown, thus we assume a plausible simple kinetic mechanism that leads Nsp5 to have a maximum constant concentration of 20 nM. We set the parameters ϕ and k_{18} to the values shown in **Table 1**:

$$\frac{d(nsp5)}{dt} = \phi - k_{18}nsp5 \quad (11)$$

where ϕ is the constant rate of production of Nsp5, and k_{18} is a rate constant (**Table 1**). The effect of the variation of parameter ϕ on the dynamics of the circuit of **Figure 2** is analyzed in **Supplementary Material S3**.

During the early stage of infection by SARS-CoV-2, the rate of variation of the concentration of IL-6 outside the lung cell depends on the rate of production of IL-6 by monocytes, leucocytes and other cells under stimulation by Tall-like Receptors (TLRs) [denoted by $\alpha(t)$] (Jafarzadeha et al., 2020; Magro, 2020), on the rate of production by lung cells due to nuclear NF κB transcriptional activity enhanced by Nsp5 (**Figure 3A**), and on the rate of degradation of IL-6 by different mechanisms. Finally, we assume that the concentration of IKK activated by IL-6 is proportional to the external concentration of the cytokine (**Eq. (2)**):

$$\frac{d(il6)}{dt} = \alpha(t) + V_{IL6}^{\max}p_{IL6}^{on}(t) - k_5 il6\cdot i\kappa bnf - k_6 il6 \quad (12)$$

where $V_{IL6}^{\max}$ is the maximum rate of translation of $IL6$, $p_{IL6}^{on}(t)$ is the probability that the $IL6$ gene is activated at time t, and k_5 and k_6 are rate constants (**Table 1**).

The rate of variation of the amount of free IκB in the system is the balance between the rate of translation of gene IκB and the rate of formation of new IκB-NF κB complexes:

$$\frac{d(i\kappa b)}{dt} = V_{I\kappa B}^{\max}p_{I\kappa B}^{on}(t) - k_4 i\kappa b\cdot nf \quad (13)$$

where $V_{I\kappa B}^{\max}$ is the maximum rate of translation of $I\kappa B$, and $p_{I\kappa B}^{on}(t)$ is the probability that the gene $I\kappa B$ is activated at time t (**Table 1**).

The rate of variation of the amount of the enzyme Cox2 in the system depends on the rate of translation of the *Cox2* gene, and its rate of inhibition by different mechanisms:

$$\frac{dcox2}{dt} = V_{Cox2}^{\max}p_{Cox2}^{on}(t) - k_{10}cox2 \quad (14)$$

where $cox2$ is the amount of the enzyme in the system, $V_{Cox2}^{\max}$ is the maximum rate of variation, $p_{Cox2}^{on}(t)$ is the probability that the gene $Cox2$ is activated at time t, k_8, k_9 and k_{10} are rate constants (**Table 1**).

The rate of variation of the amount of PGE2 in the system depends on the amount of Cox2, on the amount of IL-6, and on its rate of degradation:

$$\frac{dpge2}{dt} = k_{17}cox2 - k11pge2\cdot i\kappa bnf - k_{12}pge2 \quad (15)$$

where k_{11}, k_{12} and k_{17} are rate constants (**Table 1**).

RESULTS

In this section we present in detail and focus on the results that are relevant to understand the role of Nsp5 in the process of acute lung inflammation. The rest of the analyses and results related to the mathematical aspects of the model and its stability analysis are reported in **Supplementary Material S3**.

We solved the model using the Euler predictor-corrector and Runge-Kutta 4,5 methods with time step of 0.05 s and 720,000 integration steps to simulate a period of 10 h post infection, which is the estimated time for the first bursting of new virions into the extracellular medium (Bar-On et al., 2020; Kumar et al., 2020). We made a Boolean simulation of the circuit to confirm the dynamical behavior predicted by the ODEs model. We used the parameter values shown in **Table 1** to generate an *arbitrary reference state* (ARS) of the system for the initial conditions $i\kappa bnf$ = 5 pg ml^{-1}, and the rest of the variables equal to 0 at time $t = 0$. In this case, the input $\alpha(t) = 10$ pg ml^{-1}s^{-1} and $nsp5 = 0$ for $t \in [0, \infty)$. In this ARS, the translation velocities of all genes are set to 2 pg mL^{-1} s^{-1} (Hausser et al., 2019). In the case of the ODEs

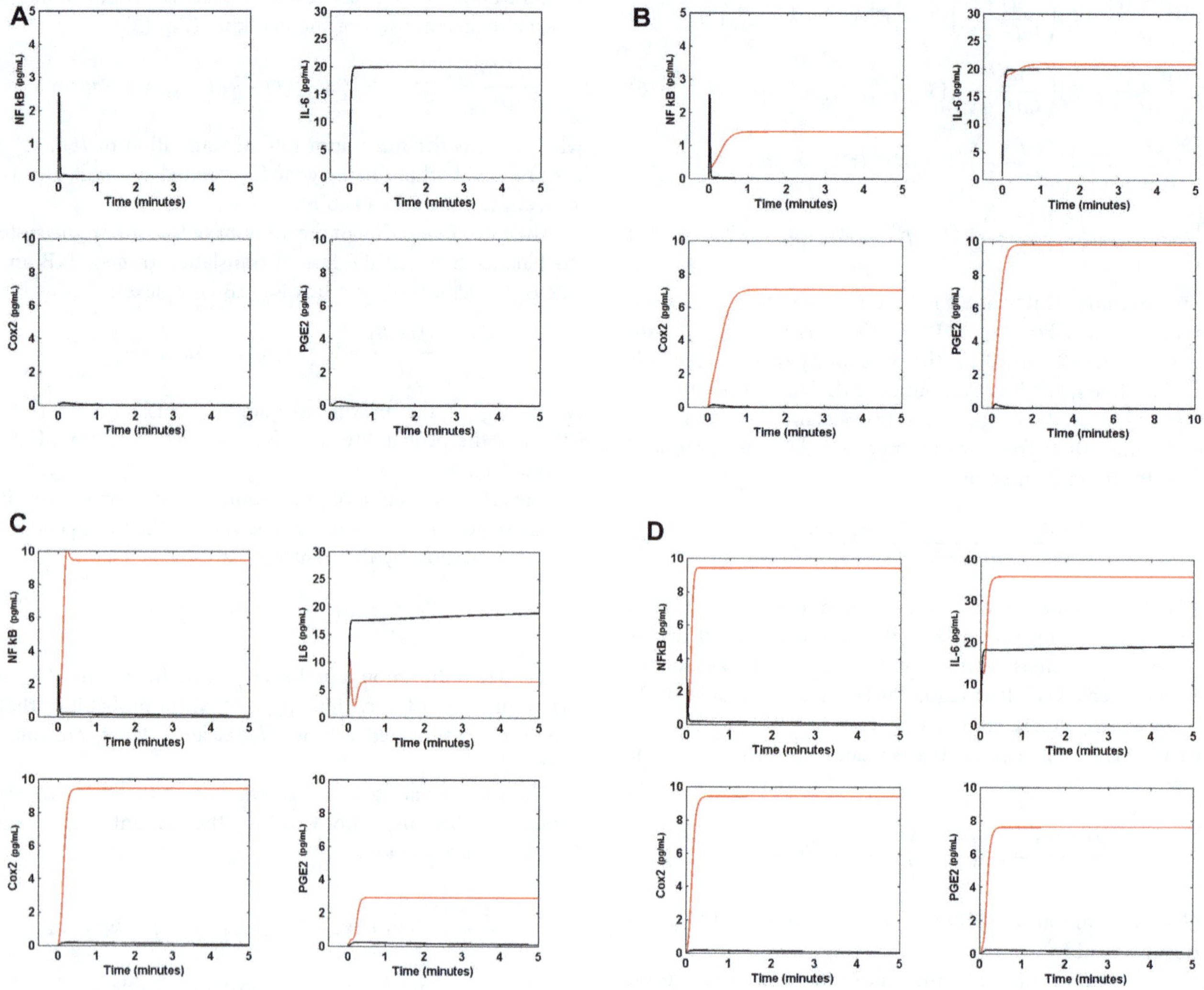

FIGURE 4 | Effect of Nsp5 on IL-6 production. **(A)** Arbitrary reference state (ARS) of the circuit of **Figure 2**. In absence of the viral protein Nsp5, the response to an external input α (t) = 10 pg $ml^{-1}s^{-1}$ is a transitory activation of NF κB, Cox2, and PGE2. In this case, IL-6 shows a steady high concentration. In this case, all the gene translation rates are set to 2 pg $ml^{-1}s^{-1}$. **(B)** In presence of Nsp5 the circuit shows steady higher concentrations of NF κB, Cox2, and PGE2 (red line) with respect to ARS (black line). IL-6 steady concentration (black line) is unaffected by the presence of the viral protein (red line). In this panel, α (t) = 10 pg $ml^{-1}s^{-1}$, and all the gene translation rates are set to 2 pg $ml^{-1}s^{-1}$. **(C)** When NF κB and IκB translation rates are V_{nf}^{max} = 10 pg $mL^{-1}s^{-1}$ and $V_{I\kappa B}^{max}$ = 15 pg $mL^{-1}s^{-1}$, respectively, and Cox2 and IL-6 translation rates are 2 nM s^{-1} the circuit shows a weak sustained activation of NF κB, Cox2, and PGE2 (black line) in response to the external input α (t) = 10 pg $ml^{-1}s^{-1}$ and in absence of Nsp5. In this case, IL-6 steady concentration does not change (black line). In presence of Nsp5 the circuit shows steady higher concentrations of NF κB, Cox2, and PGE2 (red line), although the concentration of IL-6 is lower than is absence of the virus. **(D)** In the over stimulated immune state (OSIS), the presence of Nsp5 produces an enhanced production of NF κB, Cox 2, PGE2 and IL-5 (red lines). This particular state is obtained when α (t) = 10 pg $ml^{-1}s^{-1}$, V_{nf}^{max} = 10 pg $mL^{-1}s^{-1}$,$V_{I\kappa B}^{max}$ = 15 pg $mL^{-1}s^{-1}$, V_{Cox2}^{max} = 2 pg $mL^{-1}s^{-1}$, and V_{IL6}^{max} = 20 pg $mL^{-1}s^{-1}$.

model, both numerical methods produce identical outputs indicating no bias in the predicted dynamics of the circuit due to the integration method and that the transitory sharp initial increase observed in the concentration of the proteins of the circuit are to due to the transitory initial response of the feedback loops to the input. The solution of the Boolean model confirms that the trajectories of the circuit lead to a stable node or attractor where all the nodes are in *on* state, except HDAC2 that is in state *off*, when Nsp5 is in state *on*.

Figure 4A shows that the output of the model is the transitory activation of NF κB, Cox2 and PGE2, in contrast with a sustained high activation of IL-6. In order to clarify the source of the steady activation of IL-6, we solved the model with the same initial conditions and α (t) = 0. In this case, the system does not *turn on* during all the time of simulation (data not shown), indicating that the signal from monocytes and other cells is a *necessary condition* to start the IL-6 sustained production in lung cells (**Figure 4A**). **Figure 4B** shows that when *nsp5* ≠ 0, α(t) = 0 and equal gene translation rates, the response of the system is a high sustained level of activation of NF κB, Cox2, and PGE2 with respect to the ARS. In this case, the concentration of IL-6 in the cell was only slightly affected

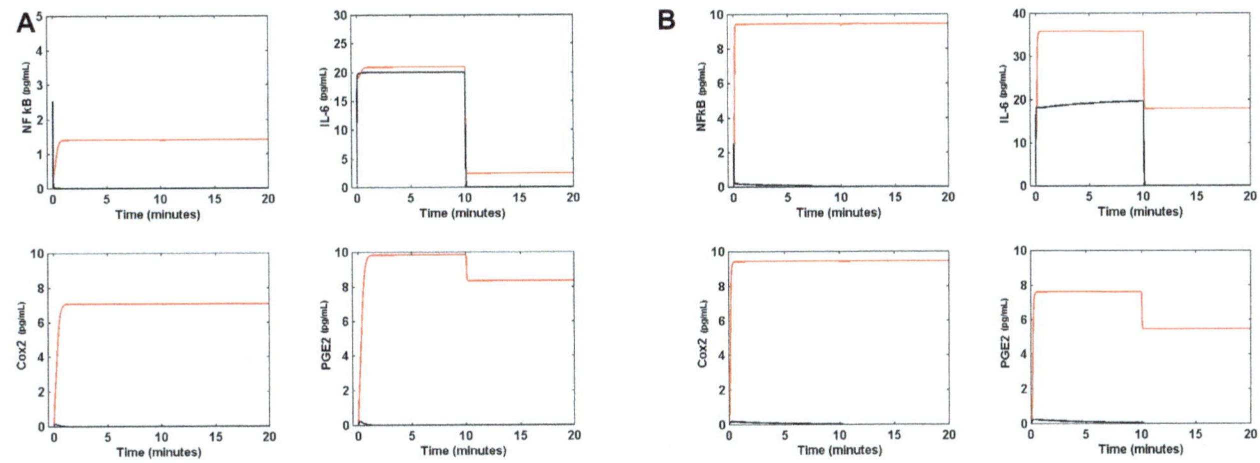

FIGURE 5 | Response of the circuit to a step function. **(A)** When the external signal α (t) is the step function of **Eq. 16** of main text and is applied to the ARS in absence of Nsp5 (black line) the level of cytokine IL-6 initially increases to a maximum value of 20 pg mL^{-1}, and becomes zero when the external signal is switched off. There is not any effect on NF κB, Cox2 and PGE2 concentrations in the circuit. However, in presence of Nsp5 (red line) the levels of NF κB, Cox2, PGE2 and IL-6 are increased in response to α t) and never become zero when the external signal is switched off. **(B)** When the step function of **Eq. 16** is applied to the circuit in absence of Nsp5 (black line) with V_{nf}^{max} = 10 pg mL^{-1}s^{-1},$V_{I\kappa B}^{max}$ = 15 pg mL^{-1}s^{-1}, V_{Cox2}^{max} = 2 pgmL^{-1}s^{-1} and V_{IL6}^{max} = 20 pg mL^{-1}s^{-1}, there is a low increase in NF κB, Cox2 and PGE2 concentrations that becomes zero when the external signal is switched *off*. IL-6 initially increases to a maximum value of 20 pg ml^{-1}, and becomes zero when the external signal is also zero. In contrast, when the circuit is in OSIS in presence of Nsp5 (red line) the concentrations of NF κB, Cox2, PGE2 and IL-6 are increased in response to α (t) and remain at a high value even the external signal is switched *off*.

by the virus. Figures from 4A to 4D show the first 5 minutes of simulation during which the circuit of **Figure 2** reaches its steady state. This result indicates that *the presence of the virus induce a sustained and persistent production of* NF κB, Cox2, *and* PGE2 in the circuit of **Figure 2**.

Translation rates of the set of genes of the model rarely have the same value, even when their activation is promoted by the same transcription factor (NF κB in this case). As shown in **Table 1**, the results of **Figures 4A,B** are obtained when the rates of translation are the same for all genes. However, in real cells this is not the case, and *Cox2*, *Il-6*, NF κB and IκB are translated at different rates. In *Homo sapiens* the estimated average rate of translation (V^{max}) of a gene is about 10^4 proteins per hour (Hausser et al., 2019). However, this average value can be increased according to the state of activity of the cell. In the present work, we arbitrary chose the value of $V^{max} = 2\,\text{pg}\,\text{mL}^{-1}\text{s}^{-1}$ for all genes in the ARF (**Table 1**). However, we made parameter variation to know how different values of this set of parameters affect the qualitative behavior of the model (**Supplementary Material S1**). **Figure 4C** shows that when in the system $V_{nf}^{max} = 10\,\text{pg}\,\text{mL}^{-1}\text{s}^{-1}$, $V_{I\kappa B}^{max} = 15\,\text{pg}\,\text{mL}^{-1}\text{s}^{-1}$, $V_{Cox2}^{max} = 2\,\text{pg}\,\text{mL}^{-1}\text{s}^{-1}$, and $V_{IL6}^{max} = 2\,\text{pg}\,\text{mL}^{-1}\text{s}^{-1}$, $\alpha(t) = 10\,\text{pg}\,\text{ml}^{-1}\text{s}^{-1}$ and *nsp5* = 0, the circuit tends to a steady state in which NF κB, Cox2, and PGE2 exhibit a constant low concentration during the time of simulation, while IL-6 steady concentration is unaffected with respect to the value shown in **Figure 4A**. When *nsp5* ≠ 0, the steady concentration of NF κB, and Cox2, are increased ~10 fold with respect to their maximum concentration in the ARS, while PGE2 concentration is increased ~4 fold; Nsp5 produces a ~4 fold decrease in IL-6 steady concentration with respect to the reference concentration shown in **Figure 4A**.

This result indicates that a the difference in translation rates between NF κB and IκB (the intensity of the inhibition of NF κB by IκB, **Figure 3A**) in absence of the virus with respect to their values in ARS induces a low sustained production of NF κB, Cox2, and PGE2 without affecting IL-6 production. However the presence of Nsp5 induces a high production of NF κB and Cox2, and a moderate increase in PGE2 concentration that decreases IL-6 concentration, *indicating that a higher rate of IκB translation with respect to* NF κB tra*nslation can decrease the concentration of the cytokine* IL-6 *in presence of the virus probably due to a lower concentration of* PGE2*in the circuit* (**Figures 2, 3A**).

Figure 4D shows that when α (t) = 10 pg ml^{-1} s^{-1}, *nsp5* = 0, $V_{nf}^{max} = 10\,\text{pg}\,\text{mL}^{-1}\text{s}^{-1}$, $V_{I\kappa B}^{max} = 15\,\text{pg}\,\text{mL}^{-1}\text{s}^{-1}$, $V_{Cox2}^{max} = 2\,\text{pg}\,\text{mL}^{-1}\text{s}^{-1}$, and $V_{IL6}^{max} = 20\,\text{pg}\,\text{mL}^{-1}\text{s}^{-1}$the circuit tends to a steady state in which NF κB, Cox2 and PGE2 exhibit a constant low concentration during the time of simulation, while IL-6 is unaffected with respect to its steady concentration in **Figure 4A**. However, when *nsp5* ≠ 0 the dynamical behavior of the circuit changes because NF κB and Cox2 show the same steady concentration that in **Figure 4C**, but PGE2 has a higher steady concentration. In this case, IL-6 shows an increase of ~2 fold with respect to the level shown in **Figure 4C**. Thus, *a high rate of IL*-6 translation can overcome the effect of an increased rate of IκB translation in presence of the virus, allowing an overproduction of the cytokine.

All these results suggest an important dynamical property of the circuit shown in **Figure 2**: a high value of the parameter V_{IL6}^{max} produces an over production of NF κB, Cox2, PGE2, and IL-6 in

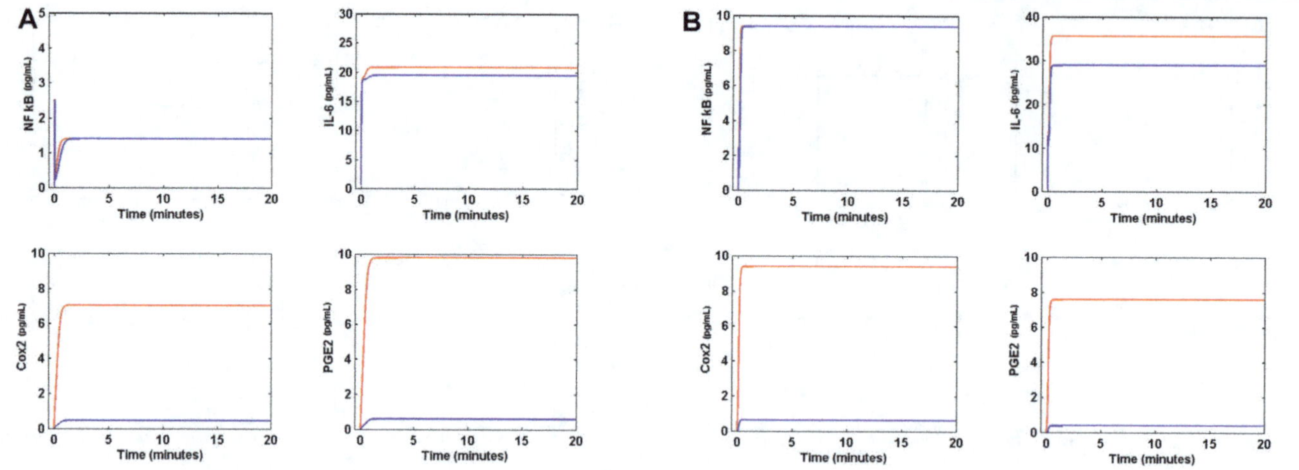

FIGURE 6 | Effect of Nimesulide on lung cell inflammation. **(A)** Effect of 14 pg mL^{-1} of Nimesulide on the levels of NF κB, Cox2, PGE2 and IL-6 when α (t) = 10 pg mL^{-1}s^{-1}, and all gene translation rates are 2 pg mL^{-1}s^{-1} in presence of Nsp5 (red line). Nimesulide decreases the concentration of Cox2 and PGE2, but has not effect on NF κB and IL-6 (blue line). **(B)** Effect of 14 pg mL^{-1} of Nimesulide on the OSIS (red line). Nimesulide significantly decreases the concentration of Cox2 and PGE2, but has not effect on NF κB, The drug has a weak effect on IL-6 concentration (blue line).

the circuit in presence of Nsp5 with respect to the ARS (**Figures 4A,D**). We name *over stimulated immune state* (OSIS) to the state of the system shown in **Figure 4D**, for which: V^{max}_{nf} = 10 pg ml^{-1} s^{-1}, $V^{max}_{I\kappa B}$ = 15 pg ml^{-1} s^{-1}, V^{max}_{Cox2} = 2 pg ml^{-1} s^{-1}, V^{max}_{IL6} = 20 pg ml^{-1} s^{-1}, *nsp5* ≠ 0 and α (*t*) = 10 pg ml^{-1} s^{-1}.

Figure 5 shows the response of the circuit to a step function defined as:

$$\alpha(t) = \begin{cases} 10 & 0 \le t < 10 \\ 0 & t > 10 \end{cases} \tag{16}$$

The latter simulates an external signal of IL-6 initially generated at a rate of 10 pg ml^{-1} s^{-1} during 10 min, and switched *off* after the 10 min. **Figure 5A** is the response of the system in ARS to the step signal, in absence and presence of Nsp5. Interestingly, in the absence of Nsp5, the circuit exhibits a low concentration of NF κB, Cox2 and PGE2, and a high concentration of IL-6, all which are zero when the external signal is switched *off.* In presence of Nsp5 the ARS is perturbed by α (t), and reaches a new steady state with high concentrations of NF κB, Cox2, and PGE2 that remain even when the external signal is switched *off.* Furthermore, the high IL-6 concentration reached when the circuit is turned *on* falls to a lower concentration different from zero when α (t) = 0.

In order to reduce the effect of Nsp5 on the circuit of **Figure 2**, we tested the effect of Nimesulide on NF κB production. Nimesulide, a Cox2 inhibitor, acts inhibiting the synthesis of Cox2 and lipooxigenase enzyme and their products (Suleyman et al., 2008). We modified **Eq. 14** to introduce an inhibition term that decreases the rate of production of Cox2 in presence of Nimesulide:

$$\frac{dcox2}{dt} = \frac{V^{max}_{Cox2} p^{on}_{Cox2}(t)}{nim + 1} - k_{10} cox2 \tag{17}$$

where *nim* is the amount of Nimesulide at time *t*, whose rate of variation of its concentration in the cell is:

$$\frac{d(nim)}{dt} = r_2 - k_{19} nim \tag{18}$$

where r_2 = 40 pg ml^{-1} s^{-1} and k_{19} = 3 s^{-1}. Solution of the modified model (**Eq. (17)**) is presented in **Figure 6**. In **Figure 6A**, Nimesulide is applied to the circuit in presence of Nsp5, and with all gene translation rates set to 2 pg ml^{-1} s^{-1}. In this case, Nimesulide has no effect on NF κB, a slightly effect on IL-6, and a significant decrease in Cox2 and PGE2 concentrations to values near to zero in presence of 14 pg ml^{-1} of the drug. The same effect is observed when the circuit is in OSIS (**Figure 6B**). Thus, Nimesulide is not an effective anti-inflammatory agent in the context of the dynamic circuit modeled here, and does not impact the concentration of IL-6 in the presence of Nsp5, even at high concentrations.

Dexamethasone (DX), is a potent synthetic glucocorticoid that inhibits NF κB transcription, and is another anti-inflammatory drug that is being used to ameliorate acute inflammatory states due to SARS-CoV-2 infection. In order to test the effect of DX on the inflammatory process in the circuit of **Figure 2**, we modified **Eq. 8** to introduce an inhibition term that decreases the probability of activation of *NF κB*:

$$\frac{dp^{on}_{NF\kappa B}(t)}{dt} = k_{15}\left(\frac{nf*}{(hd*+1)(DX+1)}\right)\left(1 - p^{on}_{NF\kappa B}(t)\right) - k_{-15} p^{on}_{NF\kappa B}(t) \tag{19}$$

where *DX* is the amount of DX at time *t*, whose rate of variation of its concentration in the cell is:

$$\frac{d(DX)}{dt} = r_3 - k_{20} DX \tag{20}$$

where r_3 = 30 pg ml^{-1} s^{-1} and k_{20} = 3 s^{-1}.

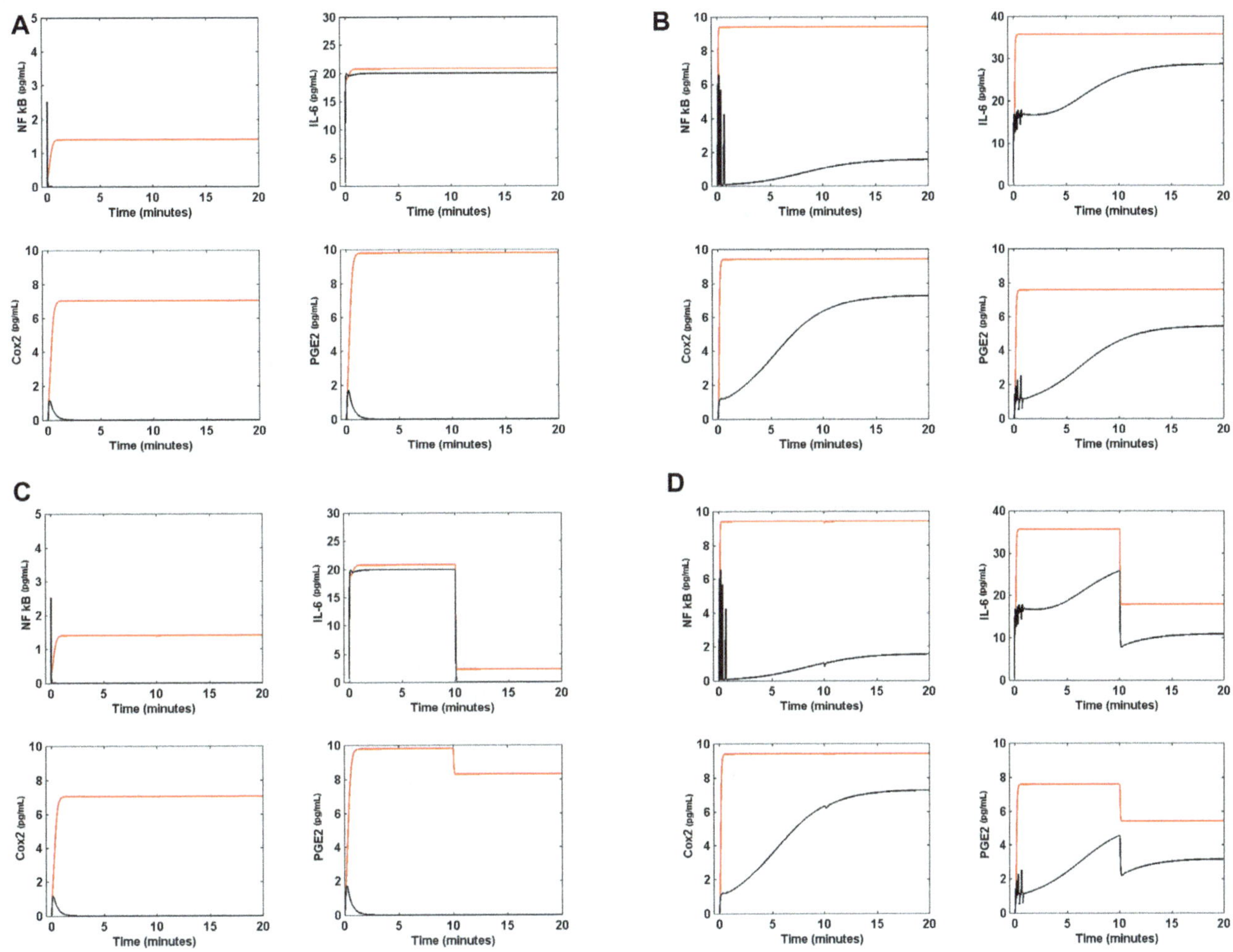

FIGURE 7 | Effect of Dexamethasone on lung cell inflammation. **(A)** Effect of 14 pg mL^{-1} of Dexamethasone (DX) on the levels of NF κB, Cox2, PGE2 and IL-6 when $a(t) = 10$ pg $mL^{-1}s^{-1}$, and all gene translation rates are 2 pg $mL^{-1}s^{-1}$ in presence of Nsp5 (red line). DX effectively decreases the concentration of NF κB, Cox2 and PGE2 to cero, but has not effect on IL-6 (black line). **(B)** Effect of 14 pg mL^{-1} of DX on the OSIS (red line). DX has a weak effect on the concentration of NF κB, Cox2, PGE2, and IL-6 (red line). **(C)** When the external signal $\alpha(t)$ is the step function of **Eq. 16** of main text and is applied to the circuit in presence of Nsp5 (red line), with all gene translation rates equal to 2 pg $mL^{-1}s^{-1}$, 14 pg mL^{-1} of DX decreases the concentration of NF κB, Cox2, PGE2 and IL-6 to zero (black line). **(D)** When the external signal $\alpha(t)$ is the step function of **Eq. 16** of main text and 14 pg mL^{-1} of DX are applied to the circuit in the OSIS, the drug has a practically null effect on the inflammation process.

Figure 7 shows the effect of DX on the circuit. **Figure 7A** shows that when DX is applied to the circuit in presence of Nsp5, and when all genes have the same translation rate of 2 pg ml^{-1} s^{-1}, the drug eliminates NF κB, Cox2 and PGE2 from the circuit, but has a null effect on the concentration of IL-6. However, when the circuit is in OSIS (**Figure 7B**), DX has little effect on the immune response in presence of Nsp5. **Figure 7C** shows that when all translation rates are the same (2 pg ml^{-1} s^{-1}), DX can shut down the immune response in presence of the virus, when the circuit input α (t) is the function of **Eq. 16**. However, DX cannot shut down the effects of Nsp5 when the circuit is in OSIS, having a little anti-inflammatory effect (**Figure 7D**). Hence, our results suggest that DX *is an effective anti-inflammatory drug during mild inflammatory states, but is less effective during critical acute lung inflammation due to SARS-CoV-2* (Horby et al., 2021). This dynamical behavior of the circuit of **Figure 2** is unaffected by higher doses of DX. When DX and Nimesulide are applied together (with 35 pg ml^{-1} of DX and 40 pg ml^{-1} of Nimesulide) to the circuit in OSIS, in which α (t) is the function of **Eq. 16**, there is also a limited anti-inflammatory effect (**Figure 8A**).

In contrast, the predicted limited effect of Nimesulide and DX on reverting the OSIS, the molecular docking of Nsp5 with a hypothetical drug like Saquinavir (Xu et al., 2020), is able to completely eliminate inflammation. We tested this hypothesis modifying Nsp5 production in **Eq. (11)** with an inhibitory term:

$$\frac{d(nsp5)}{dt} = \frac{\phi}{drug + 1} - k_{18}nsp5 \tag{21}$$

where *drug* is the amount of the hypothetical drug that can remove Nsp5 from the circuit, whose concentration at time *t* is given by:

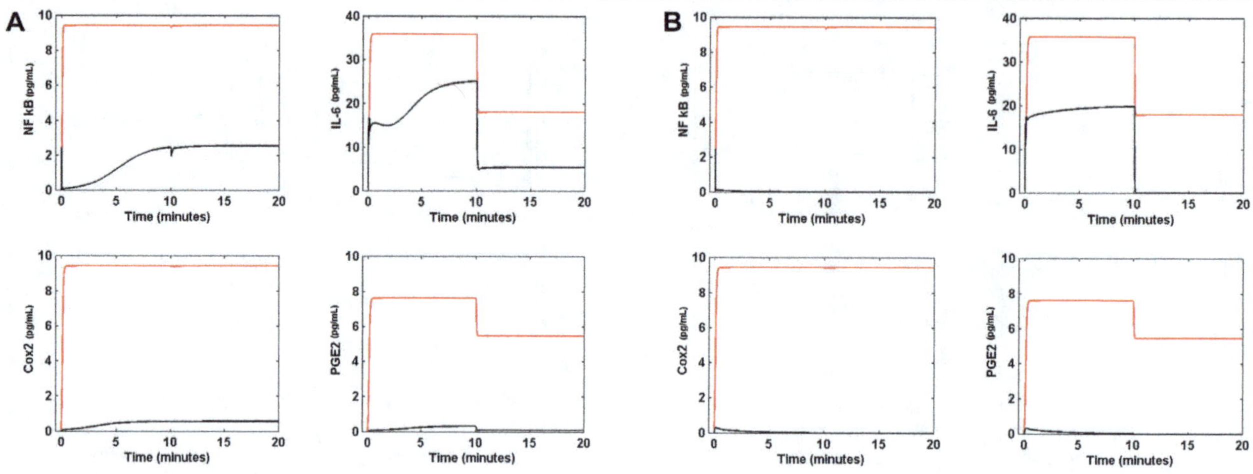

FIGURE 8 | Effect of the molecular docking of Nsp5 on lung inflammation. **(A)** When DX and Nimesulide are applied together (with 35 pg mL^{-1} of DX and 40 pg mL^{-1} of Nimesulide) to the circuit in OSIS (red line), in which α (t) is the function of **Eq. 16**, there is also a little anti-inflammatory effect. **(B)** The molecular docking of Nsp5 completely shuts down the inflammation process when the circuit is in OSIS, with α (t) given by **Eq. 16**, suggesting that Nsp5 is effectively the cause of the acute lung inflammation during SARS-CoV-2 infection.

$$\frac{d(drug)}{dt} = r_4 - k_{21}drug \tag{22}$$

with r_4 = 30 pg ml^{-1} s^{-1} and k_{21} = 3 s^{-1}.

Figure 8B shows that when the hypothetical drug is applied to the circuit in OSIS, with α (t) given by **Eq. 16**, the inflammatory process is completely shut down, *suggesting that Nsp5 is effectively the key cause of the acute lung inflammation during SARS-CoV-2 infection, and a fundamental potential target for its treatment.*

DISCUSSION

The complexity of the immune response to infections implies a complex set of different kinds of cells that involve complex regulatory networks and molecules. Together, they underlie specific responses that may lead to resolution or to inflammatory responses whose dynamical properties depend on the networks structure (i.e., the number of nodes, links, and the distribution of links between the nodes) occurring at different scales and levels (Lipniacki et al., 2004; Morel et al., 2006; Eftimie et al., 2016). The structure of such complex and dynamical network is not random due to the specific nature of its nodes and links, so that if the network has a hierarchical structure its hubs determine the overall network dynamics and the structure of its phase space (Cessac, 2010; Eftimie et al., 2016; Díaz. 2020b). In high dimensional phase spaces, steady points of diverse kinds can coexist with isolated closed curves (limit cycles), strange attractors of fractal structure, and other limit sets giving rise to a variety of biological dynamical behaviors like molecular switches, periodic and quasi-periodic oscillations, and bursting (among others). Two central problems in the analysis of this kind of dynamical systems are: 1) the structure of the phase space is strongly dependent of the value of the set of parameters of the dynamical system, and 2) the nonlinearity characteristic of biological systems such as the one treated here (**Supplementary Material S1**) (Nayak et al., 2018).

In most of the ODEs-based biological models so far studied, there is limited knowledge of the real values of the parameters, and this leads to uncertainty concerning the extent to which the model explains the real process under study. In this case, the validation of the model relied on experimental data. Nonetheless, with the exception of some particular cases (Hodgkin and Huxley, 1952), qualitative models have to be proposed and quantitative validations remain ahead (Eftimie et al., 2016). This challenge increases with the dimensionality of the model. Thus, is necessary to choose some particular properties of the network under study (inflammation network in this case) that incorporate key dynamical features of the whole system under study, and that can also aid to reduce the number of parameters of the model to the minimum possible.

In this sense, we limited the scope of this work to the study of the inflammation process of epithelial lung cells during SARS-CoV-2 infection. The epithelial lung cells form a sub-network that have two highly connected nodes: the internal signal integrator NF κB, and the external signal integrator IL-6 Receptor (IL6R) (Magro, 2020), which is activated by external IL-6 (**Figures 2, 3**). Both integrators trigger the activation of two important intermediate processes: Cox2 and PGE2 synthesis. Thus, we propose, as *a first approximation*, that the dynamical behavior of this these four nodes of the circuit of **Figure 2** reflect with certain accuracy the dynamical properties of the complex inflammation sub-network of lung cells. Thus, the dynamics of IL-6, NF κB, Cox2 and PGE2 nodes is described by a model that consist of 12 nonlinear coupled ordinary differential equations (**Table 1**), that we assume represents the central dynamical core involved in the lung cells inflammation process in response to SARS-CoV-2 infection. Such core includes three coupled feedback loops shown in **Figure 3**. We used this low-dimensionality model to explore the effect of Nsp5 in the qualitative dynamics of the inflammation circuit of **Figure 2** (Díaz, 2020b; Kumar et al., 2020).

SARS-CoV-2 main protease Nsp5 has a role as an epigenetic regulator of host DNA expression in lung cells; and thus its physical association with HADC2 (Gordon et al., 2020; Kumar et al., 2020) avoids the movement of the deacetylase from the cytoplasm to the nucleus, increasing the probability of the binding of NF κB to the promoter site of its target genes (**Eqs. 5–8**) (El Baba and Herbein, 2020). NF κB is a central integrator of the signals that initiate the inflammation process (**Figure 1**), which include IL-6 secreted by monocytes, leucocytes, macrophages, among other cells, together with signals from TLR4 and TLR7 that suppress the IκB-NF κB complex in a MyD88 independent manner (Vidya et al., 2017). NF κB enhanced transcriptional activity includes the transcription of *IL-6*, *Cox2*, IκB and NF κB itself that are key genes in the process of inflammation (**Figure 3**).

Results obtained from our model suggest that Nsp5 can effectively transform a weak inflammation response (Long et al., 2020) into a persistent sustained one that has a relative high concentration of the cytokine IL-6 (**Figure 4B**). In the example of **Figure 4B**, all genes have the same translation rate, a condition that have low probably of occurrence in the real human immune system in which every gene is subject to different processes of post transcriptional regulation (Hausser et al., 2019). When this restriction is removed, and IL-6 has a high translation rate, Nsp5 boosts the concentration of the four main proteins of the circuit with respect to their respective values in ARS, and the inflammation response becomes strongly persistent with a high IL-6 concentration. Furthermore, in this state that we named OSIS, the dynamics of the circuit of **Figure 2** becomes independent of any kind of external signal and never turns *off*, leading to the deregulation of the production of the cytokine IL-6 (**Figure 5B**). In this form, Nsp5 changes the qualitative dynamical behavior of the system, in which the trajectories that initially span around the ARS stable node now span around the OSIS stable node (**Supplementary Material S3**) (Díaz, 2020b).

An important biological consequence of this change in the qualitative dynamics of the circuit is that ACE2 receptor synthesis also becomes persistent and autonomous of any external signal to the lung cells (**Figure 2**). Furthermore, neither Nimesulide nor Dexamethasone or both can completely eliminate the OSIS *suggesting that this dynamical behavior could be the form in which the virus assures the persistence of its reproductive cycle without any perturbation from the natural defenses of the body*. This could be also a possible clue about the possible adaptive substitution of N protein used in SARS-CoV for the use of the main protease Nsp5 in SARS-CoV-2 as the switch for the inflammation process, which is necessary for ACE2 sustained production, taking into consideration that SARS-CoV N protein targets Cox2 while SARS-CoV-2 Nsp5 protein targets the master integrator NF κB. If this hypothesis is true, *this is the probable cause of the increased pathogenicity of SARS-CoV-2 with respect to SARS-CoV*.

It is of interest that the persistence of the OSIS is supported by a high translational rate of *IL-6*, which in the model must have a value of $V_{IL6}^{max} \geq 7$ pg $mL^{-1}s^{-1}$. This result pictures a probable hypothetical scenario where the external signal α (t) triggers the initial inflammation response with a low translation rate of IL-6 that can be shut down with DX. As viral infection continues, IL-6, NF κB, and IκB increase their rate of translation (V_{Cox2}^{max} value has a little weight in this process) and the dynamical behavior of the circuit of **Figure 2** becomes independent of the value of α (t), and *self-sustained*, i.e., the control of the production of the cytokine IL-6 is translated from the external immune cells to the lung cells, and cannot be completely stopped even with high doses of DX. In this form, in the model, V_{IL6}^{max} *is a bifurcation parameter* that changes the qualitative dynamical behavior of the circuit of **Figure 2** when $V_{nf}^{max} = 10$ pg $mL^{-1}s^{-1}$ and $V_{I\kappa B}^{max} = 15$ pg $mL^{-1}s^{-1}$ are constant values (**Supplementary Material S3**).

In this extreme situation (OSIS), the unique treatment possible suggested by our model is an inhibitor of Nsp5 like *Saquinavir* (Xun et al., 2020). In this case, the OSIS is completely shut down, which indirectly implies the down production of ACE2. Saquinavir is an anti-retroviral drug used against the main protease of HIV-1 (Bensussen et al., 2018; Xun et al., 2020), with some undesirable effects like diarrhea, abdominal pain, and nausea. We suggest that this drug could be a plausible treatment against the effects of SARS-CoV-2 in acute lung inflammation, and as a complement to the new vaccine against this coronavirus.

Interferon (IFN) I and III are key secretory factors in the fight against viral infections in lung cells. During the early response to SARS-CoV-2 infection, interferon pathway is blocked by viral proteins like Nsp14, Nsp16, Nsp15, Orf9b, and Nsp3, among others, that interfere with MAVS and TLRs sensing, STATS 1 and 2 activation and IFN synthesis. Experimental results show that this downregulation of IFN activity correlates with an increased severity of COVID19 symptoms (Kim and Shin, 2021). Therefore, we did not include IFN pathway in our model as a primary cause of lung inflammation. However, our model *suggest* that the initial downregulation of IFN pathway could be partially counteract by the over activation of NF κB caused by Nsp5. The master regulator NF κB targets IFNs genes (Pfeffer, 2011; Kim and Shin, 2021) probably producing a late sustained production of IFN after the initial viral infection adding a component to the cytokine storm.

In a previous work (Díaz, 2020a) the role of the viral protein Orf8 as a hub of the SARS-CoV-2 infection was suggested. This highly connected protein has as main targets those processes related to the vesicular trafficking required for the ensemble of new virions (**Figure 1**) (Gordon et al., 2020). Thus, the inhibition of the effects of Orf8 in the host cells could block the reproduction cycle of the virus but not the inflammation process because Nsp5 is not directly linked to Orf8 (Gordon et al., 2020). Rapamycin has been suggested as a drug against the effects of Orf8 but produces severe immunosuppressant effects, which, according to the results of our model, will not be of care in cases of severe lung inflammation because Nsp5 uncouple the circuit of **Figure 2** from the process of viral replication (**Figure 1** and **Figure 5B**). In this case, a treatment with Rapamycin and Saquinavir can be an alternative for patients with severe lung inflammation. This suggestion needs experimental verification and clinical evaluation.

CONCLUSION

In this work we propose a dynamical model that puts forward a novel hypothetical mechanisms underlying lung cells inflammation process in response to SARS-CoV-2. In this scenario the main protease Nsp5 effectively enhances the inflammatory process, increasing the levels of NF κB, IL-6, Cox2, and PGE2 with respect to the reference state. When the translation rates of NF κB and IκB are increased to a high constant value, and the translation rate of IL-6 is increased above the threshold value of 7 pg $ml^{-1}s^{-1}$ the circuit enters in a persistent over stimulated immune state (OSIS) with high levels of the cytokine IL-6. The OSIS never shuts down by itself, and becomes autonomous of the signals from other immune cells like macrophages and lymphocytes. Our model explains why DX or Nimesulide have little effect on the OSIS, and the only means to suppress such acute and sustained inflammation state is by inhibiting the protein Nsp5 with drugs such as Saquinavir.

In this form, the model suggests, in accordance to our hypothesis, that Nsp5 is effectively a key node underlying severe acute lung inflammation during SARS-CoV-2 infection. The persistent production of IL-6 by lung cells during infection can be one of the causes of the cytokine storm observed in critical patients with COVID19. From an evolutionary point of view, the use of Nsp5 as the switch to start inflammation, and the consequent overproduction of the ACE2 receptor, could have driven the increased pathogenicity of SARS-CoV-2 with respect to SARS-CoV.

In the absence of quantitative data on the kinetics of Nsp5 in the host cell that could give us a better overview of the dynamical behaviour of the protein in the model proposed in this work, we highlight the importance of future *in vitro* and *in vivo* experimental research. In order to experimentally validate the predictions of our model is necessary to measure the rate of production of Nsp5 during the infection of the host lung cells, and compare it with the rate of production of other viral proteins with immunomodulatory effects as Orf 7b and Orf 8, to know the real magnitude of its contribution to the inflammatory process. Furthermore, the experimental inhibition of Nsp5 could be of aid to eliminate the inhibition of HDAC2, either catalytic or mimetic, in infected cells to confirm experimentally if the predictions of the model are in concordance to the real mechanisms that contribute to the cytokines storm. The implementation of techniques as plasmid induction or transfection for the unique expression of Nsp5 and its effectors in lung epithelial tissue also promises to be a simple option to validate the proposed mathematical model, and in turn it would be an ideal platform to measure the efficacy of Nsp5 inhibitors proposed by bioinformatics and clinics.

The present theoretical work is part of the project "Dynamics of the SARS-CoV-2 network" and is based on the experimental data reported in the literature at the moment.

AUTHOR CONTRIBUTIONS

AB made the stability and sensitivity analysis of the model. JD made the model. EA-B and JD conceived the study, discussed the data, and wrote the paper.

ACKNOWLEDGMENTS

JD thanks Erika Juarez Luna for logistical support. AB, EA-B and JD thanks Dr. Antonio Valcarcel for technical support.

REFERENCES

1. Aghai, Z. H., Kumar, S., Farhath, S., Kumar, M. A., Saslow, J., Nakhla, T., et al. (2006). Dexamethasone Suppresses Expression of Nuclear Factor-kappaB in the Cells of Tracheobronchial Lavage Fluid in Premature Neonates with Respiratory Distress. *Pediatr. Res.* 59, 811–815. doi:10.1203/01.pdr.0000219120.92049.b3
2. Alexanian, A., and Sorokin, A. (2017). Cyclooxygenase 2: Protein-Protein Interactions and Posttranslational Modifications. *Physiol. Genomics* 49, 667–681. doi:10.1152/physiolgenomics.00086.2017
3. Bai, D., Ueno, L., and Vogt, P. K. (2009). Akt-mediated Regulation of NFκB and the Essentialness of NFκB for the Oncogenicity of PI3K and Akt. *Int. J. Cancer* 125, 2863–2870. doi:10.1002/ijc.24748
4. Bar-On, Y. M., Flamholz, A., Phillips, R., and Milo, R. (2020). SARS-CoV-2 (COVID-19) by the Numbers. *eLife* 9, e57309. doi:10.7554/eLife.57309
5. Bartlam, M., Yang, H., and Rao, Z. (2005). Structural Insights into SARS Coronavirus Proteins. *Curr. Opin. Struct. Biol.* 15, 664–672. doi:10.1016/j.sbi.2005.10.004
6. Bensussen, A., Torres-Sosa, C., Gonzalez, R. A., and Díaz, J. (2018). Dynamics of the Gene Regulatory Network of HIV-1 and the Role of Viral Non-coding RNAs on Latency Reversion. *Front. Physiol.* 9, 1364. doi:10.3389/fphys.2018.01364
7. Bouffi, C., Bony, C., Courties, G., Jorgensen, C., and Noël, D. (2010). IL-6- Dependent PGE2 Secretion by Mesenchymal Stem Cells Inhibits Local Inflammation in Experimental Arthritis. *PLoS ONE* 5, e14247. doi:10.1371/journal.pone.0014247
8. Breitling, R. (2010). What Is Systems Biology? *Front. Physio.* 1, 9. doi:10.3389/fphys.2010.00009
9. Cessac, B. (2010). A View of Neural Networks as Dynamical Systems. *Int. J. Bifurcation Chaos* 20, 1585–1629. doi:10.1142/S0218127410026721
10. Cho, J.-S., Han, I.-H., Lee, H. R., and Lee, H.-M. (2014). Prostaglandin E2 Induces IL-6 and IL-8 Production by the EP Receptors/Akt/NF-Kb Pathways in Nasal Polyp-Derived FibroblastsAllergy Asthma. *Allergy Asthma Immunol. Res.* 6, 449–457. doi:10.4168/aair.2014.6.5.449
11. Cohen, R., Erez, K., ben-Avraham, D., and Havlin, S. (2000). Resilience of the Internet to Random Breakdowns. *Phys. Rev. Lett.* 85, 4626–4628. doi:10.1103/PhysRevLett.85.4626
12. Danos, V., Feret, J., Fontana, W., Harmer, R., and Krivine, J. (2007). "Rule-based Modelling of Cellular Signalling," in *CONCUR 2007—concurrency Theory* (Berlin: Springer), 17–41. doi:10.1007/978-3-540-74407-8_3
13. Díaz, J. (2020a). SARS-CoV-2 Molecular Network Structure. *Front. Physiol.* 11, 870. doi:10.3389/fphys.2020.00870
14. Díaz, D. (2020b). SARS-Cov-2 Systems Biology. *Ann. Syst. Biol.* 3, 029–032. doi:10.17352/asb.000009
15. Eftimie, R., Gillard, J. J., and Cantrell, D. A. (2016). Mathematical Models for Immunology: Current State of the Art and Future Research Directions. *Bull. Math. Biol.* 78, 2091–2134. doi:10.1007/s11538-016-0214-9
16. El Baba, R., and Herbein, G. (2020). Management of Epigenomic Networks Entailed in Coronavirus Infections and COVID-19. *Clin. Epigenet* 12, 118. doi:10.1186/s13148-020-00912-7
17. Enciso, J., Mendoza, L., Álvarez-Buylla, E. R., and Pelayo, R. (2020). Dynamical Modeling Predicts an Inflammation-Inducible CXCR7+ B Cell Precursor with Potential Implications in Lymphoid Blockage Pathologies. *PeerJ* 8, e9902. doi:10.7717/peerj.9902

18. Forster, P., Forster, L., Renfrew, C., and Forster, M. (2020). Phylogenetic Network Analysis of SARS-CoV-2 Genomes. *Proc. Natl. Acad. Sci. USA* 117, 9241–9243. doi:10.1073/pnas.2004999117
19. Gordon, D. E., Jang, G. M., Bouhaddou, M., Xu, J., Obernier, K., White, K. M., et al. (2020). A SARS-CoV-2 Protein Interaction Map Reveals Targets for Drug Repurposing. *Nature* 583, 459–468. doi:10.1038/s41586-020-2286-9
20. Hamming, I., Timens, W., Bulthuis, M., Lely, A., Navis, G., and van Goor, H. (2004). Tissue Distribution of ACE2 Protein, the Functional Receptor for SARS Coronavirus. A First Step in Understanding SARS Pathogenesis. *J. Pathol.* 203, 631–637. doi:10.1002/path.1570
21. Hausser, J., Mayo, A., Keren, L., and Alon, U. (2019). Central Dogma Rates and the Trade-Off between Precision and Economy in Gene Expression. *Nat. Commun.* 10, 68. doi:10.1038/s41467-018-07391-8
22. Hekman, R. M., Hume, A. J., Goel, R. K., Abo, K. M., Huang, J., Blum, B. C., et al. (2020). Actionable Cytopathogenic Host Responses of Human Alveolar Type 2 Cells to SARS-CoV-2. *Mol. Cel* 80, 1104–1122. doi:10.1016/j.molcel.2020.11.028
23. Hennighausen, L., and Lee, H. K. (2020). Activation of the SARS-CoV-2 Receptor Ace2 through JAK/STAT-Dependent Enhancers during PregnancyAce2 through JAK/STAT-Dependent Enhancers during Pregnancy. *Cel Rep.* 32, 108199. doi:10.1016/j.celrep.2020.108199
24. Hodgkin, A. L., and Huxley, A. F. (1952). A Quantitative Description of Membrane Current and its Application to Conduction and Excitation in Nerve. *J. Physiol.* 117, 500–544. doi:10.1113/jphysiol.1952.sp004764
25. Horby, P., Lim, W. S., Emberson, J. R., Mafham, M., Bell, J. L., Linsell, L., et al. (2021). Dexamethasone in Hospitalized Patients with Covid-19. *N. Engl. J. Med.* 384, 693–704. doi:10.1056 /NEJMoa2021436
26. Jafarzadeh, A., Chauhan, P., Saha, B., Jafarzadeh, S., and Nemati, M. (2020). Contribution of Monocytes and Macrophages to the Local Tissue Inflammation and Cytokine Storm in COVID-19: Lessons from SARS and MERS, and Potential Therapeutic Interventions. *Life Sci.* 257, 118102. doi:10.1016/ j.lfs.2020.118102
27. Kim, D., Lee, J.-Y., Yang, J.-S., Kim, J. W., Kim, V. N., and Chang, H. (2020). The Architecture of SARS-CoV-2 Transcriptome. *Cell* 181, 914–921. doi:10.1016/j.cell.2020.04.011
28. Kim, Y.-M., and Shin, E.-C. (2021). Type I and III Interferon Responses in SARS- CoV-2 Infection. *Exp. Mol. Med.* 53, 750 –760. doi:10.1038/s12276-021-00592-0
29. Konwar, M., and Sarma, D. (2021). Advances in Developing Small Molecule SARS 3CLpro Inhibitors as Potential Remedy for corona Virus Infection. *Tetrahedron* 77, 131761. doi:10.1016/j.tet.2020.131761
30. Kumar, N., Mishra, B., Mehmood, A., Mohammad Athar, M., and M Shahid Mukhtar, M. S. (2020). Integrative Network Biology Framework Elucidates Molecular Mechanisms of SARS-CoV-2 Pathogenesis. *iScience* 23, 101526. doi:10.1016/j.isci.2020.101526
31. Leisman, D. E., Ronner, L., Pinotti, R., Taylor , M. D., Sinha, P., Calfee, C. S., et al. (2020). Cytokine Elevation in Severe and Critical COVID-19: a Rapid Systematic Review, Meta-Analysis, and Comparison with Other Inflammatory Syndromes. *Lancet Respir. Med.* 8, 1233–1244. doi:10.1016/s2213-2600(20)30404-5
32. Letko, M., Marzi, A., and Munster, V. (2020). Functional Assessment of Cell Entry and Receptor Usage for SARS-CoV-2 and Other Lineage B Betacoronaviruses. *Nat. Microbiol.* 5, 562–569. doi:10.1038/s41564-020-0688-y
33. Lipniacki, T., Paszek, P., Brasier, A. R., Luxon, B., and Kimmel, M. (2004). Mathematical Model of NF-Kb Regulatory Module. *J. Theor. Biol.* 228, 195–215. doi:10.1016/j.jtbi.2004.01.001
34. Long, Q.-X., Tang, X.-J., Shi, Q.-L., Li, Q., Deng, H.-J., Yuan, J., et al. (2020).
35. Clinical and Immunological Assessment of Asymptomatic SARS-CoV-2 Infections. *Nat. Med.* 26, 1200–1204. doi:10.1038/s41591-020-0965-6
36. Magro, G. (2020). SARS-CoV-2 and COVID-19: Is Interleukin-6 (IL-6) the 'culprit Lesion' of ARDS Onset? what Is There besides Tocilizumab? SGP130Fc. *Cytokine: X* 2, 100029. doi:10.1016/j.cytox.2020.100029
37. Martinez-Sanchez, M. E., Huerta, L., Alvarez-Buylla, E. R., and Villarreal Luján, C. (2018). Role of Cytokine Combinations on CD4+ T Cell Differentiation, Partial Polarization, and Plasticity: Continuous Network Modeling Approach. *Front. Physiol.* 9, 877. doi:10.3389/fphys.2018.00877
38. Masters, P. S. (2006). The Molecular Biology of Coronaviruses. *Adv. Virus. Res.* 66, 193–292. doi:10.1016/S0065-3527(06)66005-3
39. McBride, R., and Fielding, B. (2012). The Role of Severe Acute Respiratory Syndrome (SARS)-Coronavirus Accessory Proteins in Virus Pathogenesis. *Viruses* 4, 2902–2923. doi:10.3390/v4112902
40. Messina, F., Giombini, E., Agrati, C., Vairo, F., Ascoli Bartoli, T., Al Moghazi, S., et al. (2020). COVID-19: Viral-Host Interactome Analyzed by Network Based- Approach Model to Study Pathogenesis of SARS-CoV-2 Infection. *J. Transl Med.* 18, 233. doi:10.1186/s12967-020-02405-w
41. Mokuda, S., Tokunaga, T., Masumoto, J., and Sugiyama, E. (2020). Angiotensin-converting Enzyme 2, a SARS-CoV-2 Receptor, Is Upregulated by Interleukin 6 through STAT3 Signaling in Synovial Tissues. *J. Rheumato l.* 47, 1593–1595. doi:10.3899/jrheum.200547
42. Morel, P. A., Ta'asan, S., Morel, B. F., Kirschner, D. E., and Flynn, J. L. (2006). New Insights into Mathematical Modeling of the Immune System. *Ir* 36, 157–166. doi:10.1385/IR:36:1:157
43. Mukherjee, P., Shah, F., Desai, P., and Avery, M. (2011). Inhibitors of SARS-3CLpro: Virtual Screening, Biological Evaluation, and Molecular D ynamics Simulation Studies. *J. Chem. Inf. Model.* 51, 1376–1392. doi:10.1021/ ci1004916
44. Nakagawa, K., Lokugamage, K. G., and Makino, S. (2016). Viral and Cellular mRNA Translation in Coronavirus-Infected Cells. *Adv. Virus. Res.* 96, 165–192. Elsevier Inc. ISSN 0065-3527. doi:10.1016/bs.aivir.2016.08.001
45. Nayak, S. K., Bit, A., Dey, A., Mohapatra, B., and Pal, K. (2018). A Review on the Nonlinear Dynamical System Analysis of Electrocardiogram Signal. *J. Healthc. Eng.* 2018, 1–19. Article ID 6920420. doi:10.1155/2018/6920420
46. Newton, R., Seybold, J., Kuitert, L. M., Bergmann, M., and Barnes, P. J. (1998). Repression of Cyclooxygenase-2 and Prostaglandin E2Release by Dexamethasone Occurs by Transcriptional and Post-transcriptional Mechanisms Involving Loss of Polyadenylated mRNA. *J. Biol. Chem.* 273, 32312–32321. doi:10.1074/jbc.273.48.32312
47. Pan, Q., Peppelenbosch, M. P., Janssen, H. L., and de Knegt, R. J. (2012). Telaprevir/boceprevir Era: from Bench to Bed and Back. *Wjg* 18, 6183–6188. doi:10.3748/wjg.v18.i43.6183
48. Pfeffer, L. M. (2011). The Role of Nuclear Factor κB in the Interferon Response. *J. Interferon Cytokine Res.* 31, 553–559. doi:10.1089/jir.2011.0028
49. Pillaiyar, T., Manickam, M., Namasivayam, V., Hayashi, Y., and Jung, S.-H. (2016). An Overview of Severe Acute Respiratory Syndrome-Coronavirus (SARS-CoV) 3CL Protease Inhibitors: Peptidomimetics and Small Molecule Chemotherapy. *J. Med. Chem.* 59, 6595–6628. doi:10.1021/ acs.jmedchem.5b01461
50. Rahman, I., and MacNee, W. (1998). Role of Transcription Factors in Inflammatory Lung Diseases. *Thorax* 53, 601–612. doi:10.1136/thx.53.7.601 Sevajol, M., Subissi, L., Decroly, E., Canard, B., and Imbert, I. (2014). Insights into RNA Synthesis, Capping, and Proofreading Mechanisms of SARS-Coronavirus. *Virus. Res.* 194, 90–99. doi:10.1016/j.virusres.2014.10.008
51. Strogatz, S. H. (2015). *Chemistry and Engineering*. 2nd Edition. United States: CRC Press. ISBN-13 : 978-0813349107.
52. Suleyman, H., Cadirci, E., Albayrak, A., and Halici, Z. (2008). Nimesulide Is a Selective COX-2 Inhibitory, Atypical Non-steroidal Anti-inflammatory Drug. *Cmc* 15, 278–283. doi:10.2174/092986708783497247
53. Vidya, M. K., Kumar, V. G., Sejian, V., Bagath, M., Krishnan, G., and Bhatta, R. (2017). Toll-like Receptors: Significance, Ligands, Signaling Pathways, and Functions in Mammals. *Int. Rev. Immunol.* 37, 20–36. doi:10.1080/08830185.2017.1380200
54. Vilar, S., and Isom, D. G. (2020). One Year of SARS-CoV-2: How Much Has the Virus Changed? *Biology* 10, 91. doi:10.3390/biology10020091
55. Wang, L., Walia, B., Evans, J., Gewirtz, A. T., Merlin, D., and Sitaraman, S. V. (2003). IL-6 Induces NF-Kb Activation in the Intestinal Epithelia. *J. Immunol.* 171, 3194–3201. doi:10.4049/jimmun ol.171.6.3194
56. Wagner, T., Kiweler, N., and Wolff, K. (2015). Sumoylation of HDAC2 promotes NF-κB-dependent gene expression. *Oncotarget* 6, 7123–7135. doi:10.18632/ oncotarget.3344
57. Weinstein, N., Mendoza, L., and Álvarez-Buylla, E. R. (2020). A Computational Model of the Endothelial to Mesenchymal Transition. *Front. Genet.* 11, 40. doi:10.3389/fgene.2020.00040
58. Wu, A., Peng, Y., Huang, B., Ding, X., Wang, X., Niu, P., et al. (2020). Genome Composition and Divergence of the Novel Coronavirus (2019-nCoV) Originating in China. *Cell Host & Microbe* 27, 325–328. doi:10.1016/j.chom.2020.02.001
59. Xu, C., Ke, Z., Liu, C., Wang, Z., Liu, D., Zhang, L., et al. (2020). Systemic In Silico Screening in Drug Discovery for Coronavirus Disease (COVID-19) with an Online Interactive Web Server. *J. Chem. Inf. Model.* 60, 5735–5745. doi:10.1021/acs.jcim.0c00821

60. Yan, X., Hao, Q., Mu, Y., Timani, K. A., Ye, L., Zhu, Y., et al. (2006). Nucleocapsid Protein of SARS-CoV Activates the Expression of Cyclooxygenase-2 by Binding Directly to Regulatory Elements for Nuclear Factor-Kappa B and CCAAT/ enhancer Binding Protein. *Int. J. Biochem. Cel Biol.* 38, 1417–1428. doi:10.1016/ j.biocel.2006.02.003
61. Zegeye, M. M., Lindkvist, M., Fälker, K., Kumawat, A. K., Paramel, G., Grenegård, M., et al. (2018). Activation of the JAK/STAT3 and PI3K/AKT Pathways Are Crucial for IL-6 Trans-signaling-mediated Pro-inflammatory Response in Human Vascular Endothelial Cells. *Cell Commun Signal* 16, 55. doi:10.1186/ s12964-018-0268-4

Permissions

All chapters in this book were first published by Frontiers; hereby published with permission under the Creative Commons Attribution License or equivalent. Every chapter published in this book has been scrutinized by our experts. Their significance has been extensively debated. The topics covered herein carry significant findings which will fuel the growth of the discipline. They may even be implemented as practical applications or may be referred to as a beginning point for another development.

The contributors of this book come from diverse backgrounds, making this book a truly international effort. This book will bring forth new frontiers with its revolutionizing research information and detailed analysis of the nascent developments around the world.

We would like to thank all the contributing authors for lending their expertise to make the book truly unique. They have played a crucial role in the development of this book. Without their invaluable contributions this book wouldn't have been possible. They have made vital efforts to compile up to date information on the varied aspects of this subject to make this book a valuable addition to the collection of many professionals and students.

This book was conceptualized with the vision of imparting up-to-date information and advanced data in this field. To ensure the same, a matchless editorial board was set up. Every individual on the board went through rigorous rounds of assessment to prove their worth. After which they invested a large part of their time researching and compiling the most relevant data for our readers.

The editorial board has been involved in producing this book since its inception. They have spent rigorous hours researching and exploring the diverse topics which have resulted in the successful publishing of this book. They have passed on their knowledge of decades through this book. To expedite this challenging task, the publisher supported the team at every step. A small team of assistant editors was also appointed to further simplify the editing procedure and attain best results for the readers.

Apart from the editorial board, the designing team has also invested a significant amount of their time in understanding the subject and creating the most relevant covers. They scrutinized every image to scout for the most suitable representation of the subject and create an appropriate cover for the book.

The publishing team has been an ardent support to the editorial, designing and production team. Their endless efforts to recruit the best for this project, has resulted in the accomplishment of this book. They are a veteran in the field of academics and their pool of knowledge is as vast as their experience in printing. Their expertise and guidance has proved useful at every step. Their uncompromising quality standards have made this book an exceptional effort. Their encouragement from time to time has been an inspiration for everyone.

The publisher and the editorial board hope that this book will prove to be a valuable piece of knowledge for researchers, students, practitioners and scholars across the globe.

List of Contributors

Daniel R. Laucirica
Faculty of Health and Medical Sciences, University of Western Australia, Nedlands, WA, Australia
Telethon Kids Institute, University of Western Australia, Nedlands, WA, Australia

Luke W. Garratt
Telethon Kids Institute, University of Western Australia, Nedlands, WA, Australia
Telethon Kids Institute, Respiratory Research Centre, Nedlands, WA, Australia
School of Biomedical Sciences, The University of Western Australia, Nedlands, WA, Australia

Anthony Kicic
Faculty of Health and Medical Sciences, University of Western Australia, Nedlands, WA, Australia
Telethon Kids Institute, University of Western Australia, Nedlands, WA, Australia
Department of Respiratory and Sleep Medicine, Perth Children's Hospital, Nedlands, WA, Australia
School of Public Health, Curtin University, Bentley, WA, Australia
Centre for Cell Therapy and Regenerative Medicine, School of Medicine and Pharmacology, The University of Western Australia, Nedlands, WA, Australia

Jeanne Bigot, Juliette Guitard and Christophe Hennequin
Sorbonne Université, Inserm, Centre de Recherche Saint-Antoine, CRSA, AP-HP, Hôpital Saint-Antoine, Service de Parasitologie-Mycologie, Paris, France

Loïc Guillot, Manon Ruffin and Viviane Balloy
Sorbonne Université, Inserm, Centre de Recherche Saint-Antoine, Paris, France

Harriet Corvol
Sorbonne Université, Inserm, Centre de Recherche Saint-Antoine, CRSA, AP-HP, Hôpital Trousseau, Service de Pneumologie Pédiatrique, Paris, France

Jasmijn A. Schrumpf, Anne M. van der Does and Pieter S. Hiemstra
Department of Pulmonology, Leiden University Medical Center, Leiden, Netherlands

Giulio Cabrini
Center for Innovative Therapies in Cystic Fibrosis, University of Ferrara, Ferrara, Italy
Department of Life Sciences and Biotechnology, University of Ferrara, Ferrara, Italy

Department of Neurosciences, Biomedicine and Movement, University of Verona, Verona, Italy

Alessandro Rimessi and Paolo Pinton
Center for Innovative Therapies in Cystic Fibrosis, University of Ferrara, Ferrara, Italy
Department of Medical Sciences, University of Ferrara, Ferrara, Italy

Monica Borgatti, Ilaria Lampronti, Alessia Finotti and Roberto Gambari
Center for Innovative Therapies in Cystic Fibrosis, University of Ferrara, Ferrara, Italy
Department of Life Sciences and Biotechnology, University of Ferrara, Ferrara, Italy

Berengère Villeret, Brigitte Solhonne, Marjolène Straube, Flora Lemaire, Ignacio Garcia-Verdugo and Jean-Michel Sallenave
Inserm, UMR1152, Laboratoire d'Excellence Inflamex, Département Hospitalo-Universtaire FIRE (Fibrosis, Inflammation and Remodeling), Université de Paris, Paris, France

Aurélie Cazes
Inserm, UMR1152, Laboratoire d'Excellence Inflamex, Département Hospitalo-Universtaire FIRE (Fibrosis, Inflammation and Remodeling), Université de Paris, Paris, France
Assistance Publique-Hôpitaux de Paris (APHP), Hôpital Bichat, Service de Pneumologie A, Paris, France

Hong Guo-Parke, Dermot Linden, Sinéad Weldon and Clifford C. Taggart
Airway Innate Immunity Research Group, Wellcome Wolfson Institute for Experimental Medicine, School of Medicine, Dentistry & Biomedical Sciences, Queens University Belfast, Belfast, United Kingdom

Joseph C. Kidney
Department of Respiratory Medicine Mater Hospital Belfast, Belfast, United Kingdom

Bilal Alashkar Alhamwe
Institute of Laboratory Medicine, Philipps-University Marburg, Member of the German Center for Lung Research (DZL), Universities of Giessen and Marburg Lung Center, Marburg, Germany
College of Pharmacy, International University for Science and Technology (IUST), Daraa, Syria
Center for Tumor Biology and Immunology, Institute of Tumor Immunology, Philipps University Marburg, Marburg, Germany

Sarah Miethe and Holger Garn
Institute of Laboratory Medicine, Philipps-University Marburg, Member of the German Center for Lung Research (DZL), Universities of Giessen and Marburg Lung Center, Marburg, Germany
Translational Inflammation Research Division & Core Facility for Single Cell Multiomics, Philipps University Marburg, Marburg, Germany

Elke Pogge von Strandmann
Center for Tumor Biology and Immunology, Institute of Tumor Immunology, Philipps University Marburg, Marburg, Germany

Daniel P. Potaczek
Institute of Laboratory Medicine, Philipps-University Marburg, Member of the German Center for Lung Research (DZL), Universities of Giessen and Marburg Lung Center, Marburg, Germany
John Paul II Hospital, Kraków, Poland

Kevin Molloy and Noel G. McElvaney
Department of Medicine, Royal College of Surgeons in Ireland, Beaumont Hospital, Dublin, Ireland

Gerard Cagney, Eugene T. Dillon and Kieran Wynne
School of Biomolecular and Biomedical Science, University College Dublin, Dublin, Ireland

Catherine M. Greene
Department of Clinical Microbiology, Royal College of Surgeons in Ireland, Beaumont Hospital, Dublin, Ireland

Kak-Ming Ling
Paediatrics, Medical School, Faculty of Healthy and Medical Science, The University of Western Australia, Nedlands, WA, Australia
Telethon Kids Institute, Respiratory Research Centre, Nedlands, WA, Australia
Telethon Kids Institute, Centre for Health Research, The University of Western Australia, Nedlands, WA, Australia

Erin E. Gill, Amy H. Y. Lee and Robert E. W. Hancock
Centre for Microbial Diseases and Immunity Research, University of British Columbia, Vancouver, BC, Canada

Patricia Agudelo-Romero, Erika N. Sutanto, Thomas Iosifidis and Tim Rosenow
Telethon Kids Institute, Respiratory Research Centre, Nedlands, WA, Australia
Telethon Kids Institute, Centre for Health Research, The University of Western Australia, Nedlands, WA, Australia

Stuart E. Turvey
Department of Pediatrics, BC Children's Hospital, University of British Columbia, Vancouver, BC, Canada

Timo Lassmann
Telethon Kids Institute, Centre for Health Research, The University of Western Australia, Nedlands, WA, Australia

Stephen M. Stick
Telethon Kids Institute, Respiratory Research Centre, Nedlands, WA, Australia
Telethon Kids Institute, Centre for Health Research, The University of Western Australia, Nedlands, WA, Australia
School of Biomedical Sciences, The University of Western Australia, Nedlands, WA, Australia
Occupation and Environment, School of Public Health, Curtin University, Perth, WA, Australia
Department of Respiratory and Sleep Medicine, Perth Children's Hospital, Nedlands, WA, Australia
Centre for Cell Therapy and Regenerative Medicine, School of Medicine and Pharmacology, The University of Western Australia, Nedlands, WA, Australia

Andreas Frey
Division of Mucosal Immunology and Diagnostics, Research Center Borstel, Borstel, Germany
Airway Research Center North, German Center for Lung Research (DZL), Borstel, Germany

Lars P. Lunding and Michael Wegmann
Airway Research Center North, German Center for Lung Research (DZL), Borstel, Germany
Division of Asthma Exacerbation & Regulation, Research Center Borstel, Borstel, Germany

Johanna C. Ehlers
Airway Research Center North, German Center for Lung Research (DZL), Borstel, Germany
Division of Experimental Pneumology, Research Center Borstel, Borstel, Germany

Markus Weckmann
Airway Research Center North, German Center for Lung Research (DZL), Borstel, Germany
Department of Pediatric Pulmonology and Allergology, University Children's Hospital, Lübeck, Germany

Ulrich M. Zissler
Center of Allergy & Environment (ZAUM), Technical University of Munich and Helmholtz Center Munich, German Research Center for Environmental Health, Munich, Germany
Member of the German Center for Lung Research (DZL), CPC-M, Munich, Germany

Shashi P. Singh, Aryaz Sheybani and Mohan L. Sopori
Respiratory Immunology Division, Lovelace Respiratory Research Institute, Albuquerque, NM, United States

Teodora Ivanciuc and Roberto P. Garofalo
Department of Microbiology and Immunology, Galveston, TX, United States

Vernat Exil, Hemant Agarwal and Veena Raizada
Department of Pediatrics, University of New Mexico Health Sciences Center, Albuquerque, NM, United States

Hitendra S. Chand, Dinesh Devadoss and Marko Manevski
Department of Immunology and Nanomedicine, Herbert Wertheim College of Medicine, Florida International University, Miami, FL, United States

Regina Geitani and Dolla Karam Sarkis
Microbiology Laboratory, School of Pharmacy, Saint Joseph University, Beirut, Lebanon

Carole Ayoub Moubareck
Microbiology Laboratory, School of Pharmacy, Saint Joseph University, Beirut, Lebanon
College of Natural and Health Sciences, Zayed University, Dubai, United Arab Emirates

Zhengzhong Xu
Jiangsu Key Laboratory of Zoonosis, Yangzhou University, Yangzhou, China
Sorbonne Université, INSERM UMR_S 938, Centre de Recherche Saint Antoine (CRSA), Paris, France
"Mucoviscidose and Bronchopathies Chroniques", Pasteur Institute, Paris, France

Lhousseine Touqui
Sorbonne Université, INSERM UMR_S 938, Centre de Recherche Saint Antoine (CRSA), Paris, France
"Mucoviscidose and Bronchopathies Chroniques", Pasteur Institute, Paris, France

Samuel T. Montgomery
Faculty of Health and Medical Sciences, School of Biomedical Sciences, The University of Western Australia, Crawley, WA, Australia

Dario L. Frey
Department of Translational Pulmonology, Translational Lung Research Center Heidelberg, University of Heidelberg, Heidelberg, Germany
German Center for Lung Research, Heidelberg, Germany

Marcus A. Mall
German Center for Lung Research, Heidelberg, Germany
Department of Pediatric Pulmonology, Immunology and Critical Care Medicine, Charité-Universitätsmedizin Berlin, Berlin, Germany
Berlin Institute of Health, Berlin, Germany

Stephen M. Stick
Faculty of Health and Medical Sciences, School of Biomedical Sciences, The University of Western Australia, Crawley, WA, Australia
Telethon Kids Institute, The University of Western Australia, Crawley, WA, Australia
Department of Respiratory and Sleep Medicine, Perth Children's Hospital, Nedlands, WA, Australia
Centre for Cell Therapy and Regenerative Medicine, School of Medicine and Pharmacology, The University of Western Australia, Nedlands, WA, Australia

Zhixiao Sun, Ningfei Ji, Qiyun Ma, Ranran Zhu, Zhongqi Chen, Zhengxia Wang, Yan Qian, Chaojie Wu and Mao Huang
Department of Respiratory and Critical Care Medicine, The First Affiliated Hospital of Nanjing Medical University, Nanjing, China

Fan Hu
State Key Laboratory of Reproductive Medicine, Nanjing Medical University, Nanjing, China

Mingshun Zhang
NHC Key Laboratory of Antibody Technique, Department of Immunology, Nanjing Medical University, Nanjing, China

Raquel de Souza Vieira, Angela Castoldi, Paulo José Basso and Meire Ioshie Hiyane
Laboratory of Transplantation Immunobiology, Department of Immunology, Institute of Biomedical Sciences, University of São Paulo, São Paulo, Brazil

Niels Olsen Saraiva Câmara
Laboratory of Transplantation Immunobiology, Department of Immunology, Institute of Biomedical Sciences, University of São Paulo, São Paulo, Brazil
Nephrology Division, Department of Medicine, Federal University of São Paulo, São Paulo, Brazil
Renal Pathophysiology Laboratory, Department of Clinical Medicine, University of São Paulo, São Paulo, Brazil

Rafael Ribeiro Almeida
Laboratory of Transplantation Immunobiology, Department of Immunology, Institute of Biomedical Sciences, University of São Paulo, São Paulo, Brazil
Laboratory of Immunology, Heart Institute (InCor) School of Medicine, University of São Paulo, São Paulo, Brazil

Diana Feller
Department of Pharmaceutical Biotechnology, School of Pharmacy, University of Pecs, Pecs, Hungary
Department of Pharmacology and Pharmacotherapy, Medical School, University of Pecs, Pecs, Hungary
Szentagothai Research Center, University of Pecs, Pecs, Hungary

Jozsef Kun and Zsuzsanna Helyes
Department of Pharmacology and Pharmacotherapy, Medical School, University of Pecs, Pecs, Hungary
Szentagothai Research Center, University of Pecs, Pecs, Hungary

Istvan Ruzsics and Veronika Sarosi
Department of Internal Medicine, Clinical Centre and Medical School, University of Pecs, Pecs, Hungary

Judit Rapp, Krisztian Kvell and Judit E. Pongracz
Department of Pharmaceutical Biotechnology, School of Pharmacy, University of Pecs, Pecs, Hungary
Szentagothai Research Center, University of Pecs, Pecs, Hungary

Yoon-Young Sung and Ho Kyoung Kim
Herbal Medicine Research Division, Korea Institute of Oriental Medicine, Daejeon, South Korea

Seung-Hyung Kim, Won-Kyung Yang and Yang-Chun Park
Institute of Traditional Medicine and Bioscience, Daejeon University, Daejeon, South Korea

Antonio Bensussen and José Díaz
Laboratorio de Dinámica de Redes Genéticas, Centro de Investigación en Dinámica Celular, Universidad Autónoma del Estado de Morelos, Cuernavaca, Mexico

Elena R. Álvarez-Buylla
Centro de Ciencias de la Complejidad (C3), Universidad Nacional Autónoma de México, Ciudad de México, Mexico
Laboratorio de Genética Molecular, Epigenética, Desarrollo y Evolución de Plantas, Instituto de Ecología, Universidad Nacional Autónoma de México, Ciudad de México, Mexico

Index

www.ingramcontent.com/pod-product-compliance
Lightning Source LLC
LaVergne TN
LVHW082127200926
848484LV00008B/2018
* 9 7 9 8 8 8 7 4 0 5 7 7 3 *